# ANNUAL PROGRESS IN CHILD PSYCHIATRY AND CHILD DEVELOPMENT 1996

*Edited by*

**MARGARET E. HERTZIG, M.D.**

*Professor of Psychiatry*
*Cornell University Medical College*

*and*

**ELLEN A. FARBER, Ph.D.**

*Clinical Assistant Professor of Psychology in Psychiatry*
*Cornell University Medical College*

**BRUNNER/MAZEL, *Publishers* • New York**

Library of Congress Card No. 68-23452
ISBN 0-87630-828-0
ISSN 0066-4030

*Published by*
BRUNNER/MAZEL, INC.
19 Union Square West
New York, New York 10003

Manufactured in the United States of America
10  9  8  7  6  5  4  3  2  1

# CONTENTS

# Part I

# DEVELOPMENTAL ISSUES

The four papers in this section, two reviews and two empirical studies, address the capacities of young children. The first paper is a review of cognitive development in infancy. Karmiloff-Smith summarizes recent research on the phenomenal auditory, visual, and cross-modal processing capacities of newborns. Most of the studies conducted in the last decade have been done using variations on habituation and preferential looking/listening paradigms.

Some of the intriguing findings described include the following: During the last three months of intrauterine life, the fetus has the capacity for speech perception. In fact, newborns prefer listening to the mother's voice as it sounded in utero rather than ex utero. Visual discrimination of interpersonal stimuli is also apparent shortly after birth. Four-day-old children are capable of recognizing their mother's face based on the face/hair separation line. In addition, object perception studies are challenging the Piagetian view that infants initially experience the visual world as "undifferentiated and chaotic." Young infants' ability to make inferences about the movement of objects suggests that infants are equipped with domain-specific principles that enable them to process partially hidden objects as wholes. Studies of processing input intermodally also reveal infants' amazing capacities for memory and nonverbal communication of specific memories. Karmiloff-Smith notes that perceptual discriminations do not necessarily mirror cognitive discriminations. That is, while infants can make perceptual discriminations at subordinate levels (e.g., differentiating dogs) their conceptual categories are at the superordinate level (e.g., dogs versus not dogs).

The author suggests that future research should focus more on the cognitive processes involved, rather than just the presence or absence of perceptual abilities. She encourages more focus on the association of individual differences in very early infancy with domain-specific development. She suggests as well that it might be possible to do longitudinal studies to follow up abnormal phenotypes and their association with later uneven cognitive profiles. In this context, she references a paper she published in 1995 on William's syndrome. One wonders if large-scale longitudinal studies or smaller studies of children at risk (e.g., siblings of affected children) could track abnormal perception of social stimuli to the development of

1

low frequency syndromes, such as autism. In concluding, Karmiloff-Smith adds that new techniques, such as noninvasive imaging and computer simulations of early development, will bring much new information to how cognitive development proceeds from the fetus through infancy.

The second paper in this section is also a review of infant research. Thelen describes the miraculous motor skill development that occurs in the first year of life and notes that motor skill development was the first area of study in child development. In fact, Gesell's study of age norms published in the 1930s was so well received that the norms are still being used today. By the 1960s, though, researchers began to focus on social and cognitive development to the exclusion of motor development.

In recent years, new theories and tools from perceptual psychology and neurosciences have revived the field of motor development. One major area of change is recognizing advances in motor development as directly reflecting changes in brain development. For example, milestones, such as crawling and walking, have been thought to mirror a direct brain–behavior relationship. Bernstein's theory of physiology implies a more complex relationship, incorporating changes in the central nervous system, the biomechanical properties of the body, the environmental support, and the demands of the particular task. As examples, Thelen notes specific types of behaviors such as motor reflex behaviors that disappear and reappear (e.g., stepping) and hidden skills and functional activity that can be elicited under experimental circumstances (e.g., treadmill stepping).

Thelen goes on to describe how the development of "phylogenetic" skills (universal motor skills) have been misinterpreted by the maturational model. She proposes that infants learn new skills through novel tasks and that the task itself, not preprogrammed instructions, constitutes the driving force for change. Gibson's studies of infant perception using "the visual cliff" are combined with Bernstein's theory of movement and neuroscientist's theories of brain development. Advances in neuroscience highlight amazing plasticity. Edelman's theory of neuronal group selection is also described briefly. He proposes that certain connections and higher level associations are strengthened through use of motor movements and feedback.

In sum, this is a fascinating interdisciplinary integration of theories and research. Highlighting the complexities of motor development may ultimately lead to more effective interventions for children at risk for physical disabilities.

The next paper presents a study of "theory of mind" in normally developing toddlers. *Theory of mind* is defined as the understanding of others as psychological beings having mental states, such as beliefs, emotions, and intentions. Stages of theory of mind that are proposed include: 1) the mentalist stage when children begin to construe others as having psychological states that underlie behavior and 2) the representational stage when children understand that others' interpretations of the world lead to mental states that underlie behavior. Thus far, studies have identified two-and-a half to three-year-olds as mentalists. This is a much earlier age than Piaget proposed. Nonetheless, it is possible that even younger children are capable of these attributions. It is not known, however, if younger children can assign mental states because the measures available rely on verbal response.

In this well-designed set of studies, Meltzoff addresses two questions: 1) Could a procedure be developed to assess theory-of-mind in nonverbal children? and 2) Would 18-month-olds understand that others had goals and intentions that were driving their behavior? In Experiment 1, children observed an adult attempt but not complete an act. The children reenacted what the adult had intended to do. The study used four contrast groups (Total N = 40) to ensure that the children's responses were not just the natural tendency for children to respond to the demand characteristics of those objects. Children who observed an adult attempt but not successfully complete an act were just as likely to do the intended act as children who observed an adult do the completed act. In Experiment 2 (N = 60), children in one group observed an inanimate object attempt to pull apart a dowel but fail, while children in the other group observed an adult perform the same physical motion with the object. Children who observed the human attempts were much more likely to do the intended act than children who observed the inanimate object.

The behavioral reenactment is an interesting procedure for studying "theory of mind" questions in young children. It is a way for nonverbal children to tell us how they see things. Although most children are good imitators, by 18 months of age, they do not imitate direct actions if the behavior of the adult implies that the intended act was different. They are not merely responding to the behavioral acts of adults; they are ascribing intention to the adults' behavior. This procedure may be useful in studies of nonverbal autistic children for whom both "theory of mind" and imitation deficits have been found.

In his conclusion, Meltzoff discusses the varying possibilities underlying the early capacity to interpret movements of people as acts and movements of things as motions. He prefers a developmental stage model starting with some innate capacities to explain why very young children have a "folk psychology."

The last paper in this section is a study of associations among the brain, temperament, and social competence. It is intriguing because it highlights one area in which people may be "prewired" for specific developmental pathways. Fox, Rubin, Calkins, Marshall, and colleagues review the literature on the relation between frontal asymmetry assessed by EEGs and emotional disposition. Several laboratories have found that individuals exhibiting right frontal EEG asymmetry are more likely to exhibit signs of negative affect, while those exhibiting left frontal asymmetry are more likely to display positive affect. Both behaviorally inhibited and depressed individuals are more likely to exhibit right frontal asymmetry.

This study was designed to explore whether right frontal asymmetry is a marker for inhibited behavior in preschool children. The sample consisted of 48 four- to five-year-old children who were participating in a longitudinal study. Based on their response at 24 months of age in a laboratory situation designed to elicit a range of emotions, the children were assigned behavioral inhibition scores. These scores were used for their assignment to play group quartets at four years of age. Based on their behavior during free play, cleanup, and a speech, two aggregate variables were summed: social reticence–inhibition and sociability–social competence. Mothers completed the Colorado Temperament Index. Each child had an EEG recording. The EEG was scored for activity in each hemisphere and for power, a measure that acknowledges the possibility of interhemispheric communication.

Results indicated that inhibited behavior was associated with greater right frontal activation, and social competence was associated with left frontal asymmetry. EEG measures from the parietal and occipital regions were not associated with behavioral or maternal report measures. The findings are discussed in terms of brain functioning and hemispheric specialization. One wonders to what extent this pattern of inhibition can be modified by parental intervention possibly leading to changes in brain function. The authors may have additional data in a larger study from infancy that could address the question of whether children are born with this pattern of emotional responding.

# 1

# Annotation: The Extraordinary Cognitive Journey from Foetus Through Infancy

**Annette Karmiloff-Smith**
*Medical Research Council, London*

## INTRODUCTION

Cognitive development starts in the womb. During the final 3 months of interuterine life, the foetus is capable of extracting invariant patterns across the complex auditory input that is filtered through the amniotic fluid. The extraordinary cognitive journey from foetus through infancy is a period during which children learn more than at any other moment of their lives (Karmiloff-Smith, 1994). But for a long time, researchers were unaware of the extent of this early learning. In the past couple of decades, however, exciting new uses of the habituation and preferential looking/listening paradigms[1] have made it possible to bring to light hitherto unsuspected capacities of newborns and young infants. One such use has capitalized on what might be called infant "surprise". Infants are faced with situations that either violate or confirm their expectations. Take, for instance, gravity. If infants are repeatedly shown a falling ball which comes to rest on a surface, they will become habituated to the event and look at it increasingly less. If the event is then changed and the ball stops mid-air in one condition and on a higher surface in the other, two things could happen in the case of the ball violating gravity. Either infants continue to look less at the ball stopping mid-air because they don't see the event as different in any interesting way to the initial series. Or infants could dishabituate, i.e. they could

Reprinted with permission from the Journal of Child Psychology and Psychiatry, 1995, Vol. 36, No. 8, 1293–1313. Copyright © 1995 by the Association for Child Psychology and Psychiatry.

I should like to thank Gergely Csibra, Mark Johnson, Kang Lee, Jean Mandler and three anonymous reviewers for comments on an earlier version.

[1]See Bornstein (1985). A number of the infancy experimental paradigms are also described in Karmiloff-Smith (1992a), pp. 12–15, 43–45.

show renewed looking or "surprise," suggesting that the ball stopping mid-air violates their expectations of what falling objects do. Similarly, new-borns can be trained to turn their head towards a visual reward whenever there is a change from one set of phonemes to another (e.g. ba/ba/ba/ba/ga). They thereby demonstrate their capacity to discriminate between the two phonemes and to treat various forms of /ba/ as equivalent.

As exciting as these data are, the interpretation of infant behaviours remains controversial. First, it is unclear that the null hypothesis can be accepted if the infant does not dishabituate. Obviously there are many reasons why an infant might fail to make a discrimination. But even positive data are open to multiple interpretations. Theoretically the debate hinges on whether the infant is born with detailed templates of domain-specific knowledge, or whether some general learning mechanism, together with the different properties of a structured environment, suffice to explain how infants rapidly learn about the various domains of cognition. Neither of these positions in their extreme forms is correct, in my view. There is a tendency to focus on precocity rather than change. By contrast, modern cognitive neuroscience suggests a more dynamic, epigenetic view of development (Oyama, 1985) in which the timing of cortical events, together with relatively minimal predispositions, bias the infant to process certain inputs at certain times and in certain ways, and subsequently to learn about the details of each domain. This challenges the deterministic, anti-developmental nature of strong nativism. But it also questions the Behaviorist and Piagetian domain-general positions about the early period of infant cognition. Rather, during the postnatal period, predispositions orient infants' attention to different classes of input as they actively participate in the progressive structuring of their brain into increasingly specialised circuitry. So we are left with an active, constructivist, Piagetian-like infant, but with some domain-specific representational and/or processing headstarts to guide the beginnings of development to the right tracks from the outset.

This paper will review some of the exciting discoveries that have been made with respect to infant "knowledge" in a number of areas, focusing on the capacities infants have to process auditory, visual, and cross-modal inputs. I will focus on the most cognitively oriented work, without of course denying the importance of recent infancy research in domains such as motor development (Thelen & Fisher, 1983). I have purposely put the word "knowledge" in quotation marks because, whatever our interpretations of the behaviours infant development—from simple discrimination abilities to complex interpretative capacities—it clearly differs from the explicit knowledge that older children and adults can manipulate (Karmiloff-Smith, 1992a).

## PROCESSING AUDITORY INPUT

Fifteen years ago most of the work on early language focused on production, documenting the nature of early babbling, the use of single words, the so-called naming explosion, simple two- and three-word combinations, and finally the addition of morphology and grammar. Until recently there was little work on the perception of speech and language in young infants, in part because of a lack of suitable techniques. With the advances in experimental tools the picture of infants' processing of speech and language has radically changed. Here, then, I will focus on progress that has been made at the level of speech and language perception rather than early production (but see, for example, Hallé & de Boysson-Bardies, 1994; Lynch, Kimbrough Oller, Steffens & Buder, 1995; Tomasello & Olguin, 1993; Olguin & Tomasello, 1993; Woodward, Markman & Fizsimmons, 1994, with respect to some recent work on early production). And speech perception starts before birth.

A number of experiments have now demonstrated that during the last 3 months of interuterine life the foetus is actively processing incoming auditory input, and clearly distinguishing between music, language and other sounds (Wilkin, 1991). The presentation of sound to the foetus reliably elicits changes in both heart rate and motor responses (Lecanuet, Granier-Deferre & Busnel, 1988), so much so that congenital deafness can now be diagnosed during the prenatal period (Shahidullah & Hepper, 1993). Other experiments have shown that, despite the difference between the mother's voice heard *in utero* filtered through the amniotic fluid, and her voice as heard *ex utero* once the infant is born, recognition of the maternal voice is learned prenatally. Although young infants prefer to listen to mother's voice as it sounded *in utero* compared with its sound *ex utero* (Fifer & Moon, 1989), they can already discriminate at birth the mother's voice heard *ex utero* from that of other females (Hepper, Scott & Shahidullah, 1993). In other words, prior to any *ex utero* experience, newborns show that they have already extracted information about some of the invariant, abstract features of mother's voice during their period in the womb.

It is the melodic characteristics of whole prosodic units that seem to be a prime attractor of infant attention to linguistic input (Morgan, 1994). As Kuhl (1991) has pointed out, it is neither the syntax nor the semantics of "Motherese" that initially holds the attention of infants. Rather it is the rhythmic features of the acoustic signal itself, with its exaggerated prosodic contours (Kuhl, 1991; Cooper & Aslin, 1994; Kaplan, Goldstein, Huckeby & Panneton Cooper, 1995). By 4 days of age, infants use prosody to discriminate their mother tongue from other languages, but not yet the other languages amongst themselves (Mehler, Lambertz, Jusczyk & Amiel-Tison, 1986). Prosody also helps very young infants organize and remember speech information. As early as 2 months, infants recognize better the sound patterns of words that have been presented as prosodically linked together within a single clause, as opposed to the same sound patterns presented individually in a word list (Mandel, Juscyzk & Kemler-Nelson, 1994). Very rapidly infants' sensitivity extends beyond the overall prosodic patterns. Experiments have demonstrated young infants' sensitivity to relative versus absolute pitch, to vowel duration, fundamental frequency, linguistic stress, rising and falling intonation, subtle phonemic distinctions, as well as to the phonotactic patterns of the native tongue (Christophe, Dupoux, Bertoncini & Mehler, 1994; Mehler & Christophe, 1994; Eilers, Bull, Oller & Lewis, 1984, Eimas, Siqueland, Jusczyk & Vigorita, 1971; Fernald & Kuhl, 1981; Fowler, Smith & Tassinary, 1986; Jusczyk, Luce & Charles-Luce, 1994; Kuhl, 1991; Spring & Dale, 1977; Sullivan & Horowitz, 1983).

Between birth and 4 months, infants are what Kuhl (1991) has called "universal linguists," i.e., they are capable of distinguishing each of the 150 speech sounds that make up all human languages. Some phonetic discriminative abilities are not species specific; Kuhl has shown a similar capacity in chinchillas (Kuhl, 1991). However, the ability to discriminate all 150 speech sounds diminishes in the human case. Conditioned head-turning experiments have shown that with experience, (i.e. by about 10 months) infants are only able to discriminate the sounds (Jusczyk, Luce & Charles-Luce, 1994) and the words (Hallé & de Boysson-Bardies, 1994; Jusczyk, Friederici, Wessels, Svenmkerud & Jusczyk, 1993) that make up their native tongue. In other words, they seem to lose a more general biological capacity that was present at birth, and subsequently their brains become reconfigured such that they now specialise in processing the particular characteristics of their native tongue.

As a result of further experience, and as certain connections between brain cells are consolidated and others are pruned, infants progressively move to processing other characteristics of their native tongue. By 4–6 months, they attend to features such as clause boundaries, which will ultimately have syntactic value (Hirsh-Pasek, Kemler-Nelson, Jusczyk, Wright Cassidy, Druss & Kennedy, 1987; Jusczyk & Bertoncini, 1988). They prefer listening to speech samples in which pauses are inserted at clause boundaries rather than in the middle of clauses. This suggests that infants can use prosodic organization to determine some aspects of grammatical categories within a sentence, e.g. the hierarchical organization of words, phrases and clauses. Sensitivity to prosodic marking for determining clausal units is in place by 6 months of age, but the use of prosody to determine sub-clausal units at the phrasal level is only apparent at 9 months (Jusczyk, Hirsh-Pasek, Kemler Nelson, Kennedy Woodward & Pivoz, 1992).

In sum, the speech and language abilities seen in young infants are neither all present at birth nor all learned through experience. Rather, young infants actively process auditory stimuli, and their early phonemic and morphosyntactic sensitivities channel their processing of all subsequent speech input in linguistically-relevant ways.

Infants are not only sensitive to differences in the speech signal and to potential prosodic cues to syntactic organization. Before their first birthday, they start to process the subtleties of meaning also. For example, prelinguistic infants hearing the word for a common object will look longer at the picture corresponding to that word than at another picture (Plunkett, in preparation). Moreover, 17-month-olds already know something about how the presence or absence of articles affects reference. Infants will take "Dax" to refer to an individual doll (i.e. to be the equivalent of a proper name), but "a Dax" to refer to any one of a similar group of dolls (i.e. to be the equivalent of a common noun) (Katz, Baker & Macnamara, 1974). New preferential looking techniques have made further discoveries possible. Video recordings of different actions are shown on two screens. A loudspeaker placed equidistant between the two screens emits a sentence that describes the scene on one of the two screens (Hirsh-Pasek, Golinkoff, Fletcher, DeGaspe Beaubien & Cauley, 1985). The work has revealed that 17-month-old infants, who are only at the one- or two-word stage in producing language, none the less distinguish in comprehension between sentences like "Big Bird is tickling Cookie Monster" and "Cookie Monster is tickling Big Bird". In other words, rather than simply picking out the nouns and the verb, these infants are already sensitive to meaning differences conveyed by word order, even though word order is not yet used syntactically in their own input.

A common view of language acquisition was that it moves slowly from phonetic to syllabic contrasts, to words, sentences and extended discourse. However, recent work has demonstrated that language develops at many levels simultaneously, with information at each level constraining learning at other levels (Jusczyk *et al.* 1994; Gerken, Jusczyk & Mandel, 1994). Infants do not move unidirectionally from smaller to larger linguistic units, but often start by storing the larger units that they subsequently break down into component parts (Karmiloff-Smith, 1992a).

In sum, by the time they start to actually produce their first recognizable words, and well before they produce anything like a sentence, infants' brains have been actively processing the speech and language in the environment, using cues from prosody, structure and distributional patterns to construct the particularities of the system underlying their native tongue.

## PROCESSING VISUAL INPUT

Are children just as active with respect to processing the visual input around them? Clearly, unlike auditory input, visual processing cannot start in the womb, although it has been established that the foetus reacts (increased heart beat or increased movement) when a strong light is shone on the mother's abdomen (Shahidullah & Hepper, 1993). But this is an unpatterned input giving rise to gross reactions to light changes, unlike the fine auditory discriminations of which the foetus is capable. However, the moment the infant is born, visual processing starts with a vengeance.

It used to be thought that the infant saw almost nothing at birth. It has since been shown that although at certain distances visual input may appear blurred to the newborn, at others—*inter alia* roughly the distance a mother would hold her infant when feeding—many basic visual capacities are in place (Atkinson, 1984). It seems that stimulus distance (other factors held constant) is not a determinant of early discrimination abilities. Indeed, the young infant's visual capacities turn out to be considerably better than previously suspected. At birth, relatively fine spatial discriminations, including shape and size constancy, act as organizing features of perception (Slater, 1992).

The capacity to change voluntarily the focus of visual attention and ignore other competing stimuli also starts in early infancy, around 2 months of age. Studies of visual attention, visual anticipation and working memory in young infants have demonstrated surprising capacities (Gilmore & Johnson, in press; Haith, Hazen & Goodman, 1987; Hood, 1993; Johnson, 1994, 1995; Johnson, Posner & Rothbart, 1994; Johnson & Tucker, 1993). One of Johnson and collaborators' studies focuses on infants' ability to learn to predict where an interesting target will appear, and to remember that location after a delay of several seconds whilst ignoring other stimuli (Gilmore & Johnson, in press). Attractive graphic designs are presented on the centre of three computer monitor screens. When the infant's attention is captured by the central screen, one of two specific sequences of images appears in the central screen, followed by a delay period of 1–5 seconds. After the delay, a target stimulus appears on the screen on the left or on the right hand side. Over the course of the experiment, infants learn that a sequence of spiralling circles means that the target will appear on the left, while a sequence of spiralling squares means that it will appear on the right. Four-month-olds learn to process cues covertly whilst inhibiting overt gaze shifts, and then, in anticipation of the target stimulus before it actually appears, they shift their gaze towards a specific location (left or right, depending on the shapes appearing in the central screen). By varying the length of time between the cue and the target, Johnson and his colleagues have shown that 4-month-old infants' anticipatory eye movements can be used as clues to how long they can hold something in working memory and how they use that to voluntarily direct their visual attention.

Within the area of processing visual stimuli, a fundamental distinction to which young infants are particularly sensitive resides in the differences between the social and physical worlds. We will deal with each of these in turn.

### (A) Attention to Social Stimuli

Newborns are attracted to socially-relevant stimuli. For example, they preferentially track a face-like stimulus (three high contrast blobs in the location of the eyes and the mouth) over other interesting stimuli (Johnson & Morton, 1991; Vecera & Johnson, 1995). Researchers disagree as to whether the initial capacity is driven by the psychosocial features of the stimulus (Kleiner, 1987) or by the structural composition of a face-like form such as proposed by Johnson and Morton. However, as new research accumulates it seems that the latter interpretation of the newborn capacity is the favoured one. It is not until infants are about 2 months of age that they prefer a full drawing of a face (containing eyebrows, eyes, nose and mouth) over the primitive three-blob face-like stimulus. In other words, infants seem to start life with a minimal predisposition to attend to face-like stimuli, but it is only with experience that they learn about the details of the human face and prefer that over other stimuli. And by about 5 months of age, the stimulus of a static human face is no longer as attractive, because by that time, i.e. with even more experience, they prefer a face with moving internal features (Johnson & Morton, 1991).

Although recognition of mother's face has been demonstrated at 4 days of age (Field, Cohen, Garcia & Greenberg, 1984; Bushnell, Sai & Mullin, 1989; Walton, Bower & Bower, 1992), it does not appear to be based on her internal features (Pascalis, de Schonen, Deruelle, Morton & Fabre-Grenet, in press). Rather, early recognition seems to be achieved by using a general pattern processing system, rather than a face-specific one, with the infant focusing on the face/hair separation line and the outer contour of the mother's head. This is why very young infants can be disturbed when mother's hairstyle changes radically. In the first two months of life, then, recognition of individual faces calls on general pattern processing mechanisms. The early face-specific mechanism is used only to categorize stimuli as faces or nonfaces, but not yet to recognize specific ones (Johnson & Morton, 1991). It is only between 2 and 4 months that infants start to focus on the details of the internal features to recognize individual faces, at which point their recognition of mother calls on face-specific processing mechanisms and starts to resemble the way adults recognize individual faces.

It is none the less important to point to alternative interpretations. Some studies went to considerable length to match mothers for features such as hairline (Walton, Bower & Bower, 1992). Although infants may initially focus on peripheral features, the discrimination is not based on gross differences in shape, but may already be relatively subtle. Presumably, too, if the internal features were made particularly salient, e.g. by movement, then the infant's attention can be shifted to them. None the less, other things being equal, infants tend initially to use the face/hair separation line and the outer contour of the head to recognize individual faces.

That a great deal of learning goes on beyond any initial predispositions for face-like stimuli is nicely illustrated by a study on infant and adult discrimination of the faces of nonhuman primates (Sargent & Nelson, 1992). Infants up to the age of 9 months actually perform better than adults at recognizing whether a chimp face is the same as the one just seen but in another orientation, or whether it is a different chimp face. By contrast, adults have difficulty with chimp faces, although no problems arise if the faces are from the human species. In other words, with development, what starts out as a primitive, face-processing capacity gradually becomes a specialized, species-specific processing capacity, just as is the case for the consolidation of native tongue phonemic discriminations discussed earlier.

Beyond face processing in general, infants are capable of following eye gaze at about 6 months and of directing the visual attention of adults to outside entities before 12 months (Scaife & Bruner, 1975; Bates, 1976; Butterworth, 1991). A recent study by Moore and collaborators showed that under 12-month-olds will even follow the direction indicated by adult head orientation alone (with the eyes closed). Some have argued that this ability for eye gaze monitoring and joint attention underlies the later development of infants' capacity to see others as intentional agents and to build up a theory of mind (Baron-Cohen, 1989; Baron-Cohen 1994 and peer commentaries; Sigman *et al.*, 1986; Tomasello, 1994; and see Meltzoff & Gopnik, 1993, with respect to a proposed relation between imitation and a growing conception of self). But the 12-month-old's ability is limited to seeing others as intentional agents in terms of their goals and behaviours, whereas the later theory of mind capacities go beyond dyadic eye gaze monitoring and involve seeing others as mental agents in terms of their thoughts and beliefs (Baron-Cohen, 1993; Tomasello, 1994; Wellman, 1990).

Infants' attention to socially-relevant stimuli extends well beyond human faces and voices. Early on, they also seem capable of generalizing their knowledge and attributing some form of goal-directedness or intentionality to abstract stimuli (Dittrich & Lea, 1994; Gergely, Nádasdy, Csibra, & Bíró, in press; see, also, Premack & Premack, 1995). For instance, shown a large and a small circle interacting on a computer screen, 12-month-olds will interpret them as having rational, goal-directed behaviour (Gergely *et al.*, in press). In this experiment, one large red circle and one smaller yellow circle are separated by a large rectangular obstacle. The red circle expands and contracts a few times and, "in response", the yellow circle expands and contracts. Then the yellow circle appears to leap over the obstacle and come to rest next to the red circle. Infants are habituated to this scene until they show what might be termed "boredom", i.e. they look for increasingly shorter times probably because they have reached a threshold of sufficient information intake. The obstacle is then removed, and one of two things happens: either the infants see a new visual event in which the yellow circle travels along a straight trajectory (the shortest route) to the red circle, or the infants see the yellow circle move on the same trajectory as before, only this time there is no obstacle. Despite seeing a new visual event (the yellow circle moving along a straight line to the red one), the first group of infants show little recovery of interest to the display. By contrast, the infants who see the same trajectory of the yellow circle as in the previous display show significant renewed looking. The results of this experiment suggest that infants interpret the initial event in terms of the behaviour of the yellow circle being rational and goal-directed, so that in the case where it takes a detour route, where no obstacle is present, it is interpreted as behaving "irrationally". Therefore, the event is considered novel and interesting.

Why do the infants look longer at an event that is perceptually very close to what they had habituated to, and not at an event that is perceptually new? They show differential interest in the stimuli because their interpretation of the *perceptually very similar* event is *conceptually different*, in that they appear to attribute goal-directedness to the circles. Infants seem to be seeking an intentional explanation of the goal state (the yellow circle "wants" to be with the red circle) in which an action (take the shortest route to the goal) is interpreted as rational or irrational (Gergely *et al.*, in press). More recent studies suggest that the ability to generate an expectation about the most rational future action that an agent will take is in place by 9 months, but at 6 months infants are not yet able to evaluate the rationality of an agent's goal-directed actions (Gergely, Csibra, Bíró & Koós, 1994).

Of course, as with other infancy studies, these data are open to other interpretations. For example, some data in the literature suggest that there may be a developmental shift from novelty preference to similarity preference. But the design of most studies is such that, depending on the parameters of tasks, the same age infants will be expected to show novelty preference for some items and similarity preference for others. It is also possible that with older infants there is a tendency no longer to focus on total novelty, but to be interested in stimuli that have some similarity with a slight difference. This points to possible alternative explanations which are weaker than the rich conceptual interpretations offered by the authors. Such alternatives must of course always be entertained as we build up an increasingly complex picture of infant cognition.

In sum, several studies now suggest that, from early on, infants attend to stimuli that have meaningful social implications. Their early face preference creates important socially-relevant perceptual categories, and the early interpretations of behaviour in terms of rationality points to their growing conceptual knowledge of the social world.

## (B) Attention to Physical Stimuli

Infants do not only attend to social stimuli. They are also fascinated by the world of objects and learn a great deal during the first 12 months of life about the physics governing the behaviour of objects. The environment has complex structure and infant brains seem to some extent prepared to process that structure (Gibson, 1969). It has been argued that infants come into the world equipped with a number of domain-specific principles that guide their segmentation of complex visual arrays into objects (Spelke, 1991; Spelke, Vishton & von Hofsten, 1995). This challenges the long-held Piagetian view that infants initially experience the visual world as "undifferentiated and chaotic" (Piaget, 1955; Sinclair, 1971).

Spelke, Vishton and von Hofsten (1995) argue that infants' sensitivity to certain principles of physics suggests that humans begin at an early age to develop knowledge of objects and their behaviour. Object perception is guided by constraints that objects move as connected and bounded wholes, on continuous and unobstructed paths, and only on contact with other objects (i.e. they are not self-propelling). Object-directed reaching and visual tracing are guided by the constraint that objects move smoothly. The contrasting constraints, guiding object perception and object-directed actions, suggest that separate systems of knowledge underlie these different achievements. Such principles make it possible for the infant (and adult) to distinguish between the presence of a single object versus more than one, when objects are adjacent to one another or partially occlude each other. In normal visual arrays, partial occlusion is the rule rather than the exception: objects rarely present themselves in isolation against a neutral background. Hence principles for segmenting the complex array into separate objects must be called upon.

A large number of experiments have exploited these ideas. For example, infants are first habituated to a display of two identical rods moving simultaneously at the top and bottom of an occluder. After habituation, infants either see a display containing a single long rod, or one containing two separate rods. Four-month-olds are capable of inferring that if two parts are moving coherently together behind the occluder, then they belong to one and the same object (Kellman & Spelke, 1983). It is only by 7 months that infants can make the same inference if the parts are not moving together but are stationary. Adults make these inferences too. However, if the two parts are of a different colour, shape or texture, and are not moving, then 7-month-olds and adults first treat them as two different objects. Three–four-month-olds perform at chance. The moment the two parts begin to move together simultaneously, adults, 7-month-olds and 3–4-month-olds treat them as forming a single unitary object (Spelke, Breinlinger, Macomber & Jacobson, 1992). The Gestalt principles of continuation of colour, texture and shape do help the slightly older infant to discover properties of objects in stationary as opposed to moving arrays. But movement always overrides Gestalt properties for both infants and adults, because it is a better clue for segmentation.

This body of research on infant physics has shown that 3–4-month-olds store knowledge about the object world and can make inferences on the basis of perceptual input in far greater sophistication and far earlier than Piagetian theory asserts (Piaget, 1952; Sinclair, 1971). The capacity does not seem to be operative at birth, however. Slater and colleagues have demonstrated that although their visual perception (orientation discrimination, form perception, size constancy, etc.) is highly organized, newborns do not make the same inferences from perceptual input as 4-month-olds (Slater, Morison, Somers, Mattock, Brown & Taylor, 1990). So is the 3–4-month-old capacity learned? Spelke argues that, whereas other physical principles such as gravity and inertia are learned, the principles underlying object perception are innately specified and not learned. The difference between Slater's and Spelke's results can be used to suggest that the processes guiding object perception do not start out as a fully specified perceptual module, as Spelke argues, but became modularized as a product of development and experience (Karmiloff-Smith, 1992a).

Whatever the innate endowment may turn out to be, it is clear that infants go on to learn a great deal about the behaviour of objects, as further experiments have shown. Four-month-old infants were habituated to a falling ball which came to rest on a supporting surface (Spelke, 1991). They were then shown either a possible or an impossible event. The possible event was visibly different to the habituation display because the ball came to rest at a different location. In the impossible event, the ball came to rest in the same location as in the habituation display but, in order to do so, it would have had to pass through a solid surface. Now, if infants were only interested in the visual characteristics of the display, they should have found the display where the ball was in a different location novel and more interesting. But the 4-month-olds showed longer looking times at the impossible but visually similar event, i.e. they focused on the properties of the displays relevant to laws of physics. They seemed to be sensitive to and surprised by the violation of a principle that specifies that object substance is such that one solid object cannot pass through another.

Similarly, a falling object cannot stop in mid-air if there is no supporting surface. Do young infants know about this? It turns out that 4-month-olds know something about hands letting go of objects (Needham & Baillargéon, 1993), but still have a lot to learn about other principles governing kinaesthetics and gravity. For example, 4-month-olds do not show surprise when a moving object stops in mid-air (Spelke, 1991). But a couple of months later, Spelke's results show 6-month-old infants to have significantly longer looking times if a falling object does not continue its trajectory until it encounters a supporting surface. By then, infants' experiences and their perceptual analyses of events in the physical world have been sufficient to generate some new constraints on interpreting object behaviour.

Another series of ingenious experiments were designed by Baillargéon and her collaborators (Baillargéon, 1987, 1991, 1993; Baillargéon, Spelke & Wasserman, 1985). Baillargéon believes that infants first form a preliminary all-or-none concept in terms of impact/no impact, contact/no contact, etc. that captures the essence of a phenomenon but few of its details. She too used the violation of expectation method to test young infants. For example, Baillargéon habituated 3–4-month-old infants to the sight of a screen rotating 180°, until they looked for increasingly briefer times. Then, in full view of the infant, she placed a solid object behind the screen. Next, infants either saw the screen rotate to 112° (a new but normal event now that an object prevented the full rotation), or they saw the screen continue to rotate the full 180° as before (an impossible event, because the infants did not see that the object had been surreptitiously removed). As far as the visual input is concerned, the infants who saw the normal event were receiving *new* visual input (a 112° rotation), whereas the infants who saw the impossible event were receiving the *same* visual input as before (a full 180° rotation). If Piagetians were correct and young infants have no rudimentary sensitivities to the persistence of objects when out of view, then they should not expect the object which has disappeared from sight to block the screen from rotating the full 180°. However, if infants' inferences are based on some form of representation of the continued existence of objects out of sight, and if they comply with the physical principle that two objects (the screen and the object behind it) cannot occupy the same space simultaneously, then they should show increased attention with respect to the impossible event yet identical visual input. And this is precisely what happened. In other words, 3–4-month-old infants are sensitive to the fact that even when an object is occluded by a screen, it continues to exist and should therefore block the screen's rotation.

Baillargéon went on to use a similar rotating screen paradigm to demonstrate that 3–4-month-old infants can compute the relation between the height of objects and the angle of rotation that they allow, whereas it is only somewhat later that they understand rigidity and compressibility of objects (Baillargéon, 1993). Other research generated from various theoretical stances (e.g. Butterworth, 1991; Rutkowska, 1994, in press; Slater & Bremner, in press; Willatts, 1989), also challenges the Piagetian view of early infancy and shows young infants to be far more sensitive to the complexities of their physical environment than previously suspected (although see Gilmore & Johnson, in press, which suggests that in some areas of cognition, young infants turn out to be less sophisticated than the new work tends to suggest).

So have the nativists won the battle in claiming that infant cognition is to some great extent innately specified? Many developmentalists would reply in the affirmative. But this is a far from necessary conclusion from these data. Although we probably now need to invoke *some* predispositions in infant minds as they process and interpret the physical world, this does not mean that all infant capacities are specified in any detail, or even prespecified at all. Development has complex timing constraints, the environment has complex structure, and young infants are capable of very rapid learning. But it is clear that they often demonstrate surprisingly sophisticated capacities with respect to their cognitive inferences about object behaviour in the physical world, and differentiate these from the intentional and rational interpretations that they attribute to stimuli in the social world.

## PROCESSING INPUT INTERMODALLY

So far we have looked at infants' capacities to process auditory or visual input. But of course the world does not come neatly packaged for processing by isolated modalities. Information usually entails simultaneous processing by various modalities. It remains unclear whether the outputs from different modalities (e.g. vision and touch/vision and sound) are amodal and thus matched by the infant's system automatically, or whether there is a translation process between different modalities such that we can refer to cross-modal matching. None the less, a large body of research has focused on infants' capacity to process input intermodally.

It has been demonstrated that young infants can detect the correspondence between auditory speech signals and the visible articulatory movements that accompany them (Kuhl & Meltzoff, 1984). In other words, they can "lip-read". Four-month-old infants are presented with two facial images, one making the lip movement of the vowel /i/ and the other the vowel /a/ (or /i/ versus /u/). Simultaneously with the visual input, a loudspeaker located midway between the facial images produces one of the two sounds. The infants look reliably longer at the screen which corresponds to the sound they can hear, i.e. they match the auditory input onto the correct visual input (Kuhl & Meltzoff, 1984). This lip-reading capacity extends beyond single vowel discrimination. Infants also show intermodal matching with bisyllabic stimuli such as/mama/versus/lulu/, or /baby/ versus /zuzi/ (MacKain, Studdert-Kennedy, Spieker & Stern, 1983).

Language is not the only domain in which infants' capacity for processing intermodal inputs has been revealed. They are also capable of matching what they *see* another's face doing and what they *feel* their own face doing. For instance, imitation studies have shown that newborns will imitate an adult's repeated tongue protrusion (Meltzoff & Borton, 1979; Meltzoff & Moore, 1977, 1989). However, for very young infants it is essential that the tongue be moving in and out. It takes another few months before a statically presented stimulus of an already protruded tongue is imitated (Vinter, 1986). If the newborn ability cannot be explained away as a simple reflex, as some might claim, then the imitation entails a complex sequence of processes. First infants must process what they are seeing on the face of the adult. Then they must work out which part of their own face, which they cannot see but only feel, is the same as the adult's, and finally they must find a procedure to imitate the action. Infants could have opened and closed their eyes or their hands in response to the tongue protrusion, but at birth they seem already capable of matching what they see on others to what they feel on their own body.

This is one interpretation of the data, but other interpretations which attribute less to the neonate may suffice. It is a fact, for example, that the results of imitation studies are usually clearer with tongue protrusion than with any of the other stimuli presented to the infant, e.g. mouth opening, lip pursing, hand opening, etc. An alternative explanation is possible, then, in terms of stimulation always giving rise in very young infants to a form of arousal that results in the sucking response; the sucking reflex naturally involves a protrusion of the tongue. One might, therefore, predict the following: if the model were mouth opening, but when the mouth opened some attractive glittering stimuli appeared, that might generate greater arousal. In that case, tongue protrusion for mouth opening might occur more often than if the model were actually tongue protrusion. However, this alternative explanation is weakened by the fact that infant imitation improves and becomes closer to the model during the time the model is presented, suggesting that even if the imitation starts out as a reflex to general arousal, it rapidly becomes a form of imitation of the model. Such a capacity is impressive in the newborn.

The newborn capacity to imitate tongue protrusion may seem to contradict what was stated in an earlier section about the newborn's focus on hairline and head shape to recognise individual faces. This is not a necessary contradiction, however. First, the newborn imitative response could be a reflex response (like hand flapping) or releasing mechanism to an arousing stimulus (like a face), although this interpretation is weakened, as mentioned above, by the within-trial improvements. Second, as mentioned above, movement is crucial to generate neonate imitation of tongue protrusion, whereas neonate face recognition studies have demonstrated their results with static faces. Third, the newborn is *learning* about how to discriminate different faces, whereas imitation in the newborn may not involve learning. Imitation is not focused on discriminating different faces, but on using information shown on a mouth in a face, irrespective of whether the face is of the mother or a stranger. Of course the newborn can perceive internal face features; the question is whether the newborn *uses* internal features to *discriminate* particular faces from others.

Interestingly, imitation can serve the young infant as a form of nonverbal communication of memory for past events: the infant generates actions on the basis of stored representations. For instance, a group of 6-week-olds were presented with a person who pulled his tongue in and out repeatedly (Meltzoff & Moore, 1994). Then, 24 hours later each infant was brought back into the infant lab. The person seen the day before was again presented to the infant, but this time with his lips closed. The infants stared at the face with interest, and gradually started to push out their tongues, as if to say implicitly: "Hey, don't I know you? You're the one who pulled your tongue in and out when I last saw you"! They did not generate such actions in response to new faces seen for the first time. The actual status of the infant's representations remains unclear, although one-trial learning of this kind would suggest that it involves retrieval of stored knowledge. Preverbal infants are thus able to make intermodal transfer and to use behavioural reenactment to communicate their recall to others (see, also, Rovee-Collier, 1993; Perris, Myers & Clifton, 1990 on memory 2 years later for events experienced at 6 months of age; McDonough & Mandler, 1995 for illustrations of delayed imitation up to 12 months later of events seen once at 11 months of age).

Another interesting area of intermodal processing concerns touch and vision. It has been shown (Gibson & Walker, 1984; Meltzoff & Borton, 1979) that 1-month-olds are capable of intermodal matching between the shape of a dummy being sucked and pictures of dummies on a screen. This has recently been extended to newborns with simpler stimuli (Kaye & Bower, 1994). These two studies focused on the relationship between vision and exploration in the mouth. Somewhat older infants have been tested with respect to intermodal processing between vision and the hands. For example, 4-month-old infants first explored haptically (by touch only) a stimulus that they could not see because it was given to them below a screen (Streri, Spelke, & Ramiex, 1993). For one group of infants, the stimulus was composed of two independently moveable rings attached by flexible string. For another group, the rings were attached to a rigid rod forming a single object. Recall that all that the baby can feel in her hands is the existence of two rings. She must infer from exploring haptically the rigid or flexible linkage between the rings whether one or two objects are present. After habituation, infants were shown two displays, one of two rings joined by a straight rod thereby forming a single object, the other of two separate rings. Habituation to the independently moveable rings was followed by longer looking at the connected display. Similarly, habituation to the rigidly connected rings was followed by longer looking at the two separate rings. In both cases, the posthabituation displays are in a new (visual) modality, so the infants could have found either visual display novel compared to the one they had touched. But it is not the change in modality on which they focus. Rather, what they find salient are the physical principles that allow them to infer differences in objecthood. The outputs of haptic perception in 4-month-old infants can be represented in a format that is available for comparison with the outputs of visual perception.

Finally, intermodal processing has been explored in the study of infants' sensitivity to number. Initially it was shown that at birth infants can discriminate between two and three objects and at 5-months they can discriminate between three and four objects (Antell & Keating, 1983; Starkey & Cooper, 1980; Strauss & Curtis, 1981). Wynn (1992) has also argued that young infants are sensitive to elementary additions and subtractions. It also turns out that 6–8-month-old infants can detect numerical correspondence between a set of visible items and a set of audible items, i.e. intermodal matching relevant to the numerosity of displays. Thus when presented with two visual displays each with a specific number of objects, infants will focus on the one with the same number of objects as an auditory input of drum beats (Starkey, Spelke & Gelman, 1983, although see Moore, Benenson, Reznick, Peterson & Kagan, 1987, for somewhat different findings). Thus, early on infants will attend to the number-relevant properties of visual and auditory displays.

In sum, intermodal processing of input is a capacity that can be demonstrated in very young infants and serves them to make sense of the multiple overlapping stimuli in their environment. Whether this stems from a transfer of information from one modality to another, or is simply the product of amodal representations matched automatically, remains an open question for future infancy theory and research.

## PERCEIVING VERSUS CONCEIVING

Much of the research on early infancy has shown surprising discrimination capacities. For example, in the first days of life infants differentiate between circles and squares perceptually. By 3 months they can discriminate cats from dogs, cats from lions, horses from zebras, etc. (Quin, Eimas & Rosenkrantz, 1993). But such perceptual discriminations are also available to other species. They do not necessarily mirror conceptual ones. Indeed, on the basis of their perceptual discriminations, one might have thought that infants' conceptual development would start from so-called basic level categories like dog (Rosch, 1975) and gradually lead to superordinate categories like animal and subordinate categories like poodle. This is not, however, the case. Perceptual analysis, based on the visible features of objects, and conceptual analysis, based on internal representations of abstract features, seem to develop in parallel in rather different ways.

It has been shown that the earliest *conceptual* categories are at the superordinate level, despite the fact that infants are capable of *perceiving* differences at the other levels (Mandler & McDonough, 1993). For example, at 7–11 months infants categorize objects into animals and vehicles, but demonstrate no within-animal categorization. Generalization is also initially at the superordinate level and not at the basic level (Mandler & McDonough, in press). Thus 14-month-olds generalize properties such as drinking, sleeping and hopping to all animals, but not to vehicles. Likewise, they generalize key use or giving rides to all vehicles, but not to animals. In other words, a bird will be given a ride on an aeroplane along the surface of a table, whereas both actually fly! In this way, infants are demonstrating their *conceptual* knowledge of the category "animal" versus "vehicle" and ignoring the perceptual similarity between toy birds with outstretched wings and toy aeroplanes. Mandler argues that, contrary to perceptual development, conceptual development is neither constrained by visual similarity nor by basic level category membership, but by domain-level superordinate categories. Thus infants form different perceptual and conceptual categories from the outset. Once their conceptual categories are consolidated at the superordinate level, then finer perceptual analyses guide their subsequent conceptual categorization at the basic level (Mandler & McDonough, 1993).


## QUO VADIS INFANCY RESEARCH?

The past couple of decades have witnessed the discovery of capacities in newborns and young infants which were hitherto unsuspected. However, it would be a pity if future research were to be reduced solely to demonstrations of precocity, i.e. to the search for increasingly more capacities in ever younger infants. We need to know not simply whether such abilities are present, but how they are possible and what cognitive processes are involved. More focus should also be placed on individual differences in very early infancy, such as those found by Baillergéon at 3.5 months between fast habituators and slow habituators (Baillargéon, 1993) or differences in visual attention (Johnson, 1994, 1995), not only with respect to how they correlate with later IQ (Slater, 1995) but also the implications that these domain-general abilities have for different types of domain-specific development. For instance, is an infant who is a fast habituator to auditory input also fast with respect to visual input? We also need to avoid unwarranted attributions of sophisticated cognitive capacities where simpler explanations suffice. For example, what does it really mean for an infant to "know"? More precision about the actual representations underlying the early competencies is called for.

A second direction of future research concerns the relationship between early competences and later ones. There are many implicit claims in the literature that early domain-specific competences are directly linked to later capacities, yet almost no research has so far been directly focused on this issue. To be sure, research has focused on measuring correlations between later IQ and domain-general abilities in infancy (Bornstein & Sigman, 1986; Cohen & Parmelee, 1983; Colombo, Mitchell, Coldren & Freeseman, 1991; Fagan, 1984), using standardized infancy tests or measures of recognition memory, speed of habituation, preference for visual novelty, etc. (see Slater, 1995 for comprehensive review). Moreover, where such studies have demonstrated a lack of correlative relationship does not necessarily imply a lack of a developmental relationship, because individual differences may not be stable over developmental time. However, the recent spate of discoveries of what seem to be domain-specific abilities in early infancy have not, to my knowledge, been followed up longitudinally.

Theoretically, it is quite possible that there is *no* relation between the early capacity to process, say, faces and an older child's score on the Benton Face Discrimination Task or the Rivermead Face Memory Task. Likewise there may be no relation between the early capacity to match auditory to visual number displays and later abilities in counting or conservation of number. Such correlations remain to be established. In my view, however, domain-specific correlations between early infancy and later childhood are difficult to carry out in the area of normal development, because usually the domain-specific tasks are not aimed at revealing individual differences but rather at demonstrating that such abilities exist in infancy. By contrast, abnormal development offers a particularly fruitful platform from which to raise such questions (Karmiloff-Smith, 1992a, b; Karmiloff-Smith, Klima, Bellugi, Grant & Baron-Cohen, 1995). The reason for this is that if a particular syndrome is characterized by a proficiency or a deficit in a given domain, then one can seek the lack of or existence of domain-specific precursors in infancy. In the normal case, they will always both be present. It is thus essential to focus on abnormal phenotypes that can be diagnosed at birth and that give rise to uneven cognitive profiles of proficiencies and deficits (Karmiloff-Smith, 1992b). This may turn out to be a rich area of infancy research in the future, although the problems of longitudinal research with infants (e.g. high attrition rates, the state-dependent nature of achievements, measurement errors which obscure stable patterns over time, etc.) should not be underestimated. None the less, where feasible and successful, longitudinal studies starting with foetal experience through infancy could greatly add to the study of both normative change and individual differences.

In my view, infant cognition will continue to be at the centre of our endeavours to understand the workings of the human mind/brain. The use of behavioural techniques that made possible many of the discoveries discussed in this review, has recently been followed by the search for infant-friendly, noninvasive approaches to brain imaging. The next decade will undoubtedly witness many new discoveries as researchers focus on the complex relationship between the structure of the developing brain and the competencies displayed during early infancy (e.g. Bates, Thal & Janowsky, 1992; Gilmore & Johnson, in press; Janowsky, 1993; Johnson, 1990, 1994, 1995; Nelson & DeRegnier, 1992). Moreover, the growing use of computer simulations of early development (Elman, Bates, Johnson, Karmiloff-Smith, Parisi & Plunkett, in press) may also help to specify in far more detail the different ways in which things might be "innate"—predispositions in terms of computational, architectual, representational or timing biases, that constrain the way development proceeds. Despite the impressive advances in the past couple of decades in understanding the extraordinary cognitive journey from foetus through infancy, we have barely scratched the surface of this exciting area of research.

## REFERENCES

Antell, E. & Keating, D. P. (1983). Perception of numerical invariance in neonates. *Child Development, 54*, 695–701.

Atkinson, J. (1984). Human visual development over the first six months of life: a review and a hypothesis. *Human Neurobiology, 3*, 61–74.

Baillargéon, R. (1987). Young infants' reasoning about the physical and spatial properties of a hidden object. *Cognitive Development, 2*, 170–200.

Baillargéon, R. (1991). Reasoning about the height and location of a hidden object in 4.5- and 6.5-month-old infants. *Cognition, 38*, 13–42.

Baillargéon, R. (1993). The object concept revisited: new directions in the investigation of infants' physical knowledge. In C. Granrud (Ed.) *Visual perception and cognition in infancy*. Hillsdale, NJ, Erlbaum.

Baillargéon, R., Spelke, E. & Wasserman, S. (1986). Object permanence in five month old infants. *Cognition, 20*, 191–208.

Baron-Cohen, S. (1989). Perceptual role-taking and protodeclarative pointing in autism. *British Journal of Developmental Psychology, 7*, 113–127.

Baron-Cohen, S. (1993). From attention-goal psychology to belief-desire psychology: The development of a theory of mind and its dysfunction. In S. Baron-Cohen, H. Tager-Flusberg & D. J. Cohen (Eds), *Understand other minds*. Oxford: Oxford University Press.

Baron-Cohen, S. (1994). (and peer commentators) How to build a baby that can read minds: cognitive mechanisms in mindreading. *Cahiers de Psychologie Cognitive, 13*, 1–40.

Bates, E. (1976). *Language and context: The acquisition of pragmatics*. New York: Academic Press.

Bates, E., Thal, D. & Janowsky, J. S. (1992). Early language development and its neural correlates. In S. J. Segalowitz & I. Rapin (Eds), *Handbook of neuropsychology, Vol. 7, Child neuropsychology* (pp. 69–110). Amsterdam: Elsevier Science Publishers.

Bornstein, M. H. (1985). Habituation of attention as a measure of visual information processing in human infants: summary, systematization, and synthesis. In G. Gottlieb & N. A. Krasnegor (Eds) *Measurement of audition and vision in the first year of postnatal life: a methodological overview*, Norwood, NJ: Ablex.

Bornstein, M. H. & Sigman, M. D. (1986). Continuity in mental development from infancy. *Child Development, 57*, 251–274.

Bushnell, I. W. R., Sai, F. & Mullin, J. T. (1989). Neonatal recognition of the mother's face. *British Journal of Developmental Psychology, 7*, 3–15.

Butterworth, G. (1991). The ontogeny and phylogeny of joint visual attention. In A. Whiten, (Ed.), *Natural theories of mind: evolution, development and simulation of everyday mindreading.* Oxford: Blackwell.

Christophe, A., Dupoux, E., Bertoncini, J. & Mehler, J. (1994). Do infants perceive word boundaries? An empirical study of the bootstrapping of lexical acquisition. *Journal of the Acoustical Society of America, 95*, 1570–1580.

Cohen, S. E. & Parmelee, A. H. (1983). Prediction of five-year Stanford-Binet scores in preterm infants. *Child Development, 54*, 1242–1253.

Colombo, J., Mitchell, D. W., Coldren, J. T. & Freeseman, L. J. (1991). Individual differences in infant visual attention: are short lookers faster processors or feature processors? *Child Development, 62*, 1247–1257.

Cooper, P. K. & Aslin, R. N. (1994). Developmental differences in infant attention to the spectral properties of infant-directed speech, *Child Development, 65*, 1663–1677.

Dittrich, W. H. & Lea, S. E. G. (1994). Visual perception of intentional motion. *Perception, 23*, 253–268.

Eilers, R. E., Bull, D. H., Oller, K. & Lewis, D. C. (1984). The discrimination of vowel duration by infants. *Journal of the Acoustical Society of America, 75*, 1213–1218.

Eimas, P. H., Siqueland, E. R., Jusczyk, P. & Vigorito, J. (1971). Speech perception in infants. *Science, 171*, 303–306.

Elman, J. L., Bates, E., Johnson, M. H., Karmiloff-Smith, A., Parisi, D. & Plunkett, K. (in press). *Rethinking nativism: connectionism in a developmental framework.* Cambridge, MA: MIT Press.

Fagan, J. F. (1984). The relationship of novelty preferences during infancy to later intelligence and later recognition memory. *Intelligence, 8*, 339–346.

Fernald, A. & Kuhl, P. (1981). Fundamental frequency as an acoustic determinant of infant preference for motherese. Paper presented at the meeting of the Society for Research in Child Development, Boston.

Field, T. M., Cohen, D., Garcia, R. & Greenberg, R. (1984). Mother-stranger face discrimination by the newborn. *Infant Behavior and Development, 7*, 19–25.

Fifer, W. P. & Moon, C. (1989). Psychobiology of newborn auditory preferences. *Seminars in Perinatology, 13*, 430–433.

Fowler, C. A., Smith, M. R. & Tassinary, L. G. (1986). Perception of syllable timing by prebabbling infants. *Journal of the Acoustical Society of America, 79*, 814–825.

Gergley, G., Csibra, G., Bíró, S. & Koós, O. (1994). The comprehension of intentional action in infancy. Poster presented at the 9th International Conference of Infant Studies, Paris, 2–5 June 1994.

Gergley, G., Nádasdy, Z., Csibra, G. & Bíró, S. (in press). Taking the intentional stance at 12 months of age. *Cognition.*

Gerken, L. A., Jusczyk, P. W. & Mandel, D. R. (1994). When prosody fails to cue syntactic structure: Nine-month-olds' sensitivity to phonological vs syntactic phrases. *Cognition, 51*, 237–265.

Gibson, E. J. (1969). *Principles of perceptual learning and development.* Englewood Cliffs: Prentice-Hall.

Gibson, E. J. & Walker, A. S. (1984). Development of knowledge of visual-tactual affordances of substance. *Child Development, 55*, 453–460.

Gilmore, R. O. & Johnson, M. H. (in press). Working memory in infancy: six-month-olds' performance on two versions of the oculomotor delayed response tasks. *Journal of Experimental Child Psychology.*

Haith, M. M., Hazan, C. & Goodman, G. S. (1988). Expectation and anticipation of dynamic visual events by 3–5-month-old babies. *Child Development, 59*, 467–479.

Hallé, P. A. & de Boysson-Bardies, B. (1994). Emergence of an early receptive lexicon: infants' recognition of words. *Infant Behavior and Development, 17*, 119–129.

Hepper, P. G., Scott, D. & Shahidullah, S. (1993). Newborn and fetal response to maternal voice. *Journal of Reproductive and Infant Psychology, 11*, 147–153.

Hirsh-Pasek, K., Golinkoff, R., Fletcher, A., DeGaspe Baeubien, F. & Cauley, K. (1985). In the beginning: one-word speakers comprehend word order. Paper presented at the Boston Language Conference, Boston.

Hirsh-Pasek, K., Kemler-Nelson, D. G., Jusczyk, P. W., Wright Cassidy, K., Druss, B. & Kennedy, L. (1987). Clauses are perceptual units for young infants. *Cognition, 26*, 269–286.

Hood, B. M. (1993). Inhibition of return produced by covert shifts of visual attention in 6-month-old infants. *Infant Behavior and Development, 16*, 245–254.

Janowsky, J. (1993). The development and neural basis of memory systems. In M. H. Johnson (Ed.), *Brain development and cognition: a reader* (pp. 665–678). Oxford: Blackwell.

Johnson, M. H. (1990). Cortical maturation and the development of visual attention in early infancy. *Journal of Cognitive Neuroscience, 2*, 81–95.

Johnson, M. H. (1994). Brain and cognitive development in infancy. *Current Opinion in Neurobiology, 4*, 218–225.

Johnson, M. H. (1995). The development of attention: a cognitive neuroscience approach. In M. S. Gassaniga (Ed.), *The cognitive neurosciences* (pp. 735–747). Cambridge, MA: MIT Press.

Johnson, M. H. & Morton, J. (1991). *Biology and cognitive development: the case of face recognition*. Oxford: Blackwell.

Johnson, M. H., Posner, M. I. & Rothbart, M. K. (1994). Facilitations of saccades towards a covertly attention location in early infancy. *Psychological Science, 5*, 9–93.

Johnson, M. H. & Tucker, L. (1993). The ontogeny of covert visual attention: facilitatory and inhibitory effects. *Abstracts of the Society for Research in Child Development, 9*, 424.

Jusczyk, P. W. & Bertoncini, J. (1988). Viewing the development of speech perception as an innately guided learning process. *Language and Speech, 31*, 217–238.

Jusczyk, P., Friederici, A. D., Wessels, J., Svenmkerud, V. Y. & Jusczyk, A. M. (1993). Infants' sensitivity to the sound patterns of native language words. *Journal of Memory and Language, 32*, 402–420.

Jusczyk, P., Hirsh-Pasek, K., Kemler-Nelson, D., Kennedy, L., Woodward, A. & Piwoz, J. (1988). Perception of acoustic correlates of major phrasal units by young infants. Ms., University of Oregon.

Jusczyk, P. W., Luce, P. A. & Charles-Luce, J. (1994). Infants' sensitivity to phonotactic patterns in the native language. *Journal of Memory and Language, 33*, 630–645.

Kaplan, P. S., Goldstein, M. H., Huckeby, E. R. & Panneton Cooper, R. (1995). Habituation, sensitization, and infants' responses to Motherese speech. *Development Psychobiology, 28*, 45–57.

Karmiloff-Smith, A. (1992a). *Beyond modularity: a developmental perspective on cognitive science*. Cambridge MA: MIT Press.

Karmiloff-Smith, A. (1992b). Abnormal phenotypes and the challenges they pose to connectionist models of development. *Technical Report Series on Parallel Distributed Processing and Cognitive Neuroscience*, No. PDP/CNS.92.7, Carnegie Mellon University, Pittsburgh.

Karmiloff-Smith, A. (1994). *Baby it's you: a unique insight into the first three years of the developing baby*. London: Ebury Press, Random House.

Karmiloff-Smith, A., Klima, E., Bellugi, U., Grant, J. & Baron-Cohen, S. (1995). Is there a social module? Language, face processing and theory-of-mind in subjects with Williams syndrome. *Journal of Cognitive Neuroscience, 7*, 196–208.

Katz, N., Baker, E. & Macnamara, J. (1974). What's in a name? A study of how children learn common and proper names. *Child Development, 45*, 469–473.

Kaye, K. L. & Bower, T. G. R. (1994). Learning and intermodal transfer of information in newborns. *Psychological Science, 5*, 286–288.

Kellman, P. J. & Spelke, E. S. (1983). Perception of partly occluded objects in infancy. *Cognitive Psychology, 15*, 483–524.

Kleiner, K. A. (1987). Amplitude and phase spectra as indices of infants' pattern preferences. *Infant Behavior and Development, 10*, 49–59.

Kuhl, P. K. (1991). Perception, cognition, and the ontogenetic and phylogenetic emergence of human speech. In S. Brauth, W. Hall & R. Dooling (Eds), *Plasticity of development*. Cambridge, MA: MIT Press/Bradford Books.

Kuhl, P. K. & Meltzoff, A. N. (1984). The intermodal representation of speech in infants. *Infant Behaviour and Development, 7*, 361–381.

Lecanuet, J. P., Granier-Deferre, C. & Busnel, M. (1988). Fetal cardiac and motor responses to octave-band noises as a function of central frequency, intensity and heart rate variability. *Early Human Development, 13*, 269–283.

Lynch, M. P., Kimbrough Oller, D., Steffens, M. & Buder, E. H. (1995). Phrasing in prelinguistic vocalizations. *Developmental Psychobiology, 28*, 3–25.

MacKain, K., Studdert-Kennedy, M., Spieker, S. & Stern, D. (1983). Infant intermodal speech perceptions is a left-hemisphere function. *Science, 219*, 1347–1349.

Mandel, D. R., Jusczyk, P. W. & Kemler-Nelson, D. G. (1994). Does sentential prosody help infants organize and remember speech information? *Cognition, 53*, 155–180.

Mandler, J. M. & McDonough, L. (1993). Concept formation in infancy. *Cognitive Development, 8*, 291–318.

Mandler, J. M. & McDonough, L. (in press). Drinking and driving don't mix: inductive generalization in infancy. *Cognition*.

McDonough, L. & Mandler, J. M. (1995). Very long-term memory in infancy. *Memory, 2*, 339–352.

Mehler, J. & Christophe, A. (1994). Maturation and learning of language in the first year of life. In M. S. Gazzaniga (Ed.), *The cognitive neurosciences: a handbook for the field* (pp. 943–954). Cambridge, MA: MIT Press.

Mehler, J., Lambertz, G., Jusczyk, P. & Amiel-Tison, C. (1986). Discrimination de la langue maternelle par le nouveau-né. *C.R. Academie des Sciences, 303*, Serie III, 637–640.

Meltzoff, A. N. & Borton, R. W. (1979). Intermodal matching by human neonates. *Nature, 282*, 403–404.

Meltzoff, A. N. & Gopnik, A. (1993). The role of imitation in understanding persons and developing a theory of mind. In S. Baron-Cohen, H. Tager-Flusberg & D. Cohen (Eds), *Understanding other minds*. Oxford: Oxford University Press.

Meltzoff, A. N. & Moore, M. K. (1977). Imitation of facial and manual gestures by human neonates. *Science, 198*, 75–78.

Meltzoff, A. N. & Moore, M. K. (1989). Imitation in newborn infants: exploring the range of gestures imitated and the underlying mechanisms. *Developmental Psychology, 25*, 954–962.

Meltzoff, A. N. & Moore, M. K. (1994). Imitation, memory and the representation of persons. *Infant Behavior and Development, 17*, 83–99.

Moore, D., Benenson, J., Reznick, S., Peterson, M. & Kagan, J. (1987). Effect of auditory numerical information on infants' looking behavior: contradictory evidence. *Developmental Psychology, 23*, 665–670.

Morgan, J. L. (1994). Converging measures of speech segmentation in preverbal infants. *Infant Behaviour and Development, 17*, 389–403.

Needham, A. & Baillargéon, R. (1993). Intuitions about support in 4.5-month-old-infants. *Cognition, 47*, 121–148.

Nelson, C. A. & DeRegnier, R. A. (1992). Neural correlates of attention and memory in the first year of life. *Developmental Neuropsychology, 8*, 119–134.

Olguin, R. & Tomasello, M. (1993). Twenty-five-month-old children do not have a grammatical category of verb. *Cognitive Development, 8*, 245–272.

Oyama, S. (1985). *The ontogeny of information: developmental systems and evolution.* Cambridge: Cambridge University Press.

Pascalis, O., de Schonen, S., Deruelle, C., Morton, J. & Fabre-Grenet, M. (in press). Mother's face recognition in neonates: a replication and an extension. *Infant Behaviour and Development.*

Perris, E. E., Myers, N. A. & Clifton, R. K. (1990). Long-term memory for a single infancy experience. *Child Development, 61*, 1796–1807.

Piaget, J. (1952). *The origins of intelligence in children*, New York: International University Press.

Piaget, J. (1995). *The child's construction of reality*, London: Routledge and Kegan Paul.

Premack, D. & Premack, A. J. (1995). Origins of human social competence. In M. S. Gassaniga (Ed.), *The cognitive neurosciences* (pp. 205–218). Cambridge, MA: MIT Press.

Quin, P. C., Eimas, P. D. & Rosenkrantz, S. L. (1993). Evidence for representation of perceptually similar natural categories by 3- and 4-month old infants. *Perception, 22*, 463–475.

Rosch, E. (1975). Cognitive reference points. *Cognitive Psychology, 7*, 532–547.

Rovee-Collier, C. (1993). The capacity for long-term memory in infancy. *Current Directions in Psychological Science, 2*, 130–135.

Rutkowska, J. C. (1994). Scaling up sensorimotor systems: constraints from human infancy. *Adaptive Behavior, 2*, 349–373.

Rutkowska, J. C. (in press). Reassessing Piaget's theory of sensorimotor intelligence: a view from Cognitive Science. In J. G. Bremner (Ed.), *Infant development: recent advances*. Hillsdale NJ: Lawrence Erlbaum.

Sargent, P. L. & Nelson, C. A. (1992). Cross-species recognition in infant and adult humans: ERP and behavioral measures. Poster presentation, *International Conference on Infant Studies*. Miami Beach, May, 1992.

Scaife, M. & Bruner, J. (1975). The capacity for joint visual attention in the infant. *Nature, 253*, 265–266.

Shahidullah, S. & Hepper, P. G. (1993). Frequency discrimination by the fetus. *Early Human Development, 36*, 13–26.

Sigman, M., Mundy, B., Sherman, T. & Ungerer, J. (1986). Social interactions of autistic, mentally retarded and normal children and their caregivers. *Journal of Child Psychology and Psychiatry, 27*, 647–655.

Sinclair, H. (1971). Sensorimotor action patterns as the condition for the acquisition of syntax. In R. Huxley & E. Ingrams (Eds), *Language acquisition: models and methods*. London: Academic Press.

Slater, A. (1992). The visual constancies in early infancy. *The Irish Journal of Psychology, 13*, 411–424.

Slater, A. (1995). Individual differences in infancy and later IQ. *Journal of Child Psychology and Psychiatry, 36*, 69–112.

Slater, A. & Bremner, J. G. (Eds), (in press). *The psychology of infancy*. Hillsdale, NJ: Erlbaum.

Slater, A., Morison, V., Somers, M., Mattock, A., Brown, E. & Taylor, D. (1990). Newborn and older infants' perception of partly occluded objects. *Infant Behaviour and Development, 13*, 33–49.

Spelke, E. S. (1991). Physical knowledge in infancy: reflections on Piaget's theory. In S. Carey & R. Gelman (Eds), *Epigenesis of the mind: essays in biology and knowledge*. Hillsdale, NJ: Erlbaum.

Spelke, E. S., Breinlinger, K., Macomber, J. & Jacobson, K. (1992). Origins of knowledge. *Psychological Review, 99*, 605–632.

Spelke, E. S., Vishton, P. & von Hofsten, C. (1995). Object perception, object-directed action, and physical knowledge in infancy. In M. S. Gassaniga (Ed.) *The Cognitive Neurosciences* (pp. 165–180). Cambridge, MA: MIT Press.

Spring, D. R. & Dale, P. S. (1977). Discrimination of linguistic stress in early infancy. *Journal of Speech and Hearing Research, 20*, 224–232.

Starkey, P. & Cooper, R. G. (1980). Perception of number by human infants. *Science, 200*, 1033–1035.

Starkey, P., Spelke, E. S. & Gelman, R. (1983). Detection of intermodal correspondences by human infants. *Science, 222*, 179–181.

Strauss, M. S. & Curtis, L. E. (1981). Infants' perception of numerosity. *Child Development, 52*, 1146–1152.

Streri, A., Spelke, E. & Ramiex, E. (1993). Modality-specific and amodal aspects of object perception in infancy: the case of active touch. *Cognition, 47,* 251–279.

Sullivan, J. W. & Horowitz, F. D. (1983). The effects of intonation on infant attention: the role of the rising intonation contour. *Journal of Child Language, 10,* 521–534.

Thelen, E. & Fisher, D. M. (1983). From spontaneous to instrumental behaviour; kinematic analysis of movement changes during very early infancy. *Child Development, 54,* 129–140.

Thelen, E. & Smith, L. B. (1994). *A dynamic systems approach to the development of cognition and action.* Cambridge, MA: MIT Press.

Tomasello, M. (1994). Joint attention as social cognition. In C. Moore & P. Durham (Eds), *Joint attention: its origins and role in development.* Hillsdale, NJ: Lawrence Erlbaum.

Tomasello, M. & Olguin, R. (1993). Twenty-three-month-old children have a grammatical category of noun. *Cognitive Development, 8,* 451–464.

Vecera, S. P. & Johnson, M. H. (1995). Eye gaze detection and the cortical processing of faces: Evidence from infants and adults. *Visual Cognition, 2,* 101–129.

Vinter, A. (1986). The role of movement in eliciting early imitation. *Child Development, 57,* 66–71.

Walton, G. E., Bower, N. J. A. & Bower, T. G. R. (1992). Recognition of familiar faces by newborns. *Infant Behavior and Development, 15,* 265–269.

Wellman, H. (1990). *The child's theory of mind.* Cambridge, MA: MIT Press.

Wilkin, P. E. (1991). Prenatal and postnatal responses to music and sound stimuli—a clinical report. *Canadian Music Educator (Research Edition), 33,* 223–232.

Williatts, P. (1989). Development of problem-solving in infancy. In A. Slater & G. Bremner (Eds), *Infant Development,* Hillsdale, NJ: Lawrence Erlbaum.

Woodward, A. L., Markman, E. M. & Fizsimmons, C. M. (1994). Rapid word learning in 13- and 18-month-olds. *Developmental Psychology, 30,* 553–566.

Wynn, K. (1992). Addition and subtraction by human infants. *Nature, 358,* 6389, 749–750.

# 2

# Motor Development: A New Synthesis

## Esther Thelen

*Indiana University, Bloomington*

*The study of the acquisition of motor skills, long moribund in developmental psychology, has seen a renaissance in the last decade. Inspired by contemporary work in movement science, perceptual psychology, neuroscience, and dynamic systems theory, multidisciplinary approaches are affording new insights into the processes by which infants and children learn to control their bodies. In particular, the new synthesis emphasizes the multicausal, fluid, contextual, and self-organizing nature of developmental change, the unity of perception, action, and cognition, and the role of exploration and selection in the emergence of new behavior. Studies are concerned less with how children perform and more with how the components cooperate to produce stability or engender change. Such process approaches make moot the traditional nature-nurture debates.*

If one asks parents about their babies, one will almost surely hear about the child's motor milestones. "Melanie just learned to roll over." "Jason is finally sitting up alone." "I have to babyproof the house because Caitlin just started to crawl."

It is no wonder that proud parents report on these events. New motor skills are the most dramatic and observable changes in an infant's first year. These stagelike progressions transform babies from being unable even to lift their heads to being able to grab things off supermarket shelves, chase the dog, and become active participants in family social life.

Reprinted with permission from *American Psychologist*, 1995, Vol. 50, No. 2, 79–95. Copyright © 1995 by the American Psychological Association, Inc.

Frances Degen Horowitz served as action editor for this article.

This research was supported by a grant from the National Institutes of Health and a Research Scientist Award from the National Institute of Mental Health.

It is also no wonder that motor skill development was the first topic in the scientific study of infancy. Long before developmental psychologists became interested in the mental lives of infants, there was a rich tradition of careful descriptive and quasi-experimental study of how the bodies of infants grow and change. Pioneer developmental scientists such as Mary Shirley, Arnold Gesell and Myrtle McGraw spent the 1920s through 1940s conducting observations of how infants gain control of their movements. To modern developmentalists, the incredible detail of their observations and the resulting behavioral category distinctions are both amazing and somewhat excessive. Gesell, for instance, described age norms for 58 stages of pellet behavior, 53 stages of rattle behavior, and so on for 40 different behavioral series (Gesell & Thompson, 1938).

But Gesell (Gesell & Thompson, 1938) and McGraw (1943) were more than just observers and describers. They were also important theorists, interested in why infants universally pass through a series of motor milestones. Both of these early workers concluded that the regularities they saw as motor skills emerged reflected regularities in brain maturation, a genetically driven process common to all infants. Gesell was especially clear in assigning primacy to autonomous changes in the nervous system and only a secondary and supporting role to infants' experience. Some researchers claimed that this maturational urge was so strong that even restricting infant movements on cradleboards, a practice of the Hopi people of the southwest, did not deflect this timetable (Dennis & Dennis, 1940).

In some ways, these pioneers did their jobs too well. Their descriptions of motor milestones and stages were incorporated into all the textbooks. Their age norms became the bases of widely used developmental tests, and their maturational explanation was accepted as gospel and is still believed widely today. (The Hopi study, for instance, is frequently quoted in textbooks, despite many subsequent examples of experiential effects on infant motor development.) It seemed as though researchers knew everything they needed to know about motor development: It provided the universal, biological grounding for the more psychologically interesting aspects of early development—cognition, language, and social behavior. Indeed, by the 1960s, the motor field was moribund as developmentalists moved toward Piaget, behavior modification, and ethological theories of social attachment.

Now after 30 years, the cycle has again shifted, and the field is experiencing a renewed and revitalized interest in motor development. The purpose of this article is to describe this born-again field and the converging influences that shape it. What is especially exciting is not just that motor development researchers are learning more and more about how babies come to control their limbs and bodies but also that the field of motor development may again provide theoretical leadership for understanding human development in general. There are two ways in which this promise may be fulfilled. First, we seek to restore the primacy of perception and action in the evolving mental and social life of the child. Second, I hope to show in this article that the new multidisciplinary, process-oriented studies coming from this field make obsolete many old debates in developmental psychology, particularly those that pit nature against nurture.

The renaissance of motor development was marked in August 1993 by the publication of a special section of *Child Development*, a leading developmental journal, entitled "Developmental Biodynamics: Brain, Body, Behavior Connections," edited by Jeffrey J. Lockman of Tulane University and myself (Lockman & Thelen, 1993). The title captures the multiple influences that have come together to spark this new interest: dramatic advances in the neurosciences, in biomechanics, and in the behavioral study of perception and action. But most important have been new theoretical and conceptual tools that have swept away old ways of thinking and brought the promise of a developmental synthesis closer to realization.

In this article I describe these converging ideas and how they have been adapted by the contributors to this special section as well as other researchers. These influences include the pioneering work of the Russian movement physiologist N. Bernstein (1967), the extension of Bernstein's program into theories of motor behavior on the basis of physical and mathematical dynamical systems, the ecological theories of perception and perceptual development of J. J. Gibson (1979) and E. J. Gibson (1982, 1988), increased understanding of neurophysiological and biomechanical mechanisms in infants, and new theories and data on the organization and plasticity of the brain and its development. Taken together, they lead to a very different picture of the developing infant than that imagined by Gesell, Piaget, or indeed many contemporary psychologists. In the final section of the article, I outline this new view of development.

## THE BERNSTEIN REVOLUTION

To appreciate the paradigm shift engendered by Bernstein (1967), it is first useful to look at the traditional views again. Gesell (Gesell & Thompson, 1938) and McGraw (1943) described patterns and sequences of movement that emerged in lawful (if not simple) progression. They then hypothesized that the changes in behavior directly reflect changes in the brain, especially the increasing cortical control over lower level reflexes (e.g., McGraw, 1943). The brain-to-behavior causal link is an eminently plausible explanation and one that is offered by some developmentalists today (e.g., Diamond, 1990).

What then did Bernstein write (his work was first published in English in 1967) that made this explanation seriously deficient? Bernstein was the first to explicitly define movement in terms of coordination, the cooperative interaction of many body parts and processes to produce a unified outcome (see Turvey, 1990). The issue is usually stated as Bernstein's "degrees-of-freedom" problem: How can an organism with thousands of muscles, billions of nerves, tens of billions of cells, and nearly infinite possible combinations of body segments and positions ever figure out how to get them all working toward a single smooth and efficient movement without invoking some clever "homunculus" who has the directions already stored?

Having defined the issue, Bernstein (1967) then contributed foundational insights. First, he argued, researchers must reject the idea that a movement reflects a one-to-one relationship between the neural codes, the precise firing of the motorneurons, and the actual movement pattern. Movements, he recognized, can come about from a variety of underlying muscle contraction patterns, and likewise, a particular set of muscle contractions does not always produce identical movements. Why must this be? Imagine lifting your arm to shoulder height and then relaxing your muscles. Then imagine shaking your hand vigorously just at the wrist. The actual movements produced—your arm drops in the first example and your lower and upper arm vibrate in the second—are not all controlled by your nervous system. As your body parts move, they generate inertial and centripetal forces and are subject to gravity. Such forces contribute to all movements, while they are happening, and constitute a continually changing force field. Thus, the same muscle contraction may have different consequences on your arm depending on the specific context in which the contractions occur.

Bernstein (1967) saw that this meant that actions must be planned at a very abstract level because it is impossible for the central nervous system to program all of these local, contextually varying, force-related interactions specifically and ahead of time. Indeed, once a decision to move has been made, the subsystems and components that actually produce the limb trajectory are *softly assembled* (to use a term introduced later by Kugler & Turvey, 1987) from whatever is available and best fits the task. This type of organization allows the system great flexibility to meet the demands of the task within a continually changing environment, while maintaining a movement category suited to the goal in mind.

Bernstein (1967) also helped motor development researchers recognize that such an organization gives something for nothing, that is, the ability to exploit the natural properties of the motor system and the complementary support of the environment. For example, limbs have springlike properties because of the elastic qualities of muscles and the anatomical configuration of the joints. When an ordinary physical spring is stretched and released, it oscillates on a regular trajectory until it comes to rest at a particular equilibrium point. The trajectory and resting point are not monitored and adjusted (there is no "brain" in a spring) but fall out of the physical properties of the spring itself—its stiffness and damping. In a similar way, springlike limbs greatly simplify motor control. The mover only has to set the parameters of the limb spring to reach the final resting position and need not be concerned with the details of how the limb gets there. The pathway self-organizes from the properties of the components.

Likewise, the environment puts critical constraints on the degrees of freedom. For human locomotion, for example, the need to remain upright, move forward, and yet maintain an efficient periodic contact and push off from the ground limits the possible motor solutions to a restricted class. Although the system permits jumping, hopping, crawling, or dancing the tango to cross the room, organic constraints and surface properties make it more efficient for humans to walk, and this is the pattern that all nonimpaired people discover and prefer. (In the moon's reduced gravity, however, astronauts chose to jump!) Walking as a solution does not have to be preprogrammed, as it arises inevitably from constraints, given a system with many possible solutions.

In light of Bernstein's (1967) insights, the simple picture of the infant waiting for the brain to mature and then, like a marionette, executing the brain's commands is clearly untenable. For infants as well as for adults, movements are always a product of not only the central nervous system but also of the biomechanical and energetic properties of the body, the environmental support, and the specific (and sometimes changing) demands of the particular task. The relations between these components is not simply hierarchical (the brain commands, the body responds) but is profoundly distributed, "heterarchical," self-organizing, and nonlinear. Every movement is unique; every solution is fluid and flexible. How can these relations be known to the infant ahead of time? How can the timetable of motor solutions be encoded in the brain or in the genes?

## MULTICAUSAL DEVELOPMENT

An important consequence, therefore, of these new ideas of motor organization on motor development was to direct attention to the multicausality of action, including the purely physical, energetic, and physiological components traditionally thought to be psychologically uninteresting but now recognized to be essential in the final movement patterns produced.

A good example of multiple systems in motor development is the so-called newborn stepping reflex. Newborn infants, when held upright with their feet on a support surface, perform alternating, steplike movements. Newborn stepping is intriguing, first, because it is surprising to see such well-coordinated patterns at an age when infants are so motorically immature and, second, because within a few months, these movements "disappear." Infants do not step again until late in the first year, when they intentionally step prior to walking. Such regressive or U-shaped developmental phenomena are of great interest to developmentalists because they raise questions about continuity and the nature of ontogenetic precursors as well as about the function of behaviors that disappear.

The traditional explanation of the stepping response was single-causal: Maturation of the voluntary cortical centers first inhibited subcortical or reflexive movements and then facilitated them under a different and higher level of control (McGraw, 1943). This long-accepted explanation came into question when motor development researchers took a broader, systems approach. In the early 1980s, my graduate student Donna Fisher and I studied the organization of other infant leg movements, the rhythmical kicking seen when babies are on their backs or stomachs. Kicking is very common throughout infancy and, unlike stepping, does not disappear after a few months. What surprised us was that kicking and stepping appeared to be the same movement patterns. When we compared the kinematics (time-space patterns) of the joint movements and the underlying muscle activation patterns of kicking and stepping in the same infants, we found no substantial difference. They were the same movements performed in two different postures. What strained credulity was that the cortex would inhibit movements in one posture but not in another.

What else could be going on? According to the new view, movement arises from a confluence of processes and constraints in the organism and environment. A change in posture is a change in the relationship between the mass of the body and the gravitational field. Just a simple biomechanical calculation showed that it requires more strength to lift a leg to full flexion while upright than while supine, where after a certain point gravity assists in the flexion. What Fisher and I (Thelen & Fisher, 1982, 1983) also noted is that in the first two or three months, when stepping disappears, infants have a very rapid weight gain, most of which is subcutaneous fat rather than muscle tissue. Thus, their limbs get heavier but not necessarily stronger. We speculated that the "disappearing" reflex, therefore, could arise not by brain design but by the confluence of increasingly heavy legs and a biomechanically demanding posture (Thelen & Fisher, 1982). Indeed, when we experimentally manipulated mass of the legs by submerging infants in torso-deep warm water, or by adding weights, we could "restore" or "inhibit" stepping, simulating the long-term developmental changes by rather simple physical means.

I like the "case of the disappearing reflex" not because I think most developmental changes are the result of biomechanical factors but because it illustrates in rather transparent form that what may seem like a straightforward causal connection may indeed not be. Causality emerges from many factors, some of which may be rather general and nonspecific. Neither gravity nor weight gain has a prescription for stepping, yet together (and with the organic status of the infant) they help researchers understand developmental changes at a process level.

The more general implications for development are that stepping or indeed any behavior does not reside in some privileged form but emerges online within a specific context. Likewise, developmental change is not planned but arises within a context as the product of multiple, developing elements. As in Figure 1, each component has its own trajectory of change. Some elements may be fully formed early in life but unseen because the supporting subsystems and processes are not ready. Other components may be comparatively delayed, and indeed one element may act as a "rate limiter," preventing the cooperative self-organization of the other component. Only when all the components reach critical functioning and the context is appropriate does the system assemble a behavior. Although Figure 1 depicts the components as separate elements, in reality they are mutually interdependent, the activity of one subsystem changing the developmental trajectory of the others. Thus, in the stepping example, whereas muscle strength is normally a rate limiter, continued practice of stepping may strengthen both muscles and neural pathways and thus prolong the behavior beyond the time it normally regresses (Zelazo, Zelazo, & Kolb, 1972). As developmentalists, therefore, we must seek to understand how the contributing levels change by themselves and how they interact. For example, what is the role of biomechanics in early movement development, and how do the neural and biomechanical levels interact? I discuss these issues further in later sections.

### Hidden Skills

An especially intriguing (and compelling) aspect of a multicausal view of development is understanding precocial components of a behavior. These are parts of a functional activity that are normally hidden but can be elicited, usually under special experimental conditions, long in advance of

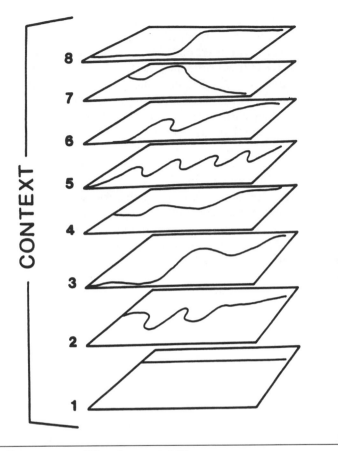

**Figure 1.** Components of Developmental Change

*Note.* Development depicted as a layered system where multiple, parallel developing components have asynchronous trajectories. At any point in time, the behavioral outcome is a product of the components within a context.

the appearance of the fully formed action. One of my favorites is Hall and Bryan's (1980) demonstration of precocial self-feeding in rat pups. Rat pups normally suckle for the first weeks of life and do not eat and drink independently until about three weeks after birth. However, when Hall and Bryan put even newborn pups in a very warm test chamber, the pups ingested liquid or semisolid food from the floor. This component of self-feeding was organically available but "waiting in the wings" for the other needed components of self-feeding (locomotion, vision, temperature regulation, etc.) to mature.

Another clear instance of precocial components, again from the human motor skill domain, is infant treadmill stepping. When infants as young as one month were held supported under the armpits so that their legs rested on a small, motorized treadmill, they performed coordinated alternating stepping movements that share many kinematic patterns with adult walking (Thelen & Ulrich, 1991). Treadmill stepping is truly a hidden skill because without the facilitating effect of the treadmill, such patterns are not seen until the end of the first year, when babies begin to walk on their own. Treadmill stepping is not a simple reflex but a complex, perceptual-motor pathway whereby the dynamic stretch of the legs provides both energetic and informational components that allow the complex pattern to emerge. Although treadmill stepping is not likely intentional, it is still exquisitely sensitive to external conditions such as the speed or direction of the belt. Indeed, infants can even maintain excellent alternation of their legs on a split-belt treadmill, when one leg is driven on a belt moving twice as fast as the other leg (Thelen, Ulrich, & Niles, 1987).

The discovery of such precocial components of later-appearing skills raises another important point for development in general. It is seductive to think that treadmill stepping or newborn pup feeding is somehow the true "essence" of the later behavior, that the stripped-down, experimentally elicited components show that the ability is there all along and that further development merely enhances performance factors. In contemporary developmental psychology, there is a fascination with finding such underlying competencies, abilities, or rules, as if they hold a more privileged causal role. Thus, there has been a trend to look for the earliest possible age at which infants have knowledge about objects, or physical laws, or language rules. Further development is then judged of lesser interest because all that develops are the factors that limit full expression of the inborn or innate knowledge.

The lesson from looking at motor skill, where the components are clearly physical and peripheral as well as central and mental, is that there is no "essence" of a behavior—an icon or structure that represents the "real" ability. It is impossible to isolate disembodied instructions to act from the actual, real-time performance of the act itself. All behavior is always an emergent property of a confluence of factors. Six-month-old infants do not step without a treadmill. Where does treadmill stepping reside, in the baby or the treadmill? Language does not develop unless infants are raised in a language environment. Where does language really exist? Just as each movement is the on-line product of complex, multiple processes, so it is that we can make no distinction between the center and the periphery, the inside and the outside, the "biological" and the experiential, the genetic and the environmental. Focusing on these dualisms diverts attention from questions of developmental process.

## THE DYNAMICS OF MOVEMENT AND ITS DEVELOPMENT

Although Bernstein has been dead for nearly 30 years, his legacy continues today in two very influential approaches to understanding movement that were spawned at the University of Connecticut in the early 1980s. In a landmark study, Kugler, Kelso, and Turvey (1980) grounded the problem of movement coordination in more general laws of physics and in particular a physical biology based on nonequilibrium thermodynamics. The natural world is composed of so-called nonequilibrium dissipative systems: complex, often heterogenous, systems that gain and lose energy. Common examples are clouds, fluid flow systems, galaxies, and of course biological systems ranging from lowly slime molds to complex ecosystems. The hallmark of such systems is the formation of patterns, often themselves complex in time and space, in an entirely self-organizing fashion. That is, there is no recipe for a cloud, or the whirlpools in a mountain stream. This organization arises only from the confluence of the components within a particular environmental context. Could human movement patterns, asked Kugler et al. (1980), arise from the same principles of self-organization that apply to other complex, dissipative systems? Could Bernstein's degrees-of-freedom problem be addressed through dynamics?

The successful application of dynamics to questions of human movement coordination has rested on studying simple rhythmic movements, especially flexions and extensions of the arms, hands, and fingers. Many human movements like walking, running, hammering, swimming, drumming, and juggling are cyclic; rhythmicity is a fundamental property of the human motor system. Even more important, however, is that the study of oscillatory movements has focused attention on new measures of time-based changes in coordination. Traditionally, psychologists have looked at performance variables, such as reaction times and accuracy measures, and have not been concerned with ongoing measures of coordination, such as trajectories and phase relations, that show not only the outcome of a movement but also its evolution. Finally, studying rhythmical movements has allowed investigators to model coordination with well-known physical and mathematical principles.

Two dynamic approaches have evolved from the original Kugler-Kelso-Turvey synthesis. The first is based on physical biology and ecological psychology and is exemplified by a book published in 1987 by Kugler and

Turvey, *Information, Natural Law, and the Self-Assembly of Rhythmic Movement*. In this theory, rhythmic movement is assembled from component oscillators, modeled as real physical pendulums and springs with particular dampness and stiffness characteristics and energetic and coupling functions. Elegant experiments where people swung hand-held pendulums demonstrated that manipulations of such physical and energetic parameters such as pendulum weight, length, and frequency resulted in changes of movement that met the model's predictions. Equally important in this view is the idea that movement is coordinated with information in the environment: indeed that people perceive this information and that principles of coupling exist just as much between perceived information and body parts as within body parts themselves.

The second line of Bernstein-inspired research is from Scott Kelso and his colleagues (Kelso, Holt, Rubin, & Kugler, 1981; Kelso, Scholz, & Schöner, 1986) and has also focused on abstract coordination dynamics and, especially, the phenomenon of phase transitions. The clearest examples of biological phase transitions are seen in quadruped gait changes: As cats, horses, dogs, and the like increase their speed of locomotion, they also change suddenly from walking to trotting to galloping. The transition is self-organizing in a fundamental sense, as it is a spontaneous shift to a more efficient footfall pattern that is emergent from the anatomical and energetic constraints of the animal. Kelso simulated such gait transitions in human experiments by having people flex and extend their index fingers either in or out of phase. When subjects began the movements out of phase (one finger flexing while the other extends) and gradually increased the movement frequency, they spontaneously shifted into an in-phase pattern, much like a horse shifts from a trot to a gallop (Kelso et al., 1981). With two physicists, Hermann Haken and Gregor Schöner, Kelso modeled this shift between the two stable phase states of the fingers as hybrid nonlinear coupled oscillators (Haken, Kelso, & Bunz, 1985; Kelso et al., 1986; Schöner & Kelso, 1988). The stable states are called *attractors* in dynamic terminology because the system settles into that pattern from a wide variety of initial positions and tends to return to that pattern if perturbed.

Additional experiments confirmed the theoretical predictions: The two stable states were both possible, but under particular frequency instructions, only one was stable. Moreover, the sudden shift occurred with the predicted loss of stability of the currently stable state, reflected in more variability and an increased responsiveness to perturbation. Movement frequency, in this case, is the control parameter, a rather nonspecific scaling of the system that nonetheless leads the system through different qualitative modes, or attractor states.

### Dynamics and Development

Although most people do not often rhythmically wiggle their fingers or swing two pendulums from their wrists, these experiments and models on relatively simple movements have uncovered principles of important generality not only for understanding the organization of movements in infants and children but also for understanding how behavior in general may change over time. In broad strokes, a developing system is a dynamic system in that patterns of behavior act as collectives—attractor states—of the component parts within particular environmental and task contexts. No privileged programs specify these patterns beforehand, but rather each mental state and motor action self-organizes from these components. Nonetheless, some patterns are preferred under certain circumstances: They act as attractors in that the system "wants" to perform them. Other patterns are possible but performed with more difficulty and are more easily disrupted. The stability of a behavioral system is a function of its history, its current status, the social and physical context, and the intentional state of the actor (Thelen, 1989, 1992).

Developmental change, then, can be seen in dynamic terms as a series of states of stability, instability, and phase shifts in the attractor landscape, reflecting the probability that a pattern will emerge under particular constraints. From dynamic principles, one can predict that change is heralded by the loss of stability. Some changing components in the system must disrupt the current stable pattern so that the system is free to explore and select new coordinative modes. The components of the system disrupting the current stability and thus engendering change can only be known through careful empirical study. This is difficult because these agents may be nonobvious and changing. For instance, growth or biomechanical factors may be important in early infancy, whereas experience, practice, or environmental conditions may become dominant later on. Once new configurations are possible and discovered, they must also be progressively tuned to become efficient, accurate, and smooth. Thus, for any particular task, a dynamic view predicts an initial high variability in configurations representing an exploration stage, a narrowing of possible states to a few patterns, and a progressive stability as patterns become practiced and reliable.

Such a view of development is illustrated by the landscape in Figure 2, which is an adaptation of the embryologist C. H. Waddington's famous epigenetic landscape (Muchisky, Gershkoff-Stowe, Cole, & Thelen, in press; Waddington, 1954). In this picture, time runs from the top to the bottom of the page. Each horizontal line is a slice of time representing the probability that the system will reside in a particular behavioral configuration as

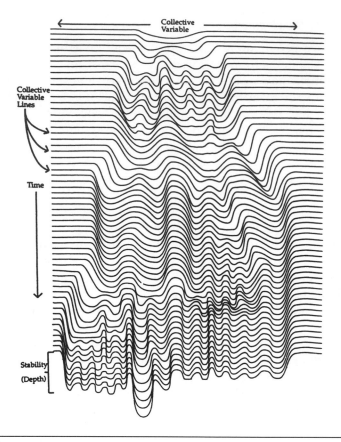

**Figure 2.** Development Depicted as a Landscape.

*Note.* Time goes from back to front. Each line represents the probability of a particular be-havioral configuration as a potential well of varying depth and steepness. *Collective variable* means that the configuration is a lower dimensional product of many interacting systems.

deep or shallow potential wells. (The line represents some behavioral vari-able that is the product of the possible configurations of the component el-ements.) A ball captured in a steep, deep potential well is stable because it takes a great deal of energy to dislodge it; when a line contains one deep well, the behavioral options are stable and limited. A shallow, flat well, in contrast, means that the system can take on many, not very stable options. Development proceeds toward many more possibilities; behavior becomes more highly differentiated. But along the way some configurations are also lost. Indeed, theory predicts that times of instability are essential to give the system flexibility to select adaptive activities. As I argue later as well, the notion of exploration and selection may be a key developmental process at both behavioral and neural levels.

## The Dynamics of Infant Leg Movements

It is not surprising that, to date, the most successful applications of dynamic principles to human development have been to rhythmic behaviors, especially walking, and the cyclic leg movements of infant kicking, stepping, and bouncing that are precursors to walking. Dynamics have been enlightening for understanding both the coordination and control of leg actions in real time and how movements change.

For example, although leg movements in early infancy are not directed toward particular task goals, they show relatively well-coordinated organization in time and space. The hip, knee, and ankle joints flex and extend in synchrony or nearly so, and the movement paths and durations are not random, but constrained. Likewise, movements between the limbs are also coordinated, often in an alternating fashion, with one leg flexing while the other extends. Remarkably, our studies showed that the patterns of muscle activation reflecting the neural control of these movements were less patterned than were the movements themselves. In particular, when legs flexed, both flexor and extensor muscle groups were active, but when legs extended, we saw little or no activity in either muscle group (Thelen & Fisher, 1983).

Such data pose problems for a view of movement as reflecting one-to-one correspondence between the neural impulses and the limb trajectory but makes more sense from a dynamic view. Indeed, Kelso, Fogel, and I (Thelen, Kelso, & Fogel, 1987) suggested that these early kicking movements were examples of rather pure spring-like oscillatory movements in human limbs. That is, the pulses of energy provided by the co-active muscle bursts, providing a forcing function for the whole-limb spring, and the resulting space-time trajectory "falls out" of these dynamic properties. In this view, then, patterns of inter-limb coordination reflect various coupling mechanisms between the single-leg oscillators.

But what happens to these whole-leg springs during development? Clearly, after a few months, infants can do more with their legs than just kick them in the air. Legs increasingly become specialized for crawling, climbing, walking, jumping, squatting, and so on. One problem for the baby is dissolving these simple, whole-leg synergies for more specific and appropriate combinations of limb control. Associated with this, of course, is assembling new and task-specific patterns within and between the joints and delivering just the right amount of muscle energy to provide sufficient but not excessive force to accomplish the task. The new approaches have begun to suggest some clues on how this might be done.

First, during the first year, infants become increasingly able to move leg joints independently. In particular, Jensen, Ulrich, Schneider, Zernicke, and I (in press) showed increasing disassociation of movement phases and progressive uncoupling of joint rotations between the newborn period and seven months, when infants begin to crawl and step. We looked specifically at how forces were generated and controlled. Newborns moved their legs primarily through power generated at the hip; later, infants could control forces at both hip and knee. This decoupling frees up degrees of freedom and provides infants with the flexibility needed to explore and discover new relations among limb patterns.

**Biomechanics of early skills.** In the previous paragraph, I discussed infants' control of forces at the joints as progressively more differentiated. This example resulted from ongoing studies—collaborations between developmental psychologists and biomechanists—looking at motor skill development at the level of the control of forces. As reviewed by Zernicke and Schneider (1993), new techniques in biomechanical analysis allow researchers to reconstruct from behavioral and anthropomorphic data the forces (torques) moving limb segments. These techniques are especially instructive because they partition the forces causing movement into those that are actively controlled by the central nervous system through muscle contraction and those that cause segments to move passively, such as gravity and inertial forces from the other moving body parts. Newborn infants, for instance, are captives of gravity and cannot even lift their heads. Yet, even in very young babies, reflex mechanisms are in place to stabilize the joints against possibly damaging inertial forces generated by fast movements in the multilinked segments (Schneider, Zernicke, Ulrich, Jensen, & Thelen, 1990). An important developmental question is how infants learn not only to protect against passive forces but also to effectively use them to reduce the demands for active muscle contraction.

## EXPLORATION AND SELECTION IN LEARNING NEW TASKS

The new views of motor development emphasize strongly the roles of exploration and selection in finding solutions to new task demands. This means that infants must assemble adaptive patterns from modifying their current movement dynamics. The first step is to discover configurations that get the baby into the "ball park" of the task demands—a tentative crawl or a shaky few steps. Then, infants must "tune" those configurations to make them appropriately smooth and efficient. Again, this tuning is discovered through repeated cycles of action and perception of the consequences of that action in relation to the goal.

Thus, the new views differ sharply from the traditional maturational accounts by proposing that even the so-called "phylogenetic" skills—the universal milestones such as crawling, reaching, and walking—are learned through a process of modulating current dynamics to fit a new task through exploration and selection of a wider space of possible configurations. The assumption here is that infants are motivated by a task—a desire to get a toy into the mouth or to cross the room to join the family—and that the task, not prespecified genetic instructions, is what constitutes the driving force for change.

Experimentally, this process of change is best seen when we give infants novel tasks and actually observe them adjusting their current dynamics to solve problems. Task novelty is important because the goal is to demonstrate a process where the outcome could not have been anticipated by phylogeny or neural codes.

A wonderful example of such a developmental study is Eugene Goldfield, Bruce Kay, and William Warren's (1993) model of infants learning to use a "Jolly Jumper" infant bouncer (Figure 3). Goldfield et al. wrote,

> Consider the situation faced by a 6-month-old when first placed in a "Jolly-Jumper" infant bouncer. The infant is hanging in a harness from a linear spring, with the soles of the feet just touching the floor. What is the "task?" What limb movements will make something interesting happen? There are no instructions or models—the behavior of the system must be discovered. (p. 1128)

Using dynamic principles, these authors modeled the bouncing infant as a forced mass spring, represented by a rather simple spring equation. Here the bouncer spring, with the infant mass attached, has particular, measurable damping and stiffness characteristics. The infant acts as the forcing function, where the baby can regulate how much force to apply and when to apply it. The model predicts that together the baby and bouncer could exhibit a specific resonant frequency where the infant gets maximal bounce for minimal energy pumps. This resonant frequency should, in turn, act as an attractor where the baby-bouncer system prefers to be. The task for the infant, then, is first to assemble the right movements to drive the spring and then to tune the spring to find the stable attractor, the most "bounce for the ounce."

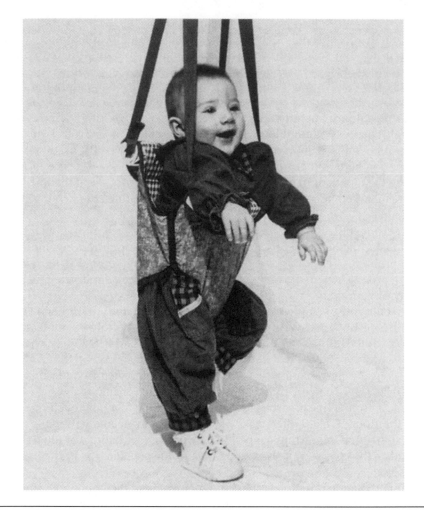

**Figure 3.** Infant in Jolly Jumper.
*Note*. Photo taken by Dexter Gormley.


Indeed, Goldfield et al. (1993) found that infants began with only a few tentative bounces, and these bounces had variable amplitudes and periods. As the weeks passed, infants increased the number of bounces and decreased their period and amplitude variability, settling in on a consistent frequency, which was a close fit to the predicted resonant frequency of the infant-bouncer spring system. Thus, infants, through vision and proprioception, sensed what force and timing parameters to adjust in their kicking to optimize their match to the characteristics of the spring, and over time, they learned and remembered these parameters.

Recently, I demonstrated infants' abilities to match their movement coordination patterns to a novel task at an even earlier age, three months (Thelen, 1994). The experimental situation was similar to one used for many years by Carolyn Rovee-Collier (1991) and her colleagues at Rutgers University to study infant memory. Three-month-old infants lay supine under an attractive crib mobile. The experimenters attached one of the baby's legs to the mobile by means of a ribbon tied around the ankle, such that the infant's spontaneous kicking movements made the mobile jiggle. Within a few minutes of such conjugate reinforcement (conjugate because the mobile provides reinforcing movement and noise in direct relation to how frequently and vigorously infants kick), infants learned the contingency and kicked faster and harder. They also remembered the motor response over several weeks and even longer if they were "reminded" of the context in which the training took place (Rovee-Collier, 1991).

My question was whether, in addition to learning to kick more, infants could also learn a novel pattern of interlimb coordination. Normally, three-month-old infants prefer either alternating kicks or kicking predominantly one favored leg. They rarely use a simultaneous double kick (the movement discovered later to operate the Jolly Jumper). To try to induce them to shift to the simultaneous, in-phase pattern, I tethered their legs together with a 5.5-centimeter piece of soft sewing elastic attached to foam ankle cuffs. The elastic allowed them to move their legs freely independently but made it much more efficient to use both legs together to get vigorous activation of the mobile (Figure 4). As predicted, infants whose legs were tethered during the reinforcement phase of the experiment learned to shift their predominant pattern to in-phase kicking. As in the Jolly Jumper experiment, infants began with a few tentative simultaneous kicks and, seeing the consequences, gradually replaced other configurations with the new form. In dynamic terms, the tethering disrupted the stability of the old attractors, allowing infants to explore the landscape and discover a more efficient leg-coupling attractor.

### Studying Processes of Change

Studies such as the mobile kicking and the Jolly Jumper are important because they move motor development researchers away from looking at only performance differences as a function of age to understanding the processes by which infants learn new skills. When researchers only test groups of in-

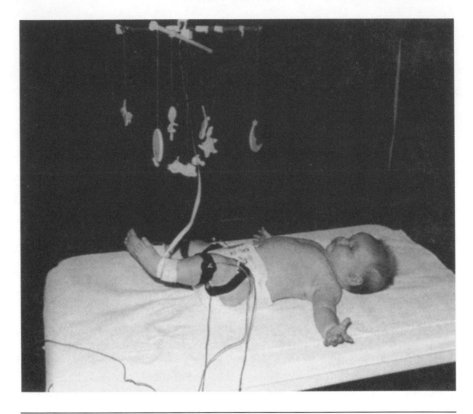

**Figure 4.** Three-Month-Old Infant in Mobile Experiment With Legs Tethered by an Elastic Cuff.

*Note*. Leg movement and muscle activation patterns recorded using electromyography. Photo taken by Dexter Gormley.

fants at different ages, they demarcate the ranges of abilities, but they cannot explain how the children moved from one performance level to another. Indeed, there are likely different pathways to the same outcome. A dynamic approach, in contrast, emphasizes these time-dependent changes. The question is always, What is changing or what is the infant doing that generates a shift into new forms? Once a transition is identified through descriptive studies, the experimenter can manipulate various factors that may move the system into new configurations, that is, to simulate the developmental change. These can be done by imposing novel tasks and creating learning experiments on a short time scale, such as the mobile experiment, or with specific enrichment or training on a longer time scale (e.g., Siegler & Jenkins, 1989). Again, it is essential that researchers know when the old forms are sufficiently unstable so that such training manipulations will be effective. Systems that are rigid have no flexibility for exploration and no ability to discover new attractors.

### Coupling Perception and Action for Learning New Skills

A central theme in the new synthesis is the inseparable coupling of perception and action in the generation and improvement of new skills. This theme is not new: Piaget (1952) believed that all representational thought had its origins in infants' repeated cycles of perceiving and acting on the world. More recently, the action-perception coupling research has been directly inspired by the theories of E. J. Gibson and J. J. Gibson on perception and perceptual development (E. J. Gibson, 1982, 1988; J. J. Gibson, 1979). In particular, these studies have demonstrated that, from the beginning, infants are continually coordinating their movements with concurrent perceptual information to learn how to maintain balance, reach for objects in space, and locomote across various surfaces and terrains (see Lockman, 1990, for a review).

The classic line of research in this domain stems directly from J. J. Gibson's (1979) concept of affordances. According to Gibson, an affordance is the reciprocal relation or "fit" between the actor and the environment that is necessary to perform functional activities. For example, adults immediately know when a chair is appropriate for sitting or a surface for walking or when an object is within reach. People and other animals directly and accurately perceive these relations by sensing information from the environment—the light or sound reflecting from the surfaces in the world—and from their own bodies through receptors in the muscle, skin, joints, and so on. The developmental question, of course, is how these relations are acquired. How do infants come to know whether they can successfully execute particular actions on the world? For example, the famous E. J. Gibson and Walk (1960) visual cliff experiment demonstrated that crawling infants understood the visual information specifying a vertical drop off and refused to cross it, even though the cliff was covered with a rigid, clear plexiglass surface. In this vein, E. J. Gibson and her colleagues subsequently found that crawlers and walkers recognized action-specific properties of surfaces as well. When faced with a rigid plywood surface or a squishy waterbed, crawlers crossed both without hesitation. Toddlers, however, hesitated and explored the waterbed and then decided to crawl rather than walk on the shaky surface (E. J. Gibson et al., 1987).

Further evidence of infants' growing abilities to detect such affordances for action was reported by Adolph, Eppler, and Gibson (1993). They provided crawlers and toddlers with a novel task, that of locomoting over a sloping surface of various degrees of steepness. (Normally, children of this age never or rarely encounter slopes.) Would these young children know when they could successfully go up or down the slope without falling? Would they be able to adjust their patterns of locomotion to the steepness of the slopes?

Going up the slope posed no problems for either the crawlers or the new walkers. Both groups tried even the steepest slopes without hesitation, even though they sometimes fell! But, as the authors noted, the consequences for falling uphill are negligible because the babies could easily catch themselves on their arms and continue. Downhill was another matter, falling downhill has serious consequences. Accordingly, as the slope steepness increased, the toddlers became increasingly wary, hesitating and touching the slopes, often refusing to go, sometimes scooting backward, but rarely falling, suggesting they understood something about how their locomotor abilities fit the task. In contrast, crawlers (who averaged 8.5 months compared with the 14-month-old toddlers) did not seem to perceive this fit. They plunged downhill rather indiscriminately and frequently had to be rescued by the experimenters. Although the crawlers evidenced some wariness by hesitating and exploring the steep slopes, many crawled down anyway, unsuccessfully. (This behavior is especially intriguing because infants plunge down slopes yet refuse the visual cliff at the same age.) Although the specific factors that convert a slope-naive crawler to a slope-smart walker are yet unknown, it is likely that the process involves infants' own continuing exploration of their action capabilities in relation to the slopes and learning and remembering about the consequences of their activities.

The primary thrust of research from a Gibsonian approach has been to understand how perception guides action. A less well-studied, but equally important, side of the equation is how action shapes perception. Motor activities are particularly critical because they provide the means for exploring the world and learning about its properties. It is only by moving eyes and head, hands and arms, and traveling from one place to another that people can fully experience the environment and learn to adapt to it. During development, then, each motor milestone opens new opportunities for perceptual discovery. Bushnell and Boudreau (1993) have provided an especially enlightening example of how important developmental accomplishments are paced by motor skills.

The skills in question involve haptics, or the ability to sense properties of objects by how they feel. Adults are adept at perceiving the shape of objects—their size, texture, weight, hardness, and temperature—by feel alone. But such perception requires that the hands perform certain particular manipulations in order to discriminate these properties. For instance, although temperature can be detected by contact with the palm or fingers, texture is determined through a side-to-side rubbing movement, volume by enclosing the object in the hand, weight by hefting, hardness by exerting finger pressure, and shape by following the contours of the object with the fingers (Lederman & Klatzky, 1987).

Newborn infants, however, cannot move their hands and arms in such discriminating fashion. They can only clutch by flexing their fingers. At about four months, their manual activities become more varied but are still comparatively limited and rhythmical: banging, scratching, rubbing, squeezing, and poking. Only at around one year do infants engage in a full range of two-handed, adapted movements, such as holding the object in one hand while manipulating it with the other. What Bushnell and Boudreau (1993) found was that infants could perceive object properties only as their manual activities permitted appropriate haptic exploration. Although earliest age limits have not been determined for many of these properties, infants appear to detect object size in the first few months and temperature likely at about the same time. These perceptions require only minimal hand skill, clutching. Discrimination of texture and hardness appears around six months, several months after the onset of the needed exploratory actions of rubbing and poking. Weight and shape are later still, as these require more differentiated finger, hand, and arm movements. Interestingly, when the mouth rather than the hands is the haptic tool, infants of much younger ages can perceive texture and hardness, as indeed in very young infants, the highly innervated and mobile mouth can perform considerably more complex exploratory movements than the hands.

## *The Unity of Perception: Action as Perception*

The distinction between perceiving and doing—the afference and the efference—is a time-honored tradition in psychology. But when researchers try to understand the intricate network of causality in early development, we must question whether this distinction is more illusory than real. People perceive in order to move and move in order to perceive. What, then, is movement but a form of perception, a way of knowing the world as well as acting on it?

In fact, recent evidence makes it seem likely that infants, from the start, understand the world from time-integrated multimodal perception. Every waking moment includes sensations not only from vision, hearing, taste, smell, and feeling but also from receptors in muscles, joints, and skin that detect position, force, and movement changes in a continually active organism. What is important is that the nervous system is built to integrate these streams of information: The senses are richly interconnected between and among many anatomically distinct areas. Conventional wisdom held that sensory modalities were processed separately until they reached high-level cortical areas of integration, where the separate tracts were combined. A view now is that multimodal information is bound together frequently and in multiple sites along the processing stream and that there is no single localized area in the brain where perceptual binding occurs (Damasio, 1989). In their book *The Merging of the Senses,* Stein and Meredith (1993) build a compelling case for sensory convergence as a fundamental and enduring characteristic of animal nervous systems, occurring at many levels. For instance, in the cat superior colliculus, a midbrain structure widely studied for its role in visual processing, a very large proportion of neurons are responsive not only to visual input but also to auditory and somatosensory input, and there are strong correspondences between the topographic maps of these modalities, a kind of common "multisensory space." These authors further suggested that motor responses are similarly integrated to produce a "multisensory—multimotor map," a mapping that may be echoed in other sites as well.

The implications for understanding development are profound and go beyond the truism that perception guides action. First, and contrary to the Piagetian belief that infants "construct" matches between their perception and their movement with development, such intermodal functioning may be basic and primitive. There are many reports in the literature demonstrating that infants can transfer between perceptual modalities at very young ages, for instance, matching the oral feel and the sight of an unusual, nubby pacifier (Meltzoff & Borton, 1979) or looking preferentially at rings moving in rigid or flexible fashion after exploring similar rings haptically (Streri & Pecheux, 1986).

Second, if infants come into the world wired to integrate information from all their senses, including their movement senses, then there is new meaning to infants' everyday experience, even the seemingly purposeless movements of the very young baby. When events happen in the world, or when people act on their environment, the information impinging on the senses from light, sound, smells, taste, and pressure are all coherent in time and space. For instance, when a mother nurses an infant, the baby is experiencing not only her perfectly synchronized voice and facial movements as she talks but also smells, tactile and vestibular cues, and eventually tastes that are all mutually correlated with those sights and sounds as well as with self-perceptions of particular postures and movements. Indeed, for all waking hours, infants are watching, listening, feeling and generating movements, and experiencing the consequences of their activities. Consider again the mobile experiment I described earlier. Each leg kick provided infants with a rich, multimodal, and coherent set of perceptions such that the infants could recognize the relationship between their own felt movement and the sights and sounds of the jiggling mobile.

But most important, it may be exactly this continual bombardment of real-life, multisensory but coherent information that fuels the engines of developmental change as infants learn to act in social and physical worlds. The key elements are the dynamic processes of exploration and selection: the ability to generate behavior that provides a variety of perceptual-motor experiences and then the differential retention of those correlated actions that enable the infant to function in the world.

## EXPLORATION AND SELECTION IN THE SERVICE OF DEVELOPMENTAL CHANGE: THE THEORY OF NEURONAL GROUP SELECTION

Exploration and selection are the fundamental processes that unite the Bernstein-inspired accounts of movement dynamics and the Gibsonian perceptual agenda into a new developmental synthesis. A third important ingredient is a theory of brain development that is consistent with the process approaches in behavioral development. It is important to know what parts of the brain change with new behavioral milestones and the cellular and chemical nature of those changes, but it is not enough. As I mentioned earlier, developmentalists usually assume that the causal link is mainly one way: The brain matures and allows new behaviors to appear. But what causes the brain to change? A burgeoning field in contemporary neuroscience deals with brain plasticity, that is, how the brain itself is molded through experience—individual perception and action. Everywhere neuroscientists look in the brain, they are finding astounding plasticity, not only in young animals but in adults as well (see reviews by Kaas, 1991; Merzenich, Allard, & Jenkins, 1990). This work makes it likely that experience is the fodder for brain change, which in turn opens up new opportunities for experience.

A brain theory consistent with the new synthesis, therefore, must account for these multiple directions of causality. One promising candidate is the theory articulated by the immunologist, developmental biologist, and neuroscientist Gerald Edelman as his theory of neuronal group selection (TNGS; Edelman, 1987; Sporns & Edelman, 1993). TNGS offers a specific neural mechanism for the acquisition of perceptual-motor skills that is consistent with both dynamic/Gibsonian behavioral perspectives and with current findings on brain function and plasticity.

TNGS is not a simple theory, and I present only the briefest outline here. TNGS begins by considering the nature of the newborn brain. The cornerstone of the theory is neural diversity. Traditionally, neuroanatomists have studied the nervous system in terms of the nuclei, tracts, layers, fissures, and circuits that are common among the members of a species. But a level down from the gross anatomy, there is enormous individual variability, from the sizes and shapes of cells and their processes, to the number, type, and degree of connections, to the grouping of the cells into layers, columns, patches and fibers, and so on. Neural diversity arises from dynamic neuroembryonic processes and means that there can be no genetically determined point-to-point wiring in the brain. Rather, the diversity provides the raw material—the rough palette—for experience-dependent selection, that is, the strengthening of certain connections—groups of neurons—through use. The second essential feature is the dense, interwoven, and overlapping pattern of connectivity within and between all areas of the brain. Edelman (1987) used the term *reentrant*, which means that every area has reciprocal and recursive signals from many other areas. Reentry is the critical process that allows integration from the multiple sensory and motor areas of the brain and that gives rise to the coordination of responses across modalities. The basis for such correlated sensations is the temporal synchrony of the signals coming from real-world things and events. Furthermore, the highly overlapping architecture of the system means that patterns of firing from two modalities extract and combine features that are held in common, a kind of mapping of maps.

Together, neural diversity and reentry thus allow the nervous system to learn to recognize and categorize sensory signals as a dynamic, self-organizing process. I make this explanation less abstract by referring again to the three-month-old infant's experience jiggling the overhead mobile. The baby initially kicks her leg spontaneously, that is, without a particular functional goal. Likewise, the infant may watch and listen to the movement and sounds of the mobile. In the experiment the correlated features of leg movement and the sights and sounds of the mobile (always perfectly coupled in real life) are reciprocally strengthened so that a higher level association emerges. As infants generate different interlimb kick patterns, the groups of neurons that receive proprioceptive, visual, and auditory input arising from simultaneous vigorous kicks and intense mobile movement and sounds are selectively activated. Over time, infants discover a class of movement patterns, a category of moving two legs together, that produces a maximal pleasing effect on the mobile. The process is self-organizing because, given the neural substrate, what is needed to get the process going are only sufficient spontaneous and exploratory movements and some general internal reinforcement value for the infant for the sights and sounds of a moving mobile. There is no genetic plan for simultaneous kicks or indeed for kicking mobiles, but the pattern can be, and is, discovered through exploration and selection. (From the dynamic view, of course, the system must be unstable enough for the patterns to shift with a change in task.) Although mobile kicking is not a human universal, the new synthesis holds that development of even the so-called phylogenetic motor skills, such as walking and reaching, occurs by a similar noninstructed process as seen in the mobile experiment. The initial state needs only the most general and high-level goal biases; simple values such as "look at complex, moving sights," "things in the mouth and in the hand are good," and so on. The specific motor actions needed to accomplish those goals "fall out," so to speak, of the correlated perceptual features of the infants' own explorations, through such neuronal group strengthening. Each new solution, each new skill, opens up new spaces for perceptual-motor exploration and discovery so that skill levels cascade from the infants' current abilities in the face of the task. Infant crawling, for instance, can be viewed not so much as an inevitable human stage as an ad hoc solution to the problem of getting desired distant objects discovered by individual infants, given a particular level of strength and postural control.

When motor development is seen the old way, as instructed from the genes through the brain, it is difficult to understand how the instructions adapt to changes in the peripheral structures. Alternatively, development as selection is an especially attractive hypothesis because it accounts for individual variability and change in activity level, body build and proportion, neural growth, and task environments. Infants, in a sense, do the best they can with what they have. Nonetheless, because humans also share anatomy and common biomechanical and task constraints, solutions to common motor problems also converge: We all discover walking rather than hopping (although our gait styles are individual and unique).

Sporns and Edelman (1993) have depicted this selectionist process as the schematic diagram shown in Figure 5. The diagram shows a developing movement repertoire carved from initial movement patterns. Each pattern is shown as a dot on the diagram in a movement space, M, specified by two variables, $\Phi1$ and $\Phi2$, where the variables might be joint angles or positions of the hand in space. The density of the dots, then, represents the frequency that movements with a particular configuration are performed. At Time 1, say birth, infants have a specified set of patterns. With growth and changing task demands at Times 2 and 3, the shape and density of the movement repertoire changes, new patterns emerge, and some old patterns lose stability, as I also showed in Figure 2. Hatched regions are patterns

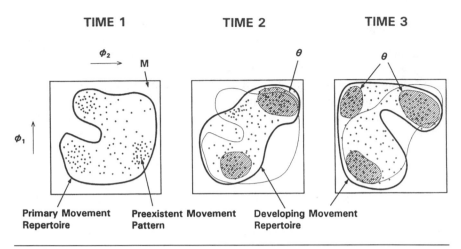

**TIME 1**          **TIME 2**          **TIME 3**

Primary Movement     Preexistent Movement     Developing Movement
Repertoire           Pattern                  Repertoire

**Figure 5.** *Schematic Diagram of Selection in Movement Repertoires.*

*Note.* M is the movement space specified by a certain combination of movement variables, $\phi 1$ and $\phi 2$. Each dot is a movement, and the density of dots signifies the frequency of movements in the space. The three frames show changes over time. The frame at the left shows the primary movement repertoire. The repertoire evolves with time to include previously unoccupied regions of M and to exclude others. Hatched regions indicate movement regions that correspond to a given task, as they emerge from the primary repertoire. From "Solving Bernstein's Problem: A Proposal for the Development of Coordinated Movement by Selection" by O. Sporns and G. M. Edelman, 1993, *Child Development, 64*, p. 970. Copyright 1993 by the Society for Research in Child Development. Reprinted by permission.

that fit particular tasks and that have thus become associated with positive value and are especially strong and stable. These areas may also evolve and change. For instance, a dense area representing the interlimb coordination pattern of crawling may become less dense with age, as crawling is replaced by other forms of locomotion.

Edelman and his colleagues have simulated noninstructed selectionist development using computer models in an aptly named "Darwin" series of automata (see Reeke, Finkel, Sporns, & Edelman, 1990; Reeke & Sporns, 1990; Reeke, Sporns, & Edelman, 1990). Again, readers are referred to detailed descriptions in the original articles; I provide here just enough background to introduce the correspondences between the simulations and data from real babies. Darwin III is an "artificial creature" that has a complex nervous system (but much simpler than a real brain), a multijointed arm, and an eye. A module in Darwin III's "brain" corresponding roughly to the cerebral cortex generates a primary repertoire of movements that are relatively unstructured. A second module, simulating the cerebellum, correlates the motor signals with current sensory inputs from the arm and the eye as well as signals from the movements produced by the motor cortex. As the arm moves around, the "neurons" in the artificial networks respond more positively when the moving hand approaches the vicinity of the target fixated by the eye. This is the "value" bias I mentioned above that works to strengthen neural groups when the arm is near the target, wherever the target is in space or whatever the joint and muscle configurations Darwin uses in that particular gesture. The networks in the brain do not initially have representations of either movements, muscle, or joint synergies; coordination arises only as gestures that get the hand closer to the target are strengthened. Thus, the automaton learns through exploring movement and its sensory consequences the subset of patterns that work.

At first, Darwin III's trajectories of arm to target show varied and tortuous pathways. With continued practice, however, the bundle of trajectories becomes much less varied and more direct (Figure 6). In dynamic terms,

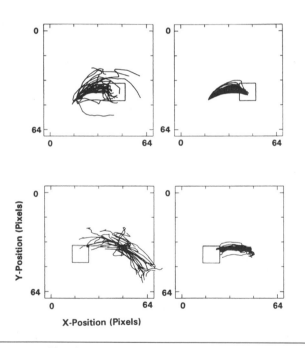

**Figure 6.** Computer Simulations of Darwin III "Learning to Reach."

*Note*. Examples of paths taken by the tip of the arm as it reaches for objects in the locations indicated by the square. Left and right panels show data sampled before and after training. The top and bottom panels give examples of motions starting at different initial conditions. From "Selectionist Models of Perceptual and Motor Systems and Implications for Functionist Theories of Brain Function" by G. N. Reeke, Jr., and O. Sporns, 1990, *Physica D, 42*, p. 359. Copyright 1990 by the Society for Research in Child Development. Reprinted by permission.

the trajectories act like a stable attractor. Likewise, the automaton "dis-
covers" particular stable patterns of coordinated joint motions. (This is
shown in Figure 7, which plots the rotation of one joint as a function of the
rotation of a paired joint, giving a trajectory in "joint space.") Recall that
there are multiple degrees of freedom in a jointed arm; there are many ways
to move the joints together to produce a particular hand path. However, as
Bernstein (1967) predicted, the possibilities become progressively reduced
as the system settles on efficient solutions. The trajectories and the joint
coordination patterns are never explicitly represented anywhere in the system; they emerge in nondeterministic fashion from a variety of starting arm
and target positions.

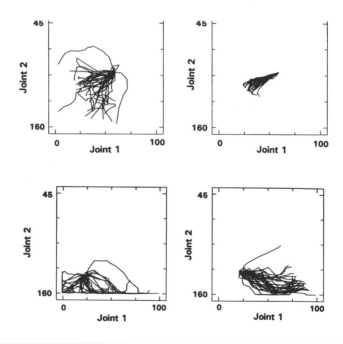

**Figure 7.** Joint Coordination Before and After Training on the Movements
Depicted in Figure 6.

*Note.* The figures plot the angular rotations of one joint as a function of the second joint. Before training, the joints do not move in relation to one another. After training, joint motions
are coordinated. From "Selectionist Models of Perceptual and Motor Systems and Implications for Functionalist Theories of Brain Function" by G. N. Reeke, Jr., and O. Sporns, 1990,
*Physica D, 42,* p 360. Copyright 1990 by the Society for Research in Child Development.
Reprinted by permission.

Human infants appear to have a similar selective process at work when they learn to reach for targets. Figure 8 is a summary of the hand path trajectories and joint coordination patterns of a single infant, Nathan, early and late in his reaching development. Nathan was one of four infants my colleagues and I followed longitudinally from 3 to 52 weeks, using sophisticated motion analysis equipment to capture their hand and joint movement trajectories (Thelen et al., 1993). In the first weeks after he started reaching, Nathan contacted the toy presented in front of him with jerky, zig-zag hand pathways (Figure 8), as did Darwin III. By the end of his first year, Nathan's hand went directly and smoothly toward the toy. He also discovered a consistent way to coordinate the lifting and extending of

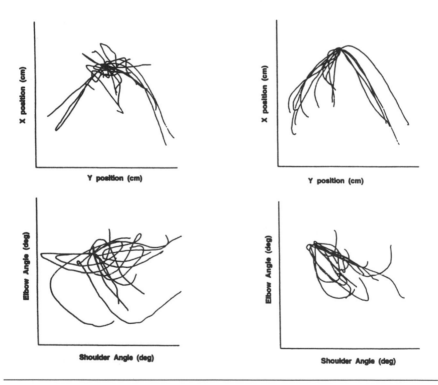

**Figure 8.** Selection in Nathan's Learning to Reach.

*Note.* Top panels: Arm trajectories, seen from an overhead view, aligned to the point of toy contact, for all of Nathan's reaches in Weeks 16, 17, and 18 (left panel; he started to reach at 12 weeks) and in Weeks 46–48 (right panel). Bottom panels: Joint coordination of shoulder and elbow for the reaches depicted in the top panels, where joint angle data were available, also, aligned to toy contact.

his arm (Figure 8). Whereas early in the year, Nathan used many different patterns of elbow and shoulder coordination, his "joint-space" envelope narrowed considerably by his first birthday. Although many patterns were possible, only some of them became stable through repeated practice cycles of reaching. The similar behavioral profiles of Nathan and Darwin III do not by themselves prove that the underlying processes are similar, of course. However, the simulation does give support to the idea that nervous systems—even very simple ones—can discover stable motor patterns through experience and that they do not have to have the detailed instructions for action built in.

## CONCLUSION: BEYOND ACTION AND PERCEPTION

It is this idea that repeated cycles of perception and action can give rise to emergent new forms of behavior without preexisting mental or genetic structures that is the link between the simple activities of the young infant and the growing life of the mind. What is new here is not that cognition grows from roots in perception and action. This was the fundamental assumption of Piaget and of many others. What is different is the rejection of the dualism between structure (in physical or mental guise) and function and the acceptance of growing humans as true dynamic systems. A current trend in developmental psychology is to look for instantiation of abilities in real and preexisting genetic instructions, stages, devices, programs, storage units, or knowledge modules to account for the fact that sometimes behavior appears to be stagelike, programmed, stored, and modular. The assumption is that the genes, stages, programs, and modules contain the instructions that direct and prescribe the performance.

What the motor studies have shown us, however, is that each component in the developing system is both cause and product. What is the ultimate "cause" if task motivates behavior while behavior enables new tasks; if biomechanical factors both limit movement and facilitate it; if diversity is the stuff of change, yet small differences have large effects; or if individuals must solve "phylogenetic" movement problems themselves, within their own limits of strength, energy, and motivation? At what point, then, can researchers partition causality into genes versus environment, structure versus function, or competence versus performance? Rather, the new synthesis sees everything as a dynamic process, albeit on different levels and time scales. Even what psychologists usually call "structure"—the tissues and organs of the body—is a dynamic process. Bones and muscles are continually in flux, although their changes may be slower and less observable than those in the nervous system.

From this new view, therefore, cognition is emergent from the same dynamic processes as those governing early cycles of perception and action. As Linda Smith and I have written (Thelen & Smith, 1994), higher order mental activities, including categorization, concept formation, and language, must arise in a self-organized manner from the recurrent real-time activities of the child just as reaching develops from cycles of matching hand to target (Thelen & Smith, 1994). And just as hand trajectories are not computed, but discovered and assembled within the act of reaching, so too does thinking arise within the contextual, historical, and time-dependent activity of the moment. The web of causality is intricate and seamless from the moment of birth.

From a dynamic point of view, therefore, the developmental questions are not what abilities or core knowledge infants and children really "have" or what parts of their behavior are truly organic or genetic but how the parts cooperate to produce stability or engender change. Such questions often require detailed longitudinal studies using individuals and their families and environmental contexts as the units of analysis. The purpose is to characterize the behavioral configuration states and measure their stabilities and their changes. Then we as researchers are in the position to identify, and perhaps manipulate, critical factors that may be moving the system into new forms. Knowing when systems are in transition is important because theory predicts that interventions can only be effective when the system has sufficient flexibility to explore and select new solutions. For developmentalists interested in providing effective and appropriate interventions for children who are at physical, emotional, or social risk, knowing that a particular trait is 25% heritable is of little use. Instead, the therapist needs to know the history of the system in all its richness and complexity, its current dynamics, and how the interventions can disrupt the stability of the current dynamics to allow new and better solutions to emerge.

## REFERENCES

Adolph, K. E., Eppler, M. A., & Gibson, E. J. (1993). Crawling versus walking infants' perception of affordances for locomotion over sloping surfaces. *Child Development, 64*, 1158–1174.

Bernstein, N. (1967). *The coordination and regulation of movements.* London: Pergamon.

Bushnell, E. W., & Boudreau, J. P. (1993). Motor development and the mind: The potential role of motor abilities as a determinant of aspects of perceptual development. *Child Development, 64*, 1005–1021.

Damasio, A. R. (1989). Time-locked multiregional retroactivation: A systems-level proposal for the neural substrates of recall and recognition. *Cognition, 33*, 25–62.

Dennis, W., & Dennis, M. (1940). The effect of cradling practices upon the onset of walking in Hopi children. *Journal of Genetic Psychology, 56*, 77–86.

Diamond, A. (1990). Developmental time course in human infants and infant monkeys and the neural bases of inhibitory control in reaching. In A. Diamond (Ed.), *The development and neural bases of higher cognitive functions* (pp. 637–676). New York: New York Academy of Sciences.

Edelman, G. M. (1987). *Neural Darwinism*. New York: Basic Books.

Gesell, A., & Thompson, H. (1938). *The psychology of early growth including norms of infant behavior and a method of genetic analysis*. New York: Macmillan.

Gibson, E. J. (1982). The concept of affordances in development: The renascence of functionalism. In W. A. Collins (Ed.), *The concept of development. Minnesota Symposium on Child Psychology* (Vol. 15, pp. 55–81). Hillsdale, NJ: Erlbaum.

Gibson, E. J. (1988). Exploratory behavior in the development of perceiving, acting, and the acquiring of knowledge. *Annual Review of Psychology, 39*, 1–41.

Gibson, E. J., Riccio, G., Schmuckler, M. A., Stoffregen, T. A., Rosenberg, D., & Taormina, J. (1987). Detection of the traversability of surfaces by crawling and walking infants. *Journal of Experimental Psychology: Human Perception and Performance, 13*, 533–544.

Gibson, E. J., & Walk, R. D. (1960). The "visual cliff." *Scientific American, 202*, 64–71.

Gibson, J. J. (1979). *The ecological approach to visual perception*. Boston: Houghton Mifflin.

Goldfield, E. C., Kay, B. A., & Warren, W. H., Jr. (1993). Infant bouncing: The assembly and tuning of action systems. *Child Development, 64*, 1128–1142.

Haken, H., Kelso, J. A. S., & Bunz, H. (1985). A theoretical model of phase transitions in human hand movements. *Biological Cybernetics, 39*, 139–156.

Hall, W. G., & Bryan, T. E. (1980). The ontogeny of feeding in rats. II. Independent ingestive behavior. *Journal of Comparative and Physiological Psychology, 93*, 746–756.

Jensen, J. L., Ulrich, B. D., Thelen, E., Schneider, K., & Zernicke, R. F. (in press). Adaptive dynamics of the leg movement patterns of human infants: III. Development. *Journal of Motor Behavior*.

Kaas, J. H. (1991). Plasticity of sensory and motor maps in adult mammals. *Annual Review of Neurosciences, 14*, 137–167.

Kelso, J. A. S., Holt, K. G., Rubin, P., & Kugler, P. N. (1981). Patterns of human interlimb coordination emerge from the properties of non-linear limit cycle oscillatory processes: Theory and data. *Journal of Motor Behavior, 13*, 226–261.

Kelso, J. A. S., Scholz, J. P., & Schöner, G. (1986). Non-equilibrium phase transitions in coordinated biological motion: Critical fluctuations. *Physics Letters A, 118*, 279–284.

Kugler, P. N., Kelso, J. A. S., & Turvey, M. T. (1980). On the concept of coordinative structures as dissipative structures. I. Theoretical lines of convergence. In G. E. Stelmach & J. Requin (Eds.), *Tutorials in motor behavior* (pp. 3–47). New York: North Holland.

Kugler, P. N., & Turvey, M. T. (1987). *Information, natural law, and the self-assembly of rhythmic movement.* Hillsdale, NJ: Erlbaum.

Lederman, S. J., & Klatzky, R. L. (1987). Hand movements: A window into haptic object recognition. *Cognitive Psychology, 19*, 342–368.

Lockman, J. J. (1990). Perceptual motor coordination in infancy. In C-A. Hauert (Ed.), *Developmental psychology: Cognitive, perceptuomotor, and neuropsychological perspectives* (pp. 85–111). New York: Plenum Press.

Lockman, J. J., & Thelen, E. (1993). Developmental biodynamics: Brain, body, behavior connections. *Child Development, 64*, 953–959.

McGraw, M. B. (1943). *The neuromuscular maturation of the human infant.* New York: Columbia University Press.

Meltzoff, A. N., & Borton, R. W. (1979). Intermodal matching by human neonates. *Nature, 232*, 403–404.

Merzenich, M. M., Allard, T. T., & Jenkins, W. M. (1990). Neural ontogeny of higher brain function: Implications of some recent neurophysiological findings. In O. Franzn & P. Westman (Eds.), *Information processing in the somatosensory system* (pp. 293–311). London: MacMillan Press.

Muchisky, M., Gershkoff-Stowe, L., Cole, E., & Thelen, E. (in press). The epigenetic landscape revisited: A dynamic interpretation. *Advances in Infancy Research.*

Piaget, J. (1952). *The origins of intelligence in children.* New York: International Universities Press.

Reeke, G. N., Jr., Finkel, L. H., Sporns, O., & Edelman, G. M. (1990). Synthetic neural modelling: A multi-level approach to brain complexity. In G. M. Edelman, W. E. Gall, & W. M. Cowan (Eds.), *Signal and sense: Local and global order in perceptual maps* (pp. 607–707). New York: Wiley.

Reeke, G. N., Jr., & Sporns, O. (1990). Selectionist models of perceptual and motor systems and implications for functionalist theories of brain function. *Physica D, 42*, 347–364.

Reeke, G. N., Jr., Sporns, O., & Edelman, G. M. (1990). Synthetic neural modeling: The "Darwin" series of recognition automata. *Proceedings of the IEEE, 78*, 1498–1530.

Rovee-Collier, C. (1991). The "memory system" of prelinguistic infants. In A. Diamond (Ed.), The development and neural bases of higher cognitive functions. *Annals of the New York Academy of Sciences, 608*, 517–536.

Schneider, K., Zernicke, R. F., Ulrich, B. D., Jensen, J. L., & Thelen, E. (1990). Understanding movement control in infants through the analysis of limb intersegmental dynamics. *Journal of Motor Behavior, 22*, 493–520.

Schöner, G., & Kelso, J. A. S. (1988). Dynamic pattern generation in behavioral and neural systems. *Science, 239*, 1513–1520.

Siegler, R. S., & Jenkins, E. (1989). *How children discover new strategies.* Hillsdale, NJ: Erlbaum.

Sporns, O., & Edelman, G. M. (1993). Solving Bernstein's problem: A proposal for the development of coordinated movement by selection. *Child Development, 64,* 960–981.

Stein, B. E., & Meredith, M. A. (1993). *The merging of the senses.* Cambridge, MA: MIT Press/Bradford Books.

Streri, A., & Pecheux, M. G. (1986). Tactual habituation and discrimination of form in infancy. A comparison with vision. *Child Development, 57,* 100–104.

Thelen, E. (1989). Self-organization in developmental processes: Can systems approaches work? In M. Gunnar & E. Thelen (Eds.), *Systems in development: The Minnesota Symposia on Child Psychology* (Vol. 22, pp. 77–117). Hillsdale, NJ: Erlbaum.

Thelen, E. (1992). Development as a dynamic system. *Current Directions in Psychological Science, 1,* 189–193.

Thelen, E. (1994). Three-month-old infants can learn task-specific patterns of interlimb coordination. *Psychological Science, 5,* 280–285.

Thelen, E., Corbetta, D., Kamm, K., Spencer, J. P., Schneider, K., & Zernicke, R. F. (1993). The transition to reaching: Mapping intention and intrinsic dynamics. *Child Development, 64,* 1058–1098.

Thelen, E., & Fisher, D. M. (1982). Newborn stepping: An explanation for a "disappearing reflex." *Developmental Psychology, 18,* 760–775.

Thelen, E., & Fisher, D. M. (1983). The organization of spontaneous leg movements in newborn infants. *Journal of Motor Behavior, 15,* 353–377.

Thelen, E., Kelso, J. A. S., & Fogel, A. (1987). Self-organizing systems and infant motor development. *Developmental Review, 7,* 39–65.

Thelen, E., & Smith, L. B. (1994). *A dynamic systems approach to the development of cognition and action.* Cambridge, MA: MIT Press/Bradford Books.

Thelen, E., & Ulrich, B. D. (1991). Hidden skills: A dynamic systems analysis of treadmill stepping during the first year. *Monographs of the Society for Research in Child Development, 56* (1, Serial No. 223).

Thelen, E., Ulrich, B., & Niles, D. (1987). Bilateral coordination in human infants: Stepping on a split-belt treadmill. *Journal of Experimental Psychology: Human Perception and Performance, 13,* 405–410.

Turvey, M. T. (1990). Coordination. *American Psychologist, 4,* 938–953.

Waddington, C. H. (1954). The integration of gene-controlled processes and its bearing on evolution. *Proceedings of the 9th International Congress of Genetics* (Caryologia Suppl.), 232–295.

Zelazo, P. R., Zelazo, N. A., & Kolb, S. (1972). "Walking" in the newborn. *Science, 177,* 1058–1059.

Zernicke, R. F., & Schneider, K. (1993). Biomechanics and developmental neuromotor control. *Child Development, 64,* 982–1004.

# 3

# Understanding the Intentions of Others: Re-Enactment of Intended Acts by 18-Month-Old Children

**Andrew N. Meltzoff**

*University of Washington, Seattle*

*Investigated was whether children would re-enact what an adult actually did or what the adult intended to do. In Experiment 1 children were shown an adult who tried, but failed, to perform certain target acts. Completed target acts were thus not observed. Children in comparison groups either saw the full target act or appropriate controls. Results showed that children could infer the adult's intended act by watching the failed attempts. Experiment 2 tested children's understanding of an inanimate object that traced the same movements as the person had followed. Children showed a completely different reaction to the mechanical device than to the person: They did not produce the target acts in this case. Eighteen-month-olds situate people within a psychological framework that differentiates between the surface behavior of people and a deeper level involving goals and intentions. They have already adopted a fundamental aspect of folk psychology—persons (but not inanimate objects) are understood within a framework involving goals and intentions.*

Reprinted with permission from *Developmental Psychology*, 1995, Vol. 31, No. 5, 838–850. Copyright © 1995 by the American Psychological Association, Inc.

This research was funded by a grant from the National Institute of Child Health and Human Development (HD-22514). I thank Alison Gopnik, Patricia Kuhl, and Keith Moore for insightful comments on drafts of this article. Ideas from each of them enriched this article. I am also indebted to John Flavell, Al Goldman, and the anonymous reviewers for making very helpful suggestions. Special thanks also go to Craig Harris and Calle Fisher for assistance in all phases of the research and to Hattie Berg, Cinda Hanson, and Eva Tejero for help in testing the children.

A central topic in developmental cognitive science is to investigate how and when children develop a folk psychology or "theory of mind," the understanding of others as psychological beings having mental states such as beliefs, desires, emotions, and intentions (Astington & Gopnik, 1991a; Flavell, 1988; Harris, 1989; Leslie, 1987; Perner, 1991a; Wellman, 1990). It would be a world very foreign to us to restrict our understanding of others to purely physical terms (e.g., arm extensions, finger curlings, etc.). Failure to attribute mental states to people confronts one with a bewildering series of movements, a jumble of behavior that is difficult to predict and even harder to explain. At a rough level of approximation, this may be something like the state of children with autism (Baron-Cohen, Leslie, & Frith, 1985; Baron-Cohen, Tager-Flusberg, & Cohen, 1993). However, normal children give elaborate verbal descriptions of the unobservable psychological states of people, indicating that they relate observable actions to underlying mental states.

Recent research on children's understanding of mind has been focused on two differentiable questions: (a) Mentalism: How and when do children first begin to construe others as having psychological states that underlie behavior? (b) Representational model of mind: How and when do children come to understand mental states as active interpretations of the world and not simple copies or imprints of it (Flavell, 1988; Forguson & Gopnik, 1988; Perner, 1991a; Wellman, 1990). One can be a mentalist without having a representational model of the mind, but being a representationalist entails being a mentalist. One has to understand that there is a mind or something like it before precise questions about the relation between mind and world can arise. A developmental ordering is suggested. It has been proposed that there is not a single "theory of mind," but rather a succession of different theories, in particular, an early mentalistic one that is replaced by a representational one (e.g., Gopnik, Slaughter, & Meltzoff, 1994; Gopnik & Wellman, 1992, 1994; Wellman, 1990, 1993).

The second question listed above has received the bulk of the empirical attention to date. The tasks used to explore it include false belief (Perner, Leekam, & Wimmer, 1987; Wimmer & Perner, 1983), representational change (Gopnik & Astington, 1988; Wimmer & Hartl, 1991), appearance-reality (Flavell, Flavell, & Green, 1983; Flavell, Green, & Flavell, 1986), level-2 perspective taking (Flavell, Everett, Croft, & Flavell, 1981), and others (C. Moore, Pure, & Furrow, 1990; O'Neill, Astington, & Flavell, 1992; O'Neill & Gopnik, 1991). Although a topic of current debate, there is growing consensus that children first adopt a representational model of mind by about 3 to 5 years of age (Flavell, 1988; Forguson & Gopnik, 1988; Perner, 1991a; Wellman, 1990, 1993).

The first question listed above concerns an earlier phase of development and has not received as much attention, but it is equally important. The experimental data that exist seem to suggest that even 2.5- to 3-year-olds are mentalists; they read below the surface behavior to understand the actions of persons. Wellman and Estes (1986) reported that 3-year-olds distinguish between mental and physical entities. Bartsch and Wellman (1989) found that 3-year-old children used beliefs and desires to explain human action. Lillard and Flavell (1990) showed that 3-year-olds have a preference for construing human behavior in psychological terms. In their study a series of pictures was shown to children and described in both behavioral and mental state terms. For example, children were shown a picture of a child sitting on the floor (back to the viewer), and this was described as a child "wiping up" and "feeling sad" about his spilled milk. A duplicate picture was then given to the child, who was asked to explain the scene in his or her own terms. The results showed that 3-year-olds were more likely to choose mentalistic descriptions than behavioral ones. This attribution of mental states by 3-year-olds is compatible with research described by Gelman and Wellman (1991) and Wellman and Gelman (1988) showing that 3- to 4-year-old children tend to postulate unobservable "insides and essences" of things earlier than classically believed (Piaget, 1929).

Philosophers have argued that among the varied mental states we ascribe to persons, beliefs are particularly complex (e.g., Searle, 1983). This is because they are the representational states par excellence. As defined by philosophers, beliefs always involve representations or interpretations of the world rather than simply attitudes toward it or relations with it; however, other mental states such as desires and intentions may easily be construed nonrepresentationally and so may be easier to understand (Astington & Gopnik, 1991b; Flavell, 1988; Gopnik & Wellman, 1994; Perner, 1991b; Wellman, 1990, 1993). Mental states such as desire and intention may be particularly good topics to investigate if one is interested in the earliest roots of children's understanding of mind.

Empirical work supports this view. Premack and Woodruff (1978) reported that a language-trained chimpanzee could correctly choose which of two pictures depicted the correct solution to a problem facing an actor, which led them to suggest at least a primitive grasp of the desires and intentions (see also Premack & Dasser, 1991). In everyday language and verbal explanations of problems set to them, children talk about desires ("I want x . . .") before they talk about beliefs ("I think x . . .") (Bartsch & Wellman, 1995; Bretherton, McNew, & Beeghly-Smith, 1981; Brown & Dunn, 1991; Moses & Flavell, 1990; Shatz, Wellman, & Silber, 1983; Wellman, 1990; Wellman & Bartsch, 1994). Moreover, laboratory studies have shown that 3-year-olds can recognize that someone has a desire even if that desire is not actually fulfilled, that is, they can differentiate desires and actions (Astington & Gopnik, 1991b). They can also distinguish between intended, unintended, and mistaken actions (Shultz, 1980; Shultz, Wells, & Sarda, 1980) and know that intentions may remain unfulfilled (Moses, 1993; see also Astington, 1991; Frye, 1991, for relevant discussions). Finally, 3-year-olds understand something about the linkage between desires, actions, and emotional reactions. They know that fulfilled desires lead to happiness and a cessation of searching, whereas unfulfilled ones lead to sadness and a continuance of search (Harris, 1989; Wellman & Banerjee, 1991; Wellman & Woolley, 1990; Yuill, 1984; also Moses, 1993).[1] Marshaling this and related philosophical, linguistic, and behavioral support, Wellman (1990, 1993; Wellman & Woolley, 1990) suggested that a "belief psychology" grows out of a prior "desire psychology," and he and others have pushed back the earliest instances of children's understanding of mind, as measured by way of desire tasks, to 2 to 3 years of age.

To date, most of the techniques for assessing children's "theory of mind" have relied on verbal report. This makes it difficult to test children before about 2- to 2.5-years old. There is a keen interest among both psychologists and philosophers (Campbell, 1994, 1995; Fodor, 1992; Goldman, 1992, 1993; Gordon, 1994) in the aboriginal roots of children's understanding of mind. Several nonverbal abilities in infancy have been proposed as candidates, including: symbolic play and metarepresentation (Leslie, 1987, 1988), joint attention and social referencing (Baron-Cohen, 1991; Butterworth, 1991; Wellman, 1990), and crossmodal representation of others as "like me" coupled with body imitation (Meltzoff, 1990a; Meltzoff & Gopnik, 1993; Meltzoff & Moore, 1995).

There is a rather large gap between these roots and the abilities examined in standard theory-of-mind experiments with 2.5- to 4-year-olds. This gap is due, in part, to the lack of a technique for exploring the relevant questions in children too young to give verbal reports. One aim of the current research is to develop a nonverbal test that can be used to pose such questions. The issue investigated here was children's understanding of the

---

[1] Other research with more complex tasks and older children also has indicated that understanding desires and intentions emerges before beliefs. Studies directly comparing beliefs to desires have revealed that children understand: (a) desires and intentions can change before they understand that beliefs can change (Gopnik & Slaughter, 1991), and (b) others have desires that differ from their own before they understand that others have beliefs that run counter to their own (Flavell, Flavell, Green, & Moses, 1990; Wellman, 1990).

intentions of others, something more akin to desires than beliefs. The test used was called the *behavioral re-enactment procedure.*

The behavioral re-enactment procedure capitalizes on toddlers' natural tendency to pick up behavior from adults, to re-enact or imitate what they see (Meltzoff, 1988a, 1988b, 1990b, 1995; Piaget, 1962). However, it uses this proclivity in a new way. In the critical test situation in Experiment 1, children were confronted with an adult who merely demonstrated an "intention" to act in a certain way. Importantly, the adult never fulfilled this intention. He tried but failed to perform the act, so the end state was never reached. It remained unobserved by the child. To an adult, it was easy to "read" the actor's intention. The experimental question was whether children interpreted this behavior in purely physical terms or whether they too read through the literal body movements to the underlying goal or intention of the act. The children, who were too young to give verbal reports, informed us how they represented the event by what they chose to re-enact. Another group of children followed the same experimental protocol and were tested in an identical fashion except that they saw the full target act. Various control groups were tested. Children's tendency to perform the target act was compared in several situations: after they saw the act demonstrated, after the target act was intended but not achieved, and after the target act was neither shown nor intended. The results suggest that 18-month-old children understand something about the intentions of others: They performed the acts the adult intended to do even though the adult's acts failed.

Experiment 2 compared children's reactions to a person versus an inanimate object. An inanimate device was built that traced the same movements through space as the human hand. The dual aims of this study were to test whether these spatial patterns might in and of themselves suggest a goal state and to explore the limits of the types of entities that may be construed as having psychological properties like intentions. The movements of the inanimate device did not lead children to produce the target acts.

Taken together, the experiments show that 18-month-old children already situate people within a psychological framework. They have adopted a key element of a folk psychology: People (but not inanimate objects) are understood within a framework that includes goals and intentions. The issue now raised for theory, and considered in the conclusions, is whether 18-month-olds impute mental states as the causes of behavior or whether they are in a transitional phase that serves to link the newborn's more embryonic notion of person (Meltzoff & Moore, 1995) to the full-blown mentalism of the 3-year-old.

# EXPERIMENT 1

## *Method*

**Children.** The participants were forty 18-month-old children ($M = 18.02$ months, $SD = .10$; range: 542–554 days old). The children were recruited by telephone calls from the university's computerized subject list. Equal numbers of boys and girls participated in the study; 37 children were White, 2 were Asian, and 1 was African American. Pre-established criteria for admission into the study were that a child be within $\pm$ 7 days of his or her 18-month birthday, have no known physical, sensory, or mental handicap, be full term (40 $\pm$ 3 weeks gestation, by maternal report), and have normal birth weight (2,500–4,500 g). No children were eliminated from the study for any reason.

**Test environment and apparatus.** The test was conducted in a room at the university that was unfurnished save for the equipment and furniture needed for the experiment. The child was tested while seated on his or her parent's lap in front of a rectangular table (1.2 $\times$ 0.8 m), the top surface of which was covered in black contact paper. A video camera behind and to the left of the experimenter recorded the infant's head, torso, and a portion of the table top in front of the child where the test objects were manipulated. A second camera behind and to the right of the child recorded the experimenter's stimulus presentations. Each camera was fed into a separate videorecorder that was housed in an adjacent room. The experiment was electronically timed by a character generator that mixed elapsed time in seconds and frames (30th of a second) onto the video records for subsequent scoring.

**Test materials.** Five objects served as test stimuli (Figure 1). The child could not have seen or played with these objects before, because they were specially constructed in the laboratory and were not commercially available. (Some parts in the stimuli were store-bought items, but these components were used in unusual ways.)

The first object was a dumbbell-shaped toy that could be pulled apart and put back together again. It consisted of two 2.5-cm wooden cubes, each with a 7.5-cm length of plastic extending from it. One tubular piece fit snugly inside the other so that it took considerable force to pull them apart (the dumbbell did not fall apart if banged on the table or shaken). The second object was a small black box (16.5 $\times$ 15 $\times$ 5.5 cm) with a slightly re-

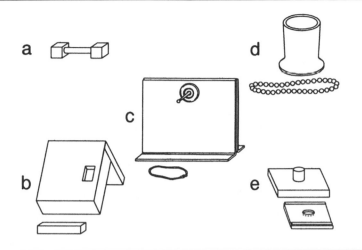

**Figure 1.** The five test objects: (a) dumbbell, (b) box and stick tool, (c) prong and loop, (d) cylinder and beads, and (e) square and post.

cessed rectangular button (3 × 2.2 cm) on the top surface. The button activated a buzzer inside the box. The box was supported by a base that tilted 30° off the table so that the front surface was facing the child. The box was accompanied by a small stick tool made of a rectangular block of wood that was used by the experimenter to push the button. The third object consisted of a horizontal prong and nylon loop. The prong was fashioned from an ornamental wooden piece with a bulbous end. It protruded horizontally from a background screen made of gray plastic (17 × 20.3 cm). The loop was made from black and yellow woven nylon tied in a circle with a diameter of 7.5 cm. The fourth object consisted of a yellow cylinder with a flared base (9.5 cm high with a 6.3-cm opening) coupled with a loop of beads (19 cm long when suspended). The fifth device was a transparent plastic square and wooden dowel. The square (10 cm) had a 2.5-cm diameter round hole cut out of the center so that it could fit over the dowel. Thin plastic strips were glued along two edges of the plastic square to raise it slightly from the table so that it could be picked up by the children. The dowel (2 cm high and 1.7 cm in diameter) was in an upright position in the center of a wooden base plate.

**Design.** The children were randomly assigned to one of four independent groups with 10 children per group. There were two demonstration groups and two control groups: Demonstration (target), Demonstration (intention),

Control (baseline), and Control (adult manipulation). Within each group the test objects were presented in five different orders such that each object occurred equally often in each position. One male and one female child were assigned to each order. Thus, order and sex of infant were counterbalanced both within and between groups.

**Procedure.** On arrival at the university, the children and their families were escorted to a waiting room where they completed the necessary forms. They were then brought to the test room where parent and child were seated at the table across from the experimenter. The experimenter handed the children an assortment of rubber toys to explore. After the infant seemed acclimated with the room and the experimenter, usually about 1–3 minutes, the warm-up toys were withdrawn and the study began.

*Demonstration (target).* For the children in this group the experimenter modeled a specific target act with each of the five objects. Each object was kept hidden before it was brought to the table for its demonstration and was returned to the hidden container before the next object was presented. For each stimulus, the target act was repeated three times in approximately 20 s and was then placed on the table directly in front of the infant. A 20-s response period was timed starting from when the infant touched the object. At the end of this response period, the first object was removed, and the second presentation was modeled following the same time procedure, and so on for the five test objects. The demonstrations were presented out of reach of the children so they could not touch or play with the toy but were confined to observing the event. The experimenter never used words related to the task such as "push button," "do what I do," or "copy me," but the experimenter was permitted to gain the child's attention by calling his or her name, saying "look over here," "oh, see what I have," or "it's your turn." The experimenter maintained a friendly demeanor throughout the demonstrations and did not express joy at successfully performing the act.

For the dumbbell, the act demonstrated was to pick it up by the wooden cubes and pull outward with a very definite movement so that the toy came apart into two halves. For the box, the act demonstrated was to pick up the stick tool and use it to push in the button, which then activated the buzzer inside the box. For the square, the act demonstrated was to pick up the plastic square and put the hole over the dowel. For the prong, the act demonstrated was to raise the nylon loop up to the prong and drape it over it. (The screen on which the prong was mounted was put perpendicular to the children on their left side.) For the cylinder, the act demonstrated was to raise the beads up over the opening of the cylinder and then to lower them down into the opening so that they were deposited on the bottom of the container.

*Demonstration (intention).* For this group the experimenter did not demonstrate the target acts. None of the final goal states was achieved. Instead, the experimenter was seen to try but fail to achieve these ends. The experimenter modeled the intention to perform these acts, but not the target acts themselves. Save for this critical difference, the remainder of the procedure for this group was identical to the group that saw the full target: The intention to produce the act was modeled three times and was followed by a 20-s response period for each test object so that the temporal factors were equated with the children who saw the target. The experimenter did not provide linguistic or facial expressions of failure. To an adult, the multiple, effortful tries effectively conveyed the intention to perform the target act, in line with Heider's (1958) descriptions of cues to intention in adult perceivers.

For the dumbbell, the experimenter picked it up by the wooden cubes, just as he had done in the Demonstration (target) condition. It appeared that the experimenter was trying to pull the ends outward. However, he failed to do so because as he pulled, one of his hands slipped off the end of the object. The direction of slippage alternated from left, to right, to left over the three stimulus presentations (the spatial terms are all referenced from the child's viewpoint). Thus there was no object transformation, and the goal state was never achieved. All that was visible were the experimenter's attempts to pull it apart.[2]

For the box, the experimenter used the stick tool and tried to push the button. However, the experimenter always missed. Thus the affordance of the box was never seen; there was no activation of the buzzer, and the goal state of touching the button with the tool was never witnessed. Each of the three misses was spatially different: First, the stick tool missed off the left, next it missed to the right, and on the third attempt it was too high. In each case the tip of the tool came down on the top surface of the box.

For the prong device, the experimenter tried but failed in his attempt to put the nylon loop over the prong. He picked up the loop, but as he approached the prong he released it inappropriately so that it "accidentally" dropped to the table surface each time. First, the loop was released slightly too far to the left, then too far to the right, and finally too low, where it fell to the table directly below the prong. The goal state of draping the nylon loop over the prong was not demonstrated.

For the cylinder, the experimenter attempted to deposit the beads into the cylinder, but failed. First, he raised the loop of beads over the cylinder

---

[2] The experimenter's demonstrations are described as if he was trying to achieve the target act. Of course, he was a confederate, and his actual intent was to give the impression that he was trying to produce the target.

and lowered them down so that just the tip of the beads crossed the edge of the top lip. The beads were then released such that they fell to the table outside the cylinder. The second attempt consisted of suspending the beads slightly too far in front of the cup so that they again fell to the table top when released. Third, the experimenter gathered the beads up into his loosely closed hand and scraped his hand over the opening of the cylinder such that the beads fell outside the cylinder instead of into it. The child thus did not see the beads deposited in the cylinder but saw three failed attempts at doing so.

For the plastic square, the experimenter picked it up and attempted to put it on the dowel. However, he did not align it properly. It was tilted slightly toward the child, and the hole was not aligned directly over the dowel. The first time the hole undershot the dowel and remained on the left, the second time it overshot it to the right, and the third time the hole was spatially in front of the dowel. The children never saw the goal state of putting the square over the dowel.

Five different acts were used, providing some assessment of generality. The dumbbell involved an "effort" to pull an object, but the object itself remained completely untransformed. The prong-and-loop device involved moving one object (the loop) in a behavioral sequence that to the adult was explained by an underlying cause—the attempt to drape the loop over the prong. It seemed possible that some tasks might be more easily understood than others. The dumbbell task might rely on perceived effort (which might be amenable to a Gibsonian analysis; Runeson & Frykholm, 1981) and may be more elementary than understanding the intent to bring about object-object relations. Furthermore, the range of stimuli investigated whether certain object-object spatial relations would be easier than others (e.g., the beads went inside the cylinder, the plastic square around the dowel, and the stick was used as an intermediary tool to poke a recessed button). The idea was to test whether any (or all) of these acts could be understood from seeing a failed attempt; the range of acts would help explore whether particular tasks were easier than others at this age.

*Control (baseline).* A baseline control group was included to assess the likelihood that the target acts used in the demonstration groups would occur in the spontaneous behavior of the children independent of the adult model. The adult demonstration was excluded, but all other aspects of the procedure remained the same: The experimenter handed the child the test stimuli one at a time and timed a 20-s response period for each object. This group controlled for the possibility that children of this age would spontaneously produce the target acts. At a more theoretical level, this group controlled for the possibility that the objects themselves have "affordances" or "demand characteristics" that are grasped by seeing the object itself. The degree that infants spontaneously engage in the target acts with these objects is evaluated, because infants are presented the same objects and are allowed to play with them for the identical response period as the other groups.

*Control (adult manipulation).* In two demonstration groups (both the target and intention) the children saw the experimenter pick up and handle the test objects. It could be argued that children may be more likely to manipulate and explore objects that the experimenter has handled. The baseline group controlled for the spontaneous production of the target actions but would not take care of controlling for any nonspecific effects of seeing the adult manipulate the objects. Therefore, a second control group was also included. In this group, the experimenter manipulated the test objects for the same length of time as in the demonstration groups. The only difference between this group and the two demonstration groups was that he neither demonstrated the target acts nor even the intention to produce them. He picked up and handled the objects but refrained from those activities. If the children produce more target behaviors in the demonstration groups than in this control it cannot be attributed to seeing the adult handle the objects, because handling time by the experimenter was equated. The combination of both baseline and adult-manipulation controls provides an excellent assessment of whether the specific content of the adult demonstration is influencing the behavior of the children.

For the dumbbell, the experimenter picked up the object by the wooden cubes and pushed both hands inward. This was shown three times in the presentation period. For the box, the experimenter held the stick and moved along the top surface of the box, with the tip of the stick passing directly next to and over the recessed button. First he held the stick horizontally and moved it from the lower edge of the surface to the upper edge and back down again, staying centered on the surface. Next, the same movement was made but with the stick aligned on the left edge of the box. Third, the same movement was repeated with the stick aligned on the right edge. For the prong, the experimenter released the loop next to the prong but did so with no evident intention of looping it over the prong. First the loop was slid along the top edge of the gray screen past the prong and was released when it reached the edge of the screen closest to the child. Second, this movement was reversed. Third, the loop was moved along the base of the screen until it was directly below the prong and was then released so that it fell to the table underneath the prong. For the cylinder, the experimenter picked up the beads and lowered them onto the table beside the cylinder (10 cm away) with no evident intent to deposit them inside it. First, the beads were lowered onto the table so that they crumpled about half way and then were released so they fell to the left of the cylinder. Next, they were raised in the air to the height needed to deposit them into the cylinder and were released so they dropped to the right of the cylinder. Third, they were gathered in a loosely held fist and then turned the fist over and released onto the table to left of the cylinder. For the plastic square, the experimenter held the square vertically so that it was standing upright on one edge and moved it along the wooden plate that held the dowel. First, the vertical plastic square was moved along the front portion of the base, then along the back, and finally along the front again. The hole was thus seen to pass directly in front and behind the dowel (the dowel could be seen right through the hole), but there was no obvious intent to fit the hole over the dowel.

**Scoring.** The response periods for all four groups were identical inasmuch as each infant had a series of five 20-s response periods. To ensure blind scoring of the data, a new videotape was made by deleting all the warm-up and presentation periods. It contained only the response periods and thus contained no artifactual clue as to the children's test group. It was scored in a random order by a coder who was kept unaware of the test group of the children.

The operational definitions of performing the target acts were the following. For the dumbbell a "yes" was scored if the infant pulled the object apart. For the box a "yes" was scored if the infant used the stick tool to push the button and activate the buzzer. For the prong a "yes" was scored if the nylon loop was put over the prong so that the prong protruded through it. For the cylinder a "yes" was scored if the beads were lowered all the way into the cylinder. For the plastic square a "yes" was scored if the infant placed the plastic square over the wooden dowel so that the dowel protruded through the hole. The scorer also recorded the latency to produce each of the target acts, timed from the moment the child first touched the toy. Latencies were measured by reference to the character generator on the video record that recorded time in seconds and frames.

The principal question was how the production of target acts varied as a function of experimental group. However, during the study it had become evident that infants sometimes duplicated the control acts that the experimenter displayed in the adult-manipulation control. The study was not designed to pursue these arbitrary acts in detail, but instances of the adults' control acts were also scored in all trials. These data are informative both for knowing whether infants reenact incidental behaviors and also whether children will perform two different actions on the test objects (one after seeing the target demonstrations and another after these control demonstrations). The operational definitions were the following: For the pull toy the infant strained to push the (unmovable) ends of the assembled dumbbell inwards, just as the experimenter had done. For the box the infant held the stick tool in a horizontal position while moving it against the face of the black box. For the prong the nylon loop was moved along the upper edge of the screen. For the cylinder the beads were suspended vertically off the table and then lowered or dropped all the way onto the table beside the cylinder without touching it. For the plastic square the infant held the piece of plastic square upright on its edge as it was moved on the wooden base as the experimenter had done.

Scoring agreement was assessed by having 25% of the children (50 trials) rescored by both the primary scorer and an independent scorer. Scoring agreement was high: Across the 50 trials, there were no intra-scorer disagreements on the production of the target acts or control acts; for the interscorer assessments, there was one disagreement for target acts and one for the control acts. The Pearson $r$ for the latency measure was .98 (mean disagreement $< 0.25$ s).

## Results and Discussion

**Main analyses.** The results suggest that 18-month-old children can understand the intended acts of adults even when the adult does not fulfill his intentions. Each child was presented with five objects, and for statistical analyses each was assigned a score ranging from 0 to 5 according to how many target acts he or she produced. Table 1 displays the mean number of target acts produced as a function of experimental group. The data were analyzed with a one-way analysis of variance (ANOVA). The results showed

TABLE 1
Number of Children Producing Target Acts
as a Function of Group

| Group | Number of target acts | | | | | |
|---|---|---|---|---|---|---|
| | 0 | 1 | 2 | 3 | 4 | 5 |
| Control (baseline) | 4 | 3 | 0 | 3 | 0 | 0 |
| Control (adult manipulation) | 3 | 4 | 3 | 0 | 0 | 0 |
| Demonstration (intention) | 0 | 0 | 2 | 0 | 4 | 4 |
| Demonstration (target) | 0 | 0 | 1 | 2 | 5 | 2 |

that the number of target acts varied significantly as a function of experimental group, with more target acts in the demonstration groups than the controls, $F(3, 36) = 22.95$, $p < .0001$. Follow-up pairwise comparisons using the Tukey honestly significant difference procedure showed that number of target acts produced by infants in the target demonstration ($M = 3.80$, $SD = 0.92$) and intention ($M = 4.00$, $SD = 1.15$) groups did not significantly differ from each other and that each group produced significantly more target acts than infants in the baseline ($M = 1.20$, $SD = 1.32$) and adult-manipulation ($M = 1.00$, $SD = 0.82$) control groups, which also did not significantly differ from each other. Nonparametric analyses of the data (Kruskal-Wallis and Mann-Whitney $U$s) yielded identical results.

It is striking that the Demonstration (target) and Demonstration (intention) groups did not significantly differ from one another. Of the 50 trials (10 s $\times$ 5 trials each) administered to the Demonstration (target) group, 38 resulted in the target act, which is similar to the 40 for the Demonstration (intention) group. A more qualitative examination of the videotapes supported this point. Infants in the intention group did not go through a period of trial and error with the test objects but directly produced the target act just as those who saw the full target had done. This can be captured by the latency to produce the target acts in the intention and target demonstration groups, which did not significantly differ from one another ($F < 1.0$) and were respectively 5.10 s ($SD = 2.74$) and 3.97 s ($SD = 2.70$). These short latencies support the impression gained from the videotapes that infants did not engage in extensive error correction and produced the targets rather directly.

Can children interpret the adult's behavior right from the first encounter? The results show that 80% of the children (8 of 10 for each demonstration group) produced the target act with the first object as compared with only 20% (5 of 20) in the control groups, $\chi^2$ (1, $N = 40$) = 10.03, $p < .005$. These data are informative because they show that prolonged exposure to these displays is not necessary; they can be interpreted even when they occur on the first trial.

Each test object was analyzed individually to assess the generality of the phenomenon and the range of events over which it works. Table 2 provides the complete data set, broken down object by object. For statistical analysis the two Demonstration groups (target and intention) were collapsed and compared with the collapsed Controls (baseline and adult-manipulation) because the expected frequencies were too small for a four-cell analysis (Siegel, 1956). The results from the 2 $\times$ 2 contingency tables comparing the number of children who produced the target response for each object (a dichotomous yes or no score) as a function of experimental treatment

TABLE 2
Proportion of Children Producing Target Acts as a Function
of Test Objects and Group

| | Group | | | |
|---|---|---|---|---|
| Test object | Control (baseline) | Control (adult-manipulation) | Demonstration (intention) | Demonstration (target) |
| Dumbbell | .20 | .40 | .80 | 1.00 |
| Box | .40 | .10 | .90 | .90 |
| Prong | .10 | .20 | .90 | .70 |
| Cylinder | .30 | .20 | .90 | .80 |
| Square | .20 | .10 | .50 | .40 |
| $M$ | .24 | .20 | .80 | .76 |

(Demonstration or Controls) showed that the demonstration was significantly more effective in eliciting the target behavior for each of the objects
considered individually. The chi-square values were as follows (all $df = 1$,
$N = 40$, one-tailed): dumbbell, 12.60, $p < .001$; box, 14.73, $p < .001$;
prong, 14.44, $p < .001$; cylinder, 12.22, $p < .001$; and square, 2.98, $p <$
.05. If one analyzes the controls versus the intention group alone, a similar
pattern emerges for each object, with significance values ranging from $p <$
.001 to $p = .056$ (for the square). The results suggest that the phenomenon
is not limited to one or two acts but is reasonably general, applying to all
five of the acts tested. The only object that seemed to cause any difficulty
was the plastic square, and re-examination of the videotapes indicated that
this task strained the manual dexterity of the 18-month-olds. The children
in both the intention and target act groups had motor skills difficulty in fit-
ting the hole over the dowel (six children failed in the Demonstration [tar-
get] group and five failed in the Demonstration [intention] group).

**Subsidiary analyses.** In the adult-manipulation control group the adult
picked up and handled the toys but did not perform the target acts. The goal
of using this control was to equate for the amount of time that the adult handled the toys with the demonstration groups. It was not intended that the
infants learn anything from these control manipulations. Nonetheless, my
impression was that children were duplicating these arbitrary acts. The data
were that 90% (9 of 10) of the children in the adult-manipulation control
group produced a control act as compared with only 6.7% (2 of 30) of the
children from the other three groups, $\chi^2$ (1, $N = 40$) = 22.11, $p < .0001$.
On average, infants in the adult-manipulation group produced 2.60 (median
= 3.00) such acts out of the five possible trials, which significantly differed
from the other groups ($M = .067$), $p < .001$, Mann-Whitney test. This re-

sult is compatible with previous reports of the imitation of novel and arbitrary acts at this age (e.g., Meltzoff, 1988a, 1995; Piaget, 1962).

## EXPERIMENT 2

The results of Experiment 1 indicated that young children can pick up information from the failed attempts of human actors. One question that arises is whether the children are responding solely to the physics of the situation (the movements that are traced in space) or whether a psychological understanding of the human actor is involved. What would children do if they saw the same movements produced by an inanimate device? Do the spatial transformations in and of themselves suggest the target act? A device was built that mimicked the movements of the actor in the Demonstration (intention) group. The device did not look human, but it had a pincer that "grasped" the dumbbell on the two ends (just as the human did) and then pulled outward. These pincers then slipped off the cubes (just as the human hand did). The pattern of movements and the slipping motions were closely matched to the human hand movements, as described below (see Figure 2).

### Method

**Children.**  The participants were sixty 18-month-old children ($M = 18.08$ months, $SD = .13$; range $= 541$–$555$ days old). Equal numbers of boys and girls participated in the study. Fifty-four children were White, 3 were Asian, and 1 each were African American, Hispanic, and Pacific Islander. The recruitment procedures and criteria for admission into the study were

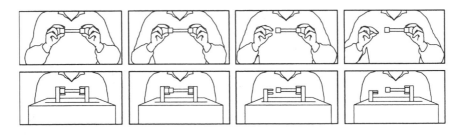

**Figure 2.** Human demonstrator (top panel) and mechanical device mimicking these movements (bottom panel) used in Experiment 2. Time is represented by successive frames left to right.

the same as in Experiment 1. One potential participant was dropped due to a procedural error.

**Test materials.** The test object was the dumbbell shown in Figure 1. For the human model group, the demonstration was performed by a human in the same way as already described in Experiment 1: Demonstration (intention). In the inanimate model group the demonstration was presented by a mechanical device (see Figure 2). This device consisted of a small box with an open back panel. Through this opening the experimenter invisibly controlled two upright mechanical arms. Each mechanical arm consisted of a vertical piece with two horizontal finger/pincers at its end. The dumbbell was held between the pincers in the same way that it was held by the human fingers. The mechanical arms traced the same movements outward as the human arms did. Like the human actor, the mechanical device failed to pull apart the dumbbell, and the pincers slid off the ends of the dumbbell just as the human fingers did. An interesting detail is that the pincers were under slight spring tension. Therefore, when the pincer slid off the end, the two pincers came together just as the human fingers did when the adult's hand slipped off the end of the dumbbell. No machine can exactly duplicate a human, and this certainly was not an attempt to construct a robot (left for future research). However, this device mimicked the pulling and slipping motion of the arms, fingers, and hands at a reasonable first approximation. It tested whether the perception of pincers slipping off the end of the dumbbell suggested the same goal state as fingers slipping off the end.

**Design.** The children were randomly assigned to one of two independent groups with 30 children per group: Human Demonstration (intention) and Inanimate Demonstration (mechanical slippage). Sex of child was counterbalanced within each group.

**Procedure.** After filling out the necessary forms, one parent and the child were escorted to the test room and acclimated as described in Experiment 1. For children in the Human Demonstration (intention) group the procedure was similar to that already described in Experiment 1, except that a female experimenter was used to present stimuli in this experiment. Briefly, the experimenter brought the dumbbell up from beneath the table with it held in her two hands. The adult then moved her arm horizontally to the left but failed to pull apart the dumbbell, because her hand slipped off (see Figure 2). This movement was repeated two more times, each time alternating the direction of the attempted pull and therefore the direction that the fingers slipped off. The same protocol was followed in the group who saw the demonstration by the mechanical device rather than by a human. The mechanical arm was moved horizontally so that the pincers slid off the dumbbell on the left side (see Figure 2). The mechanical arm was then moved in the opposite direction so that the pincers slid off on the other side and finally in the first direction again. Each time the pincers slid off the end of the dumbbell the pincers came together just as the human fingers did.

At the end of the presentation period, both groups were treated identically. The stimulus material was withdrawn and the test object put on the table directly in front of the child. A 20-s response period was electronically timed from the moment the child touched the object.

**Scoring.** The primary dependent measure was the number of children who produced the target act of pulling apart the dumbbell. This information was obtained from videotape coding by a scorer who remained uninformed about whether the previous demonstration had been shown by the person or machine. We also sought to evaluate whether children in the machine-demonstration group were frightened by the display (observations suggested not). In a separate pass (also involving "blind" scoring) the stimulus-presentation periods were scored for: infant visual attention to the presentation, social referencing to the caretaker (turning around to look at the parent), and fussing. Visual attention was measured in seconds, and the other measures were dichotomous codes of whether or not such an event occurred during the presentation period. Scoring agreement was assessed by having 25% of the children rescored by both the primary and an independent scorer. Agreement was high: There were no disagreements on the dichotomous measures; for visual attention $r = .99$ (mean disagreement $< 0.33$ s).

### Results

The children were visually riveted by both displays; visual attention to the displays exceeded 98% of the presentation period for both treatment groups. The children did not seem to be more frightened by one display than the other. There was no social referencing (turning around toward the parent) and no fussing by any of the children during the presentation periods.

Children did not seem to react differently when watching the human versus machine. The question can now be posed as to whether they interpreted the presentations differently. The data showed that they did. The groups significantly differed in their tendency to produce the target act. The children were six times more likely to produce the target act after seeing the human attempt to pull it apart (60% did so) than they were after seeing the demonstration by machine (10%). The corresponding contingency table analyzing group (human or machine) $\times$ response (yes or no) was significant, $\chi^2(1, N = 60) = 14.36, p < .0005$.

## GENERAL DISCUSSION

The goals of this research were both methodological and substantive. The first goal was to develop a procedure that could be used to pose "theory-of-mind" questions at ages younger than children could be queried through verbal means. The more substantive issues were to investigate (a) whether 18-month-olds understand the acts of others within a psychological framework that includes goals and intentions and (b) the limits of the types of entities that are interpreted within this framework. Is it tied to people?

### *Behavioral Re-Enactment Procedure*

A behavioral re-enactment procedure was developed to pose questions concerning the understanding of intention, but it would seem to have wider applicability than to intention alone. The test mandates that children formulate action plans on the basis of their interpretation of events. The response is a productive measure. Such re-presentation in action is not as informative as a verbal description, but it does entail that the children "tell" us how they saw things (rather than our making inferences from a more passive measure, such as increased or decreased attention in a habituation procedure).[3]

The re-enactment technique capitalizes on past findings that toddlers can be induced to reproduce adult's behavior (Meltzoff, 1988a, 1988b, 1993, 1995; Piaget, 1962). The normal task was modified to differentiate between a surface versus more abstract construal of an event. It asked whether infants could go beyond duplicating what was actually done and would instead enact what the adult intended to do. By analogy, if adults are asked to repeat what was said, they often paraphrase rather than quote, and we glean much from what they leave out, magnify, and transform. Like adults, infants are not little tape-recorders or videorecorders. The re-enactment procedure uses infants' nonverbal reconstructions of events to investigate their interpretive structures, here to explore their folk psychological framework.

---

[3] The habituation paradigm could be used to investigate infants' perception of intention by adapting Dasser, Ulbaek, and Premack's (1989) study of older children; converging studies using both the re-enactment and habituation procedures would enrich one's understanding of infants' notion of intention.

### Understanding Intention in Infancy

In Experiment 1, one group saw the adult perform a target act, Demonstration (target), and as expected, they re-enacted the same target. Another group provided a more novel test. They never saw the adult perform the actual target act. For example, the adult tried to pull apart a toy but failed to do so because his hand slipped off as he attempted to pull it apart. In another case the adult strove to push a button with a stick tool but failed in his attempts. In a third, the adult intended to put a loop over a prong but under- and overshot the target, and the loop ineffectually fell to the table.

The terms "tried," "strove," and "intended" are used because that is how adults would code the behavior. This is a mentalistic way of describing things. The question is whether the infants also construe it this way. Or do they see things in a less psychological manner? Perhaps in more purely physical terms?

In Experiment 1, two control groups were included. These controls assessed the likelihood that infants would produce the target acts spontaneously, through chance manipulation, or because the objects had demand characteristics that called out the response even when it was not modeled. The results showed that the target acts were not high baseline behaviors; they were not called out by the test objects themselves, or even by watching the adult perform control actions with the same test objects. Nonetheless, in the treatment groups infants accurately produced the targets. The significant difference between the treatment and control groups shows that infants' behavior was based on their perception of the adult's acts. They used the adults as a source of information about what to do with the objects, and their behavior was guided by the nature of the particular acts the adult did.

The adult's modeling of failed attempts led to a systematic effect, and the effect was extremely strong: Infants were as likely to perform the target after seeing the adult "trying" as they were after seeing the real demonstration of the behavior itself. In Experiment 1, children in the intention group performed 4.0 out of a possible 5 target acts and did so with a mean latency of 5.01 s, whereas those in the target-demonstration group performed 3.8 out of the same 5 acts with a latency of 3.97 s (statistically, these slight differences did not approach significance on either measure). These numbers are in line with my impressions in conducting the study. I did not see infants in the Demonstration (intention) condition groping toward the goal. This could have happened, and we scoured the videotapes for it, but it did not occur. It was as if children "saw through" the surface behavior to the intended act or goal.

The analysis showing that children re-enacted the incidental acts of the experimenter in the control group confirms that 18-month-olds can and do imitate fairly "meaningless" action sequences (see also Piaget, 1962). They had the motor skills to imitate the surface behavior of the adult in the Demonstration (intention) group. They could have poked the stick on the surface of the box or dropped the loop next to the prong. However, they did not re-enact what the adult literally did, but rather what he intended to do.[4] This nonverbal finding is reminiscent of Lillard and Flavell's (1990) discovery that 3-year-old children preferred to verbally describe an event in terms of underlying desire or intention rather than surface behavior ("he wants to get the cupcake" instead of "he's on tiptoes by the cupcake").

To underscore why the results reported here are relevant to the development of folk psychology, it is helpful to distinguish between seeing the behaviors of others in purely physical versus psychological terms. The former will be called *movements* or *motions* and the later human *acts*. The behavior of another person can, of course, be described at either (or both) of these levels. We can say "Sally's hand contacted the cup, the cup fell over" or "Sally intended to pick up the cup." Strict behaviorists insist on the former because what is in the respondent's mind is unobservable. Cognitive and social psychologists prefer the latter description. The current research suggests that by 18 months of age children are not strict behaviorists. They do not see the behavior of others merely in terms of "hold the dumbbell and then remove one hand quickly" but rather see an "effort" at pulling. They do not see the demonstration as "loop falls to one side of prong and then the other side," but rather as an attempt to drape it over the prong. They show us how they see or interpret these events by re-enacting them for us. Infants apparently represent the behavior of people in a psychological framework involving goals and intended acts, instead of purely physical movements or motions. Borrowing language from perceptual psychology, one might say they code human behavior in terms of the "distal

---

[4] It can be asked whether the infants performed the target by accident in the course of trying to duplicate the model's surface behavior. This seems unlikely for four reasons: (a) It was easier to miss the goal than to achieve it; for example, it's motorically easier to have the plastic square-with-hole miss the post and slide off (the observed surface behavior) than have the hole fit over the post. (b) Children succeeded on all five tasks and did so with extremely short latencies manifesting generality and speed that belie accidental behavior. (c) In the case of the dumbbell, seeing mechanical pincers slide off the toy and come together like fingers didn't prompt infants to pull apart the dumbbell, indicating that the target is not suggested simply by friction on the end of the dumbbells and movement away from the center. (d) Even in the Demonstration (intention) group, children often firmly wrapped their fingers around the ends of the dumbbell (in preparation for pulling) and visually concentrated on pulling it apart. If the dumbbell failed to come apart and the children's hands slipped off, as occasionally happened (the snug fit necessitated a considerable yank), they immediately redoubled their efforts to pull it apart. Accomplishing the target act is what terminated their behavior.

stimulus" (the intended act) instead of the "proximal cues" (the surface behavior and literal limb movements). Human behavior is seen as purposive.

Experiment 2 investigated whether there was something special about a
person, or whether 18-month-olds would make similar attributions to the
movements of an inanimate device. It is central to our adult conceptions of
the world that there are two differentiable causal frameworks: (a) a physical causality for explaining the behavior of things and (b) a psychological
causality for explaining the behavior of people. We can make errors in our
attributions, and inanimate devices can be built that strain our normal distinctions (can computers have intentional states?). However, one doesn't
generally ask the desk to move across the room—one shoves it. One doesn't
believe the car key was "trying" to hide (even if it's absent whenever
there is an important appointment). Similarly, one doesn't think that an er-
rant arrow was actually trying to hit the bullseye but failed (that ascription
is made of the archer), or that the pendulum of a grandfather clock is attempting to strike the side of the cabinet but missing. Intentions and goals
are the types of things that are used to explain the behavior of persons, not
things. In my terms, we see the bodily movements of people and interpret
them in terms of acts, and we see the movements of things and interpret
them as such, as movements or motions. Explanations for the latter lie in
the domain of physics and for the former in the domain of psychology.

The outcome of Experiment 2 was that the 18-month-olds did not tend
to produce the target act when a mechanical device slipped off the ends of
the dumbbell, but they did produce the target act when the human hand
slipped off the ends of the same toy. Evidently the goal, or to use more
careful language, the end state ("dumbbell apart") was not suggested by the
movement patterns alone when considered from a purely physical perspective. The findings provide evidence that 18-month-olds have a differentiation in the kinds of attributions they make to people versus things.

How might this tendency to treat humans within such a psychological
framework arise in the child? Two accounts can be suggested. The first is
rooted in Fodor's (1987, 1992) conjecture that humans have an innately
specified belief-desire psychology. This was elaborated in Leslie's suggestion that there is a "theory of mind module" (Leslie, 1987, 1988, 1991;
Leslie & Roth, 1993). Armed with the data reported here showing "intention-reading" in 18-month-olds, it could be proposed that there is an innate
tendency for attributing intentions to humans (see also Premack, 1990).
Fodor would certainly be comfortable with intention-reading as part of the
innate belief-desire psychology. It would be interesting if children with
autism, that is, children who have profound deficits in other aspects of understanding the minds of others (Baron-Cohen, 1990; Baron-Cohen et al.,

1985; Harris, 1993; Leslie & Roth, 1993), showed deficits on the kinds of tasks reported here.

I have previously tested newborns' reactions to human faces and discussed innate aspects of social cognition, their initial construal of what a person is, and how persons differ from things (Meltzoff & Moore, 1983, 1992, 1994, 1995). Like Fodor, I am a nativist; but I prefer a special brand of nativism that has been called starting-state nativism versus Fodorian final-state or modularity nativism (Gopnik, 1993; Gopnik & Wellman, 1994; Meltzoff & Gopnik, 1993). Starting-state nativism embraces innate psychological structure, but it also embraces development (Gopnik et al., 1994; Gopnik & Wellman, 1994; Meltzoff, 1990b; Meltzoff & Moore, 1995).

Why suggest development? First, the rudimentary understanding of human goals and intentions does not entail a grasp of more complex mental states such as "belief" (Searle, 1983), and hence not a full-blown belief-desire psychology. Others have reported a developmental progression from understanding desires to understanding beliefs (Astington & Gopnik, 1991b; Gopnik, 1993; Perner, 1991b; Wellman, 1990, 1993). The present results would add that there is some understanding of intention at 18 months, and that like the case of simple desires, this could be accomplished without understanding beliefs per se. Moreover, there are two sides to intentional action, and there may be developmental changes in understanding both. One involves the nature of the goals that are brought about, that is, the causal consequences on the world; the other involves the relation between the mind and actions.

Regarding the former, it seems likely that there are three major developmental changes within infancy in the kinds of acts that can be viewed as intentional—a progression from: (a) simple body acts, to (b) actions on objects, to (c) using one object as tool to act on a second object. At the first level, infants understand only intentions involving simple body movements such as trying to raise one's hand or making particular facial movements. Such simple actions do not refer to anything outside themselves, they are not "about" anything else. Newborns imitate simple body movements (Meltzoff & Moore, 1977, 1983), which shows an innate proclivity for re-enacting the acts of others. It is not yet known whether newborns could succeed on the type of task presented here, which distinguished between the actor's intended acts versus literal behavior—that is, whether newborns would produce the whole target after seeing a failed attempt. However, even if this were the starting state, newborns would probably not understand such tasks if they involved actions on objects, the second level described above. Younger infants attend to people, or attend to things, but not to the person-thing relation. The shift to being able to consider people in relation to things has been labeled secondary intersubjectivity (Trevarthen & Hubley, 1978), triadic interaction (Bakemen & Adamson, 1984), and other terms (Piaget, 1952, 1954). Data relevant to this transition are that at about 9 to 12 months of age infants begin to seek others as sources of information in evaluating novel objects (Campos & Stenberg, 1981; Sorce, Emde, Campos, & Klinert, 1985), perform object-related imitations (Meltzoff, 1988b), and succeed on other tasks (Baldwin & Moses, 1994; Tomasello, Kruger, & Ratner, 1993). Younger infants probably could not understand an adult's attempts to perform an action on an object because this relies on understanding a person-thing relation. Concerning the third level described above, Experiment 1 involved the intention to use a stick to push a button. There is a sharp change in infants' understanding of tools at around 15 to 18 months of age (e.g., Piaget, 1954). Because tool use itself undergoes developmental change in the child, it is likely that the understanding of tool use in others develops. Seeing another's attempt to use a tool may not be construed that way by very young infants, who would be more focused on the body transformations per se (both the arm and finger movements) than on the whole means-ends plan involving the tool. In sum, even if intention were an ontological category available to the newborn, there could still be a developmental progression in the content of this category.

Regarding the other aspect of intentional action—the relation between mind and action—a distinction needs to be drawn between (a) the end states of a purely physical pattern, (b) goals of acts, and (c) intentions as mental states. The present data allow us to infer more than (a), but do not allow us to say with assurance whether infants were using (b) or (c). Let us see what is at stake in these distinctions.

Young infants can "go beyond the stimulus," using past information to project the future. They visually extend the trajectories of moving objects in anticipating re-encounters with them (Bower, 1982; Meltzoff & Moore, 1995; M. K. Moore, Borton, & Darby, 1978; Spelke & Van de Walle, 1993). They anticipate where to look when shown an alternating pattern of flashing lights (Haith, Hazan, & Goodman, 1988). One wonders whether the infants in the experiments reported here were merely projecting the next step of a physical sequence.

The findings indicate more than this, although the argument is a delicate one. The actions in the Demonstration (intention) group did not, strictly speaking, form a progression. The infants were shown three failed attempts, but each failed in a different way (usually equidistant from the desired end) that was not incrementally related to the target act (by experimental design). This is different from anticipating that an object that was seen along a trajectory at a, b, c, will next be at d; or that a light with the alternating pattern of a, b, a, b will next flash at a. Thus, in Experiment 1 the stick missed to the left, then the right, and then too high. Couldn't the next step be a miss that was too low, to complete the pattern? If the movements qua movements specified the next step, why wasn't it suggested when the movements were traced by the mechanical device? The infants in this experiment not only went beyond the surface stimulus, but they also went beyond the stimulus in a particular way that relied on human goals or intentions, not solely physics.

We now need to consider more closely what is meant by *intention*. Searle (1983) differentiated at least two broad types of intentions. He called *prior intentions* those mental states that occur in the mind of the actor in advance of the action being performed that can be described in the form "I will do *x*." One can have a prior intention but not perform any behavior at all (e.g., if the prior intention is not actually fulfilled). These are to be distinguished from *intentions in action*, which are what is involved at the moment of purposely performing a particular bodily movement (vs. when it happens accidently or reflexively). One can have a spur of the moment intention in action, without a prior intention to have it. Every purposeful bodily movement involves an intention in action, but only some intentions in action involve prior intentions. Searle has argued that one needs at least these two varieties of intention to describe adult understanding. Astington (1991) showed that both are entailed in the 5-year-old's understanding.

It seems doubtful that 18-month-olds, let alone newborns, contemplate the prior intentions of others. These mental states are very far upstream, as it were. It is possible, however, that the 18-month-olds in these studies were manifesting an understanding of intentions in action. Infants' understanding of intention in action would allow them to make sense of what would otherwise be rather odd behavior on the part of the adult. It would organize the surface behaviors and allow the infant to see them as "failed attempts" that stemmed from one underlying cause.

However, a thoroughgoing developmental analysis must recognize that even intentions in action are, for the adult, invisible mental states imputed to the mind of the actor. Children in these studies may have imputed such states, or they may have stopped short and simply interpreted the goals of the actions. Infants may think that human acts have goals without yet ascribing underlying mental states in the mind of the actor as the cause of these goals. The results from Experiment 2 demonstrate that physical movements performed by a machine are not ascribed the same meaning as when performed by a person. Therefore, even a weak reading of the data suggests that infants are thinking in terms of goals that are connected to people and not to things. This is tantamount to saying that the infants are construing behavior in terms of a psychological framework including goals of acts, if not the intentions of actors.

The raw fact that 18-month-old children can succeed on the tasks reported here, that they can make sense of a failed attempt, indicates that they have begun to distinguish the surface behavior of people (what they actually do) from another deeper level. This differentiation lies at the core of our commonsense psychology. It underlies fluid communication (Baldwin & Moses, 1994; Bruner, 1983; Grice, 1957; Tomasello & Barton, 1994) as well as our moral judgments. This distinction is also important for understanding even very simple human behaviors. The current experiments suggest that 18-month-olds also understand the actions of others in terms of psychology, not solely physics. In this sense, 18-month-olds have already adopted the basic tenet of folk psychology.

## REFERENCES

Astington, J. W. (1991). Intention in the child's theory of mind. In D. Frye & C. Moore (Eds.), *Children's theories of mind: Mental states and social understanding* (pp. 157–172). Hillsdale, NJ: Erlbaum.

Astington, J. W., & Gopnik, A. (1991a). Developing understanding of desire and intention. In A. Whiten (Ed.), *Natural theories of mind: Evolution, development and simulation of everyday mindreading* (pp. 39–50). Cambridge, MA: Basil Blackwell.

Astington, J. W., & Gopnik, A. (1991b). Theoretical explanations of children's understanding of the mind. *British Journal of Developmental Psychology, 9*, 7–31.

Bakeman, R., & Adamson, L. B. (1984). Coordinating attention to people and objects in mother-infant and peer-infant interaction. *Child Development, 55*, 1278–1289.

Baldwin, D. A., & Moses, L. J. (1994). Early understanding of referential intent and attentional focus: Evidence from language and emotion. In C. Lewis & P. Mitchell (Eds.), *Children's early understanding of mind: Origins and development* (pp. 133–156). Hillsdale, NJ: Erlbaum.

Baron-Cohen, S. (1990). Autism: A specific cognitive disorder of 'mind-blindness'. *International Review of Psychiatry, 2*, 81–90.

Baron-Cohen, S. (1991). Precursors to a theory of mind: Understanding attention in others. In A. Whiten (Ed.), *Natural theories of mind: Evolution, development and simulation of everyday mindreading* (pp. 233–251). Cambridge, MA: Basil Blackwell.

Baron-Cohen, S., Leslie, A. M., & Frith, U. (1985). Does the autistic child have a "theory of mind"? *Cognition, 21*, 37–46.

Baron-Cohen, S., Tager-Flusberg, H., & Cohen, D. J. (1993). *Understanding other minds. Perspectives from autism.* New York: Oxford University Press.

Bartsch, K., & Wellman, H. M. (1989). Young children's attribution of action to beliefs and desires. *Child Development, 60,* 946–964.

Bartsch, K., & Wellman, H. M. (1995). *Children talk about the mind.* New York: Oxford University Press.

Bower, T. G. R. (1982). *Development in infancy* (2nd ed.). San Francisco: W. H. Freeman.

Bretherton, I., McNew, S., & Beeghly-Smith, M. (1981). Early person knowledge as expressed in gestural and verbal communication: When do infants acquire a "Theory of Mind"? In M. E. Lamb & L. R. Sherrod (Eds.), *Infant social cognition: Empirical and theoretical considerations* (pp. 333–373). Hillsdale, NJ: Erlbaum.

Brown, J. R., & Dunn, J. (1991). 'You can cry, mum': The social and developmental implications of talk about internal states. *British Journal of Developmental Psychology, 9,* 237–256.

Bruner, J. S. (1983). *Child's talk: Learning to use language.* New York: W. W. Norton.

Butterworth, G. (1991). The ontogeny and phylogeny of joint visual attention. In A. Whiten (Ed.), *Natural theories of mind: Evolution, development and simulation of everyday mindreading* (pp. 223–232). Cambridge, MA: Basil Blackwell.

Campbell, J. (1994). *Past, space, and self.* Cambridge, MA: MIT Press.

Campbell, J. (1995). The body image and self-consciousness. In J. Bermúdez, A. J. Marcel, & N. Eilan (Eds.), *The body and the self* (pp. 29–42). Cambridge, MA: MIT Press.

Campos, J. J., & Stenberg, C. R. (1981). Perception, appraisal and emotion: The onset of social referencing. In M. E. Lamb & L. R. Sherrod (Eds.), *Infant social cognition* (pp. 273–314). Hillsdale, NJ: Erlbaum.

Dasser, V., Ulbaek, I., & Premack, D. (1989). The perception of intention. *Science, 243,* 365–367.

Flavell, J. H. (1988). The development of children's knowledge about the mind: From cognitive connections to mental representations. In J. W. Astington, P. L. Harris, & D. R. Olson (Eds.), *Developing theories of mind* (pp. 244–267). New York: Cambridge University Press.

Flavell, J. H., Everett, B. A., Croft, K., & Flavell, E. R. (1981). Young children's knowledge about visual perception: Further evidence for the Level 1-Level 2 distinction. *Developmental Psychology, 17,* 99–103.

Flavell, J. H., Flavell, E. R., & Green, F. L. (1983). Development of the appearance-reality distinction. *Cognitive Psychology, 15,* 95–120.

Flavell, J. H., Flavell, E. R., Green, F. L., & Moses, L. J. (1990). Young children's understanding of fact beliefs versus value beliefs. *Child Development, 61,* 915–928.

Flavell, J. H., Green, F. L., & Flavell, E. R. (1986). Development of knowledge about the appearance-reality distinction. *Monographs for the Society for Research in Child Development, 51*, 1–68.

Fodor, J. A. (1987). *Psychosemantics: The problem of meaning in the philosophy of mind*. Cambridge, MA: MIT Press.

Fodor, J. A. (1992). A theory of the child's theory of mind. *Cognition, 44*, 283–296.

Forguson, L., & Gopnik, A. (1988). The ontogeny of common sense. In J. W. Astington, P. L. Harris, & D. R. Olson (Eds.), *Developing theories of mind* (pp. 226–243). New York: Cambridge University Press.

Frye, D. (1991). The origins of intention in infancy. In D. Frye & C. Moore (Eds.), *Children's theories of mind: Mental states and social understanding* (pp. 15–38). Hillsdale, NJ: Erlbaum.

Gelman, S. A., & Wellman, H. M. (1991). Insides and essence: Early understanding of the non-obvious. *Cognition*, 213–244.

Goldman, A. I. (1992). Empathy, mind, and morals. *Proceedings and Addresses of the American Philosophical Association, 66*, 17–41.

Goldman, A. I. (1993). The psychology of folk psychology. *Behavioral and Brain Sciences, 16*, 15–28.

Gopnik, A. (1993). How we know our minds: The illusion of first-person knowledge of intentionality. *Behavioral and Brain Sciences, 16*, 1–14.

Gopnik, A., & Astington, J. W. (1988). Children's understanding of representational change and its relation to the understanding of false belief and appearance-reality distinction. *Child Development, 59*, 26–37.

Gopnik, A., & Slaughter, V. (1991). Young children's understanding of changes in their mental states. *Child Development, 62*, 98–110.

Gopnik, A., Slaughter, V., & Meltzoff, A. N. (1994). Changing your views: How understanding visual perception can lead to a new theory of the mind. In C. Lewis & P. Mitchell (Eds.), *Children's early understanding of mind: Origins and development* (pp. 157–181). Hillsdale, NJ: Erlbaum.

Gopnik, A., & Wellman, H. M. (1992). Why the child's theory of mind really is a theory. *Mind and Language, 7*, 145–171.

Gopnik, A., & Wellman, H. M. (1994). The theory theory. In L. A. Hirschfeld & S. A. Gelman (Eds.), *Mapping the mind: Domain specificity in culture and cognition* (pp. 257–293). New York: Cambridge University Press.

Gordon, R. M. (1994, April). *Sympathy, simulation, and the impartial spectator*. Paper presented at the Mind and Morals Conference, St. Louis, MO.

Grice, H. P. (1957). Meaning. *Philosophical Review, 66*, 377–388.

Haith, M. M., Hazan, C., & Goodman, G. S. (1988). Expectation and anticipation of dynamic visual events by 3.5-month-old-babies. *Child Development, 59*, 467–479.

Harris, P. L. (1989). *Children and emotion: The development of psyhological understanding*. Oxford, England: Basil Blackwell.

Harris, P. L. (1993). Pretending and planning. In S. Baron-Cohen, H. Tager-Flusberg, & D. Cohen (Eds.), *Understanding other minds: Perspectives from autism* (pp. 228–246). Oxford, England: Oxford University Press.

Heider, F. (1958). *The psychology of interpersonal relations*. New York: Wiley.

Leslie, A. M. (1987). Pretense and representation: The origins of "theory of mind." *Psychological Review, 94*, 412–426.

Leslie, A. M. (1988). Some implications of pretense for mechanisms underlying the child's theory of mind. In J. W. Astington, P. L. Harris, & D. R. Olson (Eds.), *Developing theories of mind* (pp. 19–46). New York: Cambridge University Press.

Leslie, A. M. (1991). The theory of mind impairment in autism: Evidence for a modular mechanism of development? In A. Whiten (Ed.), *Natural theories of mind: Evolution, development and simulation of everyday mindreading* (pp. 63–78). Cambridge, MA: Basil Blackwell.

Leslie, A. M., & Roth, D. (1993). What autism teaches us about metarepresentation. In S. Baron-Cohen, H. Tager-Flusberg, & D. J. Cohen (Eds.), *Understanding other minds: Perspectives from autism* (pp. 83–111). New York: Oxford University Press.

Lillard, A. S., & Flavell, J. H. (1990). Young children's preference for mental state versus behavioral descriptions of human action. *Child Development, 61*, 731–741.

Meltzoff, A. N. (1988a). Infant imitation after a 1-week delay: Long-term memory for novel acts and multiple stimuli. *Developmental Psychology, 24*, 470–476.

Meltzoff, A. N. (1988b). Infant imitation and memory: Nine-month-olds in immediate and deferred tests. *Child Development, 59*, 217–225.

Meltzoff, A. N. (1990a). Foundations for developing a concept of self: The role of imitation in relating self to other and the value of social mirroring, social modeling, and self practice in infancy. In D. Cicchetti & M. Beeghly (Eds.), *The self transition: Infancy to childhood* (pp. 139–164). Chicago: University of Chicago Press.

Meltzoff, A. N. (1990b). Towards a developmental cognitive science: The implications of cross-modal matching and imitation for the development of representation and memory in infancy. In A. Diamond (Ed.), *The development and neural bases of higher cognitive functions. Annals of the New York Academy of Sciences. Vol. 608* (pp. 1–31). New York: New York Academy of Sciences.

Meltzoff, A. N. (1993). Molyneux's babies: Cross-modal perception, imitation, and the mind of the preverbal infant. In N. Eilan, R. McCarthy, & B. Brewer (Eds.), *Spatial representation: Problems in the philosophy and psychology* (pp. 219–235). Cambridge, MA: Basil Blackwell.

Meltzoff, A. N. (1995). What infant memory tells us about infantile amnesia: Long-term recall and deferred imitation. *Journal of Experimental Child Psychology, 59*, 497–515.

Meltzoff, A. N., & Gopnik, A. (1993). The role of imitation in understanding persons and developing a theory of mind. In S. Baron-Cohen, H. Tager-Flusberg, & D. Cohen (Eds.), *Understanding other minds: Perspectives from autism* (pp. 335–366). New York: Oxford University Press.

Meltzoff, A. N., & Moore, M. K. (1977). Imitation of facial and manual gestures by human neonates. *Science, 198*, 75–78.

Meltzoff, A. N., & Moore, M. K. (1983). Newborn infants imitate adult facial gestures. *Child Development, 54*, 702–709.

Meltzoff, A. N., & Moore, M. K. (1992). Early imitation within a functional framework: The importance of person identity, movement, and development. *Infant Behavior and Development, 15*, 479–505.

Meltzoff, A. N., & Moore, M. K. (1994). Imitation, memory, and the representation of persons. *Infant Behavior and Development, 17*, 83–99.

Meltzoff, A. N., & Moore, M. K. (1995). Infants' understanding of people and things: From body imitation to folk psychology. In J. Bermúdez, A. J. Marcel, & N. Eilan (Eds.), *The body and the self* (pp. 43–69). Cambridge, MA: MIT Press.

Moore, C., Pure, K., & Furrow, D. (1990). Children's understanding of the modal expression of speaker certainty and uncertainty and its relation to the development of a representational theory of mind. *Child Development, 61*, 722–730.

Moore, M. K., Borton, R., & Darby, B. L. (1978). Visual tracking in young infants: Evidence for object identity or object permanence? *Journal of Experimental Child Psychology, 25*, 183–198.

Moses, L. J. (1993). Young children's understanding of belief constraints on intention. *Cognitive Development, 8*, 1–25.

Moses, L. J., & Flavell, J. H. (1990). Inferring false beliefs from actions and reactions. *Child Development, 61*, 929–945.

O'Neill, D. K., Astington, J. W., & Flavell, J. H. (1992). Young children's understanding of the role that sensory experiences play in knowledge acquisition. *Child Development, 63*, 474–490.

O'Neill, D. K., & Gopnik, A. (1991). Young children's ability to identify the sources of their beliefs. *Developmental Psychology, 27*, 390–397.

Perner, J. (1991a). *Understanding the representational mind.* Cambridge, MA: MIT Press.

Perner, J. (1991b). On representing that: The asymmetry between belief and desire in children's theory of mind. In D. Frye & C. Moore (Eds.), *Children's theories of mind: Mental states and social understanding* (pp. 139–155). Hillsdale, NJ: Erlbaum.

Perner, J., Leekam, S., & Wimmer, H. (1987). Three-year-old's difficulty with false belief: The case for a conceptual deficit. *British Journal of Developmental Psychology, 5*, 125–137.

Piaget, J. (1929). *The child's conception of the world.* New York: Harcourt, Brace.

Piaget, J. (1952). *The origins of intelligence in children.* New York: International Universities Press.

Piaget, J. (1954). *The construction of reality in the child.* New York: Basic Books.

Piaget, J. (1962). *Play, dreams and imitation in childhood.* New York: W. W. Norton.

Premack, D. (1990). The infant's theory of self-propelled objects. *Cognition, 36,* 1–16.

Premack, D., & Dasser, V. (1991). Perceptual origins and conceptual evidence for theory of mind in apes and children. In A. Whiten (Ed.), *Natural theories of mind: Evolution, development and simulation of everyday mindreading* (pp. 253–266). Cambridge, MA: Basil Blackwell.

Premack, D., & Woodruff, G. (1978). Does the chimpanzee have a theory of mind? *Behavioral and Brain Sciences, 4,* 515–526.

Runeson, S., & Frykholm, G. (1981). Visual perception of lifted weight. *Journal of Experimental Psychology: Human Perception and Performance, 7,* 733–740.

Searle, J. R. (1983). *Intentionality: An essay in the philosophy of mind.* New York: Cambridge University Press.

Shatz, M., Wellman, H. M., & Silber, S. (1983). The acquisition of mental verbs: A systematic investigation of first references to mental state. *Cognition, 14,* 301–321.

Shultz, T. R. (1980). Development of the concept of intention. In W. A. Collins (Ed.), *The Minnesota Symposium on Child Psychology* (Vol. 13, pp. 131–164). Hillsdale, NJ: Erlbaum.

Shultz, T. R., Wells, D., & Sarda, M. (1980). Development of the ability to distinguish intended actions from mistakes, reflexes, and passive movements. *British Journal of Social and Clinical Psychology, 19,* 301–310.

Siegel, S. (1956). *Nonparametric statistics for the behavioral sciences.* New York: McGraw-Hill.

Sorce, J. F., Emde, R. N., Campos, J. J., & Klinert, M. D. (1985). Maternal emotional signaling; Its effect on the visual cliff behavior of 1-year-olds. *Developmental Psychology, 21,* 195–200.

Spelke, E. S., & Van de Walle, G. A. (1993). Perceiving and reasoning about objects: Insights from infants. In N. Eilan, R. McCarthy, & B. Brewer (Eds.), *Spatial representation: Problems in philosophy and psychology* (pp. 132–161). Cambridge, MA: Basil Blackwell.

Tomasello, M., & Barton, M. (1994). Learning words in nonostensive contexts. *Developmental Psychology, 30,* 639–650.

Tomasello, M., Kruger, A. C., & Ratner, H. H. (1993). Cultural learning. *Behavioral and Brain Sciences, 16,* 495–552.

Trevarthen, C., & Hubley, P. (1978). Secondary intersubjectivity: Confidence, confiding and acts of meaning in the first year. In A. Lock (Ed.), *Action, gesture, and symbol: The emergence of language* (pp. 183–229). New York: Academic Press.

Wellman, H. M. (1990). *The child's theory of mind.* Cambridge, MA: MIT Press.

Wellman, H. M. (1993). Early understanding of mind: The normal case. In S. Baron-Cohen, H. Tager-Flusberg, & D. J. Cohen (Eds.), *Understanding other minds: Perspectives from autism* (pp. 10–39). New York: Oxford University Press.

Wellman, H. M., & Banerjee, M. (1991). Mind and emotion: Children's understanding of the emotional consequences of beliefs and desires. *British Journal of Developmental Psychology, 9,* 191–214.

Wellman, H. M., & Bartsch, K. (1994). Before belief: Children's early psychological theory. In C. Lewis & P. Mitchell (Eds.), *Children's early understanding of mind: Origins and development* (pp. 157–181). Hillsdale, NJ: Erlbaum.

Wellman, H. M., & Estes, D. (1986). Early understanding of mental entities: A reexamination of childhood realism. *Child Development, 57,* 910–923.

Wellman, H. M., & Gelman, S. A. (1988). Children's understanding of the non-obvious. In R. J. Sternberg (Ed.), *Advances in the psychology of intelligence* (pp. 99–135). Hillsdale, NJ: Erlbaum.

Wellman, H. M., & Woolley, J. D. (1990). From simple desires to ordinary beliefs: The early development of everyday psychology. *Cognition, 35,* 245–275.

Wimmer, H., & Hartl, M. (1991). Against the Cartesian view on mind: Young children's difficulty with own false beliefs. *British Journal of Developmental Psychology, 9,* 125–138.

Wimmer, H., & Perner, J. (1983). Beliefs about beliefs: Representation and constraining function of wrong beliefs in young children's understanding of deception. *Cognition, 13,* 103–128.

Yuill, N. (1984). Young children's coordination of motive and outcome in judgments of satisfaction and morality. *British Journal of Developmental Psychology, 2,* 73–81.

# 4

# Frontal Activation Asymmetry and Social Competence at Four Years of Age

**Nathan A. Fox, Susan D. Calkins, and Stephen W. Porges**
*University of Maryland, College Park*

**Kenneth H. Rubin, Robert J. Coplan, and Shannon Stewart**
*University of Waterloo, Ontario*

**Timothy R. Marshall**
*Christopher Newport University, Newport News*

**James M. Long**
*James Long Company*

*The pattern of frontal activation as measured by the ongoing electroencephalogram (EEG) may be a marker for individual differences in infant and adult disposition to respond with either positive or negative affect. We studied 48 4-year-old children who were first observed in same-sex quartets during free-play sessions, while making speeches, and during a ticket-sorting task. Social and interactive behaviors were coded from these sessions. Each child was subsequently seen 2 weeks later when EEG was recorded while the child attended to a visual stimulus. The pattern of EEG activation computed from the session was significantly related to the child's behavior in the quartet session. Children who displayed social competence (high degree of social initiations and positive affect) exhibited greater relative left frontal activation, while children who displayed social with-*

Reprinted with permission from Child Development, 1995, Vol. 66, 1770–1784. Copyright © 1995 by the Society for Research in Child Development, Inc.

The research described in this article was supported by a grant from the National Institutes of Health to Nathan A. Fox (HD 17899) and by two grants from the John D. & Catherine T. MacArthur Foundation to NAF and KHR.

*drawal (isolated, onlooking, and unoccupied behavior) during the play session exhibited greater relative right frontal activation. Differences among children in frontal asymmetry were a function of power in the left frontal region. These EEG/behavior findings suggest that resting frontal asymmetry may be a marker for certain temperamental dispositions.*

Data from several sources suggest that the pattern of electroencephalographic (EEG) activation recorded over the frontal region in humans may be a marker for certain temperamental dispositions. Specifically, individuals exhibiting resting right frontal asymmetry are more likely to exhibit signs of negative affect in response to mild stress, while individuals exhibiting resting left frontal asymmetry are likely to exhibit positive affect in response to similar novel elicitors. There are both developmental and adult data that support this position (Calkins, Fox, & Marshall, in press; Davidson & Fox, 1989; Fox, Bell, & Jones, 1992).

In a series of studies with infants, Fox and colleagues (Davidson & Fox, 1989; Fox et al., 1992) found that infants exhibiting right frontal EEG asymmetry were more likely to cry to maternal separation. In addition, infants who were likely to cry consistently to maternal separation across the second half of the first year of life displayed a stable pattern of right frontal asymmetry. Calkins et al. (in press) have also reported that infants selected at 4 months of age for a high frequency of motor arousal and negative affect were more likely to display right frontal asymmetry at 9 months of age compared to infants selected for displaying positive affect. In addition, infants preselected for displaying high motor/high negative affect who exhibited right frontal asymmetry at 9 months were more likely to display signs of fear and wariness at 14 months. Calkins et al. (in press) argue that right frontal asymmetry may be an important moderator variable reflecting an infant's disposition to respond with negative affect in response to novelty.

A number of independent laboratories have confirmed the relation between frontal asymmetry and emotional disposition. Dawson et al. (Dawson, Grofer-Klinger, Panagiotides, Spieker, & Frey, 1992) reported that 10-month-old infants exhibiting right frontal asymmetry were more likely to display signs of negative affect and distress to separation than those exhibiting left frontal asymmetry. In addition, Dawson et al. (1992) reported that infants of depressed mothers evidenced this particular right frontal pattern during a face-to-face interaction with their mothers.

The asymmetry in EEG power that is reflected in the laterality index is a function of the dynamic changes in activity of both the left and right hemispheres. Traditionally, asymmetry has been indexed as the ratio of power in one hemisphere to another (R − L/R + L). The underlying assumption is that less power in one hemisphere compared to the other reflects greater relative activation in that hemisphere (Lindsley & Wicke, 1974). Thus, with the asymmetry metric, positive numbers reflect greater relative left hemisphere activation, while negative numbers reflect greater relative right hemisphere activation (Davidson, 1988). Obviously, there are a number of ways that individuals could differ in arriving at a right hemisphere asymmetry score (negative number). One individual could have more power in the left than power in the right hemisphere (an example of left hypoactivation), while one individual could have a right hemisphere asymmetry score as a result of less power in the right hemisphere (an example of right activation).

The process by which dynamic change occurs and hence whether the asymmetry index is a function of more power in one hemisphere or less power in the opposite hemisphere is of critical concern (Fox, 1994). A number of researchers have noted differences in the manner in which affective behavior is modulated as a function of either hyperactivation of one hemisphere or disinhibition of the contralateral side. One would expect behavioral differences as a function of these two different patterns of relative activation (Fox, 1994). For example, two groups of subjects may display a right frontal asymmetry score. One group's score may be the product of left frontal hypoactivation (more power in the left hemisphere), and these subjects may be expected to exhibit lack of positive affect and lack of approach (and possibly signs of depression; see Henriques & Davidson, 1991), while the scores of the second group of subjects may be the product of right frontal activation (less power in the right), and they may be expected to exhibit increased signs of negative affect and anxiety (see Calkins et al., in press; Finman, Davidson, Colton, Straus, & Kagan, 1989; Fox et al., 1992). One goal of the current study was to examine in detail differences in the dynamic nature of EEG asymmetry in relation to overt social behavior.

The notion that frontal activation may reflect an individual's disposition to respond with either positive or negative affect is derived in part from work on the relations among frontal lobe activity and the expression of emotions (see Davidson, 1983; Fox & Davidson, 1984). There is a diverse literature from cases of adults with unilateral brain damage or in response to unilateral administration of sodium amytal (WADA test) which suggests that the two hemispheres are differentially specialized for the production of different emotions. These studies have been reviewed in detail in numerous sources (Sackeim et al., 1982; Silberman & Weingartner, 1986).

In a series of papers, Fox and colleagues have demonstrated an association between left and right frontal asymmetry and emotion expression in infants (Fox & Davidson, 1986, 1987, 1988). In general, these studies indicate that infants exhibit greater right frontal asymmetry during the expression of negative emotions and greater left frontal asymmetry during the expression of positive emotions. Studies with human adults find parallel associations between facial expression of emotions and EEG asymmetry in the frontal region (Davidson, Ekman, Saron, Senulis, & Friesen, 1990).

Although the above referenced studies suggest that the two hemispheres may be differentially specialized for the production of behaviors associated with either positive or negative emotion, they do not address individual differences in the display of positive or negative affect. The conception that individual differences in the degree of frontal activation may be associated with disposition to emotional reactivity was first proposed by Davidson and Fox (1988) and is in part derived from work previously completed by Levy and colleagues (Levy, Heller, Banich, & Burton, 1983). Levy et al. (1983) were interested in understanding the variance among right-handed individuals in performance on either left or right hemisphere (verbal/ spatial) tasks. They developed a set of chimeric face tests designed to measure the degree to which individuals exhibit resting left or right hemisphere arousal. Levy et al. (1983) hypothesized an interaction between hemisphere arousal and hemispheric specialization in the performance of verbal and spatial tasks performance. They found that subjects exhibiting right hemisphere arousal when performing a right hemisphere task were better than subjects exhibiting left hemisphere arousal. Davidson and Fox (1988) argued that a similar relation might exist for affective behavior. Specifically, individuals exhibiting tonic right frontal activation may be more likely to exhibit negative affect, while individuals exhibiting tonic left frontal activation would be more likely to exhibit positive affect.

There is reason to believe that resting frontal asymmetry may be a stable within-individual characteristic that is associated with an individual's tendency to express negative affect. For example, Tomarken, Davidson, and Henriques (1990) found that subjects with resting right frontal asymmetry were more likely to rate video film clips in a negative manner, while subjects with tonic left frontal asymmetry were more likely to rate these same clips in a positive manner. Jones and Fox (1992) report a similar relation between right frontal EEG asymmetry and negative rating bias for adults selected for high positive or negative affectivity. Davidson and colleagues have also found that undergraduates who score consistently high on the Beck Depression Inventory were more likely to exhibit resting right frontal asymmetry (Schaffer, Davidson, & Saron, 1983). In a follow-up to this study, Henriques and Davidson (1990) found that adults with clinical depression exhibited greater right frontal asymmetry, and adults who had been depressed and were now in remission also exhibited this right frontal pattern. Also, Davidson and colleagues reported that children selected for characteristics of behavioral inhibition were more likely to exhibit right frontal asymmetry compared to children who were selected for extroverted behavior (Finman et al., 1989).

There is an interesting parallel between the research on social withdrawal and peer competence and the work on behavioral inhibition. Kagan and colleagues (Kagan & Snidman, 1991) have argued that wariness in the face of novel stimuli (behavioral inhibition) during the infant and toddler period is a stable characteristic that becomes associated with social wariness and solitude in the mid-years of childhood. Rubin and Lollis (1988) have suggested that among the developmental paths that might lead to social withdrawal is one in which an infant of irritable temperament who is involved in an insecure attachment relationship may evidence inhibited fearful behavior as a toddler. This fearful, anxious behavior may later be transformed to the peer setting and may be a factor in the child's inability to behave competently in social interactions.

If social withdrawal and inhibited behavior involve, in part, a disposition toward fearfulness and anxiety, it may be that children who evidence inhibited behavior in social settings also display a pattern of frontal brain electrical activity reflecting this disposition. That is, it is possible that frontal asymmetry is a marker for inhibited behavior among preschool children. The following study was designed to investigate this possibility. Forty-eight children who were part of an ongoing longitudinal study were seen at age 4 years in same-sex quartet play groups. The children's social behavior and interactive styles were observed and coded. Two weeks later, each child individually returned to the laboratory, at which time EEG was recorded while the child was presented with a computer generated stimulus. Relations among child social behaviors from the quartet session and measures of frontal asymmetry were investigated. It was predicted that children evidencing social withdrawal and inhibited behavior during the quartet session would exhibit right frontal EEG asymmetry. Similarly, it was predicted that children evidencing social competence and positive social interactive skills would exhibit left frontal EEG asymmetry. Confirmation of these predictions would suggest that frontal asymmetry may be a marker variable for affective disposition in children of preschool age.

## METHOD

### Subjects

The participants in this study were 48 preschool children (20 male, 28 female) between the ages of 49 and 62 months (mean age = 54.63 months, SD = 3.91 months). The children were primarily of middle-class background, living with their families in or near College Park, Maryland. Four of the children were African-American; the remaining 44 were Caucasian. The children were part of a larger unselected sample of 61 children who were participating in a longitudinal study (see Fox, 1989; Stifter & Fox, 1990, for details).

### Procedure

At 24 months, infants came to the lab and were exposed to a series of conditions designed to elicit a range of positive and negative affects. These conditions included presentation of an unfamiliar adult, a novel toy, and a clown, and maternal separation. Infant behaviors, including latency to approach the stranger, robot, and clown, and duration proximity to mother during the stranger, robot, and clown episodes were coded, and a standardized index of behavioral inhibition was computed from these variables.

The quartets were formed on the basis of their score on the standardized index of inhibition at 24 months. Quartets were same sex. An attempt was made to compose each same-sex quartet with one child who at 24 months was found to be inhibited, one child who at 24 months was found to be uninhibited, and two children who at 24 months were around the mean on the inhibition index. In addition, the child's age was taken into account, and an attempt was made to have children in any one quartet who were within 6 months of each other in age. Seventy-five percent of the quartets (9 of 12 quartets) met the above criteria. The remaining three quartets consisted of children whose 24-month standardized inhibition scores were more toward the mean.

The four children and their mothers came to the laboratory. Children and mothers waited in an area of the lab until all four children had arrived and all parents had been briefed and consent granted. The four children were then led into a playroom that had in it a set of attractive toys. The children were told that they were to play in this room for a while and that afterward they would participate in a set of games. The children in each quartet had never met each other. Their main point in common was that all had been born at the same local hospital and all were participants in the larger longitudinal study.

Children were given name tags, which were pinned onto their backs so that their names would be visible to the video camera. The sessions were video- and audiotaped for future coding and analysis.

The quartet session consisted of four parts. Part I was free play and lasted for 15 min. During this period of time the four children were in the room by themselves. Parents were in a waiting area and were asked, during this time, to fill out a series of questionnaires. Part II was a cleanup session that lasted up to 5 min. An experimenter entered the room and told the children that the free-play session had ended and that they were going to play a series of games. The experimenter asked the children to clean up the toys, placing them in a large cardboard box that had been placed in the center of the playroom.

Part III of the session consisted of speeches. The experimenter asked the four children to sit in a semicircle facing her (the children were facing the one-way mirror and their faces could be easily videotaped). The experimenter then told the children that they were going to play a brief game of show-and-tell during which each child would stand up and tell the rest something about their recent birthday party. The experimenter then asked for volunteers and allowed each child to stand and talk for up to 2 min. Following the speeches, the experimenter brought out to the center of the room a small table and four chairs and asked the children to sit around the table. A basket with colored cards was on the table and the experimenter asked the children to take one card of each color and make up five sets of cards (Part IV). Following this, the final 15-min free-play session began. The experimenter reentered the room, brought the box with toys, and allowed the children to play in the room by themselves for an additional 15 min.

During this visit to the laboratory, arrangements were made with each mother for an individual follow-up visit. These visits were usually within 2 weeks of the quartet session. Mothers were told that at the follow-up visit there would be a psychophysiological assessment and additional testing.

### Behavioral Coding

The videotapes of the quartet sessions were sent to the second author (KHR) for coding. Coders were blind to the assignment of the individual children and to the hypotheses of the study.

**Free-play sessions.** Behaviors in the first and second play sessions were coded with Rubin's (1989) Play Observation Scale. Ten-second intervals were coded for social participation (unoccupied, onlooking, solitary play, parallel play, conversation, group play) and the cognitive quality of play (functional, dramatic, and constructive play; exploration; games with rules). This resulted in approximately 90 coding intervals per child in each of the two free-play sessions.

Additional variables coded during the free-play sessions included (1) the proportion of observational intervals that included the display of anxious behaviors (e.g., auto-manipulatives, digit sucking, crying); (2) the latency to the child's first spontaneous utterance (first play session only); (3) the frequency of child-initiated social interactions; and (4) the frequency of social initiations from peers.

**Cleanup and ticket-sorting sessions.** During the cleanup and ticket-sorting sessions, the proportion of time each child spent *off task-unoccupied* was recorded. Behaviors were considered off-task during the cleanup if they did not involve such actions as picking up toys, or placing toys in the toy box. Off-task behaviors during the ticket-sorting session included not sorting tickets or not talking about the task at hand. Unoccupied behavior was defined similarly to the behavioral variable of the same name used during the free-play sessions. Time spent off-task but engaged in any other type of alternative activity (e.g., goofing off, continuing to play with toys, disrupting others who were trying to clean up/sort tickets) was coded as *off-task-goofing off*.

**Speeches.** The speeches were coded for (*a*) the duration of the entire speech episode, and (*b*) the percentage of time each child actually spent speaking. The duration of the episode was defined as the amount of time that each child "held the floor," from the moment he or she was asked to speak, until the researcher asked the next child to speak. The percentage of time spent talking was calculated by dividing the amount of "real time" during which each child verbally described their birthday party by the duration of their speech episode.

**Reliability.** The Play Observation Scale (Rubin, 1989) and additional observational variables were coded by four independent observers. Interrater reliability on a randomly selected group of children totaling 30% of the sample (four quartets; 16 children) was calculated between pairs of observers using Cohen's kappa. For a full variable matrix, including social and cognitive play categories, and additional observational variables, computed kappas between pairs of raters ranged between $\kappa = 0.71$ and $\kappa = 0.86$. Intercoder disagreements were resolved by review and discussion.

## Aggregate Variables

Two theoretically driven and empirically substantiated aggregate variables were computed from the variables assessed during the free-play, cleanup, ticket-sorting, and speech episodes (see also Coplan, Rubin, Fox, Calkins, & Stewart, 1994).

**Social reticence-inhibition.** The first aggregate variable was thought to represent social reticence and inhibition and was computed as the sum of the following standardized variables: (1) proportion of anxious behaviors during free play; (2) latency to first spontaneous utterance during free play; (3) proportion of reticent behavior (unoccupied and onlooking behavior) during free play; (4) proportion of unoccupied behavior during cleanup; (5) proportion of unoccupied behavior during ticket sorting; (6) the inverse of the duration of the speech episode; and (7) the inverse of total time talking during the speech episode. Intercorrelations among these indices ranged from $-.16$ to $-.47$ and from $.24$ to $.49$. All but one of the intercorrelations were statistically significant ($p < .05$).

**Sociability-social competence.** The second aggregate variable was thought to represent sociability and social competence and was computed as the sum of the following standardized free-play variables: (1) the frequency of child-initiated social interactions; (2) the frequency of initiations received from peers; and (3) the proportion of time engaged in sociodramatic play (a marker of social competence in preschoolers; Howes, 1987; Rubin, Fein, & Vandenberg, 1983). Intercorrelations among these indices ranged from $.38$ to $.60$. All of these intercorrelations were statistically significant ($p < .01$).

## Maternal Ratings

Mothers completed the Colorado Temperament Inventory (Buss & Plomin, 1984; Rowe & Plomin, 1977). This measure is composed of factors that assess maternal perceptions of various child characteristics (e.g., emotionality, activity level, shyness, soothability, sociability). Of specific interest to us were the factors assessing shyness and emotionality.

## Psychophysiological Assessment

When the child and mother returned to the lab, the child was shown the testing room, which had been decorated and designed to resemble a space shuttle. There were pictures of planets on the wall and ceiling, and a chair had been decorated as the command chair for the spaceship. In addition, a computer had been placed in the room and cardboard around the computer was set and painted to illustrate the controls of a space ship. A lycra stretch cap was placed on the child's head for EEG recording. The cap contained the electrodes for EEG recording placed in an arrangement in accordance with the 10–20 system (Jasper, 1958). A small amount of omni-prep abrasive was put into each site and the scalp gently abraded with the blunt end of a Q-tip. A small amount of electrolyte was then placed in the site and impedances were checked. Impedances were accepted if they were 5 K ohms or below.

The EEG was recorded from six sites (F3, F4, P3, P4, O1, O2, referenced to vertex, Cz). In addition, separate channels for A1 and A2 each referenced to Cz were recorded. Finally, Beckman mini-electrodes were placed on the outer canthus and supra orbit of one eye in order to record EOG. All nine channels were amplified by individual 7p511 Grass AC amplifiers with the high pass setting at 1 Hz and the low pass at 100 Hz. The data from all nine channels were digitized at 512 Hz on an IBM AT using HEM acquisition software. The digitized data were stored for later artifact editing and analysis.

After the cap was in place and impedances were checked, a computer program was started. The program consisted of a colorful building taurus and a star. The taurus and star were separate segments and each lasted for 15 to 30 sec. Each child was presented with a minimum of six taurus and star segments with the goal of collecting at least 3 min of EEG data during each condition. The child was instructed to hold still and attend to the screen when the star came on. The child was told that if he or she could attend to the star they would win a prize at the end of the session. EEG was recorded continuously during the computer session, and a separate channel indicated the onset and offset of the star section. A camera placed unobtrusively recorded the child's behavior, including visual attention to the computer monitor, during the EEG recording.

After the recording session, which lasted 10 min, the cap was removed, any excess gel was removed from the child's hair, and the child was taken to a second room for additional assessments.

The digitized EEG was transformed via software to an average reference configuration. The average reference configuration was used, as this is the preferred configuration when coherence is computed between different electrode sites (Fein, Raz, Brown, & Merrin, 1988; Lehmann, Ozaki, & Pal, 1986). The data were then scored manually for eye movement and gross motor movement artifact using software designed by James Long, Inc. The software allowed the display of all channels graphically on the computer screen. Using a cursor, the operator could underline those sections of the EEG that were contaminated by motor movement or that contained eye movements as indicated by activity in the EOG. Two coders, previously trained and tested to reliability, artifact scored the EEG data. One coder was responsible for scoring all subjects, while a second coder overlapped on 12 subjects. Cohen's kappa was computed to examine reliabilities among the coders. Kappa values ranged from 0.60 to 0.80. The artifact scored EEG was then analyzed using the same software system with a discrete fourier transform, with a hanning window of 1 sec in length and 50% overlap. Power in single Hz bins from 1 through 20 Hz was computed for each segment of the taurus and star.

**Quantification of laterality indices.** Most previous research on laterality has utilized laterality scores based on activity within each hemisphere without acknowledging the possibility of correlated activity reflecting interhemispheric communication (Wheeler, Davidson, & Tomarken, 1993). Alternatively, laterality scores could incorporate a measure of statistical dependence reflecting interhemispheric communication. One method commonly available to evaluate interhemispheric communication is to use cross-spectral analysis to generate a coherence spectrum. The coherence statistic indicates the degree that the activity (i.e., power densities) at a specific frequency or frequency band within each hemisphere is shared with the other. Coherence is independent of the amplitude of the signal (i.e., variance or power density), but is dependent upon phase. If the phase between two signals at a common frequency (or frequency band) is constant, the coherence will approach 1.0. In contrast, if the phase between two signals at a common frequency (or frequency band) is a white noise process, the coherence will approach 0. Coherence reflects the percent of shared variance between two signals at a specific frequency (or frequency band). Thus, knowledge of the coherence would enable the determination of the activity within each hemisphere that is shared with, or unique to, the activity in the other hemisphere.

There are several problems with generating a summary measure of shared and unique hemispheric EEG variance. First, coherences may not be constant across all the frequencies within the frequency band of interest (in our case, 6–8 Hz). To solve this problem, we applied the Porges method (Bohrer & Porges, 1982; Porges & Bohrer, 1990; Porges et al., 1980) to calculate a weighted coherence. The weighted coherence is determined by arithmetically weighting the coherence at each frequency within the 6–8 Hz band by its power. This method produces a ratio indicating the percent of shared variance between the two signals. Second, coherences may not be constant across time. To deal with this problem, we generalized the weighted coherence method to accumulate values across all 1-sec windows.

Although the Porges method was developed to describe the shared rhythmicity of two systems across a band of frequencies with the weighted coherence statistic, it also provides information on shared variance. Statistically, the weighted coherence is derived by the ratio of shared variance to total variance. Thus, the weighted coherence methodology provides us with a way to quantify shared variance and to use the shared variances in evaluating laterality.

As evident in Formula 1 (see the Appendix), the weighted coherence is equivalent to the sum of the products of coherence × power at each frequency within the alpha band divided by the total power within the same frequency band. The numerator of this formula provides a measure of shared power and is presented in Formula 2 (Appendix). The difference between the numerator and denominator provides a measure of unique power and is provided in Formula 3 (Appendix). These formulas were used to calculate shared and unique variances within each 1-sec window and were accumulated (i.e., added) across all available 1-sec windows to provide a measure the total shared and unique variances for each hemisphere.

Since the weighted coherence is equivalent to the percent of shared variance, multiplication of the weighted coherence by the sum of the power within the frequency band will quantify the variance shared between the two systems. Moreover, when this quantity is subtracted from the sum of the power, a measure of unshared or unique variance associated with one hemisphere is quantified. Thus, the weighted coherence methodology provides us with a method to partition power in the 6–8 Hz frequency band within each 1-sec window into shared and unique variances. To generate an estimate for shared and unique power across time, we accumulated the shared power and total power for each 1-sec window across available 1-sec windows. By subtracting the shared variance from the total power, we obtained a measure of unique variance. These procedures were calculated for each hemisphere to provide a left and right measure of shared and unique variance. The new measures of asymmetry were calculated by subtracting the natural logarithms of these variances.

In sum, the EEG analyses were computed on the standard metric of power for each electrode site, as well as on shared and unshared EEG power for each site. Laterality difference scores (Ln R − Ln L) were computed using both the traditional estimate of power and the shared and unshared power estimates.

## RESULTS

The data to be presented in this article deal specifically with relations between measures of EEG asymmetry and power and behaviors observed in the quartet session as well as relations with maternal report. The analyses that were performed were completed on the EEG data that were recorded during the "still star" conditions. There were two reasons for choosing the "still star" EEG data for subsequent analyses. First, inspection of the visual attention data revealed that subjects paid significantly more attention to the monitor during the star versus during the taurus segment. This is not surprising given that subjects were instructed that they may move around during the taurus segment but were to be still and pay attention during the star segment. Second, there were significantly more EEG data available from the star versus the taurus segment. Because subjects were allowed to move more during the taurus segment, there was more movement artifact that was edited out of the records. The greater amount of data provided a more stable estimate of individual EEG patterns. Third, preliminary analyses were completed examining relations between EEG recorded during the "taurus" phase and child social behavior. No significant relations were found. We believe this is due to the lack of subject engagement during these segments and the small amount of EEG data available for analyses. Therefore, subsequent analyses were computed on the EEG data from the "star" period.

### *EEG Asymmetry and Social Behavior*

As a first step, Pearson product correlations were computed between the two summary behavioral measures, the two CCTI factors, and the three EEG laterality measures (the traditional laterality score based on power derived from the spectral analysis, the laterality score based on shared power, and the laterality score based on unshared or unique power). As can be seen from Table 1, there were significant relations between the frontal asymmetry scores and the two behavioral summary measures as well as for one of the temperament factors. Inhibited behavior was associated with greater relative right frontal activation; the greater the inhibition score, the more negative the asymmetry score. As noted earlier, negative values on the asymmetry index reflect greater relative right activation. Social competence was associated with greater relative left frontal activation; the higher the score on social competence, the more positive the asymmetry index—positive values reflect greater relative left frontal activation. Finally, there was a trend for maternal rating of social fear/shyness to be associated with the asymmetry index. Children whose mothers rated them high on social

TABLE 1

Correlation Between Frontal Asymmetry Scores and 4-Year Behavior
and Maternal Report of Temperament

| | Traditional Frontal Asymmetry Score Ln (R) − Ln (L) | Unshared Power Asymmetry Score | Shared Power Asymmetry Score |
|---|---|---|---|
| Social competence (sociability) ....... | .47*** | .59*** | .15 |
| Inhibition (social reticence) ............ | −.16 | −.35** | −.23 |
| Social fear (CCTI Scale) .................. | −.19 | −.24* | .01 |
| Emotionality (CCTI Scale) .............. | −.13 | −.03 | −.16 |

NOTE.—$N$ = 42.
* $p$ = .06.
** $p$ = .01.
*** $p$ = .001.

fear had more negative asymmetry scores. This relation for social fear was the only significant finding among the correlations between the temperament factors and the asymmetry scores. The asymmetry scores based upon unshared or unique power were better at predicting social behavior than the traditional asymmetry measures of EEG power. None of the asymmetry measures from either the parietal or occipital regions were significantly related to any of the behavioral or maternal report measures.

Although the asymmetry index reflects relative differences in activation between the left and right hemispheres, it does not indicate the locus of within-subject differences in power. In order to examine this issue, a second set of Pearson correlations was computed between the absolute power values for each frontal lead, shared and unshared power values for the frontal leads, and the two summary behavior scores as well as the two maternal report factors. As can be seen in Table 2, there were significant associations between left frontal unshared power and the social competence and inhibition aggregate scores. Social competence was associated with less left frontal power, while inhibition was associated with more left

TABLE 2

Correlation Between Left and Right Frontal Power Values (6–8 Hz)
and 4-Year Behavior and Maternal Report of Temperament

| | Power in Left Frontal | Power in Right Frontal | Unshared Power in F3 | Unshared Power in F4 |
|---|---|---|---|---|
| Social competence (sociability) ....... | −.15 | −.13 | −.27* | −.12 |
| Inhibition (social reticence) ............ | .15 | .07 | .32** | .17 |
| Social fear (CCTI Scale) .................. | .03 | −.02 | .32** | .15 |
| Emotionality (CCTI Scale) .............. | .04 | .10 | .12 | .16 |

NOTE.—$N$ = 42.
* $p$ = .05.
** $p$ = .01.

frontal power. There were no significant associations between any of be-havioral or maternal report variables and measures of right frontal power.

As a second step to investigate the locus of effects of power, we divided children based on their standardized ($z$ transform) score of social compe-tence and inhibition. Three groups were made from each aggregate score: high ($z$ scores .5 or greater), middle ($z$ scores greater than $-.5$ and less than .5), and low ($z$ scores below $-.5$). Separate multivariate analyses of vari-ance for each score were computed with group (three levels: high/middle/low), region (three levels: frontal/parietal/occipital), and hemisphere (two levels: left/right). The dependent measures were standard EEG power in each lead, shared power, and unshared power. Across all three analyses, the only significant factor to emerge was that of region: multivariate Wilks for standard power = .255, approximate $F(2, 38) = 57.37, p = .000$; mul-tivariate Wilks for shared power = .122, approximate $F(2, 38) = 136.66$, $p = .000$; multivariate Wilks for unshared power = .609, approximate $F(2, 38) = 12.16, p = 000$.

In order to understand the effects as a function of region, we repeated the analyses on each of the behavior groups (the high, mid, and low socia-bility children and the high, mid, and low social reticence children) sepa-rately for each region (frontal, parietal, occipital). This was a group (three levels) × hemisphere (left/right) ANOVA for each of the three dependent measures (traditional power, shared power, and unshared power).

**Sociability-social competence.** There were no significant main or inter-action effects for those analyses using either traditional power or shared power as the dependent variable for any region.

For the analysis using unshared power, the two-way ANOVA for the frontal region revealed a significant two-way interaction (group × hemi-sphere), $F(2, 39) = 4.06, p = .03$. Post-hoc Newman Keuls tests compar-ing the level of unshared power in each lead between the three groups re-vealed that children exhibiting high social competence exhibited less left frontal unshared power compared to children in the low social competence group ($p < .05$) (see Figure 1). There were no significant main or interac-tion effects for the parietal or occipital data.

**Social reticence-inhibition.** There were no significant main or interaction effects for the analyses using the traditional measure of EEG power or the measure of shared power.

For the analyses using unshared power, the two-way ANOVA for the frontal region revealed a significant two-way interaction for group × hemi-sphere, $F(2, 39) = 4.19, p = .02$. Post-hoc Newman-Keuls tests revealed

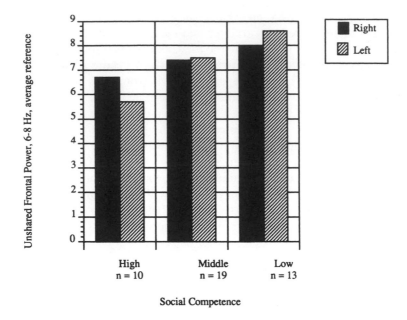

**Figure 1.** Unshared frontal power scores of children exhibiting high, medium, and low social competence at 4 years of age.

that the group of children exhibiting high social reticence displayed more left unshared power compared to the group of children exhibiting low social reticence ($p < .05$) (see Figure 2). There were no significant main or interaction effects for the parietal or occipital data.

## DISCUSSION

The data from the current study suggest that individual differences in frontal asymmetry exhibited by children may reflect, in part, their pattern of affective responsivity and consequent social competence. Children exhibiting right frontal asymmetry were less socially competent and exhibited more inhibited behaviors during a peer interaction session. Children exhibiting left frontal asymmetry were more sociable and displayed more socially competent behaviors.

Individual differences among children in EEG asymmetry were localized to the frontal region. There were no group differences among children for either the parietal or occipital scalp regions. In addition, there were no

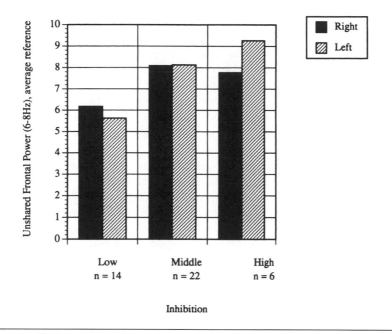

**Figure 2.** Unshared frontal power scores of children exhibiting high, medium, and low inhibition-social reticence at 4 years of age.

significant associations between parietal or occipital asymmetry scores and child behavior. This pattern of findings is similar to those of Fox et al. (1992), Davidson (Henriques & Davidson, 1991), and Dawson (Dawson et al., 1992), who have consistently found the locus of asymmetry/affect effects to be localized to the frontal scalp leads. The pattern across studies reinforces the argument that the differences among children are not a function of generalized hemispheric arousal but rather are specific to functions of the frontal region.

A number of researchers (Wheeler et al., 1993) have speculated that the pattern of asymmetry in the frontal region reflects important individual differences in affective responsivity. Davidson (Davidson, 1992), for example, has argued that the pattern of resting anterior activation (he has labeled it RAA) reflects the threshold with which individuals are likely to respond with either positive or negative affect to novelty or mild stress. He argues that these differences represent a stress diathesis. Individuals with resting greater relative right anterior activation are more likely under certain circumstances to respond with negative affect. Davidson and colleagues have found that depressed subjects or subjects in remission who had been clinically depressed were more likely to exhibit right frontal activation (Henriques & Davidson, 1991). Interestingly, they found that depression was specifically associated with reduced left frontal activation (more left frontal power or left frontal hypoactivation). There were no differences in right frontal activation between depressed and nondepressed subjects.

The current data extend these findings, suggesting that among a nonselected population of children, individual differences in their social behavior during a peer session are related to their pattern of frontal asymmetry. The current data, in addition, indicate that high degrees of sociability and social competence are also associated with frontal asymmetry.

In the studies with depressed adults, Henriques and Davidson (1991) reported that differences between depressed and control subjects were localized to the left hemisphere. That is, the pattern of right frontal asymmetry was a function of greater power in the left frontal scalp lead as opposed to less power in the right frontal lead. Henriques and Davidson (1990) suggested that higher power in the left frontal lead reflected the absence of approach behavior or absence of positive affect in these individuals. However, in these studies, differences among groups were in absolute EEG power. Since this measure is the sum of multiple sources of variance, it provides only an indirect estimate of the specific contribution of that region to the asymmetry effect. The current data, however, support these findings using a more sensitive measure of site-specific power. Right frontal asymmetry in the current study was a function of greater site-specific power in the left frontal scalp lead (left frontal hypoactivation).

Previously it had been suggested that the functional distinction between the two frontal regions in the expression of affect may involve the individual's tendency to either approach or withdraw from a novel stimulus. Fox and Davidson (1984) had suggested that the left frontal region was differentially specialized for the organization of behaviors involved in approach, while the right frontal region was specialized for the organization of behaviors involved in withdrawal. Activation of the right frontal region, therefore, would be accompanied by an increased tendency to exhibit behaviors associated with withdrawal (anxiety, negative affect). Hypoactivation of the left frontal region may be associated with the absence of approach behavior and lack of positive affect. The manner in which the two frontal regions interact, therefore, is of some importance in understanding frontal/affect behavior relations. For example, two individuals exhibiting right frontal asymmetry may in fact present with different pictures with regard to the activation of either the left or right hemispheres. One may display the asymmetry as a function of decreased right activation, while the second may display the asymmetry as a function of increased left power (decreased left activation). The asymmetry metric does not provide adequate insight into these differences, and it is therefore important to identify the specific differences between hemispheres in increase or decrease of activation.

A number of researchers have attempted to understand these changes in EEG power. One common approach has been to examine absolute power in each lead. To the extent that groups differ in the magnitude of power in one hemisphere versus another, one can infer differences in hemispheric activation. However, power in any single scalp lead is a function of multiple sources. It has thus been important to identify methods that might partial out the different sources of variance in the power measure in order to understand the unique contribution reflected at each scalp location. A number of workers have attempted regression approaches, although these methods present important statistical problems (Wheeler et al., 1993).

The approach taken in the current article (computing both shared and unshared or unique power) is an attempt at dealing with these complex issues. By computing the weighted coherence between interhemispheric electrode sites and then calculating the degree of both shared and unshared power, we can examine the degree to which asymmetry is a function of both unique and shared properties of the two sides of the brain. And we can determine with a certain degree of precision the role of each hemisphere in contributing to important behavioral differences.

It is therefore interesting to examine the relations between these different measures of EEG activation and behavior. As the data suggest, unshared power is the best discriminator of individual differences in social behavior. The magnitude of associations between asymmetry scores and behavior was greatest when this metric was used. And it best discriminated differences among high, middle, and low socially competent and socially reticent children.

Importantly, differences in frontal asymmetry between children high or low in social competence or high or low in social reticence were a function of *left*-hemisphere power. Children who were sociable, were frequent in their initiations of social interaction, and were judged to be socially competent exhibited less left frontal unshared power (hyperfrontal activation) than children exhibiting fewer of these behaviors. Children who displayed social withdrawal and anxious and onlooking behaviors exhibited greater left frontal unshared power (hypofrontal activation) compared to children who exhibited fewer of these behaviors. The pattern of these data, particularly those for the socially reticent children, is similar to that reported by Davidson and colleagues for both behaviorally inhibited children (Finman et al., 1989) and for individuals with depressive symptomatology (Henriques & Davidson, 1991). They suggest that the pattern of frontal activation recorded in these 4-year-old children reflects an important individual difference in their disposition to respond affectively to novel and mildly stressful situations.

Children exhibiting this pattern of behavior, when confronted with novel events such as interaction with unfamiliar peers in an unfamiliar environment, are likely to respond with onlooking behavior (lack of approach) and a relative absence of social interaction (lack of positive affect).

The associations found in this study between social behavior in the quartet session and left frontal power are in contrast to previous findings from Fox's laboratory, which reported an association between right frontal power and negative affect. In two studies (Davidson & Fox, 1989; Fox et al., 1992), right frontal asymmetry, a function of less right frontal power, was associated with the tendency to display distress to maternal separation. And, in a third study (Calkins et al., in press), right frontal asymmetry, again a function of less right frontal power, was associated with infants selected for a high motor/high negative affect temperamental pattern. Infants selected for this temperament display more behavioral inhibition at 14 and 24 months of age (Kagan & Snidman, 1991). There are a number of possible reasons for the apparent differences in the locus of effects between previous studies and the current data.

Previously, researchers who found a relation between right frontal asymmetry and emotional behavior indicated that the right frontal pattern was associated with the expression or disposition to express negative affect. For example, infants who cried to maternal separation or infants who cried frequently to novel stimuli were found to display less right frontal power compared to those infants who were not prone to display negative emotions in these situations. The children in the current study who exhibited a pattern of left frontal hypoactivation displayed a pattern of socially reticent behavior, including more onlooking behavior and less time talking. But there was little evidence of overt display of negative affect. It is possible that their behavior reflected one of approach/withdrawal conflict, and that this combination of both approach and withdrawal motivations is the source of the left frontal hypoactivation. Alternatively, the pattern of onlooking, unoccupied behavior and absence of overt signs of negative affect may reflect a lack of approach rather than overt withdrawal. Thus, the pattern of left frontal hypoactivation may reflect absence of approach rather than overt withdrawal.

A second possible explanation for differences in the pattern of EEG power between the current study and previous work with infants may be that there are developmental changes in the reactivity of the two hemispheres. There are data which indicate that the right hemisphere matures earlier than the left (see Bell & Fox, 1994). Differences in the locus of power may thus be a function of developmental changes in hemispheric responsivity. The right hemisphere may be more reactive at an earlier age prior to the maturation of the left hemisphere and left hemisphere functions.[1]

Another possible explanation for the different pattern of findings may involve understanding the different pathways by which infant or toddler behavioral inhibition is expressed during early and middle childhood. Previously, researchers have indicated that social withdrawal in early childhood is a risk factor for both anxiety-related disorders and depression. While the common behavioral pattern seen in infancy for these different outcomes may be behavioral inhibition, various environmental factors may influence the development (or lack of development) of different patterns of behavioral problems. It is possible that the pattern of EEG activity may change with the expression of different outcomes. At present, there are no longitudinal data that directly address this important issue. Whether the pattern of frontal EEG activity changes with the differential expression of certain behavioral styles or whether early patterns of EEG asymmetry remain stable across different paths that individuals take across development is an important question for future research.

## APPENDIX

$$C_W = \frac{\sum_{\theta 1}^{\theta 2} \text{Coh}(\theta)\hat{f}(\theta)}{\sum_{\theta 1}^{\theta 2} \hat{f}(\theta)},$$

where Coh is the coherence and $\hat{f}$ is the power at each frequency ($\theta$). In this example, ($\Theta$) includes frequency 6 Hz, 7 Hz, and 8 Hz to define the alpha band in this age group.

$$\sum_{\theta 1}^{\theta 2} \text{Coh}(\theta)\hat{f}(\theta),$$

$$\sum_{\theta 1}^{\theta 2} \hat{f}(\theta) - \sum_{\theta 1}^{\theta 2} \text{Coh}(\theta)\hat{f}(\theta).$$

---

[1] The authors would like to thank an anonymous reviewer for this suggested possible reason for the difference in the pattern of findings between the current power data and those reported for young infants.

# REFERENCES

Bell, M. A., & Fox, N. A. (1994). Brain development over the first year of life: Relations between electroencephalographic frequency and coherence and cognitive and affective behaviors. In G. Dawson & K. W. Fischer (Eds.), *Human behavior and the developing brain* (pp. 314–345). New York: Guilford.

Bohrer, R. E., & Porges, S. W. (1982). The application of time-series statistics to psychological research: An introduction. In G. Keren (Ed.), *Psychological statistics* (pp. 309–345). Hillsdale, NJ: Erlbaum.

Buss, A. H., & Plomin, R. (1984). *Temperament: Early developing personality traits.* Hillsdale, NJ: Erlbaum.

Calkins, S. D., Fox, N. A., & Marshall, T. R. (in press). Behavioral and physiological correlates of inhibition in infancy. *Child Development.*

Coplan, R. J., Rubin, K. H., Fox, N. A., Calkins, S. D., & Stewart, S. (1994). Being alone, playing alone, and acting alone: Distinguishing among reticence and passive and active solitude in young children. *Child Development, 65,* 129–137.

Davidson, R. J. (1983). Hemispheric specialization for cognition and affect. In A. Gale & J. Edwards (Eds.), *Physiological correlates of human behaviour*, London: Academic Press.

Davidson, R. J. (1988). EEG measures of cerebral asymmetry: Conceptual and methodological issues. *International Journal of Neuroscience, 39,* 71–89.

Davidson, R. J. (1992). Anterior cerebral asymmetry and the nature of emotion. *Brain and Cognition, 30,* 125–151.

Davidson, R. J., Ekman, P., Saron, C. D., Senulis, J., & Friesen, W. (1990). Approach/withdrawal and cerebral asymmetry: Emotional expression and brain physiology. *Journal of Personality and Social Psychology, 58,* 330–334.

Davidson, R. J., & Fox, N. A. (1988). Cerebral asymmetry and emotion: Developmental and individual differences. In S. Segalowitz & D. Molfese (Eds.), *Developmental implications of brain lateralization* (pp. 191–206). New York: Guilford.

Davidson, R. J., & Fox, N. A. (1989). Frontal brain asymmetry predicts infants' response to maternal separation. *Journal of Abnormal Psychology, 98,* 127–131.

Dawson, G., Grofer-Klinger, L., Panagiotides, H., Spieker, S., & Frey, K. (1992). Infants of mothers with depressive symptoms: Electroencephalographic and behavioral findings related to attachment status. *Development and Psychopathology, 4,* 67–80.

Fein, G., Raz, J., Brown, F. F., & Merrin, E. L. (1988). Common reference coherence data are confounded by power and phase effects. *Electroencephalography and Clinical Neurophysiology, 69,* 581–584.

Finman, R., Davidson, R. J., Colton, M. B., Straus, A. M., & Kagan, J. (1989). Psychophysiological correlates of inhibition to the unfamiliar in children. [Abstract]. *Psychophysiology, 26,* No. 4A, S24.

Fox, N. A. (1989). Psychophysiological correlates of emotional reactivity during the first year of life. *Developmental Psychology, 25*, 364–372.

Fox, N. A. (1994). Dynamic cerebral processes underlying emotion regulation. In N. A. Fox (Ed.), The development of emotion regulation: Biological and behavioral considerations (pp. 152–166). *Monographs of the Society for Child Development, 59* (2–3, Serial No. 240).

Fox, N. A., Bell, M. A., & Jones, N. A. (1992). Individual differences in response to stress and cerebral asymmetry. *Developmental Neuropsychology, 8*, 161–184.

Fox, N. A., & Davidson, R. J. (1984). Hemispheric specialization and the development of affect. In N. A. Fox & R. J. Davidson (Eds.), *The psychobiology of affective development*. Hillsdale, NJ: Erlbaum.

Fox, N. A., & Davidson, R. J. (1986). Taste-elicited changes in facial signs of emotion and the asymmetry of brain electrical activity in human newborns. *Neuropsychologia, 24*, 417–422.

Fox, N. A., & Davidson, R. J. (1987). EEG asymmetry in ten-month-old infants in response to approach of a stranger and maternal separation. *Developmental Psychology, 23*, 233–240.

Fox, N. A., & Davidson, R. J. (1988). Patterns of brain electrical activity during the expression of discrete emotions in ten-month-old infants. *Developmental Psychology, 24*, 230–236.

Henriques, J. B., & Davidson, R. J. (1990). Regional brain electrical asymmetries discriminate between previously depressed and healthy control subjects. *Journal of Abnormal Psychology, 99*, 22–31.

Henriques, J. B., & Davidson, R. J. (1991). Left frontal hypoactivation in depression. *Journal of Abnormal Psychology, 100*, 535–545.

Howes, C. (1987). Peer interaction of young children. *Monographs of the Society for Research in Child Development, 53* (1, Serial No. 217).

Jasper, H. H. (1958). The 10/20 international electrode system. *EEG and Clinical Neurophysiology, 10*, 371–375.

Jones, N. A., & Fox, N. A. (1992). Electroencephalogram asymmetry during emotionally evocative films and its relation to positive and negative affectivity. *Brain and Cognition, 20*, 280–299.

Kagan, J., & Snidman, N. (1991). Infant predictors of inhibited and uninhibited profiles. *Psychological Science, 2*, 40–44.

Lehmann, D., Ozaki, H., & Pal, I. (1986). Averaging of spectral power and phase via vector diagram best fits without reference electrode or reference channel. *EEG and Clinical Neurophysiology, 64*, 350–363.

Levy, J., Heller, W., Banich, M. T., & Burton, L. (1983). Are variations among right-handers in perceptual asymmetries caused by characterstic arousal differences in the hemispheres? *Journal of Experimental Psychology: Human Perception and Performance, 9*, 329–359.

Lindsley, D. B., & Wicke, J. D. (1974). The EEG: Autonomous electrical activity in man and animals. In R. Thompson & M. N. Patterson (Eds.), *Bioelectrical recording techniques* (pp. 3–83). New York: Academic Press.

Porges, S. W., & Bohrer, R. E. (1990). Analyses of period processes in psychophysiological research. In J. T. Cacioppo & L. G. Tassinary (Eds.), *Principles of psychophysiology: Physical, social and inferential elements* (pp. 708–753). New York: Cambridge University Press.

Porges, S. W., Bohrer, R. E., Cheung, M. N., Drasgow, F., McCabe, P. M., & Keren, G. (1980). New time-series statistic for detecting rhythmic co-occurrence in the frequency domain: The weighted coherence and its application to psychophysiological research. *Psychological Bulletin, 88*, 580–587.

Rowe, D. C., & Plomin, R. (1977). Temperament in early childhood. *Journal of Personality Assessment, 41*, 150–156.

Rubin, K. H. (1989). *The Play Observation Scale (POS)*. Waterloo: University of Waterloo.

Rubin, K. H., Fein, G., & Vandenberg, B. (1983). Play. In E. M. Hetherington (Ed.), P. H. Mussen (Series Ed.), *Handbook of child psychology: Vol. 4. Socialization, personality, and social development*. New York: Wiley.

Rubin, K. H., & Lollis, S. P. (1988). Origins and consequences of social withdrawal. In J. Belsky & T. Nezworski (Eds.), *Clinical implications of attachment* (pp. 219–253). Hillsdale, NJ: Erlbaum.

Sackeim, H. A., Weiman, A. L., Gur, R. C., Greenburg, M., Hungerbuhler, J. P., & Geschwind, N. (1982). Pathological laughing and crying: Functional brain asymmetry in the experience of positive and negative emotions. *Archives of Neurology, 39*, 210–218.

Schaffer, C. E., Davidson, R. J., & Saron, C. (1983). Frontal and parietal electroencephalogram asymmetry in depressed and nondepressed subjects. *Biological Psychiatry, 18*, 753–762.

Silberman, E. K., & Weingartner, H. (1986). Hemispheric lateralization of functions related to emotion. *Brain and Cognition, 5*, 322–353.

Stifter, C. A., & Fox, N. A. (1990). Infant reactivity: Physiological correlates of newborn and five-month temperament. *Developmental Psychology, 26*, 582–588.

Tomarken, A. J., Davidson, R. J., & Henriques, J. B. (1990). Resting frontal brain asymmetry predicts affective responses to films. *Journal of Personality and Social Psychology, 59*, 791–801.

Wheeler, R. W., Davidson, R. J., & Tomarken, A. J. (1993). Frontal brain asymmetry and emotional reactivity: A biological substrate of affective style. *Psychophysiology, 30*, 82–91.

# Part II

# ATTACHMENT AND PARENTING

The papers in this section deal with various aspects of parent–child relationships. The first paper by Michael Rutter is a thoughtful discussion of theoretical and clinical issues in attachment theory. In 1969, Bowlby published his first volume of a trilogy on attachment, and Ainsworth and Wittig published the first empirical test of the theory using the Strange Situation. In the decade or two following those "landmarks," many studies were designed to examine the antecedents and consequences of infant–parent attachments. More recently, there has been a growing interest in attachment across the life span and discussions of the potential implications of attachment research for clinical practice.

Rutter starts the paper by briefly discussing several modifications in the theory, including abandoning the notion of a sensitive period. He then considers some unresolved theoretical and empirical questions including the following: What is the behavioral control system underlying proximity-seeking behavior? Is the Strange Situation and its resultant discrete categories the best way to assess attachment security? Is the present concept of security, divided into three or four relationship types, adequate to cover individual variations in relationships? What is the role of temperament in children's responses to separation and reunion? How are discrepant attachment relationships experienced by a child transformed into individual characteristics that the child carries forward? Can the concept of "internal working models" be operationalized and empirically tested in different age groups? How can attachment be measured in later childhood and the adult years? What are the boundaries of attachment (i.e., What are the other important features of relationships?) What is the association of attachment with later functioning and Psychiatric Disorders? Is insecure attachment a risk factor for psychopathology?

Following his discussion of these unresolved issues, Rutter summarizes the clinical implications of attachment theory. First, more extensively than Bowlby, he dismisses psychoanalytic theories of development as inconsistent with attachment theory. He then describes the impact attachment theory has had on the provision of child care and residential care for children. There is now an appreciation of children's need for continuity in caregivers and for an opportunity to form a selective attachment. These concepts are also relevant for those who make decisions about child abuse, foster placement, and adoption. Finally, Rutter considers the importance of attachment concepts on psychotherapy, including cognitive models of relationships. In sum, Rutter reviews changes in attachment theory over the last 25 years and implications for future research and applications of this theory.

The second paper in this section, by Van Ijzendoorn, Juffer and Duyvesteyn, focuses on the clinical application of attachment theory mentioned in the Rutter chapter. Given that insecure attachment is a risk factor for later developmental problems, can intervention studies be developed that increase maternal sensitivity and decrease insecure attachments? The authors address this question in their description of 16 intervention studies that reported effects on infant–parent attachments. They divided the studies into two groups. The study was either a short-term preventive model of parent education or a longer-term therapeutic intervention. The preventive intervention was aimed at enhancing parental sensitivity through support, information, and modeling. Therapeutic approaches tried to change the intergenerational cycle of insecure attachments by changing the mental representations of relationships.

This was done by helping the mothers to relive or face their own developmental experiences and understand how these experiences were influencing their own parenting, particularly sensitivity and responsiveness to infant cues. It is worth noting that some interventions started after negative relationships were already established, while others were preventive, aiming to ensure positive relationships from the outset in samples considered at risk for difficulties.

A meta-analysis of 12 of the studies (those that had contrast groups) was done to determine if intervention affected maternal sensitivity, maternal attachment representations, or infant–parent attachment security. It was easier to increase sensitivity than it was to decrease attachment insecurity. In part, this may be a limitation of the measurement. The attachment measure is dichotomous (secure versus insecure), and the sensitivity measure is continuous. The latter measure should be more capable of demonstrating change.

It was possible to change maternal sensitivity without altering attachment security and vice versa. The authors speculate that learning new behavioral strategies for responding to infants may not be sufficient for parents to deal with attachment needs of a developing child. Finally, the authors were surprised to find that long-term interventions seemed to be less effective than short-term interventions at enhancing attachment security.

This paper highlights the difficulty in breaking the intergenerational cycle of insecure attachment among multirisk families. Overall, most of the findings were weak. Although there are numerous variables besides maternal sensitivity and attachment security that ultimately need to be considered, attachment theory provides testable hypotheses and practical applications for future intervention efforts. Potentially, the best features of some of these early efforts may be combined for more effective interventions.

This section's third paper reports on the Parenting Risk Scale, a measure developed to assess the quality of parenting. Existing measures of the quality of parenting primarily rely on observation of parent–child interaction. Mrazek, Mrazek, and Klinnert were interested in using parenting rating scales collected shortly after children's births to predict which children would develop asthma from a sample of children at genetic risk. To develop their measure, the authors reviewed the child development literature and determined five key dimensions of parenting: 1) emotional availability (e.g., warmth), 2) control (e.g., authoritative), 3) parental mental disturbance, 4) knowledge base, and 5) commitment to parenting. The Stress and Coping Interview, a 60- to 90-minute semistructured procedure, was designed to obtain ratings in each of these five areas. The interview obtained information about parent–child relationships, the marital relationship, life stressors, and social support.

The authors note that the goal of the measure was to identify parents at risk for having problems in one of the five areas that would compromise sensitive and consistent care. The scale was not designed to differentiate among degrees of good parenting. Three categories were used: Adequate Parenting, Concerns About Parenting, and Parenting Difficulties. As with most global ratings using clinical judgment, raters benefit from clinical training. Otherwise, without sufficient training, interrater reliability can be poor. The authors attempted to validate the ratings using several measures, including the MMPI for concurrent validity as well as the Behavioral Screening Questionnaire and the Strange Situation for predictive validity. The Parenting Risk Scale ratings were predictive of security of attachment at 12 months, using an observational measure, and of dysfunction on the Behavior Rating Scale, a parental report measure, at 24 months. It is worth noting that in this sample of predominantly upper middle-class families, the rates of secure attachment were significantly lower than in most samples studied. Finally, the PRS administered shortly after birth was predictive of asthma at three years of age.

The authors conclude that the structured interview and ratings could be used in clinical settings. An abbreviated version, about 30 minutes, could potentially be used in pediatric settings when specific concerns arise. Clearly, the measure has promise but needs to be used in other samples and studies before its utility can be assessed. The Parenting Risk Scale, in its current form, may prove more useful in research studies where quantitative scores are needed for analyses. Once the utility of the scale is known in other populations at risk, then it may be possible to link identified parenting difficulties with specific interventions in clinical settings.

The last paper in this section represents an approach to understanding the effects of parenting from a genetic–environmental model. The study by Reiss, Hetherington, Plomin and colleagues examines parenting differences among siblings and sibling functioning. To date most of the similarities among siblings on measures of competence and psychopathology have been found to be the result of shared genes rather than common family environments. This large-scale study examines whether siblings are treated differently by parents and whether these differences are important in the development of competence or psychopathologic outcomes. *Nonshared environment* refers to those environmental factors that produce different developmental outcomes for each sibling in a family, including differential treatment by the parents and discrepant life experiences.

A large sample was needed to investigate the effects of the shared versus nonshared environment. Families were obtained through random-digit dialing and market panels. Each family had two same gender children (no more than four years apart in age) between the ages of 10 and 18. There was a total of 708 families who varied in the genetic relatedness of the siblings ranging from monozygotic twins to genetically unrelated siblings in step-families. Interviews were conducted in the home in two sessions.

This study was well conducted. Multiple measures by multiple reporters on multiple occasions were used to assess depression and antisocial behavior. These included the Child Depression Inventory, the Behavior Problems Index (an adaptation of the Child Behavior Checklist), and a Behavior Events Inventory (child and parent report of specific behaviors during the previous week). Parenting was assessed from self-report questionnaires and ratings of videotaped interaction of each parent–child dyad.

Path analyses were used to explore the associations among parenting toward the adolescent, parenting toward the sibling, and symptoms of the adolescent and the sibling. Parental negativity and inconsistency showed strong associations with child antisocial behavior and to a lesser extent with depressive symptoms. Among the more interesting findings were that parental conflict and negative behavior directed at a sibling was associated with less psychopathology in the adolescent. The authors propose the notion of a "sibling barricade." However, the direction of effects cannot be estimated from this study. Panel data is being collected for a closer look at causality. In concluding, the authors discuss the implications of this two-child study for understanding family systems and sibling differences.

# 5

# Clinical Implications of Attachment Concepts: Retrospect and Prospect[1]

**Michael Rutter**

*Institute of Psychiatry, London*

*The key features of attachment theory are summarized and the unresolved questions considered in terms of a behavioural control system, measurement of attachment security, qualities of attachment, the role of temperament, transformation of a dyadic quality into an individual characteristic, internal working models, manifestations of attachment post infancy, how one relationship affects another relationship, boundaries of attachment, associations with later functioning, the role of parenting qualities and patterns of caregiving, adaptive value of secure attachment, and disorders of attachment. The clinical implications are discussed in terms of: the need to reject the traditional psychoanalytic theories of development, the patterns of residential care for children, the provision of child care, the assessment of parenting, the effects of parental divorce and family break-up, "maternal bonding" to infants, psychotherapy and disorders of attachment.*

## INTRODUCTION

1994 marked the 25th anniversary of the publication of the first volume of Bowlby's hugely important trilogy on attachment (Bowlby, 1969/82, 1973,

---

Reprinted with permission from the *Journal of Child Psychology and Psychiatry*, 1995, Vol. 36, No. 4, 549–571. Copyright © 1995 by the Association for Child Psychology and Psychiatry.

[1] Bowlby Memorial Lecture presented at the 13th International Congress, International Association for Child and Adolescent Psychiatry and Allied Professions, San Francisco, California, U.S.A., 24–28 July, 1994.

1980), and the 50th anniversary of his empirical study of 44 juvenile thieves, which first stimulated his interest in mother/child relationships. Along with others, his findings pointed to the likely ill-effects on personality development of prolonged institutional care and/or frequent changes of mother figure during the early years of life (Bowlby, 1988). His 1951 WHO Monograph, although it led to major improvements in the care of young children in hospitals and residential institutions, initially had quite a critical reception from academic psychologists (e.g. O'Connor & Franks, 1960) and his suggestions on the importance of attachment relationships were rejected by the psychoanalytic establishment, in a manner that was often personally hostile (see Grosskurth, 1986; Holmes, 1993a, b).

Yet, despite its initially negative reception, most of the key components of attachment concepts have received empirical support (Belsky & Cassidy, 1994; Rajecki, Lamb & Obmascher, 1978; Rutter, 1991). Moreover, attachment ideas have come to dominate writings on relationships and social development in adult life (Hazan & Shaver, 1994; Parkes, Stevenson-Hinde & Marris, 1991) as well as in childhood (e.g. Bretherton, 1990; Bretherton & Waters, 1985; Campos, Barrett, Lamb, Goldsmith & Stenberg, 1983; Greenberg, Cicchetti & Cummings, 1990; Sroufe, 1983). Finally, there has been a growing awareness of the potentially important implications of attachment concepts for clinical practice (Belsky & Nezworski, 1988). The time seems right for a reconsideration of those clinical implications. Necessarily, however, this first requires a reappraisal of the key components of attachment theory and of the extent to which they have been supported by empirical research findings.

## ATTACHMENT THEORY

The importance of Bowlby's initial writings on "maternal deprivation" lay in his emphasis that children's experiences of interpersonal relationships were crucial to their psychological development (Bowlby, 1944; 1951). The argument was that the formation of an ongoing relationship with the child was as an important part of parenting as the provision of experiences, discipline and child care. Although rejected by some at the time (see Casler, 1968), this view is now generally accepted (Dunn, 1993; Hinde, 1979; Rutter, 1981; 1991; Sameroff & Emde, 1989; Schaffer, 1990). The argument focused attention on the need to consider parenting in terms of consistency of caregivers over time and parental sensitivity to children's individuality. The trilogy on attachment took matters forward in five key ways. First, it differentiated attachment qualities of relationships from other aspects. Thus, it was noted that whereas anxiety increased attachment behaviour, it inhibited playful interactions. Second, the development of attachments were placed within the context of normal developmental processes and specific mechanisms were proposed. Most crucially, emphasis was placed on the role of attachment in promoting security and, thereby, encouraging independence. The importance of this point lay in its differentiation of attachment from dependency (Maccoby & Masters, 1970; Sroufe, Fox & Pancake, 1983) and, in so doing, underlining that the development of attachments was not just an immature phase of dependency to be "got over", but rather a feature that should serve to foster maturity in social functioning. Third, the development of attachments was placed firmly in a biological framework. The process was seen as an intrinsic feature of human development as social beings and not a secondary feature learned as a result of the rewards of feeding. Fourth, a mental mechanism, namely internal working models of relationships, was suggested as a means for both the carry forward of the effects of early attachment experiences into later relationships and also a mechanism for change. Fifth, Bowlby made various suggestions about the ways in which an insecurity in selective early attachments might play a role in the genesis of later psychopathology.

All of these key features have received substantial support from empirical research, (Belsky & Cassidy, 1994; Rajecki et al., 1978; Rutter, 1981; 1991) and, as I shall indicate, have had very important implications for both theory (Sroufe & Rutter, 1984) and practice (Holmes, 1993a,b; Schaffer, 1990). Of course, the early specification of attachment theory did not prove correct in all its details. Perhaps there are four main changes that have taken place over the years. In his early writings, Bowlby drew parallels between the development of attachments and imprinting (Bowlby, 1969/82). It became apparent that there were more differences than similarities and this parallel was dropped later on (Bowlby, 1988) and is no longer seen as helpful by most writers on attachment. Similarly, early accounts emphasized the need for selective attachments to develop during a relatively brief "sensitivity period" in the first two years of life, with the implication that even very good parenting that is provided after this watershed is too late. In keeping with the changes that have taken place in thinking about sensitive periods more generally, it has become clear that this all or nothing view required modification. There is a sensitive period during which it is highly desirable that selective attachments develop but the time frame is probably somewhat broader than initially envisaged and the effects are not as fixed and irreversible as once thought. The third change concerns abandonment of the notion of "monotropy". Bowlby's early writings were widely understood to mean that there was a biological need to develop a selective attachment with just one person and that the quality of this relationship differed from all others. The hypothesis of a high degree of selectivity (so that there is not an interchangeability among relationships) has been amply confirmed. What is now clear, however, is that although there are very definite hierarchies in selective attachments, it is usual for most children to develop selective attachments with a small number of people who are closely involved in child care. Finally, it came to be appreciated that social development was affected by later, as well as earlier relationships (Bowlby, 1988). Nevertheless, these modifications aside, the major tenets of attachment theory have been broadly confirmed. Of course, that is not to say that there is not a host of crucial questions remaining to be answered. There is. Let me deal with these by considering a round baker's dozen of issues.

## UNRESOLVED QUESTIONS

### *Behavioural Control System*

From the outset, a central feature of attachment theory concerned the proposition that attachment was under the control of a biologically based behaviour system. For a long time, there was a major problem in terminology as the same word "attachment" was used to refer to discrete patterns of behaviour (such as proximity-seeking), to a dyadic relationship, to a postulated inbuilt predisposition to develop specific attachments to individuals, and to the hypothesized internal controlling mechanisms for this predisposition (see Hinde, 1982). Few would doubt the need to invoke some such control system and helpful guidelines are available in the evidence on the conditions that promote proximity-seeking behaviour in young children. Thus, one of the important early observations was that fear intensified proximity-seeking and that, if there was no-one else to turn to, infants would cling even to an abusing parent. The monkey studies undertaken by Harlow and his colleagues (see, e.g. Harlow & Harlow, 1969) also indicated that this tendency to cling was not a function of feeding. The psychoanalytic secondary drive view could be firmly rejected. Bowlby argued that three types of features tended to activate attachment: tiredness or distress of the child, threatening features in the environment and absence or moving away of the attachment figure. Experimental work over the past two decades has also shown that there are neuroendocrine and neurobiological accompaniments of attachment responses (Kraemer, 1992; Levine, 1982). Nevertheless, substantial uncertainty remains on the sort of control system to be envisaged (should this be in neurobiological terms or in cognitive functioning?) and there is continuing uncertainty as to quite how the hypothesized system might actually work. It seems likely that the mechanisms involved in determining that proximity-seeking takes place when and how it does may well not be the same as the mechanisms involved in determining the *qualities* of a selective attachment relationship.

## Measurement of Attachment Security

A major step forward in the study of attachment relationships came with Ainsworth's recognition that the security or insecurity of an attachment relationship constituted a crucial aspect of individual differences in such relationships, together with her development of the Strange Situation procedure for assessing attachment security (Ainsworth, Blehar, Waters & Wall, 1978). In brief, it comprises a 20 minute sequence in which the young child is exposed to an unfamiliar place, an unfamiliar person, parental separation, and the experience of being alone, and, in which, the quality of reunion behaviour provides the main basis for assessment. It has worked remarkably well and it has become the standard form of measurement in attachment research. Nevertheless, it is by no means free of limitations (see Lamb, Thompson, Gardner, Charnov & Estes, 1984). To begin with, it is very dependent on brief separations and reunions having the same meaning for all children. This may be a substantial constraint when applying the procedure in cultures, such as that in Japan (see Miyake, Chen & Campos, 1985), where infants are rarely separated from their mothers in ordinary circumstances. Also, because older children have the cognitive capacity to maintain relationships when the other person is not present, separations may not provide the same stress for them. Modified procedures based on the Strange Situation have been developed for older preschool children (see Belsky & Cassidy, 1994; Greenberg et al., 1990) but it is much more dubious whether the same approach can be used in middle childhood. Also, despite its manifest strengths, the procedure is based on just 20 minutes of behaviour. It can scarcely be expected to tap all the relevant qualities of a child's attachment relationships. Q-sort procedures based on much longer naturalistic observations in the home, and interviews with mothers have been developed in order to extend the data base (see Vaughn & Waters, 1990). A further constraint is that the coding procedure results in discrete categories rather than continuously distributed dimensions. Not only is this likely to provide boundary problems, but also it is not at all obvious that discrete categories best represent the concepts that are inherent in attachment security. It seems much more likely that infants vary in their degree of security and there is a need for measurement systems that can quantify this individual variation.

### Qualities of Attachment

Following Ainsworth's extremely important and influential lead (Ainsworth, 1967; Ainsworth et al., 1978), attachment relationships have been classified as showing security (as shown by infants using the attachment figure as a secure base from which to explore, responding positively to reunions after brief separations, and returning rapidly to exploration), avoidant insecurity (in which infants explore with little reference to the attachment figure and seem to show ignoring or avoidant behaviour on reunion), and resistant insecurity (in which infants fail to move away from the attachment figure and show little exploration). The last group of infants tend to be highly distressed by separations and are difficult to settle after reunion. During the past decade, however, it became apparent that some children's behaviour did not fit readily into any of these three patterns and, moreover, that some children with a known history of abuse and neglect were classified as secure, although their behaviour outside the Strange Situation suggested abnormalities. This led to the development of an avoidant/ambivalent or disorganized category (Crittenden, 1988; Main & Solomon, 1990; Radke-Yarrow, Cummings, Kuczynski & Chapman, 1985). Even with this additional category it remains quite uncertain whether the concept of insecurity, and its classification, is adequate to cover individual variations in attachment relationships (Rutter, 1980). Thus, for example, in two studies (Rogers, Ozonoff & Maslin-Cole, 1991; Sigman & Ungerer, 1984) children with autism, who showed severe relationship deficits, did not stand out in terms of their responses to the Strange Situation, at least as traditionally measured. In a third study (Capps, Sigman & Mundy, 1994) all the autistic children showed disorganized attachment but 40% of these were subclassified as securely attached, and the overall pattern was not well captured by any of the categories. Also, children reared in institutions with an ever changing roster of numerous caregivers tend to show patterns of indiscriminant proximity-seeking that is obviously abnormal, but with qualities not well encapsulated by measures of insecurity.

### The Role of Temperament

For a long time attachment theorists were very reluctant to accept the possibility that the infants own temperamental characteristics might influence the qualities of attachment security (Sroufe et al., 1983). They emphasized that the concept applied to a dyadic relationship and not to an individual feature and that, empirically, the security shown in a child's relationship with one parent bore only a weak association with the quality shown in the relationship with the other parent (Fox, Kimmerly & Schafer, 1991). The evidence on the connections between temperament and attachment security are limited but it now seems apparent that a temperamental dimension reflecting negative emotionality is associated with insecure attachment, although it is only one of many factors that influence children's responses to separation and reunion (Thompson, Connell & Bridges, 1988; Vaughn et al., 1992).

### Transformation of a Dyadic Quality into an Individual Characteristic

The process by which a relationship quality becomes transformed into an individual characteristic remains a crucial unanswered question. There is no doubt that attachment security starts as a dyadic relationship feature, as shown by the repeated finding that the quality of a child's relationship with one person is only weakly related to the quality of relationships with other people. On the other hand, attachment theory has always argued that later relationships are strongly affected by early attachment relationships. Also, empirical findings indicate that there are continuities with later peer relationships, so that some reflection of attachment quality must be carried forward within the individual unless the continuity is merely a consequence of continuity in environmental influences (Belsky & Cassidy, 1994; Rutter, 1991). The latter cannot be a sufficient explanation in all circumstances if only because Hodges and Tizard's (1989a,b) follow-up of residential nursery children showed that the links between relationships persisted in spite of a change of environment. But, if, as has been shown, children's relationships with key figures in their environment vary in their security qualities, how are discrepant relationships dealt with in the transformation into an individual characteristic? Does the most important relationship predominate, is there a balance between differing relationships, or does one secure relationship compensate for insecurities in others? No very satisfactory explanation has been found and tested.[2]

### Internal Working Models

The prevailing view at the moment, however, is that the process resides in some form of internalized representation, or working model of relation-

---

[2] In seeking an explanation, it needs to be appreciated that the security of attachments to professional caregivers may be as important as those to parents (see e.g. Howes, Rodning, Galluzo & Myers, 1988; Aviezer, Van IJzendoorn, Sagi & Schuengel, 1994; Oppenheim, Sagi & Lamb, 1988).

ships (Bretherton, 1987, 1990; Sroufe & Fleeson, 1986; Stern, 1985). At some level, this must be the case because children are thinking, feeling beings who actively process their experiences. Necessarily, they will bring to any relationship both memories of past interactions and expectations of future ones. The difficulty comes in translating this general notion into something more specific that can lead to testable hypotheses. At the moment, the notion of internal working models is too all encompassing to have much testable explanatory power (Hinde, 1988). Furthermore, at least in so far as the processes in infancy are concerned, it would seem that the cognitive competence required to represent both sides of discrepant relationships are beyond the abilities of, say, 12-month-old infants (Dunn, 1988, 1993). The attraction of internal working models lies in its explicit recognition of the role of active thought processes in the mediation of the effects of experiences and in it providing a mechanism for both continuity and change. Nevertheless, although it is clear that they represent a reality in what is happening, so far they have failed to give any increased precision to our understanding of the processes involved.

### Manifestations of Attachment Post Infancy

One of the hallmarks of attachment theory was its claim that attachment security remained a key feature of relationships throughout the whole of life. The claim was bold but it is supported by the extensive body of evidence showing that bereavement or loss of a love relationship constitutes a potent stressor throughout life (after early infancy) and that the presence of a close confiding relationship is protective against stress in adults of all ages, as well as in children (Hazan & Shaver, 1994; Parkes et al., 1991; Rutter & Rutter, 1993). The issue that is only partially resolved concerns how to measure attachment qualities after the first few years of life. The findings certainly suggest that confiding and emotional exchange index attachment relationships during adolescence and adult life in a way that they do not in early childhood. Those features indicate which relationships include important attachment qualities but they provide a less satisfactory index of the quality of the attachment. Hazan and Shaver (1994) have provided a useful review of the features of adult relationships that are thought to reflect insecure attachment. These include both a lack of self disclosure and indiscriminant, overly intimate, self disclosure; undue jealousy in close relationships; feelings of loneliness even when involved in relationships; reluctance to commitment in relationships; difficulty in making relationships in a new setting, and a tendency to view partners as insufficiently attentive.

These characteristics make sense conceptually and they provide a good basis for further research but it remains to be determined whether these have the same meaning as the qualities of insecurity as observed in infancy.

## How One Relationship Affects Another Relationship

It is not just a matter of how attachment security is shown in varied ways over the lifespan, but also a question of how one relationship affects another relationship (Hinde & Stevenson-Hinde, 1988). Thus, strong claims have been made about the ways in which insecurity in a person's attachment relationship with parents in early childhood influences their relationships in adult life (Main, 1991; Main & Hesse, 1990; Main, Kaplan & Cassidy, 1985). This has led to Mary Main's development of the Adult Attachment Interview. This involves asking a series of apparently straightforward questions to elicit an account of childhood from which inferences are drawn about attachment and about the person's evaluation of those experiences. Attachment insecurity is identified on the basis of a tendency to deny negative experiences, to be unable to re-evoke the feelings associated with negative experiences; presentation of an over-idealized picture of parents; or a continuing precoccupation with parents associated with confused, incoherent concepts, and unresolved anger. The postulate is that it is important for healthy personality development to have access to memories of painful experiences in order to come to terms with them and to integrate them into a positive view of the self. One intriguing aspect of the connections between relationships concerns the evidence that measures of maternal attachment insecurity obtained during pregnancy predict the insecurity of the infant's attachment relationships with the mother as measured later (Fonagy, Steele & Steele, 1991; Fonagy, Steele, Steele, Higgit & Target, 1994).

Nevertheless, it would be a mistake to seek to view all connections between relationships in terms of a persistence of attachment qualities. As both Hinde and Stevenson-Hinde (1988) and Sameroff and Emde (1989) emphasized, there are many other features that require explanation. Why, for example do some women in a discordant marital relationship show more involvement (albeit with less sensitivity) with their babies than do mothers in a harmonious relationship (Engfer, 1988); why do marital relationships tend to alter after the birth of a first child (Belsky & Isabella, 1988); why do dyadic interactions tend to be different when a third party is present (Clarke-Stewart, 1978; Corter, Abramovitch & Pepler, 1983); and why do children who have a very close relationship with their mothers tend to develop a hostile relationship with their next born sibling (Dunn & Kendrick, 1982)? Whereas these compensatory and rivalry effects are in no way incompatible with the attachment theory, it is certainly not obvious that the theory provides an adequate explanation on its own (Rutter, 1991). There is a need both to consider dyadic relationships in terms that go beyond attachment concepts, and to consider social systems that extend beyond dyads (Dunn, 1993; Hinde, 1976, 1979; Nash, 1988; Sameroff & Emde, 1989).

Moreover, there is a problem in the wish of many adult attachment theorists to extend attachment concepts to sexual relationships and to parents' relationships with their young children. Thus, an absolutely key feature of secure attachment relationships in early childhood is that they provide security. This is not obviously present with respect to parent-child relationships. Thus, mothers and fathers do not usually feel more secure when their young children are with them. They *provide* security but do not *receive* it (Rutter & Rutter, 1993). Nevertheless, their early *experience* of selective attachment seems to be associated with a greater capacity to be well functioning parents. The link seems important, but it is by no means inevitable, and it is not obvious that it makes sense to equate this with an infant's attachment to its parents. Of course, the relationship is a strong committed one and it does have many features in common with attachments, but it is not identical. Similarly, sexual relationships may show strong attachment qualities but they do not necessarily do so. Thus, a person may have a strong sexual longing for someone else in the absence of a committed relationship and without that relationship bringing any sense of security. Rather than view a sexual relationship as a variety of attachment relationships it may be more useful to ask which sexual relationships show attachment qualities and which ones do not, and why there is a difference between the two.

### Boundaries of Attachment

That question leads on to the somewhat related issue of the boundaries of attachment. One of the major achievements of the initial attachment concept was the careful distinction between attachment qualities and other features of relationships. Unfortunately, the attractiveness of attachment theory has meant that there has been rather a neglect of these other features, together with an implicit tendency to discuss relationships as if attachment security was all that mattered. Both Sameroff and Emde (1989) and Dunn (1993) have drawn attention to the evidence that children's relationships with other people are complex and involve a range of different dimensions and functions. These include connectedness, shared humour, balance of control, intimacy, and shared positive emotions. If we are to understand the interconnections between relationships, it will be necessary for us to take into account the range of dimensions that seem to be involved. It seems unlikely that these will be reducible to a single process involving attachment security or any other postulated quality.

There are at least two other difficulties with the way in which attachment concepts tend to be used. First, there is a tendency to refer to relationships as if they did, or did not, reflect attachment, and as if each relationship had to be one thing or another. It is clear from the evidence that this is nonsense. To begin with, as already noted, most people have several relationships involving a strong attachment. They differ in the importance and strength of the attachment but it is a quantitative variation and not a categorical distinction. Also, however, it is obvious that any one relationship may include several different qualities. Thus, parents usually have an attachment relationship with their children but that relationship also includes caregiver qualities, disciplinary features, playmate characteristics, and other aspects. Each of these may predominate in different contexts but the overall relationship involves a complex mix of all these different features. The second major problem with the use of attachment concepts concerns the tendency to apply them to an individual, rather than to a particular relationship (Kobak, 1994). Thus, the Adult Attachment Interview classifies *individuals* as secure or insecure, rather than classifying that person's relationships with different people. This seems to have some validity in that Fonagy et al (1991, 1994) found a significant association between parental attachment security and their children's attachment security. Nevertheless, as Dunn (1993) pointed out, it is evident that parents have different relationships with different children; that children have different relationships with each of their parents; that the associations between relationships among different dyads within and outside the family are of only modest strength; and that patterns of relationships show reciprocity, rivalry, and compensation as well as generalization.

### Associations with Later Functioning

One specific issue with regard to boundaries on attachment theory concerns the predictive claims in relation to later functioning. Sroufe (1988) emphasized the need to resist the tendency to overextend predictive claims to widespread aspects of personal functioning in later life. He argued that the specific claims of attachment theory concern the child's developing sense of inner confidence, efficacy, and self worth, together with aspects of intimate personal relationships, such as the capacity to be emotionally close, to seek and receive care, and to give care to others. Thus, he suggested that attachment had no direct connections with cognitive development and that, although anxious attachment was a risk factor for psychopathology, it did not directly cause later psychiatric disorders. The empirical research findings support this caution. Significant associations have been found between insecure attachment in infancy and various forms of later psychopathology in both childhood and adult life (Belsky & Cassidy, 1994) but the associations are of only moderate strength and the findings are by no means entirely consistent across studies. The findings are such as to make it necessary to consider carefully the nature of the processes involved. Belsky and Cassidy contrasted three alternative models. First there is a narrow domain-specific model in which maternal sensitivity to attachment signals forecasts attachment security in the child, which itself predicts only outcomes directly involving the attachment system (such as later intimate relationships). According to this model, parental qualities may well be related to a much broader range of outcomes but the mechanisms involved in, say, competence in play or cognitive development are quite different and are not of attachment processes. At the other extreme, a broad general model would postulate that attachment security is directly responsible for fostering development across a wide range of domains. A third model expects to find some generality, but only because of third variables that are involved in a variety of different developmental processes. It is important to recognize that the adverse environments that predispose to attachment insecurity usually include a wide range of risk features that may have nothing much to do with attachment as such. Thus, the Harlow monkeys reared on wire surrogates showed gross problems in later sexual and parenting behaviour. But these monkeys were reared in conditions of social isolation and it cannot be assumed that the later sequelae were a result of attachment insecurity or attachment failure. Similarly, the adverse outcomes associated with an institutional rearing or child abuse are a function of environments that appear deleterious in a variety of different connections. There are good reasons for supposing that abnormalities in the development of attachment relationships play a role in these adverse outcomes but is has to be admitted that their importance in relation to alternative mediating processes has not been put to the test in a rigorous fashion as yet.

## The Role of Parenting Qualities and Patterns of Caregiving

A central tenet of attachment theory has always been that the quality of parenting is strongly influential in shaping the security of an infant's attachment relationships with parents. There is now an abundance of evidence showing the existence of significant associations. Rates of insecure attachment are substantially raised in maltreated children and in those reared by depressed mothers. With normal samples, too, measures of parental sensitivity are associated with security of attachment in the infant. Also, a therapeutic intervention in a high risk group of Dutch mothers showed that gains in maternal sensitivity were associated with a reduction in patterns of insecurity (Van den Boom, 1990). Clearly, there are associations between patterns of parenting and qualities of attachment security. Yet, it has to be said that most of the associations that have been found have been of only moderate strength. We have still to gain a full understanding of how parenting qualities interact with other variables in the development of attachment relationships.

Perhaps the greatest uncertainty concerns child care outside the home. Following Bowlby's WHO report (1951), claims were made that group daycare caused infants grave psychological damage (WHO Expert Committee on Mental Health, 1951). It is now clear that view was seriously mistaken. Most infants who experience good quality group daycare with continuity in caregiving show no detectable ill effects (Zigler & Gordon, 1982). On the other hand, there is some suggestion (albeit disputed—Clarke-Stewart, 1989; McCartney & Galanopoulos, 1988) that there *may* be elevated rates of insecurity in the case of children with early and extensive daycare experience (Belsky & Rovine, 1988). To a substantial extent, such risks as there are clearly derive from the poor quality of care rather than from the fact that it has been provided on a group basis. Nevertheless, it may be that group daycare may pose difficulties for some babies under a year old when it is on a full-time basis (Belsky & Rovine, 1988). Resolution of the issue awaits further evidence.

### Adaptive Value of Secure Attachment

Because, in ordinary circumstances, a majority of infants show secure attachments and because insecure attachments are associated with a somewhat increased risk of later psychopathology, there has been a tendency to assume that only secure attachment is normal and that it is fundamentally more adaptive in a biological sense. This represents a misunderstanding of biology, as Hinde (1982) has noted. As he commented, mothers and babies will be programmed by evolution to form a range of possible relationships that vary according to circumstances. Natural selection will tend to favour individuals with a range of potential styles, rather than those with just one style. Statistical considerations point to the same conclusion. Although secure attachments predominate in most general population samples, they are far from universal. In American samples, they average about 60% (Campos et al., 1983). It would not seem sensible to regard 40% of infants as showing biologically abnormal development. Moreover, further research is needed to determine the extent to which attachment insecurity constitutes a diagnosis-specific or general risk factor, and to delineate the mechanisms involved. The category of insecure attachment cannot be equated with psychopathology or disorder (Belsky & Nezworski, 1988).

### Disorders of Attachment

Nevertheless, there are disorders in which abnormalities in attachment features seem to constitute the predominant characteristics (Sameroff & Emde, 1989; Zeanah & Emde, 1994). Both DSM-IV (American Psychiatric Association, 1994) and ICD-10 (World Health Organization, 1992) include attachment disorders of childhood in their classification systems. Systematic evidence on these attachment disorders is distinctly limited but it appears that they may take two main forms. First, there is a variety that tends to be associated with parental abuse or neglect. There is a combination of strongly contradictory or ambivalent social responses that may be most evident at times of partings and reunions; there is emotional disturbance as evident in misery or lack of emotional responsiveness or withdrawal or aggression; and there may be fearfulness and hyper-vigilance. Second, there is a pattern that is more commonly associated with an institutional upbringing in which the children show an unusual degree of diffuseness in selective attachment during the preschool years accompanied by generally clinging behaviour in infancy and indiscriminantly friendly, attention seeking behaviour in early or middle childhood. Usually there is difficulty in forming close confiding relationships with peers. There is no doubt that these patterns occur, but Richters and Volkmar (1994) have pointed to the fact that the disorders extend beyond attachment qualities and they raise queries as to whether it is helpful to put the diagnosis in terms of a disorder of attachment *per se*.

In addition to these two postulated attachment disorders, researchers have sought to apply attachment concepts to conduct problems (Greenberg & Speltz, 1988; Greenberg, Speltz & DeKlyen, 1993; Waters, Posada,

Crowell & Keng-Ling, 1993), to patterns of social withdrawal (Rubin & Lollis, 1988), and to borderline personality disorders (Patrick, Hobson, Castle, Howard & Maughan, 1994), as well as to a range of other conditions (Parkes et al., 1991). The ideas are provocative and heuristically useful in focusing attention on the possible role of underlying relationship disturbances in conditions apparently characterized by quite different phenomonology (such as delinquent acts or depression). Further research will be needed to show how far attachment concepts are useful in gaining a better understanding of the mechanisms involved in the genesis of these disorders.

## CLINICAL IMPLICATIONS OF ATTACHMENT THEORY AND FINDINGS

Let me conclude by seeking to draw together the ideas and findings that I have reviewed in order to draw inferences about the clinical implications of attachment concepts and findings.

### *Psychoanalytic Theories of Development*

Perhaps the first implication to note is that the findings decisively reject the traditional psychoanalytic theory of development as put forward by either Freud or Klein. At first sight, that may seem a curious inference to make because in the first volume of the attachment trilogy, Bowlby stated that his frame of reference had been that of psychoanalysis and that his own early thinking on attachment had been inspired by psychoanalytic work. Also, Sroufe (1986) argued that attachment concepts had done much to advance psychoanalytic theory. Bowlby's own view, as expressed in his later papers (Bowlby, 1988) was quite different. He stated firmly that "although psychoanalysis is avowedly a developmental discipline it is nowhere weaker, I believe, than in its concepts of developmental" (p. 66). He went on to maintain that attachment theory differed fundamentally from psychoanalytic theory in its rejection of the model of development in which an individual is held to pass through a series of stages in any one of which he may become fixated or to which he may regress. He also rejected the psychoanalytic idea that emotional bonds were derivative from drives based on food or sex. He concluded that systematic and sensitive studies of human infants have rendered the psychoanalytic model of development "untenable". If the evidence requires a rejection of the psychoanalytic postulates of drive, of psychosexual stages, and of fixation and regression, there would seem to be little point in persisting with the fiction that psychoanalysis offers any useful understanding of developmental processes. It is time that the theory was given a respectful burial, but dismissed with respect to its contemporaneous value.[3]

The respect should be given, however, because historically psychoanalysis was very important. Bowlby was right in giving it credit for its role in the origins of attachment theory. Thus, it was important in suggesting a focus on relationships, despite the fact that it was hopelessly wrong in the mechanisms proposed for their development. It was also important in pointing to the role of early childhood features (although wrong in giving precedence to fantasies over life experiences—see also Stern, 1989). The focus on early life was also explicit in ethology (which played an even greater role in the development of attachment theory). But, in keeping with research findings, Bowlby in his later writings, placed a much greater emphasis on the role of later, as well as earlier experiences, and on the complex ways in which early adversities have indirect effects because of the tendency for one adversity to increase the likelihood of occurrence of another. Psychoanalytic theory was also important in its emphasis on the central role of mental mechanisms. Bowlby very firmly rejected the psychoanalytic view that childhood experiences were of only secondary importance (and the evidence supports that rejection) but he did not accept that the cognitive processing of experiences played a key role in their effects. Of course, that notion is by no means confined to psychoanalysis. For example, Kagan (1984) emphasized the same process (i.e. cognitive processing) on entirely different grounds, and internal working models are a central feature of cognitive-behavioural therapies (Beck, Rush, Shaw & Emery, 1979; Robins & Hayes, 1993; Teasdale, 1993). Although it is important not to throw out the baby with the bathwater, there is an awful lot of psychoanalytic water that needs to go down the plughole and we

---

[3] Bowlby (1988) was far from alone in considering that psychoanalytic concepts of development require radical revision (see, e.g. Emde, 1992; Zeanah, Anders, Seifer & Stern, 1989). Psychoanalysts are prone to claim that psychoanalysis paved the way in pointing to the importance of early experiences but as various reviewers have noted (see, e.g. Emde, 1992; Holmes, 1993a, b; Stern, 1989) the reverse is the case. Many Kleinian analysts still argue that object relations derive from the ontogeny of fantasy life and not from actual interactions in the family. Of course, that would not be true of most post-Freudian psychoanalytic conceptualizations. Various psychoanalytic writers (e.g. Dare, 1985, Shapiro & Esman, 1992; Wallerstein, 1988) have rightly pointed to the plurality of psychoanalystic theories, some of which are not reliant on the traditional concepts as expressed by either Freud or Klein. Nevertheless, as Wallerstein (1988) noted, the current theories do not agree on the processes involved in development (there is greater consistency on some of the key clinical concepts). Moreover, accounts of psychoanalytic views on development, in major psychiatric textbooks (e.g. Kaplan, Sadrock & Grebb, 1994), in developmental text books (Miller, 1993) and in books for a wider public (Wolff, 1981, 1989) continue to refer to the outmoded concepts listed here.

also need to appreciate that psychoanalysis is only one of the parents of the baby and that the growing infant differs in very important ways from its progenitors.

## Patterns of Residential Care for Children

The most immediate, and obvious, impact of attachment concepts was on patterns of residential care for children. Children's wards in hospitals began to allow parents to visit on a more regular basis, and to stay overnight when children were young; and there was a turning away from large institutional orphanages providing caregiving on a group basis with multiple rotating caregivers. All is not well in patterns of residential care but undoubtedly there is now a much better appreciation of children's needs. At first, there was an unfortunate emphasis on the trauma of separations so that some residential staff sought to avoid forming relationships with the children so that they would not be so upset when the staff had to change. It is now appreciated that that is not the main concern. Separations may indeed be stressful (Rutter, 1979) but the lack of an opportunity to form selective attachments is likely to be more damaging (Rutter, 1981). There is also a recognition of the need to provide continuity in caregiving for young children. Nevertheless, the problem of how to provide that is very far from solved. It is still usual in many residential nurseries for children to experience an extraordinarily large number of caregivers. In Tizard's studies (Tizard, 1977) for example, the children experienced over 50 caregivers during the preschool years.

## Provision of Child Care

It might be thought attachment concepts should have their most direct application in the field of child care, but their application here has not been free of difficulties. At first, a misleadingly concrete application of the notion of monotropy (which in itself turned out to be partially mistaken) led to recommendations that mothers should not go out to work and that all forms of group day care were necessarily harmful. It is now clear that these recommendations were misplaced (Rutter, 1991; Schaffer, 1990). Human societies have always involved several adults caring for children, as reflected in the title of Emmy Werner's (1984) excellent book "Child care; kith, kin and hired hands". Nevertheless, attachment ideas have been important in indicating some of the features that make for quality in child care and also in pointing to the importance of consistency in day care arrangements. Children cope well with having several adults look after them pro-

vided that it is the same adults over time and provided that the individuals
with whom they have a secure attachment relationship are available at
times when they are tired, distressed or facing challenging circumstances.
That much would be generally accepted. What is less clear is the extent to
which the considerations that apply to the main caregivers also apply to
subsidiary caregivers. Consistency in caregiving is clearly important but
does it have the same importance with respect to help with caregiving when
one or other of the parents constitutes the main caregiver? A satisfactory
answer to that question is not yet available.

### Assessment of Parenting

Attachment concepts, and the features involved in the use of the Strange
Situation, have been very helpful in alerting clinicians on how to assess
children's relationships with their caregivers at a time when decisions are
needed about possible child abuse, about foster placements, and about
adoption. We are now aware that just because children cling to someone
when they are stressed does not necessarily mean that they have a secure
relationship with them. It has also become apparent that separations, and
especially reunions, provide a good opportunity to assess relationships and
that we need to focus rather more on the children's use of parental presence
to have the confidence to explore than on the level of distress at the time of
separation. It has also been helpful to appreciate the difficulties experienced by young children when having to change parents in the first few
years of life, although it has been important to appreciate that they can form
new selective attachments at that age. Nevertheless, three caveats are
needed. First, as noted already, the Strange Situation itself does not constitute a diagnostic tool and the assessment of selective attachments in
older children is less straightforward than it is with infants. Second, the
original notion that children could not form initial selective attachments
after the supposed sensitive period of the first two years has proved mistaken. Hence, late adoption may be more beneficial than was once thought
(although clearly there should be a general policy of "the earlier the better"). Third, the degree of commitment of the adoptive parents seems an
important factor in success and also it is helpful for parents to have an
awareness of the types of problems that may constitute sequelae of early
adverse attachment experiences. A recognition that these need to be understood in relationship terms (see Sameroll & Emde, 1989) and not just as
signs of "naughtiness" is important.

One specific issue concerns decisions on how and when children need
to be removed from their biological parents when they are being abused or

neglected. All would accept that it is extraordinarily difficult to decide when the qualities of parental care are so bad that it is necessary to remove the child. Considerations of parent-child relationships are important but it is clear that considerations concerning safety, security and the adequacy of care are also crucial. Appreciation of the difficulties of providing all that is needed in good parenting in conditions of foster care and residential care need to be taken into account. Nevertheless, what is important is attention to the child's relationships with those who constitute his social family and not concern with some hypothetical "blood bond".

### *Parental Divorce and Family Break-up*

Early writings on the risks associated with parental divorce and family break-up focused on the role of "loss" because that had received such an emphasis in early writings on attachment. Empirical findings have made clear, however, that the main risks do not stem from loss as such but rather from the discordant and disrupted relationships that tend to precede or follow the loss. That is so with respect to risks in childhood (Block, Block & Gjerde, 1986; Cherlin et al., 1991; Rutter, 1994) and it is so with longer term risks in relation to vulnerability to depressive disorders in adult life (Harris, Brown & Bifulco, 1986; Kendler, Neale, Kessler, Heath & Eaves, 1992). These findings are, of course, entirely in line with attachment concepts. The problem lay in taking the notion of loss out of context and giving it a greater emphasis than it warranted. Loss is a risk indicator but it is not the major player in most risk mechanisms. The distinction is an important one and applies widely in the difficulties of moving from statistical associations to recommendations on policy and practice (Rutter, 1994).

### *"Maternal Bonding" to Infants*

One of the more unfortunate misapplications of attachment theory came with Klaus & Kennell's (1976) claim that mothers "bonded" with their babies during a critical period in the first few days of life and that skin to skin contact was necessary for this to take place. The empirical evidence in support of this suggestion was always weak and it did not reflect a proper understanding of attachment processes. A mother's relationship with her child is not the same thing as a child's initial selective attachments and in neither case are they dependent on a single sensory modality operating over a short time period. Kennell & Klaus (1984) in line with numerous others (Goldberg, 1983; Sluckin, Herbert & Sluckin, 1983), have now accepted that parental relationships develop over time and that there is more than one route involved. The simplistic "superglue" notion of maternal bonding has fortunately passed into oblivion. Nevertheless, it is necessary that we do not lose sight of the various important factors that may foster and facilitate the development of parents' relationships with their babies (Rutter, 1989; Rutter & Rutter, 1993).

### Psychotherapy

Thoughtful psychotherapists have sought to consider how psychotherapy may be improved by attention to attachment concepts (Holmes, 1993a, b). There is, as yet, no general agreement on the psychotherapeutic implications of attachment concepts but certain possible implications may be suggested. On the positive side, an attention to real life experiences, and not just fantasies about them, is obviously important. Equally, however, the cognitive models about such experiences and the mental models of relationships, need to be a focus. The chief shift from a traditional psychoanalytic position lies, perhaps, in attention to interpersonal, as distinct from intrapersonal, defences. Obviously, too, a recognition of the importance of the factors involved in good relationships is crucial and Holmes (1993a) suggested that this applies to the therapeutic relationships as well as to other relationships. On the negative side, as already discussed, it is important to put aside a misguided reliance on psychosexual stages and on notions of fixation and regression. These suggestions are closely related to those put forward by the psychoanalyst Peter Lomas (1987) in his book "The Limits of Interpretation: What's Wrong with Psychoanalysis?". He pointed to what he called the "dreadful, pessimistic and bizarre Freudian notion of primary narcissim" and argued that it was encouraging that psychotherapists were moving, however painfully and gradually, towards a less mechanistic idea of infantile experiences and to a greater appreciation of the importance of loving relationships. Although he was careful to note the differences between good parenting and good psychotherapy, he suggested that both need to be based on mutual warmth, respect and trust and that an undue reliance on the uninvolved, dispassionate interpretation of defences may not constitute the best way forward.

### Disorders of Attachment

Finally, it is necessary to consider the implications for psychopathological disorders. I have already noted the importance of attachment theory in drawing attention to disorders primarily characterized by abnormalities in selective attachment—so-called "reactive attachment disorders". However, three cautions are necessary. First, it is most unfortunate that DSM-IV

(American Psychiatric Association, 1994) has chosen to specify pathogenic child care as one of the diagnostic criteria. It is true that the condition came to notice in circumstances of abnormal care but the evidence is not yet available for decisions on whether the same behavioural pattern can be found in the absence of gross neglect or abuse. Second, as Richters and Volkmar (1994) pointed out, the syndrome includes a variety of psychopathological features that seem to extend well outside the bounds of an abnormality in selective attachment. Third, great care needs to be taken in the assessment of attachment qualities in children from unusual backgrounds and/or in which they have psychopathological or physical disorders (Main & Solomon, 1990; Vaughn et al., 1994). This is especially so with respect to use of the Strange Situation. Clinicians need to be aware of the necessity of not basing assessments of relationships on this one procedure, despite its many strengths. A wider range of interview and observational data are needed.

Attachment concepts have also been important in alerting clinicians to the possible role of relationship difficulties in a wider range of psychopathological disorders, but perhaps especially conduct disorders (Greenberg & Speltz, 1988; Greenberg et al., 1993), antisocial and borderline personality disorders (Patrick et al., 1994; Quinton, Pickles, Maughan & Rutter, 1993; Zoccolillo, Pickles, Quinton & Rutter, 1992) and social withdrawal (Rubin & Lollis, 1988). This fits in with the empirical evidence of the importance of poor peer relations in psychopathological disorders (Asher, Erdley & Gabriel 1994; Parker & Asher, 1987). Clearly, in some cases, abnormalities in early selective attachments with parents have played a role in etiology. Once again, however, a caution is necessary. As both Sameroff and Emde (1989) and Dunn (1993) have emphasized, attachment is not the whole of relationships and we still have much to learn about the interconnections between parent-child relationships, peer relationships, sibling relationships, and sexual relationships in adult life. Attachment concepts are clearly useful in thinking about relationship disturbances but it is important that we should not be unduly constrained by thinking only in attachment terms.

It would be reasonable to suppose that an understanding of the role of attachment difficulties in psychopathology should have implications for therapeutic interventions. It may be accepted that there are such implications but what is much less clear is just how attachment concepts should shape treatment (see Belsky & Nezworski, 1988; Sameroff & Emde, 1989, Zeanah & Emde, 1994). It is necessary that we take seriously the need to develop therapeutic approaches that build on what is known about the role of attachment disturbances but, equally it is important that we do not obtain premature closure on treatment strategies.

## CONCLUSIONS

In looking back on the 50 years since Bowlby's paper on the 44 thieves, and the 25 years since the first volume of his trilogy on attachment, it is obvious that the field has changed out of all recognition. From the early days when he was criticised by academic psychologists and ostracised by the psychoanalytic establishment, attachment concepts have become generally accepted. That they have become so, is a tribute to the creativity and perceptiveness of Bowlby's original formulations and to the major conceptual and methodological contributions of Ainsworth. It is also a function, however, of Bowlby's willingness to respond to empirical findings by modifying attachment concepts when research data indicated that changes were necessary. Inevitably, there have been instances in which attachment concepts have been overgeneralized or misinterpreted in a naive and simplistic fashion. That is unavoidable when presented with ideas that are intellectually provocative and so obviously relevant to public policy and clinical practice. As I have sought to indicate, we are very far from having reached an understanding of the development of relationships or of the ways in which distortions in relationships play a role in psychopathology. Attachment theory has been hugely helpful in bringing about progress in both areas and doubtless it will continue to do so in the future. But, if knowledge is to advance in the way that we all hope that it will, it will be necessary that we pay attention to one of the first features of attachment theory, namely that attachment is not the whole of relationships. What is needed now is a bringing together of attachment concepts and other formulations of relationships so that each may profit from the contributions of the other.

## REFERENCES

Ainsworth, M. D. S (1967). *Infancy in Uganda: infant care and the growth of love* Baltimore, MD: Johns Hopkins Press.

Ainsworth, M. D. S., Blehar, M. C., Waters, E. & Wall, S. (1978). *Patterns of attachment: a psychological study of the strange situation.* Hillsdale, NJ: Erlbaum Associates.

American Psychiatric Association (1994). *DSM-IV: diagnostic and statistical manual of mental disorders, Fourth Edition.* Washington, DC: American Psychiatric Association.

Asher, S., Erdley, C. A. & Gabriel, S. W. (1994). Peer relations. In M. Rutter & D. Hay (Eds), *Development through life: a handbook for clinicians* (pp. 456–487). Oxford: Blackwell Scientific Publications.

Aviezer, O., Van IJzendoorn, M. H., Sagi, A. & Schuengel, C. (1994). "Children of the dream" revisited: 70 years of collective early child care in Israeli kibbutzim. *Psychological Bulletin, 116*, 99–116.

Beck, A. T., Rush, A., Shaw, B. & Emery, G. (1979). *Cognitive therapy of depression.* New York: Guilford Press.

Belsky, J. & Cassidy, J. (1994). Attachment: theory and evidence. In M. Rutter & D. Hay (Eds), *Development through life: a handbook for clinicians* (pp. 373–402). Oxford: Blackwell Scientific Publications.

Belsky, J. & Isabella, R. (1988). Maternal, infant, and social-contextual determinants of attachment security. In J. Belsky & T. Nezworski (Eds), *Clinical implications of attachment* (pp. 41–94) Hillsdale, NJ: Erlbaum Associates.

Belsky, J. & Nezworski, T. (Eds), (1988). *Clinical implications of attachment.* Hillsdale, NJ: Erlbaum Associates.

Belsky, J & Rovine, M. J. (1988). Nonmaternal care in the first year of life and the security of infant-parent attachment. *Child Development, 59*, 157–167.

Block, J. H., Block, J. & Gjerde, P. F. (1986). The penalty of children prior to divorce: a prospective study. *Child Development, 57*, 827–840.

Bowlby, J. (1944). Forty-four juvenile thieves: their characters and home life *International Journal of Psycho-Analysis, 25*, 19–52.

Bowlby, J. (1951). *Maternal care and mental health.* WHO Monograph Series, No. 2. Geneva: World Health Organization.

Bowlby, J. (1969). *Attachment and loss, Vol. 1. Attachment* (2nd ed., 1982). New York: Basic Books.

Bowlby, J. (1973). *Attachment and loss, Vol 2. Separation, anxiety and anger.* London: Hogarth Press.

Bowlby, J. (1980). *Attachment and loss, Vol. 3 Loss, sadness and depression.* London: Hogarth Press.

Bowlby, J. (1988). *A secure base: clinical implications of attachment theory.* London: Routledge & Kegan Paul.

Bretherton, I. (1987). New perspective on attachment relations: security, communication, and internal working models. In J. D. Osofsky (Ed), *Handbook of infant development* 2nd edn (pp. 1061–1100). Chichester: Wiley.

Bretherton, I. (1990). Open communication and internal working models: their role in the development of attachment relationships. In R. A. Thompson (Ed), *Nebraska symposium on motivation, vol. 36. Socioemotional development* (pp. 57–113). Lincoln: University of Nebraska Press.

Bretherton, I. & Waters, E. (Eds), (1985). Growing points of attachment theory and research. *Monographs of the Society for Research in Child Development 50*, Serial No. 209, No. 1–2.

Campos, J. J., Barrett, K., Lamb, M. E., Goldsmith, H. H. & Stenberg, C. (1983). Socioemotional development. In M. M. Haith & J. J. Campos (Eds), *Infancy and developmental psychobiology, Vol. 2. Mussen handbook of child psychology* 4th edn (pp. 783–915). New York: Wiley.

Capps, L., Sigman, M. & Mundy, P. (1994). Attachment security in children with autism. *Developmental and Psychopathology, 6,* 249–261.

Casler, L. (1968). Perceptual deprivation in institutional settings. In G. Newton & S. Levine (Eds), *Early experience and behaviour.* Springfield, IL: Chas C. Thomas.

Cherlin, A J, Furstenberg, Jr, F. F. Chase-Lansdale, P. L., Kiernan. K. E. Robins, P. K., Morrison, D. R. & Teitler, J. O. (1991). Longitudinal studies of effects of divorce on children in Great Britain and the United States. *Science, 252,* 1386–1389.

Clarke-Stewart, K. A. (1978). And daddy makes three: the father's impact on mother and young child. *Child Development, 49,* 466–478.

Clarke-Stewart, K. A. (1989). Infant daycare: malignant or maligned? *American Psychologist, 44,* 266–274.

Corter, C., Abramovitch, R. & Pepler, D. (1983) The role of the mother in sibling interactions. *Child Development, 54,* 1599–1605.

Crittenden, P. M (1988) Relationships as risk. In J. Belsky & T. Nezworski (Eds), *Clinical implications of attachment* (pp. 136–174). Hillsdale. NJ: Erlbaum Associates.

Dare, C. (1985). Psychoanalytic theories of development. In M. Rutter & L. Hersov (Eds), *Child and adolescent psychiatry: modern approaches* 2nd edn (pp. 204–215). Oxford: Blackwell Scientific Publications.

Dunn, J. (1988). *The beginnings of social understanding.* Cambridge, MA: Harvard University Press.

Dunn, J. (1993) *Young children's close relationships beyond attachment.* Individual Differences and Development Series, Vol 4. Newbury Park, CA: Sage.

Dunn, J. & Kendrick, C. (1982). *Siblings, love, envy and understanding.* Cambridge, MA: Harvard University Press.

Emde, R. N. (1992) Individual meaning and increasing complexity: Contributions of Sigmund Freud and René Spitz to developmental psychology. *Developmental Psychology, 28,* 347–359.

Engfer, A. (1988). The interrelatedness of marriage and the mother-child relationship. In R. A. Hinde & J. Stevenson-Hinde (Eds), *Relationships within families: mutual influences* (pp. 104–118). Oxford: Clarendon Press.

Fonagy, P., Steele, H & Steele, M. (1991). Maternal representations of attachment during pregnancy predict the organization of infant-mother attachment at one year of age. *Child Development, 62,* 891–905.

Fonagy, P., Steele, M., Steele, H., Higgitt, A. & Target, M. (1994). The Emanuel Miller Memorial Lecture 1992. The theory and practice of resilience. *Journal of Child Psychology and Psychiatry, 35,* 231–257.

Fox, N A., Kimmerly, N I., & Schafer, W D. (1991) Attachment to mother/attachment to father. A meta-anaylsis. *Child Development, 62,* 210–255.

Goldberg, S. (1983). Parent-infant bonding: another look. *Child Development, 54*, 1355–1382.

Greenberg, M. T, Cicchetti, D. & Cummings, M. (Eds), (1990). *Attachment in the preschool years theory, research and intervention.* Chicago: University of Chicago Press.

Greenberg, M. T. & Speltz, M. L. (1988). Attachment and the ontogeny of conduct problems. In J. Belsky & T. Nezworski (Eds), *Clinical implications of attachment* (pp. 177–218). Hillsdale, NJ: Erlbaum Associates.

Greenberg, M. T., Speltz, M. L. & DeKlyen, M. (1993). The role of attachment in the early development of disruptive behaviour problems. *Development and Psychopathology, 5*, 191–213.

Grosskurth, P. (1986). *Melanie Klem. her world and her work.* London: Hodder & Stoughton.

Harris, T., Brown, G. W. & Bifulco, A. (1986) Loss of parent in childhood and adult psychiatric disorder the role of lack of adequate parental care. *Psychological Medicine, 16*, 641–659.

Harlow, H. F. & Harlow, M. K. (1969). Effects of various mother-infant relationships on rhesus monkey behaviours. In B. M. Foss (Ed.) *Determinants of infant behaviour* Vol 4 (pp. 15–36) London: Methuen.

Hazan, C. & Shaver, P. R. (1994). Attachment as an organizational framework for research on close relationships. *Psychological Inquiry, 5*, 1–22.

Hinde, R A. (1976). Interactions, relationships and social structure. *Man, 11*, 1–17.

Hinde, R A (1979). *Towards understanding relationships.* London: Academic Press.

Hinde, R. A. (1982). *Ethology* Oxford: Oxford University Press.

Hinde, R. A. (1988). Continuities and discontinuities. Conceptual issues and methodological considerations. In M. Rutter (Ed), *Studies of psychosocial risk the power of longitudinal data* (pp. 367–383). Cambridge: Cambridge University Press.

Hinde, R. & Stevenson-Hinde, J. (Eds), (1988). *Relationships within families: mutual influences.* Oxford: Clarendon Press.

Hodges, J. & Tizard, B. (1989a). IQ and behavioural adjustment of ex-institutional adolescents. *Journal of Child Psychology and Psychiatry, 30*, 53–75.

Hodges, J. & Tizard, B. (1989b). Social and family relationships of ex-institutional adolescents. *Journal of Child Psychology and Psychiatry, 30*, 77–97.

Holmes, J. (1993a). Attachment theory: a biological basis for psychotherapy? *The British Journal of Psychiatry, 163*, 403–438.

Holmes, J. (1993b). *John Bowlby and attachment theory.* London/New York: Routledge.

Howes, C., Rodning. C., Galluzzo, D. C. & Myers, L. (1988). Attachment and child care: relationships with mother and caregiver *Early Childhood Research Quarterly, 3*, 403–416.

Kagan, J. (1984) *The nature of the child.* New York: Basic Books.

Kaplan, H. I., Sadock, B J. & Grebb, J. A. (1994). *Kaplan and Sadock's synopsis of psychiatry*, 7th edn. Baltimore, MD: Williams and Wilkins.

Kendler, K. S., Neale, M. C., Kessler, R. C., Heath. A. C. & Eaves, L. J. (1992). Childhood parental loss and adult psychopathology in women: a twin study perspective. *Archives of General Psychiatry, 49*, 109–116.

Kennell, J. H. & Klaus, M. H. (1984). Mother-infant bonding: weighing the evidence. *Developmental Review, 4*, 275–282.

Klaus, M. H. & Kennell, J. H. (1976). *Maternal-infant bonding: the impact of early separation or loss on family development*. Saint Louis, MO: C. V. Mosby.

Kobak, R. (1994). Adult attachment: A personality or relationship construct? *Psychological Inquiry, 5*, 42–44.

Kraemer, G. W. (1992). A psychobiological theory of attachment. *Behavioral and Brain Sciences, 15*, 493–541.

Lamb, M. E., Thompson, R A., Gardner, W., Charnov, E L & Estes, D. (1984). Security of infantile attachment as assessed in the "Strange Situation": its study and biological interpretations. *Behavioral and Brain Sciences, 7*, 127–147.

Levine, S. (1982). Comparative and psychobiological perspectives on development. In W. A. Collins (Ed.), *The concept of development. The Minnesota Symposia on Child Psychology* Vol. 15 (pp. 29–63). Hillsdale, NJ: Erlbaum Associates.

Lomas, P. (1987). *The limits of interpretation: what's wrong with psychoanalysis?* Harmondsworth, Middlesex: Penguin.

Maccoby, E. & Masters, J. C (1970). Attachment and dependency. In P. H. Mussen (Ed.), *Carmichael's manual of child psychology* Vol 2, 3rd edn (pp. 73–157). New York: Wiley.

Main, M. (1991) Metacognitive knowledge, metacognitive monitoring and singular (coherent) vs multiple (incoherent) models of attachment findings and directions for future research. In Parkes C., Stevenson-Hinde J. & Morris P. (Eds), *Attachment across the life cycle*. London: Tavistock, Routledge Press.

Main, M. & Hesse, E. (1990). Parents' unresolved traumatic experiences are related to infants in disorganized attachment status: is frightened and/or frightening parental behavior the linking mechanism? In M. T. Greenberg, D. Cicchetti & E. M. Cummings (Eds), *Attachment in the preschool years theory, research and intervention* (pp. 161–184) Chicago. IL: University of Chicago Press.

Main, M., Kaplan, N. & Cassidy, J. (1985) Security in infancy, childhood and adulthood: A move to the level of representation. In I. Bretherton & E. Waters (Eds), Growing points of attachment theory and research. *Monographs of the Society for Research in Child Development. 50*, Serial No. 209, 66–104.

Main, M. & Solomon, J. (1990) Procedures for identifying disorganized/disoriented infants in the Ainsworth Strange Situation. In M. T. Greenberg, D. Cicchetu & E. M. Cummings (Eds), *Attachment in the preschool years, theory, research and intervention* (pp. 121–160). Chicago: University of Chicago Press.

McCartney, K. & Galanopoulos. A. (1988). Child care and attachment: a new frontier the second time around. *American Journal of Orthopsychiatry, 58*, 16–24.

Miller, P. (1993) *Theories of developmental psychology* 3rd edn. New York. W. H. Freeman.

Miyake, K. Chen, S. & Campos, J. J. (1985) Infant temperament, mother's mode of interaction and attachment in Japan: an interim report. In I. Bretherton & E. Waters (Eds), Growing points of attachment theory and research. *Monographs of the Society for Research in Child Development, 50*, Serial no. 209, 276–297.

Nash, A. (1988). Ontogeny, phylogeny and relationships. In S. W. Duck (Ed.), *Handbook of personal relationships* (pp. 121–141). Chichester: Wiley.

O'Connor, N & Franks, C. M. (1960). Childhood upbringing and other environmental factors. In H. J. Eysenck (Ed.), *Handbook of abnormal psychology*. London: Pitman.

Oppenheim, D., Sagi, A. & Lamb, M. (1988). Infant-adult attachments on the kibbutz and their relation to socio-emotional development four years later. *Developmental Psychology, 24*, 427–433.

Parker, J. G. & Asher, S. R. (1987) Peer relations and later personal adjustment: are low-accepted children at risk? *Psychological Bulletin, 102*, 357–389.

Parkes, C. M., Stevenson-Hinde, J. & Morris, P. (Eds), (1991). *Attachment across the life cycle*. London: Tavistock/Routledge.

Patrick, M., Hobson, P., Castle, D., Howard, R. & Maughan, B. (1994). Personality disorder and the mental representatives of early social experience. *Development and Psychopathology, 6*, 375–388.

Quinton, D., Pickles, A., Maughan, B. & Rutter, M. (1993). Partners, peers, and pathways: assortative pairing and continuities in conduct disorder. *Development and Psychopathology, 5*, 763–783.

Radke-Yarrow, M., Cummings, E. M., Kuczynski, I., & Chapman, M. (1985). Patterns of attachment in two-and three-year-old normal families with parental depression. *Child Development, 56*, 884–893.

Rajecki, D. W., Lamb, M. E. & Obmascher, P. (1978) Toward a general theory of infantile attachment: a comparative review of aspects of the social bond. *Brain and Behavioral Sciences, 1*, 417–436.

Richters, M. M. & Volkmar, F. R. (1994). Case study: reactive attachment disorder of infancy or early childhood. *Journal of the American Academy of Child and Adolescent Psychiatry, 33*, 328–332.

Robins, C. J. & Hayes, A. M. (1993). An appraisal of cognitive therapy. *Journal of Consulting and Clinical Psychology, 61*, 205–214.

Rogers, S. J., Ozonoff, S. & Maslin-Cole. C. (1991). A comparative study of attachment behavior in young children with autism or other psychiatric disorders. *Journal of the American Academy of Child and Adolescent Psychiatry, 30*, 483–488.

Rubin, K. H. & Lollis, S. P. (1988) Origins and consequences of social withdrawal. In J. Belsky & T. Nezworski (Eds), *Clinical implications of attachment* (pp. 219–252). Hillsdale: NJ: Erlbaum Associates.

Rutter, M. (1979). Separation experiences: a new look at old topic. *Journal of Pediatrics, 95*, 147–154.

Rutter, M. (1980). Attachment and the development of social relationships. In M. Rutter (Ed.), *Developmental psychiatry* (pp. 267–279). Washington, DC: American Psychiatric Press.

Rutter, M. (1981). *Maternal deprivation reassessed* 2nd edn. Harmondsworth, Middlesex: Penguin.

Rutter, M. (1989). Intergenerational continuities and discontinuities in serious parenting difficulties. In D. Cicchetti & V. Carlson (Eds), *Child maltreatment* (pp. 317–348). New York: Cambridge University Press.

Rutter, M. (1991) A fresh look at "maternal deprivation". In P. Bateson (Ed), *The development and integration of behaviour* (pp. 331–374). Cambridge: Cambridge University Press.

Rutter, M. (1994). Family discord and conduct disorder: cause, consequence or correlate? *Journal of Family Psychology, 8,* 170–186.

Rutter, M. (1994). Beyond longitudinal data, causes, consequences, changes and continuity, *Journal of Consulting and Clinical Psychology.*

Rutter, M. & Rutter, M. (1993). *Developing minds: challenges and continuities across the lifespan.* Harmondsworth, Middlesex: Penguin, New York: Basic Books.

Sameroff, A. J. & Emde, R. N. (Eds), (1989). *Relationship disturbances in early childhood: a developmental approach.* New York: Basic Books.

Schaffer, H. R. (1990). *Making decisions about children: psychological questions and answers.* Oxford: Basil Blackwell.

Shapiro, T. & Esman, A. (1992) Psychoanalysis and child and adolescent psychiatry. *Journal of the American Academy of Child and Adolescent Psychiatry, 31,* 6–13.

Sigman, M. & Ungerer, J. (1984). Attachment behaviors in autistic children. *Journal of Autism and Developmental Disorders, 14,* 231–244.

Sluckin, W., Herbert, M. & Sluckin, A. (1983) *Maternal bounding.* Oxford: Blackwell Scientific.

Sroufe, L. A. (1983). Infant-caregiver attachment and patterns of adaptation in the preschool the roots of maladaptation and competence. In M. Perlmutter (Ed.), Development and policy concerning children with special needs. *Minnesota Symposia in Child Psychology* Vol. 16 (pp. 41–83). Hillsdale, NJ: Erlbaum Associates.

Sroufe, L. A. (1986). Bowlby's contribution to psychoanalytic theory and developmental psychology. *Journal of Child Psychology and Psychiatry, 27,* 841–849.

Sroufe, L. A. (1988). The role of infant-caregiver attachments in development. In J. Belsky & T. Nezworski (Eds), *Clinical implications of attachment* (pp. 18–38). Hillsdale, NJ: Erlbaum Associates.

Sroufe, L. A. & Fleeson, J. (1986). Attachment and the construction of relationships. In W. Hartup & Z. Rubin (Eds), *Relationships and development* (pp. 51–71). Hillsdale, NJ: Erlbaum Associates.

Sroufe, L. A., Fox, N. & Pancake, V. (1983) Attachment and dependency in developmental perspective. *Child Development, 55*, 17–29.

Sroufe, L. A. & Rutter, M. (1984). The domain of developmental psychopathology. *Child Development, 55*, 17–29.

Stern, D. N. (1985). *The interpersonal world of the infant: a view from psychoanalysis and developmental psychology*. New York: Basic Books.

Stern, D. N. (1989). The representation of relational patterns: Developmental considerations. In A. J. Sameroff & R. N. Emde (Eds), *Relationship disturbances in early childhood: a developmental approach* (pp. 52–68). New York: Basic Books.

Teasdale, J. (1993). Emotion and two kinds of meaning: therapy and applied cognitive science. *Behaviour Research and Therapy, 31*, 339–354.

Tizard, B. (1977). Varieties of residential nursery experience. In J. Tizard, I. Sinclair & R. V. G. Clark (Eds), *Varieties of residential experience* (pp. 102–121). London: Routledge & Kegan Paul.

Thompson, R. A., Connell, J. P. & Bridges, L. J. (1988). Temperament, emotion, and social interactive behavior in the strange situation: an analysis of attachment system functioning. *Child Development, 59*, 1102–1110.

Van den Boom, D. (1990). Preventive intervention and the quality of mother-infant interaction and infant exploration in irritable infants. In W. Koops et al. (Eds), *Development psychology behind the dikes* (pp. 249–270) Amsterdam Eburon.

Vaughn, B. E., Goldberg, S., Atkinson, I., Marcovitch, S., MacGregor, D. & Seifer, R. (1994). Quality of toddler-mother attachment in children with Down Syndrome: limits to interpretation of strange situation behavior. *Child Development, 65*, 95–108.

Vaughn, B. E., Stevenson-Hinde, J., Waters, E., Kotsaftis, A., Lefever, G. B., Shouldice, A., Trudel. M & Belsky, J. (1992) Attachment security and temperament in infancy and early childhood: some conceptual clarifications. *Development Psychology, 28*, 463–473.

Vaughn, B. E. & Waters, E. (1990). Attachment behavior at home and in the laboratory. *Child Development, 61*, 1965–1973.

Wallerstein, R. S. (1988) One psychoanalysis or many? *International Journal of Psychoanalysis, 69*, 5–21.

Waters, E., Posada. G., Crowell, J. & Keng-Ling, L. (1993). Is attachment theory ready to contribute to our understanding of disruptive behavior problems? *Development and Psychopathology, 5*, 215–225.

Werner, E. F. (1984). *Child care: kith, kin and hired hands*. Baltimore, MD: University Park.

Wolff, S. (1981). *Children under stress* 2nd edn. Harmondsworth, Middlesex: Penguin.

Wolff, S. (1989). *Childhood and human nature: the development of personality*. London/New York: Routledge.

World Health Organization (1992). *The ICD-10 classification of mental and behavioural disorders: clinical descriptions and diagnostic guidelines.* Geneva: World Health Organization.

World Health Organization Expert Committee on Mental Health (1951). *Report of the second session 1951* Geneva: WHO.

Zeanah, C H., Anders, T. F., Seifer, R. & Stern, D. M. (1989) Implications of research on infant development for psychodynamic theory and practice. *Journal of the American Academy of Child and Adolescent Psychiatry, 28,* 657–668.

Zeanah, C. H. & Emde, R. N. (1994) Attachment disorders in infancy and childhood. In M. Ruter, E. Taylor & I. Hersov (Eds), *Child and adolescent psychiatry modern approaches* 3rd edn (pp. 490–504). Oxford: Blackwell Scientific Publications.

Zigler, E. F. & Gordon, E. W. (Eds), (1982). *Day care: scientific and social policy issues.* Boston, MA: Auburn House.

Zoccolillo, M., Pickles, A., Quinton, D. & Rutter, M. (1992). The outcome of childhood conduct disorder: implications for defining adult personality disorder and conduct disorder. *Psychological Medicine, 22,* 971–986.

# 6

# Breaking the Intergenerational Cycle of Insecure Attachment: A Review of the Effects of Attachment-Based Interventions on Maternal Sensitivity and Infant Security

**Marinus H. van IJzendoorn, Femmie Juffer
and Marja G. C. Duyvesteyn**
*Center for Child and Family Systems, Leiden, The Netherlands*

*In this paper the effectiveness of preventive or therapeutic interventions aiming at enhancing parental sensitivity and children's attachment security is addressed. Sixteen pertinent studies have been reviewed, and 12 studies have been included in a quantitative meta-analysis (N = 869). Results show that interventions are more effective in changing parental insensitivity (d = .58) than in changing children's attachment insecurity (d = .17). Longer, more intensive, and therapeutic interventions appear to be less effective than short-term preventive interventions. Interventions which are effective at the behavioral level may not necessarily lead to changes in insecure mental representations of the parents involved. The implications of changes at the behavioral level (sensitivity; attachment) without accompanying changes at the representational level will be discussed.*

Reprinted with permission from the *Journal of Child Psychology and Psychiatry*, 1995, Vol. 36, No. 2, 225–248.

Preparation of this paper was supported by a PIONEER award of the Netherlands' Organization for Scientific Research to Marinus van IJzendoorn (NWO; grant no. PGS 59-256). The authors acknowledge the comments of Marian Bakermans-Kranenburg on an earlier draft of this paper.

## INTRODUCTION

In the past few decades attachment research has documented the causes and consequences of insecure infant-parent attachment in some detail. Several studies have shown that insecure attachment in infancy is associated with a higher risk of malfunctioning in the socio-emotional domain during the preschool years (Bretherton, 1985; Sroufe, 1988). Although insecure attachment cannot be considered 'pathological' *per se* (Van IJzendoorn & Bakermans-Kranenburg, in press), its status as a risk factor has urged researchers and clinicians to reflect on potentially preventive and corrective measures (Belsky & Nezworski, 1988). Recently, several intervention studies aiming at the prevention or the correction of insecure attachment have been performed, but their effectiveness appeared to be equivocal. One of the purposes of this review is to distill some uniform trend or estimate of the average effect from those studies.

The intervention studies are based on hypotheses about causal factors influencing the development of secure attachment. Many studies have shown that parental sensitivity has to be considered a key factor (Goldsmith & Alansky, 1987). Ainsworth and her colleagues (1978) defined sensitivity as the ability to accurately perceive and interpret the infants' attachment signals, and to respond to them promptly and adequately. A persistent lack of sensitivity and an inconsistent display of sensitivity were found to stimulate the development of an insecure bond between infant and parent. Furthermore, recent studies on the intergenerational transmission of attachment have shown that parental sensitivity and children's attachment were both associated with parents' mental representations of attachment, that is, their perception of their attachment biography (Main, Kaplan & Cassidy, 1985; Van IJzendoorn, in press). Insecure representations of attachment were found to be associated with insensitive responses to the infant's attachment signals, and with an insecure infant-parent attachment relationship. For intervention studies two—complementary—approaches to the problem of preventing or correcting the development of insecure attachments seem to be indicated: First, the intervention efforts may be directed at parental sensitivity, that is, at the behavioral level. Second, interventions may also focus on the parents' mental representations of attachment, that is, on the representational level, in order to pave the way for subsequent behavioral changes. In a simplified form, the model underlying most intervention studies is the following (Figure 1).

The two types of intervention—the behavioral and the representational approach—are different in design and focus. An example of the first approach is the Anisfeld, Casper, Nozyce and Cunningham (1990) study in

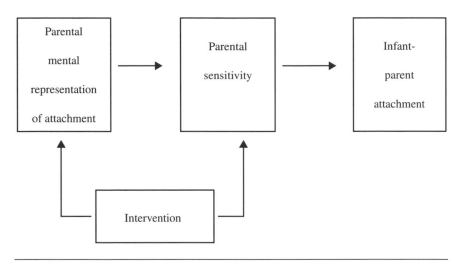

**Figure 1.** A model of interventions in attachment.

which mothers are provided with soft baby carriers to carry their babies during the first months in order to enhance the physical contact between parent and infant. The presupposition is that carrying the baby leads to prompt responses to attachment signals such as crying behavior, and thereby stimulates feelings of security in the infant. The second approach is often modeled after Fraiberg et al.'s (Fraiberg, Aldelson & Shapiro, 1975) infant-mother psychotherapy in which the parent is enabled to discuss her 'ghosts' of the past, that is, her childhood experiences with insecure attachments, and their influence on the interactions with the child. The intervention study of Lieberman, Weston and Pawl (1991) is an example of this approach. In weekly unstructured sessions at home the intervenors provided support and therapy for the mothers during a year, with the object of enhancing their empathy for the affective and developmental needs of their children.

Intervention studies aiming at attachment are extremely important, not only from an applied viewpoint but also from a theoretical perspective. By means of carefully designed intervention studies, empirical evidence for cause-effect relations might be found. Most research on attachment is correlational—cross-sectional or longitudinal—and it remains complicated to derive causation from correlation (Lamb, Thompson, Gardner & Charnov, 1985). In many studies the correlation between parental sensitivity and children's attachment on the one hand, and between parental attachment representations and children's attachment on the other hand, has been established; but even on the basis of longitudinal designs one can only speculate about causal relations and the absence of third factors (Van IJzendoorn, 1992). The manipulation of the alleged cause, e.g. sensitivity, and observation of predicted changes in the effect, e.g. attachment, constitute a much more direct way of confirming causal hypotheses. Against this background the intervention studies gain even more weight, and their evaluation is important as a test of some core issues in attachment theory.

Several issues and questions may be derived from the various approaches of the intervention studies. First, the intervention studies all focus on changing the quality of the infant-parent attachment relationship. Their object is to change insecure attachments into secure attachments, or to prevent insecure attachments from developing. The studies pursue this objective by influencing parental sensitivity or parental mental representations of attachment. An important question then is, whether a change of sensitivity or representation does indeed result in a change of infant attachment insecurity, and whether this latter change is comparable to the former in terms of effect size. Because the associations between sensitivity and attachment representations on the one hand, and between sensitivity and infant attachment security on the other hand are far from perfect, it may be hypothesized that intervention studies might more easily reach their proximal goal of changing sensitivity than their ultimate goal of changing attachment security. However, if intervention studies do influence sensitivity but if, at the same time, they do not result in similar changes in attachment security, some doubts about the causal relation between sensitivity and attachment would arise. In Figure 2 the possible results of intervention studies are presented.

In Figure 2 eight possible outcomes of intervention studies on attachment have been depicted. The possibilities (c) and (g) constitute falsifica-

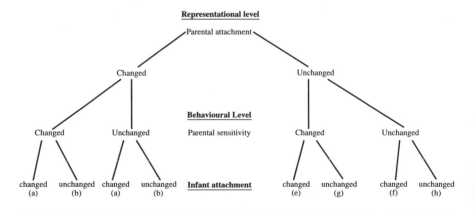

**Figure 2.** Hypothetical outcomes of intervention studies on attachment.

tions of the connection between sensitivity and attachment, because changes in sensitivity are not accompanied by changes in attachment security. Possibilities (d) and (h) mean that the interventions failed to reach their goal of changing infant-parent attachment although, in alternative (d), at least the parental representation of attachment was changed. Possibility (a) is of course the perfect outcome of any intervention study: the change of parental attachment representations is accompanied by a change of sensitivity which results in a changed attachment security. Alternative (b) would mean that changed attachment representations may effect changes in another behavioral domain than sensitivity, and through that channel influence the infant-parent attachment security. Elsewhere, we have shown that the concept of sensitivity cannot carry the whole weight of the intergenerational transmission of attachment, and that other aspects of the parent-child interactions must be responsible for part of the transmission ('the transmission gap', Van IJzendoorn, in press). In alternative (e) the intervention is effective on the behavioral level (sensitivity and attachment) but not on the representational level, and in alternative (f) the change in infant attachment cannot be explained on the basis of changes in parental representations or in sensitivity.

Most intervention studies included in this review do not report on changes in attachment representations. One of the most intriguing issues in this area, however, is the issue of generalizability: If the parent's sensitivity for the infant's attachment cues has been changed, how firmly is this change rooted in the parent's personality and how long will its influence last? It can be imagined that teaching a parent to be sensitive to the infant's attachment signals is effective in the short run, but that it does not generalise to the type of sensitivity required in a next phase of the infant's development. For example, a baby carrier is not useful for toddlers anymore, but they still might need (different kinds of) physical contact for which the intervention has provided no specific training. It may be hypothesized that outcome (e) is even counterproductive in that tensions are created between the parents' representations and their behavior, and in that the children's expectations of sensitive interactions with their parents may not be fulfilled at a later stage, e.g. in toddlerhood.

In this paper we will address the following issues: First, how effective are intervention studies on attachment on average? Is the effectiveness of intervention studies dependent on intervention characteristics such as duration and focus? Second, do intervention studies show similar effects on parental sensitivity as they do on infant-parent attachment security? We expect intervention studies to be somewhat more effective in the proximal domain of sensitive parental behavior. Third, how deeply rooted in personality are changes of sensitivity, that is, are changes at the behavioral level always accompanied by changes at the representational level or can there be a discrepancy which might restrict the generalizability of the changes?

To answer these questions we will review the extant literature, and perform a meta-analysis. The combination of a narrative review and a quantitative meta-analysis provides the most complete overview of the state of the art of intervention. In a narrative review we are able to describe idiosyncratic characteristics of each study and to evaluate their strengths and weaknesses. In the meta-analysis we are able to trace general trends and to test some hypotheses about differential effects.

## A NARRATIVE REVIEW OF INTERVENTION STUDIES

Through PsychLit, Dissertation Abstracts, ERIC, consultation of experts, and the 'snowball' method (Mullen, 1989) we have collected 16 intervention studies which at least reported effects (or the absence thereof) on infant-parent attachment. We did not include intervention studies focusing on parental sensitivity, and which did not report on attachment data. The studies may be divided into preventive and therapeutic interventions, and we will discuss these two subsets in two separate sections. In Table 1, we have presented an overview of the basic characteristics of the intervention studies.

### Preventive Interventions

This type of intervention study is based on the model of parent education programs and programs for parental support. Some preventive studies are of quite short duration, of a few months, with a relatively small number of personal contacts between intervenors and subjects. Other preventive studies are, however, more laborious. The interventions are often particularly focused on the behavioral level, that is, they try to enhance parental sensitivity.

Anisfeld et al. (1990) designed their experiment to test the hypothesis that increased physical contact would promote more maternal sensitivity and more secure attachment between infant and mother in a low SES, predominantly Hispanic and African-American sample. Newborn infants were randomly assigned to an experimental group ($N = 23$) that received soft baby carriers leading to more physical contact, or to a control group ($N = 26$) that received plastic infant seats. Most mothers used the baby carrier quite intensively (half of them daily) for the first 8.5 months. At 3.5 months a global sensitivity rating was completed; the authors used Crnic's scale for sensitivity to the baby's cues, state, and rhythm. At 13 months the Strange Situation procedure (Ainsworth et al., 1978) was used to assess the quality of infant-mother attachment. Experimental mothers received higher ratings on the sensitivity scale but the difference was not significant. In the experimental group, however, 83% of the infants appeared to be securely attached, whereas in the control group only 38% was secure. This difference was significant. The authors conclude that the process of being carried close to the mother seemed to have had an effect on the infant's attachment security above and beyond that attributable to increased maternal sensitivity as measured by the Crnic scale (Anisfeld et al., 1990).

Barnard, Magyary, Sumner, Booth, Mitchell and Spieker (1988) recruited pregnant women with low social support. Subjects were randomly assigned to either the Mental Health Model ($N = 68$) or the Information/Resource Model ($N = 79$). This latter model was a regular support program for disadvantaged young mothers, and it served as the 'dummy' treatment in this experiment. The Mental Health Model focused on developing a supportive relationship with the pregnant women through a series of home visits. Nurses with graduate training supported the women in daily life situations, provided a role model and tried to increase the mother's social competence. The treatment was completed at the end of the baby's first year. Parental sensitivity was measured with the Nursing Child Assessment Teaching Scale (NCATS) at intake, 1, and 2 years. Infant-mother attachment was measured with the Ainsworth Strange Situation procedure at 13 and 20 months. The mothers in the experimental group were rated as more sensitive and competent on the NCATS, but there were no differences on the security of attachment classifications at 13 months; overall only 45% of the infants demonstrated a secure attachment relationship.

Jacobson and Frye (1991) studied the effects of social support to newly delivered low-SES mothers participating in the federally funded Women, Infants and Children food supplementation program. Pregnant women were randomly assigned to either an experimental ($N = 23$) or a control ($N = 23$) group. Subjects in the experimental group were regularly visited at home by a 'volunteer coach', starting visits during pregnancy and continuing throughout the first year of life. The coach talked with the mother about the pregnancy, and about preparations for the coming baby; she also talked with the mother about her expectations, developmental milestones and health concerns, and the kinds of activities mothers and infants enjoy together. The Home Observation for Measurement of the Environment (HOME; Caldwell & Bradley, 1984) was administered at 13 months to assess maternal involvement with the child, and security of attachment was

TABLE 1

Characteristics of Intervention Studies

| Authors | Sample | Age Child at Start | Intervention | Intensity | Design | Post-test attachment | | Procedure/ age of child |
|---|---|---|---|---|---|---|---|---|
| Anisfeld et al. (1990) | low SES N = 49 | immediately after birth | soft baby carrier | 8.5 mo. | post-test only contr. group | exp. group: control group: | 83% secure 38% secure | SSP*/13 mo. |
| Barnard et al. (1988) | women with low social support N = 95 | during pregnancy | supportive relation with home-visitor | > 1 yr. | exp. + contr. group dummy-interv. | exp. group vs. contr. group | no difference | SSP/13 mo. |
| Barnett et al. (1987) | highly anxious middle class N = 52 | immediately after birth | general support anti-anxiety measures | 1 yr. | post-test only control group | exp. group: control group: | 59% secure 74% secure | SSP/12 mo. |
| Beckwith (1988) | low SES sick prematures N = 70 | immediately after birth | supportive relation with home-visitor | 1 yr. | pre-test–post-test control group | exp. group: control group: | 51% secure 51% secure | SSP/13 mo. |
| Brinich et al. (1989) | nonorganic failure-to-thrive | 5 mo. | three kinds of support during home-visits | 1 yr. | no control group | 3 groups: | no difference | SSP/12 mo. |
| Erickson et al. (1992) | low SES first borns N = 154 | during pregnancy | multiservice program M-C psychotherapy | 1 yr. | pre-test–post-test control group | exp. group: control group: | 46% secure 67% secure | SSP/13 mo. |
| Jacobson et al. (1991) | low income first borns N = 46 | during pregnancy | supportive relation with home-visitor | > 1 yr. | exp. + contr. group | exp. group vs. contr. group: | $p < .005$ | Q-sort†/14 mo. |
| Juffer (1993) | adopted first children N = 90 | 6 mo. | video-intervention/ written information | 3 sessions | pre-test–post-test control group | exp. group: control group: | 90% secure 70% secure | SSP/12 mo. |

| Study | Sample | Age | Intervention | Sessions/Duration | Design | Comparison | Results | Assessment/Age |
|---|---|---|---|---|---|---|---|---|
| Juffer et al. (1994) | insecure low SES mother $N = 1$ | 11 mo. | video/written information biographical discussions | 4 sessions | case-study | change from insecure→secure | | SSP/14 mo. AAI/14 mo. |
| Lambermon and Van IJzendoorn (1989) | mothers with large or small network first borns $N = 32$ | 6 wks. | parent education | 4 times (by mail) | randomized block-design | exp. group: base-line | 50% secure 38% secure | SSP/15 mo. |
| Leifer et al. (1989) | depressive mother $N = 1$ | 7 mo. | individual therapy + M-C psychotherapy | 2 yrs. | case-study | change from insecure→secure | | SSP/20 mo. |
| Lieberman et al. (1991) | low SES insecure children $N = 82$ | 12 mo. | M-C psychotherapy | 1 yr weekly | randomized block-design | exp. versus control group | not significant | Q-sort/24 mo. |
| Lyons-Ruth et al. (1990) | low SES multirisk mothers $N = 28$ | 5 mo. | supportive home-visits | 47 visits | exp. + contr. group | exp. group: control group: | 57% secure 20% secure | SSP/12 mo. |
| Meij (1992) | low SES first borns $N = 78$ | 6 mo. | video-intervention/ written information | 3 sessions | pre-test-post-test control group | exp. group: control group: | 88% secure 77% secure | SSP/12 mo. |
| Murray et al. (in press) | insecure child $N = 1$ | 18 mo. | M-C psychotherapy | 8 weekly sessions | case-study | change from insecure→secure | | SSP/20 mo. |
| Van den Boom (1988) | low SES irritable first borns $N = 100$ | 6 mo. | supportive home-visits | 3 sessions | four-group design (Solomon) | exp. group: control group: | 68% secure 28% secure | SSP/12 mo. |

*SSP = Strange Situation Procedure
†Q-sort = Waters' Attachment Q-sort

assessed using Waters and Deane's (1985) Attachment Q-Sort procedure at home at 14 months. Mothers in the two groups did not differ on the HOME inventory or on any of the HOME subscales at 13 months. Nevertheless, the two groups differed significantly on the Attachment Q-Sort: Children in the experimental group appeared to be more secure on the Summary Attachment Ratings scale.

In the same line, Beckwith (1988) reports on a preventive intervention project designed to provide supportive home-visitor services to parents of infants who were at double jeopardy, both biologically and socially, that is, sick preterm infants being raised by low-income parents. The intervention started in hospital and was continued throughout the first year; 35 families were visited at home regularly by a professional home-visitor who tried to develop a trusting, supportive relationship, and provided concrete assistance as well as helping the parent to develop observational skills towards their infants. A matched comparison group of 35 families participated in measures for quality of mother-infant interaction and security of attachment. Beckwith found that the intervention was associated with increased maternal involvement and an increased level of reciprocal interactions at 9 months. Intervention was not associated with an increase in security of attachment at 13 months. A small majority of the infants in both groups were securely attached (51%). The author suggested that because of differential attrition (more mothers discontinued participation in the control group) the intervention group was at higher risk on the continuum of caretaking casualty (Sameroff & Chandler, 1975), which might have decreased the intervention effect.

Lyons-Ruth, Connell, Grunebaum and Botein (1990) assigned weekly home-visiting services to 31 infants at high social risk due to the combined effects of poverty, maternal depression and caretaking inadequacy. The goals of the services were: providing an accepting and trustworthy relationship; increasing the family's competence in assessing resources to meet basic needs; modelling and reinforcing more interactive, positive and developmentally appropriate exchanges between mother and infant; and decreasing social isolation. A control group was established by a similar clinical referral process as was used to identify the intervention group, but this group of 10 families was referred at 18 months and was assessed prior to any intervention. We consider that group to be the control group (the authors mention a community group of 35 families which they use as a second comparison group). The Ainsworth sensitivity scale was used to assess maternal sensitivity to infant's attachment cues at 18 months, as well as a Covert Hostility scale, an Interfering Manipulation scale, and a Flatness-of-Affect Scale. The scales loaded high on a factor labeled Maternal Involvement, which was used here as an adequate approximation of sensitiv-ity. Infant-mother attachment security was assessed with the Strange Situ-ation procedure. The authors found no significant effects of treatment on maternal sensitivity or involvement. The intervention was successful, how-ever, in affecting attachment security: Among untreated high-risk infants there was a very high rate of insecure infants (80%) as compared to the high-risk infants who did receive treatment (43%). The authors suggest that their measures for maternal sensitivity did not tap the specific interactive patterns in a high-risk group. The nonrandomized design might provide an-other explanation for the differential effects on sensitivity and attachment.

Barnett, Blignault, Holmes, Payne and Parker (1987) collected Strange Situation data in an Australian, nonclinical sample of 134 infant-mother pairs. A few days after delivery, mothers were screened on state and trait anxiety measures and the high-anxiety subjects were randomly assigned to a professional intervention ($N = 29$), to a nonprofessional intervention ($N = 28$), or to a control group ($N = 23$). The professional intervention was provided for 12 months by female social workers who offered general support and specific anti-anxiety measures, promoted self-esteem, and en-couraged appropriate maternal sensitivity to infant cues. For the non-professional intervention, an experienced mother was asked to offer the support. Only the professional intervention resulted in a significant anxi-ety-reducing effect, and here we will compare the professional intervention with the untreated high-anxiety group. The intervention was not effective in changing attachment security: In the control group 74% of the infants were securely attached, whereas in the intervention group only 59% of the infants were securely attached. The negative effect might be caused by the high percentage of security in the control group: a ceiling effect cannot be excluded as an alternative interpretation.

In The Netherlands, several intervention studies have been carried out, and their common characteristic is the short duration, three or four contacts between a supportive coach and the mothers. Van den Boom (1988; 1991) focused on a 100 highly irritable infants from lower-class families, and her intervention aimed at enhancing maternal sensitivity between the sixth and ninth month of the baby's life. The intervenor visited the mothers three times at home, and assisted them to adjust their behaviors to the infants' unique cues, in particular to negative signals such as crying. But the inter-venor also paid attention to stimulating playful interaction. The interven-tion was continuously monitored by means of the same observational sys-tem that was used in the pre- and post-tests. The quality of mother-infant interactions was observed at the age of 6 (pre-test) and 9 months (post-test). Several sensitivity ratings and frequency scores were included in an overall measure for maternal responsiveness. The quality of the infant-mother attachment relationship was measured by the Strange Situation procedure at 12 months. A Solomon four-group randomized design was used to control for potential pre-test effects. Mothers who participated in the intervention were significantly more responsive on the post-test than the control mothers. Furthermore, the intervention was successful in changing attachment insecurity. In the experimental group 68% of the infants appeared to be secure, whereas only 28% of the infants in the control group were securely attached to their mother. The majority of the untreated irritable infants were avoidantly attached (56%).

Two replications have been carried out to test the stability and generalizability of the results of this highly effective and efficient parent education program. Meij (1992) studied the effects of a comparable intervention program in a sample of 78 lower-class families. In this case, the intervention, aiming at enhancing the quality of parental sensitivity, appeared to be less effective. In one subsample ($N = 26$) the parents participated in a similar intervention as Van den Boom's (1988). In a second subsample ($N = 26$) only a booklet was provided with information about parent-infant interaction. The third subsample was the control group. No short-term or long-term effects were found for maternal sensitivity as measured by the Ainsworth sensitivity scale. With regard to the quality of attachment it was found that neither at the age of 12 months nor at the age of 18 months were the intervention programs effective. The author noted that a relatively high number of infants in this sample were securely attached (77%) which may have caused a ceiling effect.

The second replication was carried out in a sample of 90 Dutch adoptive families (Juffer, 1993). The infants came from Sri Lanka and South Korea and were adopted at a very early age (within a few months after birth). There were two types of interventions aimed at enhancing parents' sensitivity and infants' attachment security: the first type consisted of written information only and the second type combined written information with three visits of video home-trainers who gave feedback on the mother-infant interaction videotaped at home. Although a large majority of the control infants were securely attached (70%), the most intensive intervention program with video-feedback resulted in a significant increase of securely attached infants (90%). The intervention was also effective in enhancing maternal sensitivity as measured with the Ainsworth sensitivity and cooperation scales.

Lambermon (1991; Lambermon & Van IJzendoorn, 1989) studied the effects of two types of parent education programs—videotaped and written information about sensitive parenting—in a sample of 35 families with extremely small or extremely large social networks. The design was a pre-test- post-test design with two factors: experimental condition (written or videotaped information) and size of social network (small or large). The pre-tests were performed between the 6th and 8th week, the intervention took 4 weeks, and the post-tests were performed between the 13th and 16th week after birth. Maternal sensitivity was rated on several scales developed by Ainsworth, and by Belsky. At 15 months the Strange Situation procedure was completed. The results of the study have demonstrated that the written material was superior to the videotaped information in influencing maternal sensitivity. Videotaped models of 'strange' mothers and infants caused identification problems for several participating mothers. The intervention groups did not differ significantly in percentage of secure infant-mother dyads, and in both groups 50–62% were insecurely attached. Because the written information appeared to be more effective than the videotaped information, and because there were no reasons to suspect that the videotaped information would have led to negative effects (Lambermon, 1991), the videogroup was considered to provide the base-line for evaluating the effects of the written information.

Brinich, Drotar and Brinich (1989) studied the effects of three types of intervention on the security of attachment in 59 children with early histories of nonorganic failure to thrive (NOFT). All children (33 African-American) were from economically disadvantaged families, the majority of whom received Aid to Dependent Children. The infants were randomly assigned to one of three time-limited intervention plans with an average duration of 1 year, that were conducted at home. The type of intervention was not expected to influence patterns of attachment at 12 months while intervention was still going on (Brinich et al., 1989). Interventions were terminated when the children were at an average age of 14 months. The three interventions—family centered; parent centered; and advocacy—did indeed not affect security of attachment differentially. A small majority of the total sample (51%) was securely attached. A control group was absent for ethical reasons so no treatment group received a dummy treatment.

### Therapeutic Interventions

Whereas preventive interventions aim at enhancing parental sensitivity through support, information, feedback and modelling, therapeutic approaches start with the idea that parents have to remember and reexperience their childhood anxieties and sufferings (the 'ghosts in the nursery') in order to be sensitive to their infants' attachment signals (Fraiberg et al., 1975). In fact, more than preventive interventions, parent-infant psychotherapy emphasizes the representational level in trying to break the cycle of intergenerational transmission of insecure attachments (Carter, Osofsky & Hann, 1991; Cramer et al., 1990; Wright, 1986). Therapeutic interventions are, of course, not exclusively focused on the representational level, but include many behavioral components as well.

Lieberman et al. (1991) studied the effects of therapeutic intervention in a sample of 93 low-SES, Spanish-speaking mothers recently immigrated from Mexico or Central America to the U.S.A. At 12 months the Strange Situation procedure was completed, and 59 insecurely attached dyads were randomly assigned to the intervention ($N = 34$) and a control group ($N = 25$). The securely attached dyads formed a second 'control' group which we have not included in our review. The intervention started immediately after the Strange Situation assessment, and continued throughout the second year of life with unstructured home visits taking place weekly. The intervention was meant to provide the mother with a corrective attachment experience and to enable her to explore her own attachment biography as well as her current feelings of anger and ambivalence towards others (including the child and the intervenor). The intervenor also provided appropriately timed developmental information, but she abstained from didactic teaching. At 24 months, security of attachment was assessed using Waters and Deane's (1985) Attachment Q-Sort which was completed by the intervenor. During a free-play session, maternal emphatic responsiveness was rated on a scale using criteria based on body orientation, postural and facial expression, and timing and context of responses. Experimental mothers appeared to have higher scores on emphatic responsiveness, whereas there were no group differences on the Attachment Q-Sort. Although the authors also report on another attachment measure, we selected this measure of attachment security because it is a widely used and validated instrument (Vaughn & Waters, 1990).

Egeland and Erickson (1993; Erickson, Korfmacher & Egeland, 1992) report on the preliminary results of their STEEP project (Steps Toward Effective Enjoyable Parenting) for high-risk mothers and infants. STEEP is aimed at enhancing the quality of the infant-mother attachment relationship through the modification of the mother's mental representation of attachment. STEEP helps mothers to face their own developmental history, to examine its effects on parenting, and to express the (anxious) feelings arising from past and present attachment relationships. The study involved 154 high-risk mothers who were pregnant with their first child at the time of recruitment. They were at risk because of poverty, lack of education, single status, social isolation and unstable life arrangements in general. Seventy-four mothers were randomly assigned to STEEP which started with home visits and group meetings before birth and continued throughout the first year after birth. Experimental mothers were more sensitive to the infants' attachment signals, were more stimulating (as indicated by the HOME), and were generally more competent in managing their daily life. Unfortunately, at 13 months only 46% of the STEEP intervention infants appeared to be securely attached, whereas 67% of the controls were securely attached. The authors speculate that the 'insight'-oriented approach to intervention may not be effective in a group of mothers with serious behavioral, intellectual and adjustment problems. Another possibility might be that this approach needs more time to trickle through (the so-called 'sleeper'-effect).

Murray and Cooper (in press) present a case-study on the effects of a short-term mother-infant psychotherapy. The infant was insecurely attached to her mother at 18 months. The intervention of eight weekly sessions aimed at enhancing this relationship. The Adult Attachment Interview (Main & Goldwyn, 1985–1993) to assess the representation of the attachment biography was completed by the mother before the start of the sessions to direct the psychotherapy. After the sessions, the Strange Situation procedure was completed to assess infant-mother attachment security. The infant was securely attached at the post-test, and the authors also report a change of mental representation of attachment in the mother. They found a shift from dismissing to autonomous attachment. The latter finding, however, was not based on a second Adult Attachment Interview but on the discourse with the mother as part of the evaluation.

Another interesting case-study is presented by Leifer, Wax, Leventhal-Belfer, Fouchia and Morrison (1989). They describe a quantitative single case study to illustrate how an early intervention program used two therapeutic modalities to treat a depressed mother and her 2-month-old son. The first treatment started when the infant was 7 months old and lasted for a period of 8 months (15 sessions). The second treatment started when the infant was 15 months old and continued for almost another year. The treatment modalities included psychodynamically oriented individual therapy and parent-infant relationship treatment in which the dyad was also seen by a second therapist. The authors found that at 12 months the maternal sensitivity continued to be low, and the quality of the infant-mother attachment relationship was anxiously-avoidant. At 18 months, the mother began to show more sensitivity and less intrusiveness. At 20 months the attachment relationship was evaluated to be secure with some traces of avoidance. Anecdotally the authors describe changes in mental representation of attachment: the mother began to connect her current fear of dealing with her child's attachment needs to her own attachment experiences as a child. She was also able to reflect on some positive features of her childhood. Her life-long fear of dependence which had affected her attachment to her child, was finally examined within the safety of the therapeutic relationship and this seemed to lead to a more balanced attachment representation.

Juffer, Duyvesteyn and Van IJzendoorn (1994) present a case-study in which an insecure-dismissing mother with her 11-month-old daughter participated. The case is part of a larger pre-test/post-test control group design. The Adult Attachment Interview and Ainsworth's sensitivity measure were used as pre- and post-tests, and the Strange Situation procedure was included in the post-test. The intervention was implemented between the 11th and 13th month after the birth of the firstborn baby. In four intervention sessions the mother received written information about sensitive interaction with infants, feedback on video-taped interactions with her child, and the intervenor involved the mother in discussions about her childhood attachment experiences in relation to the current interaction with the baby. At the pre-test the mother appeared to be insecure-dismissing (Main & Goldwyn, 1985–1993), and her sensitivity rating was rather low (3.3 on the Ainsworth nine-point scale). At the post-test the mother again had to be classified as insecure-dismissing, but her sensitivity rating was almost 2 scale points higher. This change on the behavioral level was reflected in the Strange Situation assessment. At 14 months the child was classified as securely attached to her mother. In sum, at the time of recruitment the mother demonstrated an insecure-dismissing representation of her attachment biography, and she appeared to be extremely insensitive to the infant's attachment cues. After four intervention sessions in which the mother received concrete feedback on her interactions with her daughter, and talked intensively about her past attachment experiences, she showed much more sensitivity, and her child appeared to be securely attached. Nevertheless, the mother's representation of attachment still remained insecure.

## A META-ANALYSIS OF INTERVENTION STUDIES

From the intervention studies we derived the relevant statistics to determine the effects on parental sensitivity and on infant-mother attachment security. In the case of parental sensitivity we chose those (composite) measures that were most closely associated with the original Ainsworth scale for sensitivity. In most studies the same measure for quality of attachment was used, i.e. the Strange Situation procedure. In the meta-analysis we addressed the following questions: (1) Do interventions enhance the parent's sensitivity to infant's attachment cues, and, if so, how large is the average effect? (2) Do interventions enhance the quality of the infant-mother attachment relationship, and if so, how large is the average improvement? We defined improvement here as a change from an insecure to a secure attachment relationship.

We have presented the relevant statistics in Table 2. For meta-analytic purposes we have had to exclude the case-studies and the study by Brinich et al. (1989), in which an untreated control group was lacking. Twelve studies were included in this meta-analysis. Earlier meta-analyses in the area of attachment were based on similar number of studies (Goldsmith & Alansky, 1987; Fox, Kimmerly & Schafer, 1991). The statistics for sensitivity and attachment have been presented separately. Because the statistics are quite divergent, we have computed a common meta-analytic indicator for effect size: Cohen's $d$, that is the standardized difference between the means of the experimental and control group (Mullen, 1989; Rosenthal, 1991). On this basis, we have computed the combined effect sizes for sensitivity and for attachment, for which the separate effect sizes were weighted by the size of the samples (Mullen, 1989).

Although intervention studies are time-consuming and expensive, almost 900 mother-infant dyads have participated in this type of study. They have profited from the interventions: the combined effect size for sensitivity is $d = .58$, which is highly significant. Against the background of Cohen's (1988) criteria for weak ($d = .20$), medium ($d = .50$), and strong ($d = .80$) effect sizes, the interventions have been rather successful in enhancing parents' sensitivity to infants' cues. The effectiveness of the studies is, however, quite heterogeneous. The intervention by Van den Boom (1988) was by far the most effective ($d = 2.62$), whereas its replication by Meij (1992) did not show any effect at all. We have already mentioned the possibility of a ceiling effect in the case of Meij's study.

The combined effect size for quality of attachment is considerably weaker: $d = .17$ which is significant at the $p = .036$ level. According to Cohen's (1988) criteria this effect size is weak. Cohen equals $d = .17$ to a correlation coefficient of $r = .09$, which is less than 1% explained variation in attachment security. Rosenthal (1991), however, introduced the so-called 'binomial effect size display' (BESD) as a more adequate indicator of size and relevance of the effect, and demonstrated that even $d = .17$ can be of great practical importance. Rosenthal (1991) mentions several studies in the medical sciences showing effect sizes smaller than $d = .17$ which nevertheless provided important practical (and theoretical) applications.

The combined effect size seems to be an adequate indicator of the global trend in this set of 12 studies because outlying studies are lacking. The negative effects of Lieberman et al. (1991), Erickson et al. (1992), and Barnett

## TABLE 2
### Intervention Studies on Sensitivity and Attachment: Meta-Analytic Data

| Study | Year | N | Measure | Sensitivity Statistic | d | Attachment* Measure | Statistic | d |
|---|---|---|---|---|---|---|---|---|
| 1. Anisfeld et al. | 1990 | 49 | sensitivity (Crnic) | $F(1,42) = 2.96$ | .53 | SSP | $p = .019$ | .62 |
| 2. Barnard et al. | 1988 | 95 | NCATS | $p < .05$ | .34 | SSP | $p = .50$ | .00 |
| 3. Barnett et al. | 1987 | 52 | — | — | — | SSP | $\chi^2 = 1.32$ | −.32 |
| 4. Beckwith | 1988 | 70 | involvement | $p = .05$ | .40 | SSP | $p = .50$ | .00 |
| 5. Erickson† | 1992 | 135 | HOME | $p = .05$ | .29 | SSP | $p = .008$ | −.42 |
| 6. Jacobson and Frye | 1991 | 46 | involvement | $p = .50$ | .00 | Q-Sort | $t = 3.21$ | .97 |
| 7. Juffer‡ | 1993 | 90 | sens/coop. (Ainsworth) | $p = .03$ | .50 | SSP | $\chi^2 = 3.75$ | .42 |
| 8. Lambermon and Van IJzendoorn§ | 1989 | 32 | responsive involvement | $F(1,31) = 5.34$ | .83 | SSP | $\chi^2 = 0.51$ | .25 |
| 9. Lieberman‖ et al. | 1991 | 82 | empathic responsiveness | $t(51) = 2.506$ | .70 | Q-Sort | $t(51) = -.445$ | −.12 |
| 10. Lyons-Ruth et al. | 1990 | 40 | involvement (composite) | $p = .50$ | .00 | SSP | $p\P = .04$ | .58 |
| 11. Meij‡ | 1992 | 78 | sensitivity (Ainsworth) | $t(49) = -.028$ | −.01 | SSP | $\chi^2(1;51) = 1.076$ | .29 |
| 12. Van den Boom | 1988 | 100 | sensitivity (composite) | $F(1,90) = 154.95$ | 2.62 | SSP | $p = .001$ | .65 |
| Total | | | $N = 869$ | | $d = .58$ | | | $d = .17$ |

* In case of more than one measurement, the first is included; SSP = Strange Situation procedure; † estimated data for sensitivity; ‡ cumulative intervention versus control group; § attachment data derived from Lanbermon (1991); ‖ intervention group versus insecure control group; ¶ exact Fisher p-values for forced classifications.

174

et al. (1987) should, however, be noted. Although these negative effects are quite weak, they nevertheless represent the possibility of counterproductive results and 'iatrogenic damage'. It is puzzling that the interventions with negative effects were therapeutic and intensive (Cramer et al., 1990). In fact, the combined effect size for the long-term interventions ($N = 7$) was $d = .00$, whereas the combined effect size for the short-term interventions was $d = .48$. Maybe the narrow scope of the behaviorally oriented short-term interventions is a key factor in changing the infant-mother attachment relationship.

The difference between the combined effect size for sensitivity and for attachment is rather large. Of course, one would expect interventions aiming at enhancing maternal sensitivity to be most successful in reaching this proximal goal. In most interventions, secure attachment is the distal goal, to be reached through a change of sensitivity. We should also note that, in that case, the effect of interventions on attachment is dependent on the influence of a change in sensitivity on the quality of the attachment relationship. This influence cannot be stronger than the association between sensitivity and attachment. The intervention studies presuppose that sensitivity is the most important and strongest determinant of attachment, but meta-analytic data show that the association is modest (Goldsmith & Alansky, 1987). Furthermore, there might be other ways in which infant-mother attachment is influenced (Van IJzendoorn, in press). Therefore, interventions aiming at enhancing sensitivity may only have modest effects on attachment. Although the difference between effect sizes for sensitivity and attachment is rather large, it might be somewhat inflated for two reasons. First, several measures for sensitivity exist and some researchers might have chosen to report on the measures with the strongest effects. For attachment, only two generally accepted measures exist—the Strange Situation procedure and the Attachment Q-Sort. Second, attachment security as measured by the Strange Situation procedure is a dichotomous variable (insecure versus secure), which might restrict the intervention effects. The sensitivity measures are continuous, and restriction of range is not plausible here.

## DISCUSSION

The intervention studies presented above have a common goal: to enhance the quality of the infant-mother attachment relationship. Their intervention strategies, designs, and effectiveness are quite divergent.

The scope of the interventions differs widely between studies. Many studies aim at enhancing physical contact between mothers and infants (soft baby carriers) or sensitive interactions in general, because these factors are considered to be crucial in shaping the infants' attachment relationship to their mothers. Some studies also aim at the maternal attachment representation, and try to offer the mothers a supportive, therapeutic relationship that serves as a safe base to explore the 'ghosts' of the past. Both types of intervention, however, use similar criteria for effectiveness: change of insensitivity and infant attachment insecurity. For studies focusing on the representational level, though, the proximal goal of changing maternal attachment representations might be reached without accompanying changes at the behavioral level—which may come later in time. Although the Lieberman et al. (1991) and Egeland and Erickson (1993) studies did not show significant positive effects on infant attachment security, they might have been effective in changing maternal attachment representations, but the authors have not (yet) collected or reported data on the representational level.

In addition, the interventions differ strongly in terms of focus. Some studies use a very narrow scope and are only designed to change a concrete aspect of mother-infant interactions (Anisfeld et al., 1990; Van den Boom, 1988). If these interventions are successful, it is exactly clear what part of the intervention programme is responsible for the effective change. Other studies, however, use a very wide scope and offer general, supportive services to help disadvantaged mothers to survive in a poor environment. The Egeland and Erickson (1993) intervention program is, in fact, a multi-service package addressing not only childrearing problems but also financial, insurance, housing and other practical issues. In multi-problem samples it may even be impossible to focus only on enhancing mother-infant interactions without taking the social context into account. But when urgent 'survival' needs dominate the intervention, it may well be at the cost of the effectiveness at the level of maternal sensitivity. And even if the broad-band approach is effective in changing attachment relationships it will be difficult to trace this effect back to specific facets of the program.

The interventions also differ strongly in terms of intensity, that is, the number and kind of contacts between intervenors and subjects. Some studies did not provide personal interaction between staff and subjects at all, but offered a soft baby carrier (Anisfeld et al., 1990), or written information about sensitive parenting (Lambermon, 1991). Other studies included three home visits (Juffer, 1993; Van den Boom, 1988) and still other studies provided more than 50 personal contacts between coaches and families (Lieberman et al., 1991; Lyons-Ruth et al., 1990). Considering the broad range of intervention contacts, it is puzzling to see that long-term interventions do not seem to be more effective than short-term interventions in reaching the same goal: enhancing the child's attachment security. One of the explanations may be that the more intensive interventions were carried out in groups with multiple, and more serious problems. In terms of attachment security, though, some short-term interventions were effective in groups with only about 30% securely attached children (control group; Van den Boom, 1988), whereas some long-term interventions were ineffective in groups with more than 60% securely attached infants (control group; Egeland & Erickson, 1993). If personal interaction between intervenor and subject is used to teach adequate parenting strategies or to provide feedback on videotaped behavior, the interventions seem to be more successful than in the case of therapeutic assistance—which again is puzzling. We should not exclude the possibility, however, that in the long run therapeutic interventions will be more effective because they affect the roots of insecure attachments in the parent's own childhood attachment experiences.

The designs of the intervention studies range from randomized pre-test/post-test control group designs to single case-studies. The majority of the studies use one or the other form of randomized experimental designs, and this type of design allows, in principle, for valid conclusions. Nevertheless, in some studies differential attrition is an important drawback, (e.g. Egeland & Erikson, 1993) because the similarity of experimental and control group may be jeopardized. In the long-term, intensive intervention studies, parents in the control group may become demotivated, in particular when they experience many problems for which they do not receive help. At the post-test the control group may seem to function better, only because the families with the most serious problems stopped participating. In short-term intervention studies it may be much easier to prevent attrition, and to avoid its differential effects on the experimental and control groups. Therefore, they may seem to be more effective than long-term interventions. In line with the problem of attrition is the possibility of a ceiling effect. If the control group shows an overrepresentation of securely attached infants at the post-test, it will be very difficult for any intervention to prove its effectiveness. It may, in fact, even be ethically debatable whether to intervene in families without insecure attachments (e.g. Meij, 1992), because positive effects cannot be expected and counterproductive effects might not be excluded.

Lastly, the generalizability of the results may be difficult to establish. Many intervention studies did not only include insecurely attached infant-mother dyads, but dyads at risk for many reasons, such as physical, socio-economic, or mental reasons. Every sample seems to be characterized by a very complex constellation of depriving factors, and it may be impossible to outline the population from which they have been drawn. For the time being it seems safest to assume that interventions may only be effective in families with an overrepresentation of insecure attachments, but there may be limits to the severity of the problems for which attachment-oriented interventions can provide solutions. The generalizability of the results may also be restricted to the behavioral level, and to the short-term. On the basis of the current studies we do not know whether the interventions affect the parents' attachment representations; because longitudinal intervention studies are still missing, we do not know whether behavioral changes in the first phase of attachment formation will be stable throughout the preschool years.

## CONCLUSIONS

From our narrative review and meta-analysis we may derive the following conclusions: (1) Interventions are effective in enhancing maternal sensitivity to infant's attachment cues; (2) Interventions may be effective in enhancing the quality of the infant-mother attachment relationship, but the size of the effect is small; (3) Short-term interventions with a clear focus appear to be more effective than long-term broad-band interventions; (4) Enhancing maternal sensitivity and infant attachment security does not necessarily imply a change in maternal attachment representation.

The intervention studies represent almost all hypothetical outcomes as described in Fig. 2. The case-studies of Murray and Cooper (in press), and Leifer et al. (1989) seem to represent the most optimal outcome of changes in maternal attachment representations, maternal sensitivity, and infant attachment security (a). In contrast, Barnett et al. (1987) and Meij (1992) did not effect any change, but they did not measure attachment representations (d or h). Three studies were successful in enhancing maternal sensitivity and infant attachment security (a or e), but attachment representations were not measured (Anisfeld et al., 1990; Juffer, 1993; Van den Boom, 1988). Five studies were successful in changing maternal sensitivity only (c or g) (Barnard et al., 1988; Beckwith, 1988; Erickson et al., 1992; Lambermon, 1991; Lieberman et al., 1991). Two studies resulted in some change of attachment security only (b or f) without accompanying change of sensitivity (Jacobson & Frye, 1991; Lyons-Ruth et al., 1990). Our case-study (Juffer et al., 1994) was an example of possibility (e): changes in maternal sensitivity and infant attachment security without changes in maternal attachment representations.

From our meta-analysis we may conclude that the association between maternal sensitivity and infant attachment security indeed is a causal relation. Overall, enhancing maternal sensitivity implied a (small) improvement in infant attachment security. Sensitivity is, however, not a necessary nor a sufficient condition for attachment security. Some studies were able to enhance attachment security without changing sensitivity (not a necessary condition), whereas other studies effected increased sensitivity without accompanying improvement of infant attachment security (not a sufficient condition). In this respect we want to emphasize two conclusions: first, the empirical impact of sensitivity on attachment appears to be only modest and not in accordance with its central position in attachment theory. Second, there must be other ways in which parents influence their children's attachment formation than through sensitive interactions (cf. Van IJzendoorn, in press). In attachment theory, the search for alternative pathways to attachment (in-) security should be opened.

Our case-study showed that interventions may create discrepancies between the representational and the behavioral level, that is, they may be effective in enhancing parental sensitivity and infant attachment without influencing parental attachment representations (Juffer, et al., 1994). If parents only acquire new behavioral strategies to interact with their infant, they may not be able to find ways to deal with the attachment needs of the developing child. Because they are still dismissive of, or preoccupied with, their own attachment biography, they might be less creative and flexible, and more defensive than secure parents in interacting with toddlers or older children who are exploring the boundaries of their physical and social environment. The generalizability of the intervention might, therefore, be restricted. In the long run, the discrepancy between the representational and the behavioral level may even be counterproductive because the child may experience a discontinuity between the sensitive parent in the early years, and the lack of parental responsiveness later on.

Another interpretation of the discrepancy would be more optimistic: the change at the behavioral level may, after some time, induce a change at the representational level ('sleeper-effect'). It may take more time to change mental representations than to learn new behavioral strategies. Furthermore, a securely attached child may provoke positive interactions with the parent, not only in infancy but also in toddlerhood. Bowlby (1982) emphasized the stability of interaction patterns that become self-fulfilling prophecies: from a transactional perspective (Sameroff & Chandler, 1975), the child may reinforce the mother's sensitive behavior, even at a later stage of development. The child may help to break the intergenerational cycle of insecure attachment, because the current positive attachment experiences may enable the mother to re-enact her negative attachment experiences of the past (Fraiberg et al., 1975).

Our review has shown that behaviorally oriented, short-term interventions may be most effective in enhancing infants' attachment security, but these interventions may not break the intergenerational cycle of insecure attachment by changing infants' as well as parents' attachment insecurity. In the long run, interventions that also enhance parents' secure attachment representations may be more effective. More research is needed to test this hypothesis. Future intervention studies should compare the effectiveness of a behavioral approach with a representational type of intervention. In a longitudinal experimental design, it is possible to study the long term consequences of each intervention modality for both the behavioral and representational dimension of attachment formation in parents and in their children.

# REFERENCES

Ainsworth, M. D. S., Blehar, M. C., Water, E. & Wall, S. (1978). *Patterns of attachment, a psychological study of the Strange Situation.* Hillsdale, NJ: Erlbaum Associates.

Anisfeld, E., Casper, V., Nozyce, M. & Cunningham, N. (1990). Does infant carrying promote attachment? An experimental study of the effects of increased physical contact on the development of attachment. *Child Development, 61,* 1617–1627.

Barnard, K. E., Magyary, D., Sumner, G., Booth, C. L., Mitchell, S. K. & Spieker, S. (1988). Prevention of parenting alterations for women with low social support. *Psychiatry, 51,* 248–253.

Barnett, B., Blignault, I., Holmes, S., Payne, A. & Parker, G. (1987). Quality of attachment in a sample of 1-year-old Australian children. *Journal of the American Academy of Child and Adolescent Psychiatry, 26,* 303–307.

Beckwith, L. (1988). Intervention with disadvantaged parents of sick preterm infants. *Psychiatry, 51,* 242–247.

Belsky, J. & Nezworski, T. (1988) (Eds), *Clinical implications of attachment.* Hillsdale, NJ: Erlbaum Associates.

Bowlby, J. (1982). *Attachment and loss (Vol.1). Attachment.* New York: Basic Books.

Bretherton, I. (1985). Attachment theory: retrospect and prospect. In I. Bretherton & E. Waters (Eds), Growing points of attachment theory and research. *Monographs of the Society for Research in Child Development, 50,* 66–104.

Brinich, E., Drotar, D. & Brinich, P. (1989). Security of attachment and outcome of preschoolers with histories of nonorganic failure to thrive. *Journal of Clinical Child Psychology, 18,* 142–152.

Caldwell, B. M. & Bradley, R. H. (1984). *Administration manual. Home observation for measurement of the environment.* Little Rock, Arkansas.

Carter, S. L., Osofsky, J. D. & Hann, D. M. (1991). Speaking for the baby: a thera-peutic intervention with adolescent mothers and their infants. *Infant Mental Health Journal, 12*, 291–301.

Cohen, J. (1988, revised edition). *Statistical power analysis for the behavioral sciences*. New York: Academic Press.

Cramer, B., Robert-Tissot, C., Stern, D. N., Serpa-Rusconi, S., De Muralt, M., Besson, G., Palacio-Espasa, F., Bachmann, J. P., Knauer, D., Berney, C. & D'Arcis, U. (1990). Outcome evaluation in brief mother-infant psychotherapy: a preliminary report. *Infant Mental Health Journal, 11*, 278–300.

Egeland, B. & Erickson, M. F. (1993). Attachment theory and findings: implications for prevention and intervention. In S. Kramer & H. Parens (Eds), *Prevention in mental health: now, tomorrow, ever?* Northvale, N.J.: Jason Aronson, Inc.

Erickson, M. F., Korfmacher, J. & Egeland, B. (1992). Attachments past and present. Implications for therapeutic intervention with mother-infant dyads. *Development and Psychopathology, 4*, 495–507.

Fox, N. A., Kimmerly, N. L. & Schafer, W. D. (1991). Attachment to mother/attachment to father: a meta-analysis. *Child Development, 62*, 210–225.

Fraiberg, S., Adelson, E. & Shapiro, V. (1975). Ghosts in the nursery. A psyhonanalytic approach to the problems of impaired infant-mother relationships. *Journal of the American Academy of Child Psychiatry, 14*, 387–423.

Goldsmith, H. H. & Alansky, J. A. (1987). Maternal and infant temperamental predictors of attachment. A meta-analytic review. *Journal of Consulting and Clinical Psychology, 55*, 805–816.

Jacobson, S. W. & Frye, K. F. (1991). Effect of maternal social support on attachment: Experimental evidence. *Child Development, 62*, 572–582.

Juffer, F. (1993). *Verbonden door adoptie. Een experimenteel onderzoek naar hechting en competentie in gezinnen met een adoptiebaby.* [Attached through adoption. An experimental study on attachment and competence in families with an adopted baby]. Amersfoort: Academische uitgeverij.

Juffer, F., Duyvesteyn, M. G. C. & Van IJzendoorn. M. H. (July 1994). *Intervention in transmission of attachment across generations: a case study.* Poster presented at the Biennial Meeting of the International Society for the Study of Behavioral Development, 27 June–2 July 1994, Amsterdam (The Netherlands).

Lamb, M. E., Thompson, R. A., Gardner, W. & Charnov, E. L. (1985). *Infant-mother attachment: the origins and developmental significance of individual differences in Strange Situation behavior.* Hillsdale, NJ: Erlbaum Associates.

Lambermon, M. W. E. (1991). *Video of folder? Korte- en lange-termijn-effecten van voorlichting over vroegkinderlijke opvoeding.* [Videotaped or written information?]. Leiden: DSWO Press.

Lambermon, M. W. E. & Van IJzendoorn, M. H. (1989). Influencing mother-baby interaction through videotaped or written instruction: evaluation of a parent education program. *Early Childhood Research Quarterly, 4*, 449–459.

Leifer, M., Wax, L., Leventhal-Belfer, L., Fouchia, A. & Morrison, M. (1989). The use of multitreatment modalities in early intervention: a quantitative case study. *Infant Mental Health Journal, 10*, 100–116.

Lieberman, A. F., Weston, D. R. & Pawl, J. H. (1991). Preventive intervention and outcome with anxiously attached dyads. *Child Development, 62*, 199–209.

Lyons-Ruth, K., Connell, D. B., Grunebaum, H. U. & Botein, S. (1990). Infants at social risks: maternal depression and family support services as mediators of infant development and security of attachment. *Child Development, 61*, 85–98.

Main, M., Kaplan, N. & Cassidy, J. (1985). Security in infancy, childhood and adulthood. A move to the level of representation. In I. Bretherton & E. Waters (Eds), Growing points of attachment theory and research. *Monographs of the Society for Research in Child Development, 50*, 66–104.

Main, M. & Goldwyn, R. (1985–1996). *Adult Attachment Classification System.* Unpublished manuscript. Berkeley: University of California.

Meij, J. Th. H. (1992). *Sociale ondersteuning, gehechtheidskwaliteit en vroeg-kinderlijke competentieontwikkeling.* [Social support, attachment, and early competence]. Nijmegen, The Netherlands: Catholic University (dissertation).

Mullen, B. (1989). *Advanced basic meta-analysis.* Hillsdale, NJ: Erlbaum Associates.

Murray, L. & Cooper, P. (in press). Clinical application of attachment theory and research: Change in infant attachment with brief psychotherapy. *Journal of Child Psychology and Psychiatry.*

Rosenthal. R. (1991). *Meta-analytic procedures for social research.* Beverly Hills, CA.: Sage Publications.

Sameroff, A. & Chandler, M. J. (1975). Reproductive risk and the continuum of caretaking casualty. In F. D. Horowitz (Ed.), *Review of child development. Vol. 4* (pp. 187–244). Chicago: University of Chicago Press.

Sroufe, L. A. (1988). The role of infant-caregiver attachment in development. In J. Belsky & T. Nezworski (Eds), *Clinical implications of attachment* (pp. 18–40). Hillsdale, NJ: Erlbaum Associates.

Spangler, G. & Grossmann, K. E. (1993). Biobehavioral organization in securely and insecurely attached infants. *Child Development, 64*, 1439–1450.

Van den Boom, D. (1988). *Neonatal irritability and the development of attachment: observation and intervention.* Unpublished doctoral dissertation, Leiden University, Leiden (The Netherlands).

Van den Boom, D. (1991). Preventive intervention and the quality of mother-infant interaction and infant exploration in irritable infants. In W. Koops, H. Soppe, J. L. van der Linden, P. C. M. Molenaar & J. J. F. Schroots (Eds), *Developmental psychology behind the dykes. An outline of developmental psy-*

*chological research in the Netherlands* (pp. 249–269). Delft (The Netherlands): Eburon.

Van IJzendoorn, M. H. (1992). Intergenerational transmission of parenting: a review of studies in non-clinical populations. *Developmental Review, 12,* 76–99.

Van IJzendoorn, M. H. (in press). Adult attachment representations, parental responsiveness, and infant attachment. A meta-analysis on the validity of the Adult Attachment Interview. *Psychological Bulletin.*

Van IJzendoorn, M. H. & Bakermans-Kranenburg, M. J. (in press). Attachment representations in mothers, fathers, adolescents, and clinical groups: a meta-analytic search for normative data. *Journal of Consulting and Clinical Psychology.*

Vaughn, B. E. & Waters, E. (1990). Attachment behavior at home and in the laboratory: Q-sort observations and strange situation classifications of one year-olds. *Child Development, 61,* 1965–1973.

Waters, E. & Deane, K. E. (1985). Defining and assessing individual differences in attachment relationships: Q-methodology and the organisation of behavior in infancy and early childhood. In I. Bretherton & E. Waters (Eds), Growing points of attachment theory and research. *Monographs of the Society for Research in Child Development, 50,* (1–2, serial no. 209), 41–65.

Wright, B. M. (1986). An approach to infant-parent psychotherapy. *Infant Mental Health Journal, 7,* 247–263.

# 7

# Clinical Assessment of Parenting

**David A. Mrazek**

*Children's National Medical Center and George Washington University
School of Medicine, Washington, D.C.*

**Patricia Mrazek**

*Institute of Medicine, Washington, D.C.*

**Mary Klinnert**

*National Jewish Center for Immunology and Respitory Medicine and
University of Colorado Health Sciences Center, Denver*

*Objective: This report describes the Parenting Risk Scale and
reviews previous approaches to the systematic assessment of
parenting. Five key dimensions of parenting are described as
well as the method for rating the occurrence of difficulties and
concerns about parenting using a semistructured interview
methodology. **Method:** The Parenting Risk Scale was developed
with two cohorts of young children. One cohort consisted of 150
children at increased genetic risk for developing asthma but
who were physically healthy during the initial periods of assessment of parenting. A second cohort of healthy children at no
elevated risk for asthma was similarly studied. **Results:** Reliability of the parenting ratings was found to be acceptable with
appropriate training, and both concurrent and predictive va-*

Reprinted with permission from the *Journal of the American Academy of Child and Adolescent Psychiatry*, 1995, Vol. 34, No. 3, 272–282. Copyright © 1995 by the American Academy of Child and Adolescent Psychiatry.

This work was supported through grant 88-1013-85 from the W.T. Grant Foundation, grant 2KO2-
MH00430 from the National Institute of Mental Health, grant 1 RO1 MH44729 from the National Institute of Mental Health, grant NIH HL-36577 from the National Jewish Center Clinical Investigation Committee, and a grant from the Developmental Psychobiology Research Group. The authors thank Laura
Hodder and David McCormick for their help in the preparation of the data, data analysis, and preparation of the manuscript.

*lidity were demonstrated to be excellent. High stability in the ratings of adequacy of parenting was documented. Specifically, ratings made during the prenatal assessment were highly significantly associated with completely independent ratings of parenting made more than 4 years after the birth of the index child (r = .42, p < .0001). The appropriateness of this method for the assessment of the quality of parenting in clinical settings is highlighted. **Conclusions:** The Parenting Risk Scale is a reliable and valid measure for the systematic assessment of five key dimensions of parenting.*

It is self-evident that under usual circumstances, good parenting contributes to the development of normal children. The issue of what constitutes being a good parent has been discussed in numerous scientific and lay publications and is a practical issue for pediatric care providers who must rely on parents to administer their prescriptions and follow their instructions. This report describes the Parenting Risk Scale (PRS), which is an interview methodology that has been designed to identify parenting difficulties. The scale can be used as an adjunct to the pediatric care of children with chronic illnesses as well as for the assessment of their risk for subsequent developmental psychopathology.

The trials and triumphs of parents have been a persistent literary theme. The Bible provides text that illustrates classic parenting dilemmas, and Shakespeare not only captured many of the intense conflicts that occur between parents and their children, but also cunningly mocked the pretentious and often awkward efforts of the older generation in such scenes as the comical soliloquy of Polonius.

Throughout the history of psychology, the quality of parenting has been a central component of most child developmental theories. Similarly, poor parenting has been considered to be a risk factor for the development of psychopathology throughout the history of child psychiatry. Surprisingly, parenting has remained an extraordinarily difficult construct to measure. The assessment of parenting, and particularly of the quality of parenting, is explicitly a part of every child psychiatric evaluation. Similarly, in pediatrics there is at least an implicit expectation that an assessment of parenting is a critical aspect of the overall evaluation of the family. The reality of clinical practice is that parental behaviors and attitudes are routinely classified as good or bad despite diplomatic communications that frame these parental characteristics as more effective or less supportive. Yet, despite numerous attempts to develop straightforward methodologies to assess the construct of parenting, there is still no generally accepted approach for defining the quality of parenting other than the traditional clinical evaluation based on systematic interviews with both parents and their children coupled with observations of family interactions. In many ways, a large component of "family" assessments is the assessment of appropriate parenting, despite the relabeling of this component using a variety of oblique strategies. While the jargon of family assessments often focuses on "dyadic" or "triadic" elements of the family's interactions or examples of dysfunctional communication (Minuchin et al., 1978), it is the parents who play the dominant role in creating the structure of the family and who establish the customary pattern of family communication.

Child psychiatrists and pediatricians have special access to understanding the process of parenting. Even during this era of mobile and complex medical care systems, pediatric clinicians often have the opportunity to develop a longitudinal perspective of the development of children. They are also exposed to a full range of parenting abilities as they care for children with superlative parents as well as families who have serious problems. The PRS lends itself well for use in both child psychiatric and pediatric settings as it focuses on assessing a parent's response to both acute and chronic illnesses. Furthermore, its narrative format allows its inclusion within the context of a comprehensive evaluation of the family. However, as the full Stress and Coping Interview usually requires at least 60 minutes to administer, the PRS is not an appropriate screening instrument for routine pediatric visits.

One problem that has plagued the development of parenting measures has been a persistent defensiveness on the part of parents. Universally, parents have rejected attempts to focus on their shortcomings. This understandable but unfortunate posture has often been explained as an appropriate reaction to what are now accepted as "unfair parent-blaming" attributions that were made by a generation of psychodynamic clinicians. It is true that some parents have been incorrectly targeted as having played a central role in the development of their children's illnesses. This previously misguided view is most vividly illustrated by syndromes that have been eventually shown to have powerful biological origins. The classic example of this phenomenon is the belief that the "refrigerator parents" of infantile autistic children played a causal role in the development of the severe social and emotional difficulties of their children (Kanner, 1935). A similar misperception was that "schizophrenogenic" mothers were primarily responsible for the development of schizophrenia in their ill-fated offspring. With the advent of better genetic and neurochemical understandings of these syndromes, these earlier attributions have been shown to be incorrect and quite unfair to the parents of these severely ill children.

On the other hand, there is little doubt that the quality of early parenting is critical for the development of well-adjusted children who are self-confident and socially competent. Evidence for the link between problematic parenting and developmental psychopathology has been found in many studies but is most vividly illustrated by studies of children who have been severely physically or emotionally abused (Mrazek, 1993). From early in their development, these children show aberrant patterns of emotional regulation (Gaensbauer and Mrazek, 1981), and their early abuse is associated with a higher incidence of later emotional dysfunction (Carlson et al., 1989; Martin and Beezley, 1977). While it is encouraging that some children can survive even quite overwhelming maltreatment without developing psychiatric disturbances (Mrazek and Mrazek, 1987), abusive parenting is still one of the most potent predictors of later psychopathology.

A major problem for the mental health clinician is how to effectively define inappropriate parenting in the absence of straightforward and easily administered instruments designed to capture this dimension. This is particularly true in pediatric settings for two reasons. First, assessments must be made quickly. Second, documenting the ability of parents to appropriately care for their children plays a critical role in the medical team's judgment of the optimal treatment strategy to manage the child's pediatric symptoms or initiate a plan designed to prevent the onset of subsequent illness.

We have focused on the concept of parenting risk as part of a research protocol designed to monitor the early development of children at risk for physical and emotional disturbances. Using this system, parenting risk does not refer exclusively to overtly destructive or incompetent parenting behaviors but includes more subtle judgment that requires the rater to make an assessment of the probability that the evaluated parents will make decisions regarding the care of their children that place these children at increased risk for the development of either emotional or medical difficulties. In that regard, the appraisal of the presence of parenting risk must involve the consideration of a broad range of behaviors and attitudes.

The objective of this article is to review briefly the issues related to the assessment of parenting. We emphasize those issues that are particularly appropriate for the assessment of the parenting of young children and children evaluated in clinical settings. We describe a new semistructured interview methodology that has been developed as part of the W.T. Grant Asthma Risk Study and discuss its reliability, concurrent validity, and predictive validity. Finally, we discuss the advantages and limitations of this interview strategy within a clinical setting and we consider new directions for the development of more discrete measures of parenting function that will have both clinical and research implications.

## METHODS FOR THE ASSESSMENT OF PARENTING

The use of questionnaires to measure parenting has a long history in the study of child development. Early work highlighted multiple dimensions of parenting, and this strategy has remained as one standard approach that has been used to categorize parents (Schaefer, 1959; Sears et al., 1957). The primary dimension that Sears used to characterize parenting was based on the warmth versus the aloofness that parents demonstrated. The second dimension that he considered to be central was the degree of parental control. While these early studies were influential in the development of the understanding of critical aspects of parenting, they were not well integrated into clinical practice. A third dimension of parenting that has been conceptualized to be associated with psychopathology is the presence of parental mental disturbance (Rutter, 1966) or coercive parental actions (Dowdney et al., 1984; Mrazek et al., 1982). A fourth dimension of parenting that has been well appreciated in pediatrics, but which has been somewhat minimized in psychiatric formulations of parenting competence, is the parents' capacity to understand the basic knowledge base required to care appropriately for their child. These cognitive components include their having a basic awareness of the emotional and physical needs of young children. A fifth dimension of parenting is the degree of commitment of time and energy that parents are willing to make in order to enhance the development of their children. The recent focus on "quality time" that sometimes occurs in the absence of an appreciation of the need for absolute time with children illustrates this dimension. It is obvious that for the time parents spend with their children to be effective, parents must relate with their children. Being in close proximity is a necessary but not sufficient component of good parenting. The five key dimensions of parenting that can be derived from the child developmental literature are summarized in Table 1.

TABLE 1
Key Dimensions of Parenting

| | |
|---|---|
| Emotional availability | Degree of emotional warmth |
| Control | Degree of flexibility and permission |
| Psychiatric disturbance | Presence, type, and severity of overt disorder |
| Knowledge base | Understanding emotional and physical development as well as basic child care principles |
| Commitment | Adequate prioritization of child care responsibilities |

The work of Baumrind (Baumrind, 1971; Baumrind and Black, 1967) has specifically focused on qualities of parenting along the dimension of control. This work has provided convincing evidence that authoritative parents tend to be more effective than either rigid authoritarian parents or parents who are considered to be permissive. This work has been further developed by evidence demonstrating the shifts in parenting behavior required of parents at different stages in the development of their children. The skills that are required to be sensitive and responsive to a newborn infant are very different from those skills that are helpful in negotiating the separation and individuation of a young adolescent.

Scarr (1992) has shown that the parents' genetic endowment has a strong influence on the quality of their parenting. Although it is true that familial interactions (Baumrind, 1993) and cultural imperatives (Jackson, 1993) shape the formation of a child's identity, the importance of the parents' genetic contributions to the child's emotional development continues to be underestimated despite strong empirical evidence (Scarr, 1993). To clarify the ongoing debate focusing on the relative contributions of genes and environment, empirical data are needed that include both greater precision of the genetic loci responsible for parental behavior and more sensitive methodologies to quantify phenotypic expression of behavioral traits. Whereas extensive models have been put forward (Belsky, 1984), no methodologies that effectively capture variations in parenting effectiveness have been available.

## METHOD

### *Parenting Risk Scale*

**Sample.** The PRS was initially used to evaluate a sample of 180 families. One hundred fifty of these families had a child who was at increased genetic risk for the development of asthma because at least one parent had asthma. Parents with a full range of asthma severity participated. Thirty comparison families who had healthy infants at no increased risk for asthma were also studied. Most of the 180 families were referred to participate in our longitudinal study from obstetric practices in the Denver metropolitan area. A small number were referred from allergists or independently heard about the study. Ninety percent of the families were Caucasian and a large majority were middle or upper class. A more extensive sociodemographic description of the sample has been reported elsewhere (Mrazek et al., 1991).

**Scale characteristics.** The PRS was developed to capture systematically the broad range of parenting behaviors that are represented by the five parenting dimensions. Ratings were made after conducting a semistructured interview with the parent which is described in this report. Its primary goal is to identify parents who demonstrate overt difficulties or who exhibit behaviors that indicate that they are at potential risk for having problems in the provision of consistent and sensitive care for their children because of a problem in at least one of the five major dimensions of parenting.

The scale was patterned after a clinical global rating scale that had been developed at the National Institute of Mental Health by the Radke-Yarrow team and was used in her depression study to quantify early risk of disturbance in preschool children (Radke-Yarrow et al., 1992). Three categories were conceptualized in the development of the National Institute of Mental Health scale. One category was used to indicate the presence of a problem that required clinical intervention. An intermediate category representing subclinical rather than overtly pathological symptoms allowed clinicians to identify children at risk. A normal category was used to classify a broad range of behavior, none of which was believed to be pathogenic. We have used a similar strategy (Table 2).

TABLE 2
Parenting Risk Scale

| Category | Definition |
| --- | --- |
| Parenting Difficulties | Serious problems that would alert a clinician that family intervention was needed (e.g., punitive parenting, major parental psychopathology, inadequate child care arrangements) |
| Concerns about Parenting | Less serious problems that would not elicit the need for immediate intervention but would suggest the need for seeking follow-up (e.g., intermittent maternal rejection of the child, parental psychopathology that is being ineffectively treated and is interfering with child care, exposure of the child to intense marital conflict) |
| Adequate Parenting | No ongoing problems; within this range of functioning there would be both average and exceptional parenting |

While this approach appears straightforward, what makes it an effective strategy is its ability to combine complex classes of behaviors based exclusively on the single characteristic of risk for negative impact on child development. Although this approach is promising for the examination of pathogenic parenting, it is of relatively little use in the assessment of optimal parenting. The scale follows an old clinical tradition of trying to identify the "good enough" mother (Winnicott, 1957) but adds a dimension of "almost good enough." This is exactly the threshold that is critical for assessing parents in the pediatric setting, where differentiating sensitive mothers from very sensitive mothers is of little practical relevance. Furthermore, this focus on the relevant negative parental behaviors and attitudes associated with disturbance allows for the identification of relationships that would otherwise be obscured if the entire spectrum of parenting behavior was coded. An analogy is the force required to break a twig. There is no correlation between amount of effort and the snap. All of the levels of effort before the break are associated with the stick's being intact, whereas all of the greater levels of force are associated with it's being broken. The level of force that is required to snap a particular type of twig can eventually be rather well determined.

One of the major advantages of the PRS is that it can be used to reliably quantify clinical impressions in pediatric or psychiatric diagnostic settings because the relevant data are derived as part of a systematic semistructured interview rather than as a result of an elaborate research paradigm. The Stress and Coping Interview focuses on (1) current or potential rejection, neglect, or abuse of the child; (2) a review of any difficulties that the child is experiencing; (3) a discussion of the quality of the parents' marriage; (4) the life stressors that have occurred in the previous 12 months; (5) the occurrence of any overt parental psychopathology; (6) quality of the parents' social support network; (7) conflicts between child care responsibilities and maternal employment, professional, or educational objectives; (8) child care and medical emergencies; and (9) a brief medical history of the child (Table 3).

The interviewer is encouraged to use verbal probes to ascertain sufficient information to be able to rate the quality of the marriage, the severity of recent stressors, and level of maternal coping. This interview procedure has been previously described as it pertains to gathering data relevant to the coding of the "quality" of the parents' marital relationship (Klinnert et al., 1992). The entire Stress and Coping Interview requires between 60 to 90 minutes to complete, depending on the complexity of the life events that have occurred, but the interview can be conducted in an abbreviated form to target a particular construct. The time frame of inquiry has usually been

TABLE 3
Content Areas of the Stress and Coping Interview
Required to Make the Judgment of Parenting Risk

---

1. Any sign of current or potential rejection, neglect, or abuse
2. A review of any difficulties that the child will be experiencing
3. A discussion of quality of the parents' marriage
4. The life stressors that have occurred in the previous 12 months
5. The occurrence of any overt parental psychopathology
6. Quality of the parents' social support network
7. Potential maternal employment, professional, and educational conflicts
8. Child care and medical emergencies
9. Medical history

---

determined to extend back for 12 months, but it can be modified to define any time frame of particular interest (e.g., 9 months in the case of reflecting back on the course of a pregnancy). Both parents can be interviewed together, but an interview with only the mother has proved to be an effective strategy. For example, in the Asthma Risk Study, only the mother was interviewed when the child was 3 weeks old. These maternal assessments proved to be highly predictive of later difficulties as is demonstrated in the "Results" section of this article. It is not necessary to record interview sessions if the interview is being used clinically in a pediatric setting, but videotaping or audiotaping these interview sessions does provide a valuable method for periodically ensuring interrater reliability when the interview is used to assess a large research sample.

The following parental attitudes and behaviors were documented during the interview: (1) the emotional climate in the home, (2) attributions of negative traits to the child, (3) using the child to meet parental emotional needs, (4) inappropriate expectations for the child, (5) lack of support for the child's increasing autonomy, (6) competitiveness with the child for spousal attention, and (7) lack of knowledge or concern about health maintenance or behavioral difficulties.

The PRS ratings were designed to classify parents into one of three categories. Parents in the first category of the scale, Parenting Difficulties, were determined to have at least one problem in one of the five dimensions that was sufficiently serious to warrant the need for clinical intervention. The second category, Concerns about Parenting, was used to designate parents who were functioning on a higher level but where there was some concern about one of the five dimensions of parenting that was specifically noted during the interview and prompted the rater to recommend monitoring the family for future signs of more overt disturbance. The third category was designated to be Adequate Parenting. These parents were noted to be affectively available, sensitive to appropriate limit-setting, free of any overt psychopathology that might affect the child, aware of the developmental needs of the child, and committed to a lifestyle that would allow them to sufficiently support their child's emotional development. The PRS classified two thirds of the parents as functioning at an adequate level.

## Measures Used to Examine Validity

**Stress and Coping Interview.** A set of clinical judgments concerning key family characteristics was documented using 5-point scales designed to categorize different levels of functioning (Klinnert et al., 1992; Mrazek et al., 1991). An appraisal of the mother's ability to modulate distress for her baby, maternal role conflict, general coping, a judgment regarding the presence and severity of postpartum depressive symptoms, and a rating of the quality of the parents' marriage were made. More practical judgments, such as the degree to which health precautions are being taken by the parents, were also made at all points.

**Minnesota Multiphasic Personality Inventory (MMPI).** The MMPI (Hathaway and McKinley, 1970) is a 566-item paper-and-pencil test that is used to measure 10 dimensions of personality. It contains 3 validity scales, 10 clinical scales, and 4 special scales. Currently, the MMPI is the most widely used personality measurement instrument in psychological research and has been used extensively for both clinical and research purposes.

**Behavioral Screening Questionnaire.** This semistructured interview was designed to document the occurrence of commonly encountered early behavioral disturbances in 12 specific areas (Richman and Graham, 1971). The maximum score is 24. A score of 10 or more is indicative of clinically significant behavioral disturbance (Richman et al., 1982). Good interrater reliability has been established. The Behavioral Screening Questionnaire has been used widely as a screening questionnaire and was validated in a large American sample by a team from Harvard on Martha's Vineyard, Massachusetts (Earls et al., 1982). In addition, this instrument was used in assessing severely asthmatic preschool children who were found to have more early difficulties than healthy comparison children (Mrazek et al., 1985).

**Ainsworth strange situation.** The Strange Situation is a widely used method of assessing early infant attachment and is based on the coding of a highly structured paradigm that involves two maternal separations and reunions (Ainsworth et al., 1978; Ainsworth and Wittig, 1969). A rating of the quality and security of attachment is derived; this rating has been associated with later emotional adjustment and relationships (Sroufe et al., 1984).

## RESULTS

### *Reliability*

The interrater reliability of the PRS has been assessed consistently over the course of the Asthma Risk Study. Original interrater reliability assessed when the children were 3 weeks old was calculated to be 76% (Mrazek et al., 1991). Subsequent reliability of the coding of the adequacy of parenting was found to be 74% during the evaluations that occurred when study children were 6 months of age. Reliability was calculated using two methods. The first was the review of videotapes by a second rater. The alternative method was direct observation of the interview by a second clinician and simultaneous rating. Percent agreement was calculated by examining the frequency of exact agreement over the total number of paired codings. Like all interview ratings assessments, the level of reliability is enhanced by regular reliability checks. When two raters worked closely together, levels of reliability approached 90%. Conversely, if raters are allowed to work in isolation, rater drift can result in interrater reliability of less than 70% After considerable experience with this measure, it is clear that it can be used in a highly reliable manner, but rating is substantially enhanced by clinical training in a mental health discipline. Good reliability between psychiatrists, psychologists, social workers, and postdoctoral clinical students was achieved after focused training sessions. The duration of training varied from 3 to 4 sessions for experienced clinicians to approximately 10 sessions for graduate student raters.

It was conceptualized that quality of parenting would be stable but that some variability in parenting would occur over time for a variety of reasons. First, it is reasonable to expect that parenting will improve with experience. A second consideration is that severe stressors can occur that have a negative impact on the capacity of parents to care for their children. Third, protective factors such as the arrival of a grandmother to help with child care can occur and result in an improvement in the ability of young parents to cope with early challenges of child rearing. Fourth, therapeutic interventions such as the introduction of a course of antidepressant medication can improve depressed parents' capacity to respond sensitively to their children. Fifth, the demands of parenting vary with the developmental stage of the child such that the skills and abilities that are required to adequately care for an infant are clearly different from those required to care for a 2-year-old who is beginning to establish greater autonomy.

Despite these factors that can lead to changes in the quality of parenting, it has been clinically observed that the quality of parenting is usually very stable. Furthermore, some powerful components of parenting are certainly the result of parental genetic endowment, the child's primary temperament, and early familial experiences that include the parenting that the child's parent received many years before the conception of the child. Demonstrations of the stability of maintained relationships have included studies of intergenerational patterns of attachment. The results of assessments using the Adult Attachment Interview demonstrate that the patterns of attachment that children form with their mothers are often similar to the coded category of attachment that their mother had with her own mother. High rates of continuity for intergenerational patterns of attachment have been reported (Main et al., 1985).

### Concurrent Validity

**Association with interview scale scores.** Seven interview rating scales were scored during the maternal interview that occurred 3 weeks after the birth of the index child (Klinnert et al., 1992; Mrazek et al., 1991). Four of these ratings were significantly associated with the rating of parenting risk and provide some insight into the range of problems represented by the PRS (Table 4). For example, mothers who were rated as having parenting difficulties were much more likely to be coded as coping poorly than were those rated under parenting concerns or adequate parenting ($p < .0001$). Similarly, problematic marital satisfaction and difficulties in modulating the child's affect were highly significantly associated with the PRS. Postpartum depression was rare in this sample, but when it did occur, depressed mothers were always coded as having either parenting concerns or parenting difficulties.

**Association with *MMPI* scales.** Of the nine standard MMPI scales, five were significantly associated with the PRS. In every case, the significant difference was that the parents with problematic parenting had elevated scale scores. However, the absolute levels of these elevations were modest, and none of the mean MMPI scores for the group that was coded as

TABLE 4

Association Between Parenting Risk Categories and Four Other Interview Rating Scales, Using $\chi^2$ Analysis

| Problems Identified Using Interview Rating Scales | Parenting Risk Categories[a] | | | | Significance (p Values) |
| --- | --- | --- | --- | --- | --- |
| | Adequate Parenting | Parenting Concerns | Parenting Difficulties | | |
| Problematic maternal coping | 24 | 81 | 87 | | .0001 |
| Problematic marital adjustment | 10 | 53 | 79 | | .0001 |
| Poor maternal modulation | 1 | 16 | 67 | | .0001 |
| Postpartum depression | 0 | 8 | 13 | | .005 |

[a] Values are percentages.

having problematic parenting would be considered to be overtly patholog-ical. This pattern of elevated scale scores had not been predicted. First, the most significantly related scales (i.e., psychopathic deviance, schizophre-nia, paranoia, and depression) are among the most clearly associated with psychopathology at extreme elevations. However, less dramatic personal-ity dysfunction in these areas could also interfere with adequate parenting. The fifth scale that was associated with the PRS was psychasthenia, which is a measure of anxiety level and rigidity. Elevated scores on this scale may represent a potential problem related to adaptability or may be an indica-tion of psychopathology. Given that all ratings of parenting risk were made with no awareness of the MMPI scores, these multiple significant associa-tions provide support for the concurrent validity of the PRS (Table 5).

## Predictive Validity

**Prediction of later behavioral problems.** Given the long-standing clini-cal association between parenting dysfunction and behavioral difficulties, a reasonable test of a measure of parenting is its ability to accurately pre-dict these problems. The 3-week ratings using the PRS were significantly associated with the overall behavioral questionnaire scores based on ma-ternal interviews that were conducted when the children were 24 months of age. Sixty percent of the children whose mothers had been rated as having parenting difficulties in the perinatal period were documented to have de-

TABLE 5

Association Between Parenting Risk
and Prenatal Maternal Minnesota Multiphasic Personality
Inventory (MMPI) Scale Scores Determined
Before the Birth of the Child

| MMPI Scale | Adequate Parenting | Inadequate Parenting | Significance |
|---|---|---|---|
| Psychopathic Deviance | 52.2 | 57.4 | .001 |
| Schizophrenia | 51.8 | 55.1 | .005 |
| Paranoia | 54.7 | 58.4 | .008 |
| Depression | 50.0 | 54.1 | .009 |
| Psychasthenia | 51.4 | 54.0 | .033 |
| Social Introversion | 51.9 | 53.5 | .372 |
| Hypochondriasis | 53.6 | 54.9 | .404 |
| Hypomania | 54.0 | 54.9 | .604 |
| Hysteria | 56.3 | 56.8 | .742 |

TABLE 6
Association Between Parenting Risk
and Behavioral Disturbance at 24 Months

| Parenting Risk Category | Percent with Behavioral Disturbance |
|---|---|
| Parenting Difficulties | 60 |
| Concerns about Parenting | 49 |
| Adequate Parenting | 31 |

*Note:* $\chi^2 = 7.13$, $p = .03$.

veloped a sufficient number of behavioral problems to place them in the clinical range of dysfunction on the Behavioral Screening Questionnaire (Richman and Graham, 1971) (Table 6).

**Prediction of attachment at 12 months.** Security of attachment has been shown to be associated with both sensitive and responsive parenting. The PRS was predicted to identify mothers with problematic parenting styles whose children would be predicted to have a greater likelihood of developing insecure attachments as ascertained by the Strange Situation. Children of mothers who had been coded as having parenting difficulties when their children were 3 weeks of age were significantly more likely to develop insecure attachments than were children of mothers who had been rated as demonstrating adequate parenting (71% versus 36%) (Table 7).

**Prediction of the later onset of asthma.** Problematic parenting has long been hypothesized to be associated with a greater risk for the development of asthma in children who have a genetic vulnerability for the development of this illness. The PRS was designed to provide a sensitive method of

TABLE 7
Association Between Parenting Risk and Security
of Attachment at 12 Months

| Parenting Risk Category | Insecure Attachment | Secure Attachment |
|---|---|---|
| Parenting Difficulties | 71 | 29 |
| Concerns about Parenting | 51 | 49 |
| Adequate Parenting | 36 | 64 |

*Note:* Values are percentages. $\chi^2 = 7.56$, $p = .02$.

quantifying the full range of parenting difficulties and concerns that were conceptually believed to be associated with the onset of asthma in these children. Preliminary analyses of the association of the PRS with the onset of asthma, using maternal report methodology to establish the occurrence of wheezing, revealed a positive association when the children were 2 years of age (Mrazek et al., 1991). Subsequent analyses using stricter criteria for the diagnosis of asthma based solely on medical records confirmed this initial relationship when the children were 3 years of age. Children of parents who had been determined to have parenting difficulties when they were 3 weeks of age were significantly more likely to have developed asthma by the time they were 3 years old than were children at the same level of genetic risk but whose parents had been assessed as demonstrating adequate parenting (20% versus 5%) (Table 8).

**Stability of parenting risk score.** Just as the quality of mother-child attachment tends to be fairly stable over time, so does the parental pattern of relating to the child. Similarly, while the quality of an attachment is subject to change based on the dyad's exposure to intervening risk factors or the introduction of protective factors, the parenting risk score similarly is affected by major intervening factors as demonstrated by the parenting risk assessments that were completed over the first 4 years of the Asthma Risk Study. Two types of analyses were completed to examine the stability of the scale. First, the full scale was considered. Using both repeated $\chi^2$ analyses or Spearman rank-ordered correlations, significant stability was demonstrated. All $\chi^2$ analyses between time points showed significant stability at levels that varied from $p < .02$ to $p < .0001$. Spearman rank-ordered correlations were similarly stable, with comparable levels of significance. Of considerable interest were the results of the analyses comparing ratings of parenting risk made based on the prenatal interviews;

TABLE 8
Association Between Parenting Risk
and the Onset of Asthma

| Parenting Risk Category | Percent Who Develop Asthma by 3 Years of Age |
|---|---|
| Parenting Difficulties | 20 |
| Concerns about Parenting | 16 |
| Adequate Parenting | 5 |

*Note:* $\chi^2 = 6.16$, $p = .05$.

these were highly correlated with rates of parenting risk made by an independent clinician who was blind to all previous coding when the children were 4 years of age ($r = .42, p < .0001$). Second, when the scale was used to dichotomize the sample into adequate parents and those with some level of parenting concern or difficulties, both statistical methods still resulted in entirely comparable high levels of significant stability.

## DISCUSSION

The PRS is well suited for use in clinical settings as it is based on a systematic semistructured interview that is designed to clarify highly relevant diagnostic data that are generally accepted as appropriate areas of inquiry regarding the care and development of children. The interview is sufficiently flexible to be able to assess the parents of children with a wide range of psychiatric or pediatric conditions. The full Stress and Coping Interview requires 60 to 90 minutes to conduct, but an abbreviated version that primarily targets the content areas relevant to coding the PRS can be completed in approximately 30 minutes. Although even this abbreviated version may be too long to be adopted by pediatricians as a component of a routine pediatric history, the interview is an entirely appropriate method for a member of the pediatric team to use to explore family concerns that arise during the medical evaluation.

The Stress and Coping Interview provides a useful organizational structure to collect and sort through the complex parental behaviors and emotions that contribute to competent parenting. The evaluation and monitoring of the five dimensions of parenting (Table 1) not only serves as a useful method for ensuring a comprehensive approach to the evaluation of the family but also provides a consistent framework that has proven to be a particularly useful strategy for working with multidisciplinary teams on both child psychiatric inpatient services and inpatient pediatric units. One specific advantage of using the PRS routinely in clinical settings is that problematic parenting behaviors that affect a single discrete dimension of parenting can be designated as a focal problem on the problem list of the medical record. These more discrete parenting difficulties can be more effectively monitored than more obscure entries (e.g., "psychosocial problems") that all too often appear in the problem list of the chart. With a more precise designation of the problem, it is also often easier for the clinical team to develop a therapeutic action plan.

Having residents routinely use the Stress and Coping Interview to collect data from parents and then score the PRS to evaluate the quality of parenting provides an efficient didactic strategy for conveying basic family assessment skills. For example, incorporating the stress and coping questions as part of the standard clinical diagnostic interview often leads to rapid identification of problematic family interactions that are associated with symptomatic behavior in the child patient. Early recognition of behavioral and emotional problems subsequently increases the probability of implementing quite specific interventions designed to resolve the target concerns. Optimally, early indicated preventive interventions, as defined by the recent Institute of Medicine report on prevention, may result in the avoidance of the onset of subsequent psychiatric disorders (Mrazek and Haggerty, 1994).

While the identification and documentation of adequate parenting may seem to be a less critical objective than identifying problematic parenting, the assessment of competent parents using the Stress and Coping Interview frequently yields important information to the clinician that can be used in the development of a care plan for the medical and nursing teams. Similarly, the designation of either concerns about parenting or parenting difficulties provides important information that can be used effectively by pediatric and social work staff to identify children who need special services as well as providing some quantification of a previously elusive risk factor for the subsequent development of early behavioral difficulties.

Given the critical role that parenting plays in both normal child development and in the theoretical underpinnings of developmental psychopathology, an obvious question is why no generally accepted method for coding the quality of parenting has become a standard for the field. While there are many reasons, two issues are undeniably important: evaluating parents is difficult, and it entails some liability.

Methods for the evaluation of parenting have been proposed by some of the most creative researchers in fields of child psychiatry (Anthony and Benedik, 1970; Cohen, 1977) and child psychology (Baumrind, 1971; G.R. Patterson, R.S. Ray, D.A. Shaw, J.A. Cobb, unpublished, 1969). Although interesting methods for the assessment of parenting have been developed, the complex multidimensional characteristics of parent-child interactions have proven to be very difficult to capture without obtaining an extensive data set that includes documentation of the affective state of the parent and the quality of the interactions of the parent with the child. Just as in the initial development of the attachment of the infant to the parent and the reciprocal bonding of the parent to the child, characteristics such as parental sensitivity and responsivity are critical and are extremely difficult to capture within the context of a questionnaire. It is also generally accepted that a wide range of parenting dimensions contribute to the competence of a parent. Consequently, the assessment of parenting requires a complex algorithm to appropriately assign relative significance to the disparate cognitive, emotional, and behavioral components of interactions of the parent with the child. Two of the many variables that contribute to the assessment of parenting are how difficult the child is to care for and the available resources of the family. It is self-evident that there is enormous variability in the temperament, cognition, competencies, affect regulation, and health of siblings, who have a probability of a sharing 50% of their respective genomes but this critical factor of individual differences is rarely considered in questionnaires that have been designed for the assessment of parenting. The PRS has the advantage of evaluating many dimensions of parenting within the context of the extended family and community as well as capitalizing on the clinical experience of the rater in weighing the data. It also narrowly focuses the raters' judgments to the task of identifying concerns about parenting and parenting difficulties that are believed to be risk factors for the development of early psychopathology. Consequently, the PRS does not allow for the differentiation of adequate, good, excellent, and superlative parenting, which would require a different data set to be able to discriminate reliability. However, methods to accomplish this objective could be developed by using the same conceptual dimensions that were used to design the PRS.

Clinicians are often reluctant to make judgments about parenting. There are many explanations for this phenomenon that include the limited demonstrated validity of previous methods for the assessments of parenting and the medical/legal liabilities associated with documenting disturbances of parenting in the current litigious health care environment. Furthermore, the changing role of women in society, coupled with the persistent social expectation that mothers act as the primary caretakers of their children, has contributed to the high emotional valence associated with negative parenting assessments. This issue is well illustrated by the controversial debate related to the potential impacts on child development of the range of currently utilized child care alternatives.

While the ratings derived for the PRS do not provide quantification of the range of severity of specific salient parenting deficits, they do effectively identify children at risk for negative outcomes. Consequently, the PRS score promises to be a useful research instrument for the documentation of parental dysfunction. The predictive capability of the PRS is greater than that of currently available questionnaires (Abidin, 1990a,b) or card sort methodologies (J.H. Block, unpublished, 1980; Davies et al., 1991), and its use is more practical than complex interactive paradigms (Cox et al., 1989). However, the PRS scores do not provide insight into which parenting characteristics are linked to which specific subsequent childhood conditions. In this regard, a next step in the development of appropriate and more precise instruments for the assessment of parenting would be to conduct a comprehensive study of parents that could reliably document levels of competency for each of the five specific parenting dimensions described in this article. This quantification would lead to the capability of linking variable patterns of parenting to differential outcomes in groups of children at risk for the development of specific emotional or behavioral disturbances. During the conduct of prospective studies, relevant parental risk and protective factors could be monitored in an ongoing manner to interpret variability in developmental outcomes of the index children. This research strategy will become increasingly practical when cohorts of children at risk for specific illnesses can be identified by determining the presence of specific genetic alleles that require exposure to environmental stressors to serve as releasers and trigger the expression of the disease. Better definition of such parental risk factors will provide the opportunity to develop more specific and effective familial interventions targeted at decreasing the incidence of childhood disturbances.

## REFERENCES

Abidin RR (1990a) The stresses of parenting. *J Clin Child Psychol* 19:298–301.

Abidin RR (1990b), *Parenting Stress Index.* Charlottesville, VA: Pediatric Psychology Press.

Ainsworth MDS, Blehar MD, Waters E, Wall S (1978), *Patterns of Attachment.* Hillsdale, NJ: Lawrence Erlbaum and Associates

Ainsworth M, Wittig BA (1969), Attachment and exploratory behavior of one-year-olds in a strange situation. In: *Determinants of Infant Behavior IV*, Foss BM, ed. London: Methuen, pp 111–136.

Anthony EJ, Benedik T, eds. (1970), *Parenthood: Psychology and Psychopathology.* Boston: Little, Brown Publishers

Baumrind D (1971), Current patterns of parental authority. *Dev Psychol Monogr* 4(1):1–103.

Baumrind D (1993), The average expectable environment is not good enough: a response to Scarr. *Child Dev* 64:1299–1317.

Baumrind D, Black AE (1967), Socialization practices associated with dimensions of competence in preschool boys and girls. *Child Dev* 38:291–327.

Belsky J (1984), The determinants of parenting: a process model. *Child Dev* 55: 83–96.

Carlson V, Cicchetti D, Barnett D, Braunwald KG (1989), Finding order in disorganization: lessons from research on maltreated infants' attachments to their caregivers. In: *Child Maltreatment: Theory and Research on the Causes and*

*Consequences of Child Abuse and Neglect*, Cicchetti D, Carlson V, eds. New York: Cambridge University Press, pp 494–528.

Cohen D (1977), Parental style. Mothers' and fathers' perceptions of their relations with twin children. *Arch Gen Psychiatry* 34:445–51.

Cox MH, Owen MT, Lewis JL, Henderson VK (1989), Marriage, adult adjustment, and early parenting. *Child Dev* 60:1015–1024.

Davies WH, Noll RB, DeStefano L, Bukowski WM, Kulkarni R (1991), Childhood cancer and parental child-rearing practices. *J Pediatr Psychol* 16:295–306.

Dowdney L, Skuse D, Rutter M, Quinton D, Mrazek D (1984), Parenting qualities: concepts, measures, and origins. *J Child Psychol Psychiatry* 26(suppl 4): 599–625.

Earls F, Jacobs G, Goldfein D, Gilbert A, Beardslee W, Rivinus T (1982), Concurrent validation of a behavior problems scale to use with 3-year-olds. *J Am Acad Child Psychiatry* 21:47–57.

Gaensbauer TJ, Mrazek D (1981), Differences in the patterning of affective expression in infants. *J Am Acad Child Psychiatry* 20:673–691.

Hathaway SR, McKinley JC (1970), *Minnesota Multiphasic Personality Inventory*. Minneapolis: University of Minnesota Press.

Jackson JF (1993), Human behavioral genetics, Scarr's theory, and her views on interventions: a critical review and commentary on their implications for African-American children. *Child Dev* 64:1318–1332.

Kanner L (1935), *Child Psychiatry*. Springfield, IL: Charles C Thomas.

Klinnert MD, Mrazek P, Mrazek DA (1992), Quality of marital relationship: a clinical rating scale. *Psychiatry* 55:132–145.

Main M, Kaplan N, Cassidy J (1985), Security in infancy, childhood, and adulthood: a move to the level of representation. *Monogr Soc Res Child Dev* 50: 66–104.

Martin HP, Beezley P (1977), Behavioral observations of abused children. *Dev Med Child Neurol* 19:373–387.

Minuchin S, Rosman BL, Baker L (1978), *Psychosomatic Families*. Cambridge, MA: Harvard University Press.

Mrazek PJ (1993), Maltreatment and infant development. In: *Handbook of Infant Mental Health*, Zeanah CH Jr, ed. New York: Guilford Press, pp 159–170.

Mrazek D, Anderson I, Strunk R (1985), Disturbed emotional development of severely asthmatic preschool children. In: *Recent Research in Developmental Psychopathology. Journal of Child Psychology and Psychiatry Book Suppl 4*, Stevenson J, ed. Oxford, England: Pergamon Press, pp 81–94.

Mrazek DA, Dowdney L, Rutter ML, Quinton DL (1982), Mother and preschool child interaction: a sequential approach. *J Am Acad Child Psychiatry* 21: 453–464.

Mrazek PJ, Haggerty RJ, eds. (1994), *Reducing Risks for Mental Disorders*. Washington, DC: National Academy Press.

Mrazek DA, Klinnert MD, Mrazek P, Macey T (1991), Early asthma onset: consideration of parenting issues. *J Am Acad Child Adolesc Psychiatry* 30: 277–282.

Mrazek PJ, Mrazek DA (1987), Resilience in child maltreatment victims: a conceptual exploration. *Child Abuse Negl* 11:357–366.

Radke-Yarrow M, Nottelmann E, Martinez P, Fox MB, Belmont B (1992), Young children of affectively ill parents: a longitudinal study of psychosocial development. *J Am Acad Child Adolesc Psychiatry* 31:68–77.

Richman N, Graham P (1971), A behavioral screening questionnaire for use with three-year-old children. *J Child Psychol Psychiatry* 12:5–33.

Richman N, Stevenson JE, Graham PJ (1982), *Pre-School to School: A Behavioral Study*. London: Academic Press.

Rutter ML (1966), *Children of Sick Parents*. London: Oxford University Press.

Scarr S (1992), Developmental theories for the 1900's: development and individual differences. *Child Dev* 63:1–19.

Scarr S (1993), Biological and cultural diversity: the legacy of Darwin for development. *Child Dev* 64:1333–1353.

Schaefer ES (1959), A circumplex model for maternal behavior. *J Abnorm Soc Psychol* 59:226–235.

Sears RR, Maccoby E, Levin H (1957), *Patterns of Child Rearing*. Evanston, IL: Row, Peterson & Company.

Sroufe LA, Schork E, Motti E, Lawroski N, LaFreniere P (1984), The role of affect in emerging social competence. In: *Emotion, Cognition, and Behavior*, Izard C, Kagan J, Zajonc R, eds. New York: Cambridge University Press, pp 289–319.

Winnicott DW (1957), *The Child and the Family*. London: Tavistock Publications; New York: Basic Books.

# 8

# Genetic Questions for Environmental Studies: Differential Parenting and Psychopathology in Adolescence

**David Reiss, George W. Howe, Samuel J. Simmens, and Danielle A. Bussell**

*George Washington University School of Medicine and Health Sciences, Washington, D.C.*

**E. Mavis Hetherington, Sandra H. Henderson, Thomas J. O'Connor, and Tracy Law**

*University of Virginia, Charlottesville*

**Robert Plomin**

*Pennsylvania State University, University Park*

**Edward R. Anderson**

*Texas Tech University, Lubbock*

**Background:** *Recent genetic evidence suggests that the most important environmental influences on normal and pathologic development are those that are not shared by siblings in the same family. We sought to determine the relationship between differences in parenting styles and depressive symptoms and antisocial behavior in adolescence, and to compare the influence of these nonshared experiences with genetic influences.* **Methods:** *We studied 708 families with at least two same-sexed adolescent siblings who were monozygotic twins (93 families), di-*

Reprinted with permission from *Archives of General Psychiatry*, 1995, Vol. 52, 925–936. Copyright © 1995 by the American Medical Association.

This research was supported by grant 5-ROI-MH43373 from the National Institute of Mental Health, Rockville, MD, and by a grant from the William T. Grant Foundation, New York, NY.

*zygotic twins (99 families), ordinary siblings (95 families), full siblings in step families (181 families), half siblings in step families (110 families), and genetically unrelated siblings in step families (130 families). Data on parenting style were collected by questionnaire and by video recording of interaction between parents and children.* **Results:** *Almost 60% of variance in adolescent antisocial behavior and 37% of variance in depressive symptoms could be accounted for by conflictual and negative parental behavior directed specifically at the adolescent. In contrast, when a parent directed harsh, aggressive, explosive, and inconsistent parenting toward the* sibling, *we found* less *psychopathologic outcome in the adolescent.* **Conclusions:** *Parenting behavior directed specifically at each child in the family is a major correlate of symptoms in adolescents. Furthermore, harsh parental behavior directed at a sibling may have protective effects for adolescents, a phenomenon we call the "sibling baricade."*

Recent genetic studies have suggested that siblings raised in the same family differ on a broad range of measures of competence and psychopathologic outcome. Whatever similarities siblings show mostly result from shared genes rather than common family environments.[1,2] These findings from genetic studies have posed two questions to researchers of the family environment. First, are siblings treated differently by their parents or do they experience themselves as being treated differently? Second, do these differences play an important role in the development of either competence or psychopathologic outcome?

The term *nonshared environment* refers to those environmental factors that produce different developmental outcomes for each sibling in a family. Examples of shared environmental influences are social class, neighborhood decay, and maternal depression. Examples of nonshared environment are differential treatment of the siblings by the parents, highly discrepant life experience within any sibship, and differences in the quality of marriage of two siblings when they become adults.

To estimate the importance of the nonshared environment in depression and antisocial behavior, some investigators have examined variations in dimensions of depressive symptoms and antisocial behavior in nonclinical populations. In studies of depressive symptoms in adults[3] and child twins,[4] environmental influence is predominantly of the nonshared type. Studies of antisocial behavior[5-8] showed a more equal influence of shared and non-shared influences. With clinical populations, adoption studies of conduct disorders and antisocial personality disorder yield little evidence of shared environmental influences,[9] but twin studies show a substantial effect.[10] For diagnosed affective disorders, the evidence of the importance of nonshared environmental factors, in sharp contrast to shared environmental factors, is clear. For example, twin studies show concordance well below 100%,[10-12] and adoption studies show little difference between the adopting parents of depressed or manic-depressed patients and the adopting parents of index subjects without affective disorders.[10-13]

Unfortunately, these genetic studies cannot specify which specific non-shared environmental factors are important. These factors may be biologic (such as toxins or intrauterine viruses) or social. Furthermore, they may not be general influences: influential differences may be unique for each family. Recent preliminary studies have directly measured specific nonshared factors in the family environment by sampling families with two or more children and have studied the effects of differential parenting or other sibling differences in family and social factors. Dunn et al[14] showed that children who received more maternal affection and less maternal control than their siblings showed less internalizing symptoms. Siblings who received more control showed more externalizing behavior.[15] Other investigators have shown that more parental punishment is associated with more suicidal ideation and oppositional behavior.[16]

More conventional studies, involving only one child per family, suggest that parental warmth and support buffers children against externalizing and antisocial behavior[17] and is positively associated with a child's self-esteem.[18] Conflictual and coercive parenting is positively associated with externalizing, including disruptive and deceitful behavior, in general[17] and with more narrowly defined antisocial behavior in particular.[19,20] However, where parents can track the behavior of their children—both inside and outside the home—and can exert effective discipline, the risk of antisocial behavior in children and adolescents is reduced.[19,20] These findings suggest that three domains of parental behavior influence adolescent depression and antisocial behavior: (1) warmth/support, (2) conflict and coercion, and (3) monitoring/control. The present study seeks to assess whether parents treat their children differently and, if they do, whether these differences are associated with offspring psychopathologic development. Subsequent reports will detail the role of genetic factors in these associations.

## SUBJECTS AND METHODS

### *Types of Families Studied*

The sample included families in two broad classes. The first class consisted of those with no divorce after the birth of the oldest child in our sample (nondivorced families); thus, both children were biologic offspring of both parents. This class had three groups: 93 families with identical (monozygotic) twins, 99 with fraternal (dizygotic) twins, and 95 with full nontwin siblings. Eighty-five of the families with monozygotic twins, 87 of those with dizygotic twins, and 90 full-sibling families had no history of marriage before the current one for the mothers, and 85, 81, and 87 families, respectively, had no history of previous marriage for the fathers. Twin zygosity was determined by the research staff interviewer and parent report of physical similarity by means of a modified form of a questionnaire designed to determine zygosity in adolescent twins.[21] This questionnaire, when compared with blood tests of single-gene markers, is accurate in greater than 90% of cases. Zygosity could not be determined in 6% of the twins with this questionnaire, a rate comparable with that in other studies.

The second class included step families, also divided into three groups: 181 families with full siblings, brought into the current marriage by the mother from a previous marriage (sibling pairs share approximately 50% of their genes); 110 families with half siblings in which the mother brought one child from a previous marriage and had the second child with her current spouse (sibling pairs share approximately 25% of their genes); and 130 families with genetically unrelated siblings in which the father and mother each brought a child to the current family from a previous marriage. In our total sample, 70% of the families had one or more other siblings, with the total number of children from those families ranging from three to 10. In 238 families (33%), the siblings tested were the only two children in the family, in 272 (38%) there were only younger children than those tested, in 141 (20%) there were only older children, and in 69 (10%) there were both younger and older children. (Twelve twin pairs were excluded from analysis because of uncertain zygosity.)

Each family, to be included in the sample, must have had two children of the same gender, no more than 4 years apart in age and no younger than 10 years or older than 18 years. To be sure that none of the step families were in the early stages of family formation, the current marriage had to be of at least 5 years' duration. The tested siblings in each family had to be residents in the household at least half of each week.

According to the 1980 Current Population Survey, only 0.04% of house-holds met our sampling requirements for unrelated siblings, and 0.12% met requirements for half siblings.[22] Thus, we screened 675,000 households, by means of a combination of random digit dialing and market panels, to meet the minimum sample size of 100 families of blended and unrelated siblings.

All remarried families of unrelated siblings and of half siblings drawn from the market panels were approached, since these were the rarest types. The participation rates were 44% and 48%, respectively. This rate com-pares favorably with sampling procedures in other family studies that have used community or national registers and that required three or four mem-bers of a family to be recruited for joint testing and assessment (30.5%[23] and 41%).[24] We do not have enough information on nonparticipant fami-lies to estimate the bias in our test sample, if any. Both families of twins and remarried families of full siblings were sampled until a targeted group size was reached, with some attempt to select families that matched those of unrelated siblings and half siblings with respect to age and age spacing of children. Families of twins were also sampled until a targeted group size was reached. Since we did not approach all eligible families in these groups, no true response rate can be computed. Nondivorced families of full siblings were obtained by the random digit dialing procedure.

The mean age of children in the sample was 13.8 years; the mean age for mothers and fathers was 38.1 and 41.0 years, respectively. As a conse-quence of their identical age, the older twin in the twin families was younger than the older siblings in other families, whereas the younger twin was older than the younger siblings in other families. There were few dif-ferences in demographic variables across the six groups. The mean dura-tion of marriage was, as expected, significantly greater for the nondivorced sample (18.4 years) than it was for the step families (8.9 years). Again, as expected, the families with half siblings had a longer mean ($\pm SD$) duration of marriages (13.2 $\pm$ 2.76 years) than did the full (7.5 $\pm$ 2.76 years) or un-related-sibling (7.2 $\pm$ 2.7 years) step families. The mean number of years of education was 13.6 for mothers and 14.0 for fathers, with families of half siblings showing significantly lower scores, for both, in comparison with the other five groups. Family income (mean for the total sample ranged between \$25,000 and \$35,000) was also significantly lower in the half-sibling families. The Hollingshead four-factor indicator of socioeconomic status showed that step families were significantly lower than the nondi-vorced families. Ninety-four percent of the women and 93% of the men were white, with the remainder consisting of other ethnic groups. The relatively high proportion of whites in our sample of families with long marital duration reflects their lower divorce and higher remarriage rates, when compared with African Americans and nonwhite Hispanics.[25]

Our sample scored approximately the same on several measures of psychopathologic outcome as other non-psychiatric samples of children of approximately the same age.[4,26–28]

## Procedure

Families were studied during a 15-month period in all states, with the exception of South Dakota, Alaska, and Hawaii. Thirty-seven interviewer teams, unaware of the study's hypotheses and under the supervision of four full-time field managers, conducted all interviews in the families' homes. Most interviews were conducted by two member teams, but for some families with older children, they were conducted by single interviewers. Data were collected in two 3-hour sessions in the home no more than 2 weeks apart. Family members also completed simple questionnaires between the two sessions. Interview teams collected videotaped family interaction during the interviews, about half from each of the two sessions. These consisted of nine 10-minute interactions of each parent with each of the two siblings. Each dyad discussed and attempted to resolve a problem they had previously selected as a problem for them.

## Measures of Depressive Symptoms and Antisocial Behavior

We measured depressive symptoms and antisocial behavior as continuous variables rather than making categorical distinctions between "cases" and "noncases." This strategy was more likely to yield analyzable distributions in an ordinary-risk population. It has been used to predict concurrent adaptive functioning in adolescents,[22,29–31] to make concurrent distinctions between cases and noncases[32] as well as more specific syndromes,[26] and to assess adolescents' risk for adult psychopathologic development and maladaptive functioning.[33]

We used three measures of depressive symptoms in the adolescents: the Child Depression Inventory[26] (27 symptom items, including feelings of loneliness, sadness, poor appetite and sleep, and thoughts about suicide during the past 2 weeks) and a comparable parent version of the Child Depression Inventory;[34] the Behavior Problems Index[35] (adapted from the Child Behavior Checklist,[36] this is a 32-item scale that covers a full range of psychopathologic development during the past 3 months with six items concerning depression); and the Behavior Events Inventory.[17,20] This last measure asked each parent and both children to report the presence or absence of specific depressive behaviors, such as "cried" or "been withdrawn" during the past week.

Antisocial behavior was measured by a six-item scale from the Behavior Problems Index and nine items from the Behavior Events Inventory, such as "stole," "lied or cheated," or "skipped school." In addition, coders rated videotapes of the child's interaction with both parents, on a single five-point scale, for antisocial behavior, including instances of disruptive, rude, coercive, and aggressive behavior. Weighted κ for the reliability of this coding judgment was 0.77,[37] and the intraclass correlation coefficient between coders was .86. Separate coders were always used for each of the two children in a family.

The Child Depression Inventory and Behavior Events Inventory were administered twice at least a week apart. Thus, combined scores are less likely to reflect transient mood or behavioral disturbances.

### Measures of Parenting

Three domains of parenting were measured by means of coding of videotaped interaction and self-report questionnaires: conflict/negativity; warmth/support; and monitoring/control.[17] Twenty-one undergraduate and graduate students served as coders of parenting measures. We used 21 global scales from the Global Coding System.[17] Each rating required judging a 10-minute videotaped segment of interaction on a five-point scale. Coders were trained until they reached a criterion level of 60% exact agreement with a criterion coder. After they met that criterion, an average of 48% of all subsequent coding was checked for reliability. Where reliability fell below 60% perfect agreement, coding was redone.

The self-report and observer rating scales used to assess parenting are summarized in Table 1.[38]

### Analytic Strategy

**Operationalizing differential parenting effects.** We framed hypotheses concerning differential parenting in two ways. First, we examined certain patterns of simple correlations between parenting and adolescent symptoms. The relationships between these patterns and our hypotheses concerning differential parenting are summarized in Table 2. When parenting and outcome were substantially correlated for each child, but parenting to-

TABLE 1
Measures of Parenting and Their Reliabilities

| Domains and Scales | Focus of Measurement | Coefficient α | | Intraclass |
| --- | --- | --- | --- | --- |
| | | Child | Parent | |
| **Conflict/Negativity** | | | | |
| Self-report | | | | |
| Parent-child disagreement | Frequency of disagreements on specific issues (eg, telephone use) | .78–.91 | .83–.85 | . . . |
| Punitiveness | Frequency of yelling and punishing | .89–.90 | .89–.91 | . . . |
| Yielding to coercion | Surrendering to concompliant and disruptive behavior | .57–.61 | .63–.73 | . . . |
| Verbal aggression[38] | Swearing, threatening, stomping out of room | .72–.75 | .73–.74 | . . . |
| Open conflict | Frequency of severe conflict and fights | .70–.72 | .70–.78 | . . . |
| Observer ratings | | | | |
| Anger and rejection | Verbal and nonverbal criticism and denigration | . . . | . . . | .81 |
| Coercion | Manipulative control, including whining and threat | . . . | . . . | .78 |
| Transactional conflict | Reciprocate and escalated argument and conflict | . . . | . . . | .79 |
| **Warmth/Support** | | | | |
| Self-report | | | | |
| Closeness and rapport | Pleasure in closeness and involvement | .90–.92 | .85–.90 | . . . |
| Expression of affection | Overt signs of affection and pleasures in joint activity | .69–.85 | .73–.88 | . . . |
| Observer ratings | | | | |
| Warmth and support | Positive feelings, affection | . . . | . . . | .79 |
| Assertiveness | Positive expressions of needs; self-confidence and patience | . . . | . . . | .75 |

*(continued)*

TABLE 1 (*Continued*)

| Domains and Scales | Focus of Measurement | Coefficient α | | Intraclass |
|---|---|---|---|---|
| | | Child | Parent | |
| Communication | Ability to listen, explain, and elicit other's view | . . . | . . . | .62 |
| Involvement | Own initiative and encouraging other's participation | . . . | . . . | .68 |

**Monitoring/Control**

| Domains and Scales | Focus of Measurement | Child | Parent | Intraclass |
|---|---|---|---|---|
| Self-report | | | | |
| Knowledge | Information about child's activities | .88–.90 | .90–.91 | . . . |
| Attempted control | Efforts to control child's activities | .92–.93 | .91–.91 | . . . |
| Actual control | Successes in controlling child's activities | .95–.94 | .93–.94 | . . . |
| Observer ratings | | | | |
| Child monitoring | Parent knows about child's activities | . . . | . . . | .64 |
| Influence | Parent attempt at control | . . . | . . . | .68 |
| Parental authority | Successful influences on child's behavior and opinions | . . . | . . . | .64 |

ward each of the children was not correlated, then the lack of sibling correlation of symptom patterns was likely to result in part from differential parenting for this particular parenting variable. To test for this pattern, the relevant correlations were estimated for the three parenting domains and the two sets of outcomes, antisocial behavior and depressive symptoms.

Second, it seemed likely that most findings would not necessarily fit exactly any of the cells in Table 1. For example, it is possible that the correlation between parenting toward the adolescent and parenting toward the sibling would be moderate, but the correlation between parenting and outcome could still reflect effects specific to each adolescent. Regression analyses were used to test this hypothesis, by estimating parameters reflecting the relationship between parenting toward an adolescent and that adolescent's outcome while controlling for the level of parenting directed toward that adolescent's sibling. In this case the effects of differential parenting are measured directly, as indicated by this coefficient. We refer to

TABLE 2
Interpreting the Possible Patterns of Correlations Among Parenting
and Adolescent Outcome Variables

| Correlation Between Parenting and Outcome | Correlation Between Parenting Toward Child X and Child Y | Interpretation |
|---|---|---|
| Low | Low | Parenting is different for the 2 children and is also unrelated to outcome |
| Low | High | Parenting of the 2 children is highly correlated and is unrelated to outcome |
| High | Low | Clearest indication of non-shared effects: parenting is both different for each child and highly associated with outcome |
| High | High | Parenting is correlated for both children and strongly associated with outcome; non-shared parenting effects are impossible to detect |

this as the *specific effect*, since only variance in parenting that is specific to the child is related to variance in that child's symptoms. Figure 1 presents a path diagram depicting these regression analyses.

**Aggregating symptom measures.** Seven aggregate measures of symptoms for each child in a family were used. These reflect depressive symptoms as reported by mother, father, and child, and antisocial behavior as reported by mother, father, child, and observer. Aggregation was accomplished in the following way. First, each measure administered twice over the set of interviews was averaged across the two administrations (The correlations between session 1 and session 2 on all measures of psychopathologic outcome were invariably high.) Next, each measure from each respondent or source was standardized across all 1440 siblings in all families. Finally, all standardized measures of depressive symptoms and antisocial behavior from a particular respondent were averaged.

**Composting measures of parenting.** We examined patterns of intercorrelations among all measures of parenting to verify that each measure was

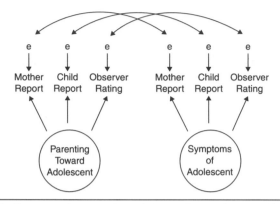

**Figure 1.** Path diagram of regression analyses for testing specific relationships between parenting and outcome, the *specific effects* as well as the relationship of parenting to siblings on the outcomes for the adolescents, the *cross-sibling effects*.

properly assigned to its correct domain. First, for the self-report scales, we performed a confirmatory factor analysis with the use of a three-factor solution on all parenting scales from the oldest child's report of the mother's parenting. Scales were constrained to load only on one factor. The same analysis was repeated for each child's report of parenting toward the mother, each child's report of parenting toward the father, and each parent's report of his or her parenting toward each child. All eight analyses achieved a satisfactory fit, with Bentler's[39] nonnormed fit index ranging from 0.79 to 0.88 across all analyses. That is, our hypotheses about three parenting variables—conflict/negativity, warmth/support, and monitoring/control—fit the observed correlations among the 14 measures of parenting for each reporter and each parent.

We used the same approach to test the dimensionality of the observer ratings. Four analyses were done on four different sets of ratings, reflecting the mother's observed behavior toward her oldest and youngest child and the father's observed behavior toward his oldest and youngest child (Bentler's nonnormed fit index, 0.89 to 0.92)

These findings justified aggregating measures within dimensions for each respondent. Each measure was standardized across all 1440 children, and standardized measures were averaged to create an index of each parenting domain as reported by each respondent and by observers. This resulted in 18 variables: three domains of parenting (conflict/negativity, warmth/support, and monitoring/control) for each parent (mother and father) as reported by that parent, by the child, and by observers.

## Testing Hypotheses Concerning Differential Parenting

**Dealing with response bias.** Preliminary analyses indicated that simple aggregation across respondents (parent, child, and observer) might introduce biases into analyses testing hypotheses about the link between parenting and child symptoms. For example, mothers may consistently see their parenting as less conflictual and negative than it really is. Moreover, this reporting bias may also influence reports of outcome variables, such that mothers who see their own parenting as less negative may also report their children as less depressed than they actually are.

Thus, we used structural equation modeling techniques that allow for aggregation of such reports independent of respondent bias. This algebraic procedure fits an observed set of correlations among many variables with a model of how those variables might be related.[40] The two components of the model are (1) a "measurement model," which specifies that certain measured variables are all indicators of an underlying or "latent variable," and (2) a specified set of relationships among the latent variables. In these analyses, measures of each parenting domain are considered as indicators of the underlying latent variable for that domain. Similarly, measures of each set of symptoms are considered as indicators of latent variables reflecting that symptom group.

We can also specify a relationship between the errors of measurement of two or more of the measured variables. If we expect errors of measurement from the same respondent (eg, the mother) to be correlated between her report of parenting and her report of her children's psychopathologic outcome, this is similar to partialing these errors or biases from our estimate of the relationship between the latent variable of parenting and of psychopathologic outcome (Figure 2).[41]

**Correlation and regression analyses.** With the use of all 1440 children, structural equation models with correlated errors were used to calculate the correlations between latent variables reflecting parenting toward a child, parenting toward his or her sibling, and symptoms reported for a child and for the sibling (Table 2) Data concerning each child were entered twice, once to represent the parenting toward that child and once to represent that child as the sibling of the other child in the family. This required us to restrict our model by (1) constraining the path "parenting toward adolescent" and path "parenting toward sibling" to be equal and (2) adjustment of the *df* for each analysis because of the redundancy introduced by including data from all individual children in measuring each latent variable.

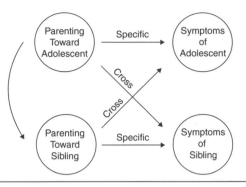

**Figure 2.** Partial structural equation model showing correlated error method of eliminating respondent bias effects.

Regression analyses (Figure 1) were conducted in a similar fashion. The only difference involved a respecification of the structural model such that both parenting variables (parenting toward adolescent and parenting toward sibling) were included as exogenous variables predicting each of the outcomes (symptoms for adolescent and symptoms for sibling).

## RESULTS

### *Conflict/Negativity*

Data concerning parents' engagement in conflict/negativity were analyzed at three levels. At the most general level, all conflict/negativity measures reporting behavior of both mother and father were used as indicators of a general conflict/negativity latent variable. We saw this latent variable as reflecting the general atmosphere of parenting as directed toward a particular adolescent by both parents. This seemed reasonable, since structural equations that included separate mother and father latent variables reflecting conflict/negativity indicated a high correlation between these two ($r = .85$, SE $= .19$). At the next lower level, the measures for mother's and father's behavior were analyzed separately. Finally, we repeated our analyses for each particular measure of conflict/negativity for each parent, to clarify our more general findings.

Table 3 summarizes findings from the regression models for general parental conflict/negativity in relation to antisocial behavior and depressive symptoms. Since this table format will be used to present data from most analyses, we will discuss Table 3 in some detail.

TABLE 3
Relationships Between Parental Conflict/Negativity, Depression,
and Antisocial Behavior for Mothers and Fathers Combined*

| Relationship of Conflict/Negativity | Antisocial Behavior Coefficient ± SE | Depression Coefficient ± SE |
|---|---|---|
| Between parenting toward adolescent and sibling | 0.56 ± 0.08 | 0.55 ± 0.07 |
| Between parenting and outcome, *specific* | 0.79 ± 0.06 | 0.62 ± 0.05 |
| Between parenting and outcome, *cross* | −0.05 ± 0.03 | −0.14 ± 0.04 |
| $\chi^2$/df | 309/63 | 236/53 |
| Bentler's NNFI | 0.89 | 0.90 |

* See Figure 1 for illustration of notation. NNFI indicates nonnormed fit index.

In Table 3, row 1 provides an estimate of the correlation of general parental conflict/negativity directed toward each child with general parental conflict/negativity directed toward his or her sibling. This is equivalent to an intraclass correlation coefficient. Estimates for this correlation, for any parenting variable, should be equal in all models; the slight differences in these tables result from minor fluctuations in the estimation procedures used. These correlations address our first primary question: how similarly do parents treat two children of the same gender close in age? These data demonstrate a substantial correlation between sibling environments as measured by parental conflict/negativity.

Row 2 of Table 3, labeled "specific," reports the standardized regression coefficient estimating the relationship between parental conflict/negativity toward each child adjusted for the level of conflict/negativity toward each child's sibling. As noted earlier, we consider this regression coefficient to provide an adjusted estimate of the association of parenting specific to a child with that child's symptoms. The regressions in Table 2 suggest that this effect is substantial for parental conflict/negativity, as it has an association with antisocial behavior and depressive symptoms in adolescents. This provides strong support for the interpretation that parental conflict/negativity specific to each child, as indexed by this partialing approach, is strongly associated with adolescent antisocial behavior and depressive symptoms.

Row 3, labeled "cross," contains the standardized regression coefficient estimating unique cross-sibling effects. That is, these measure the indirect association of parenting toward a sibling with outcomes in the adolescent.

While the cross correlations, not shown in Table 3, are significant for antisocial behavior (0.39) and depressive symptoms (0.21), the regression coefficients (which are adjusted for the level of parental conflict/negativity toward the adolescent whose symptoms are being predicted) are small, suggesting that the simple cross correlations are attributable mostly to the strong correlation between siblings on this parenting variable.

Rows 4 and 5 provide summary statistics for the structural equation models used to estimate the correlations in this table. These indicate that the fit between model and data are good. Correlations among errors estimated by the model are not reported herein to conserve space, but in general most of these correlations were substantial, indicating that much of the variance in our measures involved observer bias and providing strong support for the need to remove this variance by means of this method of modeling.

Table 4 presents data on antisocial behavior and depressive symptoms separately for mothers and fathers. Coefficients for mothers and fathers were similar and did not differ greatly from those in analyses of general parental conflict/negativity. Regression coefficients estimating unique cross-sibling effects were negligible for fathers but showed a small but significant negative relationship for mothers.

Table 5 reports results of separate scales used as indicators of parental conflict/negativity for antisocial behavior and depressive symptoms. The regression coefficients are reported in Table 5. In an occasional instance in this table, as well as others, we display regression coefficients that are greater than 1.0 and/or SEs that are very high. These are the results of very high correlations of measures of parenting toward the adolescent with measures of parenting toward the sibling. The very high coefficients or SEs reflect uncertainty in the estimation procedure and are interpreted as nonsignificant findings.

Five of these scales involve self-report measures. Since each was completed by the parent and the child about that parent, structural equation modeling with latent variables and correlated errors to remove respondent bias effects could be used. However, this is not true for the observer coding of parental conflict/negativity, which was based on only one reporter, the coder. Thus, comparisons of coefficients are valid across the five self-report measures but must be somewhat tentative when these measures are compared with the observer data.

Correlations between parenting toward adolescent and that toward sibling (row 1) showed striking differences among the scales. Yielding to coercion showed much higher correlations than did symbolic aggression or conflict, particularly for fathers. Standardized regression coefficients re-

TABLE 4

Relationship Between Conflict/Negativity, Warmth/Support, and Monitoring/Control and Antisocial Behavior or Depressive Symptoms*

| | Coefficient ± SE | | | | | |
| --- | --- | --- | --- | --- | --- | --- |
| | Conflict/Negativity | | Warmth/Support | | Monitoring/Control | |
| Relationships | Mother | Father | Mother | Father | Mother | Father |
| **Antisocial Behavior** | | | | | | |
| Between parenting toward adolescent and sibling | 0.52 ± 0.05 | 0.61 ± 0.10 | 0.61 ± 0.06 | 0.67 ± 0.04 | 0.80 ± 0.04 | 0.89 ± 0.03 |
| Between parenting and outcome, *specific* | 0.75 ± 0.06 | 0.82 ± 0.07 | −0.30 ± 0.05 | −0.37 ± 0.05 | −0.12 ± 0.05 | −0.15 ± −0.07 |
| Between parenting and outcome, *cross* | −0.04 ± 0.04 | −0.04 ± 0.05 | −0.03 ± 0.05 | 0.10 ± 0.05 | −0.09 ± 0.05 | −0.04 ± 0.06 |
| $\chi^2/df$ | 139/30 | 157/30 | 131/30 | 115/30 | 62/30 | 89/30 |
| Bentler's NNFI | 0.91 | 0.89 | 0.89 | 0.91 | 0.97 | 0.95 |
| **Depressive Symptoms** | | | | | | |
| Between parenting toward adolescent and sibling | 0.50 ± 0.07 | 0.57 ± 0.11 | 0.60 ± 0.06 | 0.66 ± 0.04 | 0.79 ± 0.04 | 0.88 ± 0.03 |
| Between parenting and outcome, *specific* | 0.56 ± 0.05 | 0.64 ± 0.06 | −0.26 ± 0.06 | −0.37 ± 0.06 | −0.03 ± 0.06 | −0.17 ± 0.08 |
| Between parenting and outcome, *cross* | −0.12 ± 0.04 | 0.01 ± 0.04 | 0.10 ± 0.06 | 0.20 ± 0.05 | −0.09 ± 0.06 | 0.09 ± 0.09 |
| $\chi^2/df$ | 97/22 | 150/22 | 85/22 | 75/22 | 59/22 | 78/22 |
| Bentler's NNFI | 0.91 | 0.84 | 0.91 | 0.93 | 0.95 | 0.94 |

* See Figure 1 for illustration of notation. NNFI indicates nonnormed fit index.

TABLE 5

Relationship of the Six Component Scales of Conflict/Negativity
and Antisocial Behavior or Depressive Symptoms*

| | Coefficient ± SE | | | | | |
| | Disagreement | | Punitiveness | | Yielding to Coercion | |
| Relationship | Mother | Father | Mother | Father | Mother | Father |
|---|---|---|---|---|---|---|
| **Antisocial Behavior** | | | | | | |
| Between parenting toward adolescent and sibling | 0.53 ± 0.09 | 0.52 ± 0.12 | 0.67 ± 0.10 | 0.73 ± 0.13 | 0.75 ± 0.31 | 0.96 ± 0.23 |
| Between parenting and outcome, *specific* | 0.70 ± 0.06 | 0.74 ± 0.08 | 0.71 ± 0.09 | 0.80 ± 0.14 | 0.66 ± 0.37 | 1.92 ± 6.9 |
| Between parenting and outcome, *cross* | 0.00 ± 0.04 | 0.02 ± 0.07 | −0.21 ± 0.08 | −0.28 ± 0.13 | −0.26 ± 0.37 | −1.63 ± 7.1 |
| $\chi^2/df$ | 90/22 | 83/22 | 83/22 | 92/22 | 69/22 | 89/22 |
| Bentler's NNFI | 0.93 | 0.93 | 0.93 | 0.92 | 0.93 | 0.91 |
| **Depressive Symptoms** | | | | | | |
| Between parenting toward adolescent and sibling | 0.52 ± 0.08 | 0.52 ± 0.11 | 0.60 ± 0.10 | 0.64 ± 0.12 | 0.51 ± 0.42 | 0.92 ± 0.20 |
| Between parenting and outcome, *specific* | 0.49 ± 0.06 | 0.54 ± 0.07 | 0.56 ± 0.07 | 0.62 ± 0.10 | 0.27 ± 0.09 | 1.17 ± 2.6 |
| Between parenting and outcome, *cross* | −0.15 ± 0.05 | −0.16 ± 0.06 | −0.21 ± 0.06 | −0.18 ± 0.08 | 0.10 ± 0.09 | −1.04 ± 2.5 |
| $\chi^2/df$ | 65/12 | 62/12 | 63/12 | 53/12 | 56/12 | 54/12 |
| Bentler's NNFI | 0.90 | 0.90 | 0.91 | 0.92 | 0.89 | 0.90 |

* See Figure 1 for illustration of notation. NNFI indicates nonnormed fit index.

flecting the specific effects of parenting all tended to be similar across measures (row 2). These findings again support the interpretation that parental conflict/negativity specific to a particular child has a strong relationship with that child's antisocial behavior.

Punitiveness, for mothers and fathers, showed moderate levels of unique cross-sibling effects as reflected in standardized regression coefficients. These data suggest that the *greater* the parental punitiveness that is shown to the sibling, the *less* antisocial behavior that is shown by the adolescent.

Observer measures of parental conflict/negativity show lower correlations between parenting toward adolescent and toward sibling, and lower correlations between parental conflict/negativity and child antisocial behavior, in correlational and regression analyses. Although muted, these data show general patterns similar to those of self-report data, with specific conflict/negativity being significantly associated with adolescent behavior and cross-sibling regression coefficients showing little or no effect. Patterns of coefficients for analyses involving depressive symptoms, reported

| | Coefficient ± SE | | | | |
|---|---|---|---|---|---|
| Symbolic Aggression | | Conflict | | Observer Coding Coefficient | |
| Mother | Father | Mother | Father | Mother | Father |
| 0.45 ± 0.10 | 0.39 ± 0.14 | 0.36 ± 0.11 | 0.51 ± 0.14 | 0.39 ± 0.03 | 0.41 ± 0.03 |
| 0.57 ± 0.07 | 0.63 ± 0.09 | 0.61 ± 0.07 | 0.68 ± 0.08 | 0.26 ± 0.03 | 0.22 ± 0.03 |
| −0.01 ± 0.05 | 0.04 ± 0.08 | 0.00 ± 0.06 | −0.08 ± 0.07 | 0.10 ± 0.03 | 0.03 ± 0.03 |
| 68/22<br>0.94 | 64/22<br>0.94 | 93/22<br>0.91 | 95/22<br>0.91 | 38/10<br>0.95 | 46/10<br>0.94 |
| 0.40 ± 0.11 | 0.35 ± 0.14 | 0.36 ± 0.11 | 0.44 ± 0.14 | 0.39 ± 0.03 | 0.41 ± 0.03 |
| 0.54 ± 0.07 | 0.56 ± 0.08 | 0.46 ± 0.07 | 0.49 ± 0.07 | 0.10 ± 0.03 | 0.12 ± 0.03 |
| −0.03 ± 0.06 | 0.10 ± 0.07 | −0.12 ± 0.06 | −0.04 ± 0.06 | 0.04 ± 0.03 | 0.01 ± 0.03 |
| 58/12<br>0.89 | 48/12<br>0.91 | 74/12<br>0.87 | 59/12<br>0.91 | 49/10<br>0.91 | 41/10<br>0.93 |

in Tables 4 and 5, were similar to those found for antisocial behavior, except that cross-sibling effects were more frequent.

### Warmth/Support

Structural equations including separate mother and father latent variables reflecting warmth/support indicated only a moderate correlation between these two ($r = .50$, SE = .14). For this reason, analyses were not conducted for general parental warmth/support, but only for mothers and fathers separately.

Table 4 reports the results of structural equation estimates of regression coefficients relating parental warmth/support to adolescent antisocial behavior and depressive symptoms. Considering the correlation between sibling environments on the dimension of parental warmth/support, these data were similar to those for conflict/negativity, showing substantial correlations for parental warmth/support. However, regression coefficients between parental warmth/support and both types of symptoms were smaller, although still significant. As Table 4 shows, this pattern was generally true for the standardized regression coefficients reflecting the specific effects of parental warmth toward a particular child. These data provide support for the importance of parental warmth/support specific to each child, but the effects appear to be much lower than those found for conflict/negativity. The cross-sibling effects in Table 4 also show that the *more* warmth/support that is shown to the sibling, the *more* the adolescent shows depressive symptoms.

We examined, in greater detail, the four component measures of warmth/support. The following specific regressions were significant for the components of warmth/support and antisocial behavior: mother's and father's closeness and rapport ($-0.27$; $-0.34$), mother's and father's expressive affection ($-0.27$; $-0.27$), and mother's observed warmth ($-0.14$). The following were significant for depressive symptoms: mother's and father's closeness and rapport ($0.33$; $-0.26$) and father's instrumental affection ($-0.20$). None of the cross-sibling regressions were significant.

### Monitoring/Control

Structural equations including separate mother and father latent variables reflecting monitoring/control indicated a strong correlation between these mothers and fathers ($r = .75$, SE $= .27$). Because of high correlations, as shown in Table 4, between parents' scores, we report analyses only for mothers and fathers separately. These tables also show that the effects of specific parental monitoring/control on adolescent symptoms were not significant. Cross-sibling regression coefficients also show low or no significant effects.

Analyses of the specific scales from the monitoring/control composites, presented in Table 6, essentially replicated these findings in the case of depressive symptoms, with one exception: the regression coefficient for maternal control attempts was significant, indicating that attempts specific to a particular adolescent are related to increased depressive symptoms. A more interesting picture emerges for antisocial behavior: knowledge and actual control appear to have the predicted effect; they are inversely related to antisocial behavior. Control attempts, which may reflect ineffective monitoring, are positively related to antisocial behavior. These contrasting effects are almost certainly responsible for the null findings, shown in Table 3, when all four measures of monitoring/control are aggregated.

Cross-sibling correlations provide evidence that *higher* father's knowledge of sibling activities is significantly associated with *lower* antisocial behavior in the other adolescent. However, *higher* father's successful con-

# TABLE 6

## Relationship Between the Four Components of Monitoring/Control and Antisocial Behavior or Depressive Symptoms*

| | Coefficient ± SE | | | | | | | |
| --- | --- | --- | --- | --- | --- | --- | --- | --- |
| | Knowledge | | Control Attempts | | Actual Control | | Observer Coding Coefficient | |
| Relationships | Mother | Father | Mother | Father | Mother | Father | Mother | Father |
| **Antisocial Behavior** | | | | | | | | |
| Between parenting toward adolescent and sibling | 0.86 ± 0.21 | 0.85 ± 0.19 | 0.80 ± 0.22 | 0.81 ± 0.18 | 0.79 ± 0.24 | 0.85 ± 0.20 | 0.30 ± 0.03 | 0.42 ± 0.03 |
| Between parenting and outcome, *specific* | −0.30 ± 0.10 | −0.16 ± 0.07 | 0.21 ± 0.08 | 0.18 ± 0.07 | −0.21 ± 0.05 | −0.40 ± 0.11 | −0.02 ± 0.02 | 0.04 ± 0.03 |
| Between parenting and outcome, *cross* | −0.09 ± 0.09 | −0.17 ± 0.07 | −0.22 ± 0.07 | −0.20 ± 0.07 | 0.01 ± 0.04 | 0.22 ± 0.11 | −0.01 ± 0.03 | 0.01 ± 0.03 |
| $\chi^2/df$ | 65/22 | 71/22 | 48/22 | 47/22 | 65/22 | 59/22 | 37/10 | 46/10 |
| Bentler's NNFI | 0.95 | 0.96 | 0.97 | 0.98 | 0.95 | 0.96 | 0.95 | 0.93 |
| **Depressive Symptoms** | | | | | | | | |
| Between parenting toward adolescent and sibling | 0.83 ± 0.16 | 0.86 ± 0.17 | 0.81 ± 0.22 | 0.80 ± 0.16 | 0.78 ± 0.22 | 0.82 ± 0.17 | 0.30 ± 0.03 | 0.42 ± 0.03 |
| Between parenting and outcome, *specific* | −0.12 ± 0.10 | −0.15 ± 0.08 | 0.22 ± 0.10 | 0.09 ± 0.07 | −0.16 ± 0.06 | −0.10 ± 0.07 | 0.04 ± 0.03 | 0.07 ± 0.03 |
| Between parenting and outcome, *cross* | 0.01 ± 0.09 | 0.09 ± 0.09 | −0.29 ± 0.08 | −0.13 ± 0.07 | 0.02 ± 0.05 | 0.01 ± 0.05 | 0.01 ± 0.03 | −0.01 ± 0.03 |
| $\chi^2/df$ | 53/12 | 45/12 | 36/12 | 43/12 | 39/12 | 42/12 | 43/10 | 45/10 |
| Bentler's NNFI | 0.93 | 0.96 | 0.96 | 0.96 | 0.95 | 0.95 | 0.92 | 0.92 |

* See Figure 1 for illustration of notation. NNFI indicates nonnormed fit index.

225

trol of the sibling is associated with *higher* antisocial behavior in the other adolescent.

### Influence of Gender, Social Class, and Age of Children

We compared the effects of sibship genders for all the models presented in Tables 3 through 6. We estimated statistical significance by comparing models in which the two genders were constrained to have equal coefficients with those in which the models were free to vary.[39] There were no gender differences for any of the specific effects. We also examined the effects of social class, mean education level of the parents, and mean age of the two children by recomputing the regressions shown in Table 4 after controlling for these variables. Of the 36 regressions shown in these tables, only two were changed by more than 0.10 (father's warmth/support, specific association with depressive symptoms, $-0.26$; father's warmth/support, cross-sibling regression with depressive symptoms, 0.08). At this level, where scale scores are aggregated, there were no more effects than would be expected by chance, so we did not examine these effects on the component scales of the three main parenting variables.

## COMMENT

### Limitations

At the outset, the reader should be aware of two major limitations. First, direction of effects cannot be estimated: variation among adolescents in symptoms may lead to variation in correlated parental response, or the reverse relationship may hold. The literature using the traditional single-sibling design indicates that, for families of preadolescents and adolescents, either is possible.[17,20,39,42,43] We recently collected a second panel of data from this sample; this will help to resolve which of these influences are most important and will explore between-group differences—if any—in causal direction.

Second, the mechanisms linking parenting practices and psychiatric symptoms may not be purely psychosocial. There may be a substantial influence of heritable characteristics of the child on parenting practices.[44] Moreover, our outcome measures—depressive symptoms and antisocial behavior—also show significant heritabilities; for antisocial behavior, $h^2 = 0.55$, and for depressive symptoms, $h^2 = 0.44$. Where independent and dependent measures are heritable, genetic influences common to both may explain part or all of any associations observed.[45] Using other data in this study, we are currently testing models to parse out these common genetic influences.

## Specific Association Between Parenting and Adolescent Adjustment

Conflict/negativity showed strong associations with antisocial behavior and, to a lesser extent, with depressive symptoms. These associations were roughly the same in magnitude for mothers and fathers. Furthermore, all five subscales for the self-report measures showed strong associations with psychopathologic outcome. It is not simply aggressiveness or punitiveness by the parent that plays a role, but also the parent's yielding to coercion by the child. Thus, what may lie at the core here is a toxic combination of sustained negative and disruptive affect and inconsistency in parental authority and direction. As such, our findings may relate to those single-child family studies of both Baumrind,[46] who reported the importance of parental consistency for competent adolescent adjustment, and Elder,[47] who reported the disruptive effects of emotionally explosive parental behavior.

The large magnitude of these effects, particularly for conflict/negativity, is notable. For antisocial behavior, this variable accounted for 56% of variance for fathers and 69% for mothers. For depressive symptoms, it accounted for 31% for fathers and 41% for mothers. The multiagent, multimethod measurement strategy permits a more reliable estimate of an underlying true score for independent and dependent measures and thus may increase variance explained. Studies using somewhat comparable research strategies and analytic methods with adolescents, parenting measures, and antisocial behaviors have produced large effect sizes of 21% to 27%,[17] 30% to 40%,[20] and 42% to 53%, respectively.[30] However, the latter two studies used a broader band of parenting measures and for this reason probably showed large effect sizes. It is fair to say that our results account for nearly twice as much variance as those of previous studies of a single domain of parenting variables and antisocial behavior.

Thus, some factor other than our statistical and measurement procedure must be responsible for the large effect sizes. The presence of a second sibling in our design does not fully account for these unusual effect sizes. While informative, the unique cross correlations were, for the most part, small and did not alter the specific effect sizes much. Thus, it might be argued that the unique, specific effects are those that could have been measured in any study that used the conventional one-child-per-family design if a researcher concentrated on just those parenting behaviors that were directed at the child in question. However, as noted, one-child studies have not shown effect sizes this large. It is possible that, in our study, inclusion of two siblings in the research design was usefully reactive. The central feature of this research design may alert parents and children that the research team is interested in contrasts and comparisons. Indeed, many of our self-report measures for parents regularly asked the parents to rate their behavior toward one child on a large number of items and then rate the second child on the same items, a procedure that must call attention to contrasts and comparisons. Children are asked to compare directly how they are treated by each parent with the treatment received by the other child by means of a unique instrument called the Sibling Inventory of Differential Experience.[48] These explicit techniques, plus the welter of demand characteristics, may act to bring out in the open those contrasting environmental experiences whose validity is confirmed by their predictable association with outcome variables.

In contrast, the relatively small associations between observed parenting and adolescent symptoms may, as noted, result from one or more of a set of factors. First, we observed only a brief 10 minutes of interaction between a parent and each child. Second, there is only one type of observer— by definition and design—in observer coding, so we cannot correct for observer bias. Third, observer coding may be examining a different domain of parenting than do the self-report scales. The correlation among all self-report scales, within a domain, were high. However, those between self-report and observer ratings, within a domain, ranged from only 0.11 ($P < .01$) to 0.27 ($P < .001$).

Findings for warmth/support show a different pattern. The associations of parental warmth/support specific to each child with outcome measures are much lower for parental warmth/support. Where it does show significant associations, it is inversely related to psychopathologic outcome as predicted. Warmth/support is more strongly and positively associated with positive outcomes in adolescents, particularly social responsibility.[49]

Data on monitoring/control show yet another pattern. Parenting behavior toward the siblings is much more highly correlated. This allows less opportunity for specific effects to emerge (Table 2). Nonetheless, this domain shows an interesting difference among the component subscales. Two measures, the parents' knowledge about the adolescents and their behavior and the parents' successful control of that behavior, show modest negative correlations with antisocial behavior as predicted. These two domains of monitoring may be thought of as competent monitoring. However, the scale measuring attempted control probably reflects attempts that fail; if this is the case, it is not surprising that it shows modest positive associations with antisocial behavior.

The correlation between antisocial behavior and depressive symptoms in our data was .43 and was consistent with previous findings.[50–52] Thus, it is not surprising that we did not find specific family correlates for each.

## Effects of Parenting Toward Siblings on Adolescent Symptoms

For the aggregated variables shown in Table 4, the unique cross correlations are small, suggesting that—at the aggregated level—there are virtually no indirect effects of parenting, via treatment of the sibling, on adolescent antisocial behavior or depressive symptoms.

However, analysis of the component scales of conflict/negativity shows an interesting pattern: for punitiveness, the *more* conflict/negativity is aimed at the sibling, the *less* antisocial behavior is shown by the adolescent. A similar effect is apparent for disagreement and punitiveness and for depressive symptoms. The effect sizes for some of these unique cross correlations are comparable with the specific effects for warmth/support and antisocial and depressive symptoms. In other words, an adolescent is less likely to show antisocial behavior and depressive symptoms as much by having his or her sibling be the focus of parent conflict/negativity as by being the direct recipient of parental warmth/support.

The cross correlations of the monitoring/control scales add a dimension to this pattern. The *more* control attempts and knowledge of sibling behavior is directed at the sibling, the *less* likely that the adolescent will show abnormal behavior. If we can read the father's knowledge of sibling behavior as signifying his preoccupation with the sibling, all of the significant cross correlations fall into a pattern. The *more* harsh, aggressive, explosive, inconsistent, ineffective, and preoccupied behavior is shown toward the sibling, the *less* psychopathologic outcome is seen in the adolescent.

Apparently, adolescents are least likely to show antisocial behavior or depressive symptoms if they receive little conflict/negativity and much warmth directly from their parents *and* their sibling receives a good deal of problematic parenting. We may refer to this profile of effects as a *sibling barricade*. Evidence of a sibling barricade as a socialization phenomenon cannot be obtained in an ordinary single-child design.

The possible connection between sibling barricade and conflict/negativity is supported by the correlation between mothers and fathers for conflict/negativity, which was the highest of three domains of parenting ($r_{c/n} = .84$, SE $= .19$; $r_{w/s} = .50$, SE $= .14$; and $r_{m/c} = .74$, SE $= .27$, where c/n indicates conflict/negativity; w/s, warmth/support; and m/c, monitoring/control). In families in which an adolescent is receiving high levels of conflict/negativity, he or she is getting it more or else equally from both parents.

Furthermore, we found that conflict/negativity from both parents is equally associated with the child's symptoms. Other studies suggest that it is likely that there is considerable conflict between husbands and wives in those families in which at least one child is the recipient of parental conflict/negativity.[17,30,53,54] Whether the child's behavior is cause or effect, the data suggest a tangled triad of family members—mother, father, and the child who is the target of problematic parenting. This triad shows relationships filled with tension, aggression, inconsistency, and ineffectiveness. A child who is not protected by the barricade gets a double dose of conflict/negativity from both parents, who also may be in a state of war with one another. It becomes more understandable, therefore, why a child who is, for whatever reason, barricaded from this troubled family subsystem may be much less likely to show symptoms.

### Correlation of Parenting Toward Adolescent with That Toward Sibling

These correlations form the hub for subsequent searches for nonshared effects. It has not been known whether parents treat same-sex similar-aged children alike. If their treatment is similar, then it is unlikely that parenting is a source of nonshared environmental influence. As already suggested, it is critical to understand who is reporting these differences parents, children, or observers. For example, parents may be biased by a strong desire to treat both children equally. Children, on the other hand, may be exquisitely sensitive to differences in how they and siblings are treated, this may start early in the second year of life.[15] In our study, for conflict/negativity, parents were most likely to report that they treat children similarly. The mean correlation across all the component scales for parent reports was .64. On the other hand, the correlation between the adolescent and siblings on their reports on the same parent was only .23 averaged across all scales and both parents. Observer ratings were midway between the parents' and children's reports; for conflict/negativity, the correlation was .30. Similarly, findings have been reported in previous studies.[55]

The striking contrasts between parents' and children's perceptions of parenting have two implications for family systems and the impact of uncorrelated experiences on development. First, the differing parental and child sensitivities may—in healthy families—operate to keep actual differences in parenting relatively low. The parents' bias toward reporting consistency may reflect their investment in maintaining equity. Thus, while they may be relatively blind to actual inconsistencies across children, they would be sensitive to complaints about it. Children, probably from the earliest ages, develop capacities not only to observe these differences but also to complain about them.[56] This two-generational dipole may function to keep actual differences to a relative minimum. We previously reported that the magnitude of these differences is associated with maladjustment in adolescent siblings.[22]

Second, the high level, of children's sensitivities to differences may mean that relatively small differences—as detected by either parents or casual outsiders—may make a big difference in the psychological life of children. Indeed, this generational dipole directs our attention to differences among children in how they perceive family process; these differences may play a large role in their psychological development.

Taken together, these data represent an early effort, using sensitive measures of psychosocial process, to explore a hypotheses generated by research on behavioral genetics. The genetic data, without direct measures of environmental data, suggested that environments specific for each sibling in the family have the biggest impact on normal and pathologic psychological development. The findings reported herein, using a broad range of direct measures of the environment, support this environmental hypothesis derived from genetic studies.

## REFERENCES

1. Plomin R, Daniels D. Why are children in the same family so different from one another? *Behav Brain Sci.* 1987; 10:1–16.

2. Plomin R, Emde RN, Braungart JM, Campos J, Corley R, Fulker DW, Kagan J, Reznick JS, Robinson J, Zahn-Waxler C, DeFries JC. Genetic change and continuity from fourteen to twenty months: the MacArthur Longitudinal Twin Study. *Child Dev.* 1994;64:1354–1376.

3. Kendler KS, Heath A, Martin NG, Eaves LJ. Symptoms of anxiety and depression in a volunteer twin population. *Arch Gen Psychiatry.* 1986,43:213–221.

4. Wierzbicki M. Similarity of monozygotic and dizygotic child twins in level and lability of subclinically depressed mood. *Am J Orthopsychiatry.* 1987;57:33–40.

5. Rowe DC. Biometrical genetic models of self-reported delinquent behavior: twin study. *Behav Genet.* 1983;13:473–489.

6. Rowe DC. Genetic and environmental components of antisocial behavior: a study of 255 twin pairs. *Child Dev.* 1986;54:473–489.

7. Rowe DC, Rodgers JL, Meseck-Bushey S, St John C. Sexual behavior and non-sexual deviance: a sibling study of their relationship. *Dev Psychol.* 1989; 23:61–69.

8. Plomin R, Chipuer HH, Neiderhiser J. Behavioral genetic evidence for the importance of the nonshared environment. In: Hetherington EM, Reiss D, Plomin

R, eds. *Separate Social Worlds of Siblings: Impact of the Nonshared Environment on Development*. Hillsdale, NJ: Lawrence Erlbaum Associates; 1993: 1–33.

9. Cadoret RJ, O'Gorman TW, Troughton E, Heywood E. Alcoholism and antisocial personality: interrelationships, genetic and environmental factors *Arch Gen Psychiatry*. 1986;42:161–167.

10. Cloninger CR, Gottesman II. Genetic and environmental factors in antisocial behavior disorders. In: Mednick S, Moffitt T, Stack S, eds. *The Causes of Crime*. New York, NY: Cambridge University Press; 1987:92–109.

11. Bertelsen A, Harvald B, Hauge M. A Danish twin study of manic-depressive disorder. *Br J Psychiatry*. 1977;130:330–351.

12. Nurnburger JI, Gershon ES. Genetics of affective disorders. In: Friedman E, ed. *Depression and Antidepressants. Implications for Course and Treatment*. New York, NY: Raven Press; 1981:23–39.

13. Wender PH, Kety SS, Rosenthal D, Schulsinger F, Ortmann J, Lunde I. Psychiatric disorders in the biological and adoptive families of adopted individuals with affective disorders. *Arch Gen Psychiatry*. 1986;43:923–929.

14. Dunn J, Stocker C, Plomin R. Nonshared experiences within the family: correlates of behavioral problems in middle childhood. *Dev Psychopathol*. 1990;2:113–126.

15. Dunn J, McGuire S. Young children's nonshared experiences: a summary of studies in Cambridge and Colorado. In: Hetherington EM, Reiss D, Plomin R, eds. *Separate Social Worlds of Siblings: Impact of the Nonshared Environment on Development*. Hillsdale, NJ: Lawrence Erlbaum Associates; 1993.111–128.

16. Tejerina-Allen M, Wagner B, Cohen P. A comparison of across-family and within-family parenting predictors of adolescent psychopathology and suicidal ideation. In Hetherington EM, Reiss D, Plomin R, eds. *Separate Social Worlds of Siblings: Impact of the Nonshared Environment on Development*. Hillsdale, NJ Lawrence Erlbaum Associates;1994:143–158.

17. Hetherington EM, Clingempeel WG. Coping with marital transitions, a family systems perspective. *Mongr Soc Res Child Dev*. 1992;57 (serial no 227).

18. Bell DC, Bell LG. Parental validation and support in the development of adolescent daughters. In: Grotevant HD, ed. *Adolescent Development in the Family*. San Francisco, Calif: Jossey Bass Inc; 1983:27–42.

19. Patterson G. *Coercive Family Process: A Social Learning Approach*. Eugene, Ore: Castalia; 1982.

20. Patterson GR, DeBaryshe BD, Ramsey E. A developmental perspective on antisocial behavior. *Am Psychol*. 1989;44:329–335.

21. Nichols RC, Bilbro WC. The diagnosis of twin zygosity. *Acta Genet*. 1966;16:265–275.

22. Reiss D, Plomin R, Hetherington EM, Howe G, Rovine M, Tryon A. The separate social worlds of teenage siblings. In Hetherington EM, Reiss D, Plomin

R, eds. *Separate Social Worlds of Siblings: Impact of the Nonshared Environment on Development.* Hillsdale, NJ: Lawrence Erlbaum Associates; 1993: 63–109.

23. Fisher L, Ransom DC, Terry HW, Lipkin M, Weiss R. The California family health project, I: introduction and description of family health. *Fam Process.* 1992;31:231–250.

24. Olson DH, McCubbin H, Barnes HL, Larsen AS, Muxen MJ, Wilson MA. *Families, What Makes Them Work.* Beverly Hills, Calif: Sage Publishers Inc; 1989.

25. Sweet JA, Bumpass LL. *American Families and Their Households.* New York, NY: Russell Sage Foundation; 1987.

26. Kovacs M. The Children's Depression Inventory (CDI). *Psychopharmacol Bull.* 1985;21:995–998.

27. Glyshaw K, Cohen LH, Towbes LC. Coping strategies and psychological distress: prospective analyses of early and middle adolescence *Am J Community Psychol.* 1989;17:607–623.

28. Peterson JL, Zill N. Marital disruption, parent-child relationships and behavior problems in children. *J Marr Fam.* 1986;48:295–307.

29. Faust J, Baum CG, Forehand R. An examination of the association between social relationships and depression in early adolescence. *J Appl Dev Psychol.* 1985;6:291–297.

30. Fauber R, Forehand R, Thomas AM, Wierson M. A mediational model of the impact of conflict on adolescent adjustment in intact and divorced families: the role of disrupted parenting. *Child Dev.* 1990;61:1112–1123.

31. Slotkin J, Forehand R, Fauber R, McCombs A, Long N. Parent-completed and adolescent-completed CDIs: relationship to adolescent social and cognitive functioning. *J Abnorm Child Psychol.* 1988;16:207–217.

32. Achenbach TM, Edelbrock C. Behavioral problems and competencies reported by parents of normal and disturbed children aged four to sixteen. *Mongr Soc Res Child Dev.* 1981;46(serial no. 188).

33. Kandel DH, Davies M. Adult sequelae of adolescent depressive symptoms. *Arch Gen Psychiatry.* 1986;43:255–262.

34. Panak WF, Garber J, Schwartz D. Parent report on the Child Depression Inventory: reliability and validity. Presented at the American Psychological Association Annual Meeting; August 11–15, 1989; New Orleans, La.

35. Zill N. *Behavior Problems Scale Developed for the 1981 Child Health Supplement to the National Health Interview Survey.* Washington, DC: Child Trends Inc; 1985.

36. Achenbach TM, Edelbrock C. *Manual for the Child Behavior Checklist and Revised Child Behavior Folder.* Burlington, Vt: University of Vermont; 1983.

37. Cohen J. Weighted kappa nominal scale agreement with provision for scaled disagreement or partial credit. *Psychol Bull.* 1968;70:213–222.

38. Straus MA. Measuring intrafamily violence and conflict: the Conflict Tactics (CT) Scale. *J Marr Fam.* 1979;41:75–85.

39. Bentler PM. *EQS Structural Equations Program Manual.* Los Angeles, Calif BMDP Statistical Software Inc; 1989.

40. Loehlin JC. *Latent Variable Models: An Introduction to Factors, Path and Structural Analysis* Hillsdale, NJ: Lawrence Erlbaum Associates; 1987.

41. Bank L, Dishion T, Skinner M, Patterson GR. Method variance in structural equation modeling: living with 'glop.' In: Patterson GR, ed. *Depression and Aggression in Family Interaction.* Hillsdale, NJ: Lawrence Erlbaum Associates; 1990:247–279.

42. Gjerde PF, Block J, Block JH. The preschool family context of 18 year olds with depressive symptoms: a prospective study. *J Res Adolesc.* 1991;1:63–92.

43. Patterson GR, Capaldi D, Bank L. An early starter model for predicting delinquency. In: Pepler DJ, Rubin KH, eds. *The Development and Treatment of Childhood Aggression.* Hillsdale, NJ: Lawrence Erlbaum Associates; 1991:139–168.

44. Plomin R, Reiss D, Hetherington EM, Howe G. Nature and nurture: genetic influence on measures of family environment. *Dev Psychol.* 1994;30:32–43.

45. Plomin R, Bergeman CS. The nature of nurture: genetic influence on 'environmental' measures. *Brain Behav Sci.* 1991;14:373–427.

46. Baumrind D. The influence of parenting style on adolescent competence and substance abuse. *J Early Adolesc.* 1991;11:56–95.

47. Elder GH Jr. Problem behavior and family relationships: life course and intergenerational themes. In: Sorensen AM, Weinert FE, Sherrod LR, eds. *Human Development and the Life Course: Multidisciplinary Perspectives.* Hillsdale, NJ: Lawrence Erlbaum Associates, 1986:293–342.

48. Daniels D, Dunn J, Furstenberg F, Plomin R. Environmental differences within the family and adjustment differences within pairs of adolescent siblings. *Child Dev.* 1985;56:764–774.

49. Anderson E, Reiss D, Plomin R, Hetherington EM. The effects of differential parental treatment on personality development during adolescence. *J Fam Psychol.* 1994;8:303–320.

50. Geller B, Chestnut EC, Miller MD, Price DT, Yates E. Preliminary data on *DSM III* associated features of major depressive disorders in children and adolescents. *Am J Psyhiatry.* 1985;142:643–644.

51. Puig-Antich J. Major depression and conduct disorder in prepuberty. *J Am Acad Child Psychiatry.* 1982;21:118–128.

52. Woolston JL, Rosenthal SL, Riddle MA, Sparrow SS, Cicchetti D, Zimmerman LD. Childhood comorbidity of anxiety/affective disorders and behavior disorders. *J Am Acad Child Adolesc Psychiatry.* 1989;28:707–713.

53. Capaldi DM. Co-occurrence of conduct problems and depressive symptoms in early adolescent boys, I: familial factors and general adjustment at grade 6. *Dev Psychopathol.* 1991;3:277–300.

54. Conger RD, Conger KJ, Elder GH Jr, Lorenz FO, Simons RL, Whitbeck LB. A family process model of economic hardship and adjustment of early adolescent boys. *Child Dev.* 1992;63:526–541.

55. Daniels D, Plomin R. Differential experiences of siblings in the same family. *Dev Psychol.* 1985;21:747–760.

56. Dunn J, Munn P. Development of justification in disputes with mother and sibling. *Dev Psychol.* 1987;23:791–798.

# Part III

# ASPERGER'S DISORDER AND AUTISM

The papers in this section reflect the continuing interest and concern of investigators and clinicians alike with the pervasive developmental disorders. In the first paper in this section, Klin, Volkmar, Sparrow, Cicchetti, and Rourke utilize information derived from recent neuropsychological studies of individuals with developmental disorders as the basis for examining the validity of the diagnosis of Asperger's Disorder.

Although Asperger's Disorder has been included in both the ICD-10 and DSM-IV diagnostic systems, the validity of the diagnosis as distinct from other conditions, most particularly the other pervasive developmental disorders, remains controversial. First published in 1944, only one year after Kanner's initial paper on Autistic Disturbances of Affective Contact, Asperger's work was essentially unknown in the English literature until the early 1980s. As documented in a growing number of case reports, common clinical features include a paucity of empathy; naive, inappropriate, one-sided social interaction; limited ability to form friendships; social isolation; pedantic and poorly intonated speech; poor nonverbal communication; and intense absorption in circumscribed topics, such as the weather, and motor awkwardness, generally occurring in individuals of normal intelligence.

Despite the clarity of the clinical description, Asperger's Disorder has been used inconsistently by clinicians to refer to autistic persons with higher levels of intelligence, adults with autism, or as a broader term for children whose function is "atypical" but who do not meet full criteria for autism. Recent progress in the nosology of Asperger's Disorder, reflected in the defining criteria of ICD-10 and DSM-IV, provides the opportunity to examine the validity of distinguishing between Asperger's Disorder and autism.

In a highly innovative approach, Klin and colleagues, base their examination of validity on observed similarities between individuals diagnosed as having Asperger's Disorder and those with a particular subtype of learning disability, Nonverbal Learning Disabilities syndrome (NLD). A relatively unknown concept among psychiatrists, NLD is defined on the basis of a cluster of deficits affecting such nonverbal aspects of functioning, including tactile–perception, psychomotor coordination, visual–spatial organization, nonverbal problem solving, and appreciation of incongruities and humor. While the rote verbal capacities and verbal memory skills of individuals with the NLD profile are described as well developed, affected persons are noted to exhibit poor pragmatics and prosody of speech, as well as significant deficits in social perception, social judgment, social interaction skills, and deficits in the appreciation of subtle, and sometimes even fairly obvious, nonverbal aspects of communication. While the neuropsychological profile of individuals with NLD suggests greater right hemisphere dysfunction, the typical neuropsychological profile obtained for individuals with high functioning autism suggests left hemisphere dysfunction.

In this study, the neuropsychological profiles of 21 individuals with Asperger's Disorder and 19 with high-functioning autism, all meticulously diagnosed in accordance with ICD-10 research criteria and who were of comparable age and IQ, are compared. The groups differed significantly in 11 neuropsychological areas, with the profile obtained for individuals with Asperger's Disorder coinciding closely with the cluster of neuropsychological assets and deficits captured by the NLD designation.

The findings have both theoretical and practical implications. There may well be two (if not more) types of conditions at the higher end of the spectrum of severe social disability, one type with predominantly left hemisphere involvement and the other with right hemisphere involvement, which can be distinguished on the basis of neuropsychological profile. Regardless of whether Asperger's Disorder and high-functioning autism are truly different diagnostic entities, the neuropsychological pattern of assets and liabilities elucidated in this study suggest that intervention strategies for Asperger's Disorder should be designed with this pattern specifically in mind.

In the second paper in this section, Capps, Sigman, and Yirmiya consider the phenomenology of high-functioning autism from a social/emotional perspective. A review of the rapidly expanding body of literature on the emotionality of autistic individuals serves to underscore that older, nonretarded individuals with autism display considerable understanding of their own emotions and the emotions of others. Rather than simply revising conceptualizations of autism to fit the abilities of higher-functioning individuals or questioning the accuracy of the diagnosis, it is important to attempt to understand what may contribute to the development of emotional strengths. To this end, the study reported by Capps et al. had three objectives: 1) to examine the extent to which awareness of peculiarities might be mediated by intelligence and by the ability to read and share the emotions of others, 2) to investigate the relationships between high-functioning autistic children's perceptions of their own social abilities and their parents' perceptions of the children's social adaptation, and 3) to examine parents' perceptions of their children's emotional experiences over the course of daily life.

Subjects included 18 children and adolescents with DSM-III autism who were between 9 and 16 years of age and whose Verbal, Performance and Full-Scale WISC-R IQs were all at or above 75. Children completed the Perceived Competence Scale for Children, as well as measures designed to assess ability to communicate about emotional experience and empathy: The Vineland Adaptive Behavior Scales and an Emotion Behavior Checklist were administered to parents.

Analysis of the data revealed a complex set of associations between intellectual, social, and emotional competencies. Children who perceived themselves as less socially competent demonstrated stronger intellectual capabilities, greater understanding of the emotional experiences of others, and were better able to access their own emotional experiences than those who perceived themselves as more socially competent. Parents reported that children who considered themselves less socially competent displayed more socially adaptive behavior and expressed more interest and less sadness and fear than those who considered themselves as more socially competent.

These findings have implications for the design of both educational and social interventions. Moreover, in emphasizing the importance of understanding both subjective experience as well as objective behavior, the authors underscore the importance of continued attention to individual differences, even among individuals with a common diagnosis.

Howlin, Wing, and Gould's paper on the recognition of autism in children with Down syndrome adds to previous reports of the coexistence of these two disorders. Although autism is a relatively rare occurrence in people with Down syndrome, it has been suspected in epidemiologic surveys that utilized the Medical Research Council's Handicaps, Behavior, and Skills interview schedule to occur in 9 to 10 percent of autistic children.

The four case studies serve to acquaint readers with features of phenomenology, as expressed in dually diagnosed children, and underscore the importance of correcting the frequently held, but clearly mistaken, belief that the two conditions *never* co-occur. The authors emphasize that late diagnosis, or the failure to diagnose at all, may have long-term detrimental effects on the lives of affected children and their families. As such children fall further and further behind others with Down syndrome, their additional problems are frequently misinterpreted as a reflection of willfulness, poor motivation, or lack of cooperation. Parents may feel increasingly responsible for their children's deficiencies, an experience not dissimilar to that of parents of children with high-functioning autism or Asperger's Disorder. In both instances, correct diagnosis is often welcomed, as it provides a coherent explanation for observed behavioral difficulties, identifies more appropriate strategies for intervention, and affords some measure of relief from guilt.

In the final paper in this section, Quintana, Birmaher, Stedge, Lennon, Freed, Bridge, and Greenhill report the results of a study of the effectiveness of methylphenidate in the treatment of autistic children. In addition to their pervasive impairments in communicative, cognitive, and social development, autistic children often display myriad associated symptoms, including lability of mood, impulsiveness, short attention span, stereotypic and repetitive movements, and hyperactive behavior, which pose significant difficulty in educational and social situations. Pharmacological interventions directed towards the amelioration of associated symptoms have included neuroleptics, naltrexone, and more recently the serotonin reuptake inhibitors. Although there have been few systematic studies of the use of stimulants in autistic children, it has long been thought that administration was contraindicated because of associated increases in irritability, disorganization, and stereotypic movements.

Ten children between the ages of 7 and 11, with a DSM-III-R diagnosis of Autistic Disorder, participated in a double-blind crossover study using placebo and two methylphenidate doses, 10 mg or 20 mg BID. Behavioral measures included the Childhood Autism Rating Scale, the Conner's Abbreviated Parent Questionnaire, and the Aberrant Behavior Checklist. Side effects were measured by the Side Effects Checklist for Stimulant Medication, which assessed irritability, headaches, stomachaches, tics, lack of appetite, weight loss, insomnia, and hallucinations, the Abnormal Involuntary Movement Scale, and the Aberrant Behavior Checklist. Results indicated that subjects showed a modest but statistically significant reduction in hyperactivity and other aberrant behaviors when receiving methylphenidate, as contrasted with placebo. There were no age, dose, or developmental quotient effects, and there were no statistically significant side effects. The study was limited to the treatment of a small group of children, and further studies with larger samples are clearly warranted. Nevertheless, the improvement in hyperactivity without the development of side effects suggests that methylphenidate may have a role in the treatment of hyperactive children with Autistic Disorder.

# 9

# Validity and Neuropsychological Characterization of Asperger Syndrome: Convergence with Nonverbal Learning Disabilities Syndrome

A. Klin, F. R. Volkmar, S. S. Sparrow, D. V. Cicchetti
and B. P. Rourke

*Yale University School of Medicine, New Haven*

*The authors investigated the validity of Asperger Syndrome (AS) by comparing the neuropsychological profiles in this condition and Higher-Functioning Autism (HFA). Diagnostic assignment followed a stringent procedure based on ICD-10 research criteria for the two disorders. The groups had comparable age and Full Scale IQ distributions. The groups differed significantly in 11 neuropsychological areas. The profile obtained for individuals with AS coincided closely with a cluster of neuropsychological assets and deficits captured by the term nonverbal learning disabilities, suggesting an empirical distinction from HFA.*

## VALIDITY AND NEUROPSYCHOLOGICAL CHARACTERIZATION OF ASPERGER SYNDROME

Although autism has been widely recognized as the prototypic pervasive developmental disorder (PDD), various other diagnostic concepts with features somewhat similar to autism have been described (Klin & Volkmar, 1995). In contrast to autism, these conditions have been less intensively

Reprinted with permission from the *Journal of Child Psychology and Psychiatry*, 1995, Vol. 36, No. 7, 1127–1140. Copyright © 1995 by the Association for Child Psychology and Psychiatry.

studied and their validity is more controversial (Volkmar et al., 1994). One of these conditions has been termed Asperger syndrome (AS) (Asperger, 1944), after the Austrian physician who described a number of cases whose clinical features resembled Kanner's (1943) description of autism (e.g. problems with social interaction and communication, and circumscribed and idiosyncratic patterns of interest). However, Asperger's description differed from Kanner's in that speech was less commonly delayed, motor deficits were more common, the onset appeared to be somewhat later, and all the initial cases occurred in boys (Wing, 1981). Asperger also suggested that similar problems could be observed in family members, particularly fathers.

Asperger's work was essentially unknown in the English literature for many years. An influential review and series of case reports by Wing (1981) increased interest in AS and since then, both the usage of the term in clinical practice and the number of case reports has been steadily increasing (Gillberg, 1991; Klin, 1994; Szatmari, Tuff, Finlayson & Bartolucci, 1990). The commonly described clinical features of the syndrome include (a) paucity of empathy; (b) naïve, inappropriate, one-sided social interaction, little ability to form friendships, and consequent social isolation; (c) pedantic and poorly intonated speech; (d) poor nonverbal communication; (e) intense absorption in circumscribed topics, such as the weather, facts about TV stations, railway timetables or maps; these are learned in rote fashion and reflect poor understanding, conveying the impression of eccentricity; and (f) clumsy and ill-coordinated movements and odd posture (Wing, 1981). Prevalence rates of 1–10 cases in 10,000 have been suggested (Wing, 1981; Gillberg, 1991), although the lack of generally agreed upon definitions, at least until recently, complicates the interpretation of available research on this point (Tantam, 1988). Although the syndrome was originally reported only in boys, reports of girls with the syndrome have now appeared; it does, however, appear that as in autism, males are significantly more likely to be affected (Szatmari et al., 1990; Volkmar, Szatmari & Sparrow, 1993; Wing, 1991). Although most individuals with the condition function in the normal range of intelligence, some have been reported to be mildly retarded (Wing, 1991). The apparent onset of the condition, or at least its recognition, is probably somewhat later than autism; this may reflect the relatively more preserved language and cognitive abilities (Volkmar & Cohen, 1991). The condition tends to be highly stable (Asperger, 1979), and the higher intellectual skills observed suggest a better long-term outcome than is typically observed in autism (Tantam, 1991).

## Validity of Asperger Syndrome

The validity of AS as distinct from other conditions, notably the other pervasive developmental disorders, remains controversial (Rutter, 1985; Wing, 1991). Disagreements about the validity of the category and the absence until recently of "official" definitions of AS have meant that the concept has often been used inconsistently by clinicians, who have employed it to refer to autistic persons with higher levels of intelligence, adults with autism, or even as a broader term for all "atypical" children who do not fulfill criteria for autism (Klin, 1994). A lack of uniformity in usage of the term also characterizes definitions adopted for the purpose of research, as different sets of diagnostic criteria have been used by different researchers, with resulting complications for interpretation of research (Ghaziuddin, Tsai & Ghaziuddin, 1992a).

Relative to other pervasive developmental disorders, the validity of AS as distinct from "high functioning autism" (HFA) (i.e. autism associated with overall normal intelligence) has been the topic of greatest debate (Wing, 1991).

There is little disagreement regarding the fact that AS is on a phenomenological continuum with autism, particularly in relation to the problems in the areas of social and communication functioning (Rutter, 1989). For example, within the DSM-III-R diagnostic system, persons with AS would either meet criteria for autistic disorder or would be said to exhibit PDD-NOS (Tsai, 1992). What is less clear is whether the condition is qualitatively different from, rather than just a milder form of, autism unaccompanied by mental retardation (Volkmar & Cohen, 1991). Several studies (Szatmari et al., 1990; Ozonoff, Roge & Pennington, 1991) have attempted to identify discriminating criteria between the two conditions with only mixed results to date. Two factors appear to have contributed to this state of affairs: first, a lack of operationalization and systematic and consensual assignment of the AS diagnosis; and second, a great degree of circularity involved as findings often reflected the criteria adopted in the assignment of a diagnosis of AS and HFA in the first place (Klin, 1994).

On the basis of the available research data, AS was included in both the ICD-10 (WHO, 1990) and DSM-IV (American Psychiatric Association, 1994) diagnostic systems; the two definitions are largely compatible although the ICD-10 system explicitly notes that the validity of the condition apart from HFA remains controversial. However, the advent of the ICD-10 (WHO, 1990) research definition of AS has recently made possible the use of consensual diagnostic criteria. The ICD-10 definition focuses on the differences between AS and autism and takes a more stringent approach than have others adopted by some prominent researchers (Ghaziuddin et al., 1992a), e.g. in ICD-10 the social deficits and unusual behaviors subsumed under the "resistance to change/restricted interest" criteria are the same as for autism but for a diagnosis of AS early language must be near normal.

In the recent DSM-IV Autism/PDD Field Trial (Volkmar et al., 1994), an analysis of cases diagnosed with AS by experienced clinicians yielded some limited evidence for the validity of the condition and its ICD-10 categorical definition. When compared to individuals with HFA (full scale IQ > 85), individuals with AS were less likely to have exhibited delays in the development of spoken language or currently exhibit language/communication deviance; motor delays and "clumsiness" were more variable; isolated special skills (often related to abnormal preoccupations) were more frequent; social, communicative and "resistance to change" symptoms were less frequent; finally, individuals with AS were more likely to exhibit verbal IQ scores greater than performance IQ scores, while the opposite trend was obtained for individuals with HFA. The present study utilizes this recent progress in the nosology of AS and adopts a stringent diagnostic assignment following ICD-10 defining criteria of AS and autism in the investigation of the neuropsychological profiles in these two conditions.

It is also important to note that there are several diagnostic concepts, other than the pervasive developmental disorders, which share, to a great degree, the phenomenological aspects of AS (Bishop, 1989; Denckla, 1983; Rourke, 1989; Voeller, 1986; Weintraub & Mesulam, 1983; Wolff & Chick, 1980). In neuropsychology, a particular subtype of learning disabilities termed the Nonverbal Learning Disabilities syndrome (NLD), has been recently given a great degree of attention (Rourke, 1989). NLD is defined on the basis of a cluster of deficits affecting the nonverbal aspects of the child's functioning including deficits in tactile perception, psychomotor coordination, visual-spatial organization, nonverbal problem-solving, and appreciation of incongruities and humor. Individuals with the NLD profile are also reported to exhibit well developed rote verbal capacities and verbal memory skills, difficulty in adapting to novel and complex situations and overreliance on rote behaviors in such situations, relative deficits in mechanical arithmetic as compared to proficiencies in single word reading, poor pragmatics and prosody in speech, and significant deficits in social perception, social judgment, and social interaction skills. There are marked deficits in the appreciation of subtle and even fairly obvious nonverbal aspects of communication, which often result in social disdain and rejection by others. As a result, individuals with NLD exhibit a marked tendency toward social withdrawal and are at risk for development of serious mood disorders. Many of the clinical features clustered together in NLD have also been described in the neurological literature as a form of *Developmental Learning Disability of the Right Hemisphere* (Denckla, 1983; Weintraub & Mesulam, 1983). Children presenting with this condition have also been shown to exhibit profound disturbances in interpretation and expression of affect and other basic interpersonal skills (Voeller, 1986). A familial link has also been suggested (Weintraub & Mesulam, 1983).

Whereas the phenomenological similarities between AS and developmental right-hemisphere dysfunction have been alluded to in the literature (Molina, Ruata & Soler, 1986; Tsai, 1992), NLD has been a relatively unknown concept among psychiatrists (Klin, 1994). The importance of the NLD and related concepts lies in the fact that the neuropsychological profile obtained for individuals so described exhibits a greater right hemisphere dysfunction (Rourke, 1989), whereas the typical neuropsychological profile obtained for individuals with HFA indicates a greater left hemisphere dysfunction (Dawson, 1983; Rumsey, 1992). This would suggest that, based on neuropsychological profiles, there might be at least two types of conditions at the higher end of the spectrum of severe social disabilities: one type with predominantly left hemisphere involvement and the other with right hemisphere involvement (Tsai, 1992). The phenomenological similarities between AS and NLD suggest the use of the NLD profile as a neuropsychological model of AS.

This study was concerned with comparing the neuropsychological profiles of carefully diagnosed individuals with AS and higher-functioning autism (HFA). The neuropsychological profiles obtained for the two groups were hypothesized to differ, with the NLD cluster of assets and disabilities serving as a closer neuropsychological model of AS than HFA. The present exploration of a neuropsychological distinction between the two conditions is the first attempt to explore the validity of AS vis-à-vis HFA while utilizing a stringent application of the ICD-10 defining criteria of AS and autism.

## METHOD

### Subjects

Potential subjects (N = 73) were recruited from a consecutive case series of individuals seen at the Developmental Disabilities Clinic of our Center and from the membership of the Learning Disabilities Association of America (LDAA). To be eligible for inclusion, each subject had to have extensive records, including developmental and behavioral history and comprehensive neuropsychological data. Of the 73 potential subjects, 24 had been evaluated at the Child Study Center while the remaining 49 had undergone similar evaluations elsewhere. Inclusionary criteria included a Full Scale IQ of over 70 as well as a diagnosis of AS or autism according to both experienced clinicians (FV and AK) and ICD-10 research criteria.

From the potential subject pool, 33 cases were eliminated from subsequent analysis because either one or more Full Scale IQ scores of below 70 had been obtained in the individual's lifetime or, more commonly, because a diagnosis of either AS or HFA could not be unequivocally confirmed. The remaining subjects, 21 with AS and 19 with HFA, constituted the final sample. The groups did not significantly differ in terms of age, sex, and Full Scale IQ distributions A summary of sample characteristics is given in Table 1.

**Diagnostic assignment.** Psychiatric diagnosis was assigned without knowledge of the subjects' neuropsychological characterization, after a thorough review of records by two of the authors (AK and FRV) who also completed the ICD-10 rating criteria for autism and AS (see Table 2). As noted above, potential subjects for whom there was no concordance between clinician-assigned diagnosis and ICD-10 ratings were excluded from the study. To ensure that the diagnosis of AS was made on the strictest possible basis, the draft ICD-10 research definition was modified in some respects Firstly, consistent with the results of the DSM-IV Autism/PDD field trial (Volkmar et al., 1994), only one item in the symptom cluster of "restricted interests and activities" was required, and (2) the associated features in ICD-10 of "delayed motor milestones and presence of motor 'clumsiness'," and "isolated, unusual all-absorbing skill or activity", that are considered suggestive (but not required) for an ICD-10 diagnosis of AS, were necessary diagnostic criteria. This most stringent approach appeared

TABLE 1
Sample Characteristics

| Age | Sex | Full Scale IQ | |
|---|---|---|---|
| HFA ($N = 19$) | Mean = 15.36 ($SD = 9.12$) | 17 males and 2 females | Mean = 95.63 ($SD = 8.27$) |
| AS ($N = 21$) | Mean = 16.11 ($SD = 8.27$) | 19 males and 2 females | Mean = 96.76 ($SD = 18.19$) |

$N = 40$ (24 from Yale, 16 contacted through the LDAA).

TABLE 2
Defining Criteria for HFA and AS

**Childhood Autism** (ICD-10 DRAFT Research Criteria)
  (1)  1 out of 3 onset criteria
  (2)  3 out of 5 criteria involving "qualitative impairments in reciprocal social interaction"
  (3)  2 out of 5 criteria involving "qualitative impairments in communication"
  (4)  2 out of 6 criteria involving "restricted, repetitive, and stereotyped patterns of behavior, interests and activities
  (5)  Exclusion of other disorders

**Asperger Syndrome** (ICD-10 DRAFT Research Criteria)
  (1)  "A lack of clinically significant general delay in language or cognitive development" + onset criteria
  (2)  "Qualitative impairments in reciprocal social interaction" (criteria as for autism)
  (3)  "Restricted, repetitive, and stereotyped patterns of behavior, interests and activities" (criteria as for autism) + 1 endorsed item sufficient (rather than the required 2)
  (4)  Exclusion of other disorders (e.g. autism, PDD-NOS)
  (5)  Delayed motor milestones and presence of motor "clumsiness"
  (6)  Isolated, unusual all-absorbing special skill or activity

to us to be most consistent with the particularly distinctive features of AS as described in the literature (Klin, 1994).

The interrater reliability for both clinician-assigned diagnosis and ICD-10 rating criteria were examined by the random selection of half of the sample (i.e. 20 subjects) and having their records reviewed and their diagnostic procedure completed by an additional experienced clinician unaware of previous diagnostic assignment. The interrater reliability, as measured by the chance-corrected coefficient Kappa ($K$) and proportion of observed agreement ($PO$) (Siegel & Castellan, 1988) was excellent for clinician-assigned diagnosis ($K = .799$, $SE = .095$; $PO = 90$), and fair to excellent for the diagnosis criteria (range of $K$ .50 − .80; range of $PO$ .75 − .95) (Cicchetti & Sparrow, 1981).

**Neuropsychological characterization.** Twenty-two items (see Table 3), including seven areas of assets and 15 areas of deficits that define the condition of Nonverbal Learning Disabilities (NLD) (Rourke, 1989) were rated by an experienced neuropsychologist on the basis of a thorough review of neuropsychological records. These criteria were rated in terms of assets or deficits, depending on whether results in normed instruments or clinical observations were described as relative assets or clinically signif-

TABLE 3
Defining Criteria for Nonverbal Learning Disabilities (NLD)

| Assets | Deficits |
|---|---|
|  | Fine motor skills |
|  | Gross motor skills |
|  | Visual-motor integration |
| Auditory perception | Visual-spatial perception |
| Rote material | Novel material |
| Auditory/verbal memory | Visual memory |
|  | Verbal concept formation |
|  | Nonverbal concept formation |
| Phonology | Prosody |
| Vocabulary |  |
| Verbal output | Verbal content |
|  | Pragmatics |
| Word decoding/spelling | Reading comprehension |
|  | Mechanical arithmetic |
|  | Social competence |
|  | Emotional competence |

icant deficits in the various areas examined. A conservative algorithm for the NLD+ or NLD− characterization was defined, with the former requiring the concordance of at least 10 of the 15 deficits *and* five of the seven assets. Deficits in tactile perception were excluded from this rating system because of the low frequency with which such deficits were mentioned in the reports of neuropsychological assessments. It should be noted that the following items were rated on a basis of, mostly, clinical observations rather than normed instruments: Gross Motor skills (as observed or measured during the evaluation, rather than reported on the basis of the subject's "clumsiness" in real-life situations, e.g. performance at sports or use of equipment requiring a minimal degree of motor coordination); phonology (i.e. articulation), and prosody (primarily intonation and modulation of volume, although, in some cases, also pitch and rhythm); verbal output (frequency and length of utterances), verbal content (coherence of utterances and ability to convey logical thoughts), pragmatics (e.g. relevance and quantity of utterances, reciprocity, topic management—i.e. demarcation of beginning and ending of topic); social competence (e.g. understanding and conformity to rules and conventions of social interaction, friendships, and so forth), and emotional competence (e.g. empathy, affect modulation).

The interrater reliability of ratings of neuropsychological criteria was examined by randomly selecting one-half of the sample (i.e. 20 subjects) and having their neuropsychological records reviewed and their ratings completed by an additional neuropsychologist. The interrater reliability for the NLD+/NLD− characterization was very good ($K$ = .749, $SE$ = .105; $PO$ = .90), and fair to excellent for the rating criteria (range of $K$ .48 − .80; $PO$ .75 − 1.00) (Cicchetti & Sparrow, 1981).

## *Procedures*

The neuropsychological data for the AS and HFA groups were compared in terms of Verbal IQ—Performance IQ difference, overlap between psychiatric diagnosis (i.e. AS and autism), neuropsychological characterization (i.e. NLD+/NLD−), and presence of deficits in the 22 neuropsychological areas defining the NLD syndrome.

## RESULTS

Although the AS and HFA groups did not differ in terms of Full Scale IQ, the Verbal and Performance IQ (VIQ and PIQ), and particularly the VIQ-PIQ differential (i.e. VIQ-PIQ) were significantly different. The AS group exhibited a higher VIQ and lower PIQ in comparison to the HFA group (see Table 4). The IQ distribution of the AS group indicates that, for this sample, a higher VIQ than PIQ was a universal finding. A repeated measures analysis of variance of clinical group (i.e. AS and HFA) by IQ type (i.e. verbal and performance) revealed a significant interaction between clinical diagnosis and IQ type ($F_{(1,38)}$ = 16.05, $p$ < .001).

When the degree of overlap between psychiatric diagnosis (i.e. AS/HFA) and neuropsychological characterization (i.e. NLD+/NLD−) was examined, a high degree of concordance between AS and NLD+ was observed. This suggests that the NLD profile was indeed an adequate model of neuropsychological assets and deficits encountered in individuals with AS. As can be seen in Table 5, this was not the case for individuals with HFA.

In order to compare the neuropsychological profile of the two groups in more detail, the frequency of subjects exhibiting *deficits* on the 22 areas defining the NLD characterization was examined. As can be seen in Table 6, 11 of the 22 items discriminated between the AS and HFA groups. Of these 11 items, six were found to be predictive of a diagnosis of AS, whereas five were predictive of a diagnosis of "Not—AS" (Table 7).

TABLE 4
Differential Patterns of Verbal IQ, Performance IQ, and Verbal–Performance IQ
Discrepancy for the HFA and AS Groups

| | IQ Distribution | | |
| | HFA Mean *(SD)* | AS Mean *(SD)* | Statistical Significance |
| --- | --- | --- | --- |
| Full Scale IQ | 95.63 (14.66) | 96.76 (18.19) | NS |
| Verbal IQ (VIQ) | 94.63 (22.53) | 108.95 (18.52) | $p < .001$ |
| Performance IQ (PIQ) | 96.68 (12.56) | 85.14 (18.81) | $p < .01$ |
| VIQ-PIQ | −2.05 (25.69) | +23.81 (14.07) | $p < .001$ |

It should be noted that four areas were found to be deficient for the great majority of subjects in both AS and HFA groups: three of these ("prosody", "social and emotional competence") are subsumed under the diagnostic definition of AS and autism, whereas one ("verbal content") is not. Of the remaining 18 areas, only deficits in "Gross Motor Skills" and "Fine Motor Skills" could possibly be subsumed under the diagnostic criterion for AS "motor clumsiness", although the latter has rarely been operationally defined or systematically described (Ghaziuddin, Tsai & Ghaziuddin, 1992b). Therefore, with the possible exception of five items (gross and fine motor skills, prosody, and social and emotional competence), the remaining areas of neuropsychological characterization appeared to be independent of the initial psychiatric diagnostic assignment. Of these five items, three areas (prosody and social and emotional competence) did not differ between the AS and HFA groups.

Finally, as shown in Table 3, the operational definition of *NLD+* was made in terms of an *a priori* decision regarding the required number of concordant assets and deficits as predicted by the NLD model (i.e. ≥ 5 out of 7 assets, and ≥ 10 out of 15 deficits, see Table 3. As this decision had been

TABLE 5
Overlap Between Psychiatric Diagnoses
(HFA and AS) and Neuropsychological
Characterization (NLD+ and NLD−)

| | NLD+ | NLD− |
| --- | --- | --- |
| HFA | 1 | 18 |
| AS | 18 | 3 |

Fisher's exact $p = .000$ ($p < .001$).

TABLE 6
Frequency of Subjects Exhibiting Deficits on the 22 NLD Items

| Item | HFA | AS | Fisher's $p$ |
|---|---|---|---|
| Fine motor skills | 6/19 | 19/21 | .001*** |
| Gross motor skills | 12/19 | 21/21 | .003** |
| Visual-motor integration | 8/19 | 19/21 | .002** |
| Visual-spatial perception | 5/19 | 16/21 | .004** |
| Auditory perception | 10/19 | 1/21 | .001** |
| Novel material | 11/19 | 15/21 | .510 |
| Rote material | 2/19 | 0/21 | .219 |
| Verbal memory | 11/19 | 5/21 | .049* |
| Visual memory | 9/19 | 19/21 | .005** |
| Verbal concept formation | 10/19 | 10/21 | 1.000 |
| Nonverbal concept formation | 5/19 | 16/21 | .004** |
| Articulation | 11/19 | 1/21 | .001*** |
| Vocabulary | 8/19 | 0/21 | .001** |
| Verbal output | 11/19 | 1/21 | .001*** |
| Verbal content | 18/19 | 20/21 | 1.000 |
| Prosody | 17/19 | 19/21 | 1.000 |
| Pragmatics | 16/19 | 20/21 | .331 |
| Word decoding | 7/19 | 2/21 | .060 |
| Reading/comprehension | 10/19 | 10/21 | 1.000 |
| Arithmetic | 8/19 | 9/21 | 1.000 |
| Social competence | 19/19 | 21/21 | 1.000 |
| Emotional | 19/19 | 21/21 | 1.000 |

\* $p < .05$; \*\* $p < .01$; \*\*\* $p < .001$.

made on a theoretical basis prior to data collection, we explored the utility of this cut off point for a prediction of a diagnosis of AS in the case of the present sample of individuals with AS and HFA. However, the adopted cut off point was only one of 128 possible cut off points (i.e. 0–7 out of 7 assets, AND 0–15 out of 15 deficits, hence $8 \times 16 = 128$). In order to obtain an empirically-derived *optimal* cut off point, it was necessary to analyze the utility of the *a priori* cut off point vis-à-vis all other possible cut off points. The sensitivity, specificity and coefficient of agreement *Kappa* for all 128 combinations were calculated (Kraemer, 1988). Eight combinations were associated with a *Kappa* $\geq .75$ ("excellent" agreement (Cicchetti & Sparrow, 1981). The sensitivity and specificity for these combinations ranged from .76 to .90 and .95 to 1.00, respectively. The *a priori* combination (i.e. $\geq 5$ out of 7 assets, and $\geq 10$ out of 15 deficits) exhibited a sensitivity of .86, a specificity of .95, and a *Kappa* of .80. The highest *Kappa* (.85) was exhibited by the combination including $\geq 3$ out of 7 assets, and

TABLE 7
Eleven Neuropsychological Deficits Discriminated
Between HFA and AS

| Predictive of AS<br>[items ranked by $r_{(phi)}$] | $r_{(phi)}$ |
|---|---|
| Fine motor skills | .61*** |
| Visual motor integration | .52** |
| Visual spatial perception | .50** |
| Nonverbal concept formation | .50** |
| Gross motor skills | .48** |
| Visual memory | .47** |
| Predictive of not-AS<br>[items ranked by $r_{(phi)}$] | $r_{(phi)}$ |
| Articulation | −.58*** |
| Verbal output | −.58*** |
| Auditory perception | −.54** |
| Vocabulary | −.53* |
| Verbal memory | −.35* |

$*p < .05; **p < .01; ***p < .001.$
$r_{(phi)}$ = extent of association between item and diagnosis and level of
significance.

$\geq 10$ out of 15 deficits (sensitivity of .90 and specificity of .95). These results suggest that (a) the *a priori* decision regarding the operational definition of *NLD+* proved to be highly predictive of a diagnosis of AS in the
present sample; and (b) as a number of variations of the *NLD+* operationalization were highly predictive of a diagnosis of AS in the present
sample, the present results also suggest that the overlap between *NLD+*
and AS is a rather robust phenomenon.

## DISCUSSION

This study examined the neuropsychological profiles of a group of AS and
HFA individuals whose diagnostic assignment was made of following
stringent criteria and an algorithm based on ICD-10 research criteria for the
two conditions. A comparison of neuropsychological profiles revealed that
11 areas discriminated between the two conditions, nine of which were apparently independent from the psychiatric diagnostic assignment. The high
level of concordance between AS (but not HFA) and a neuropsychological

characterization of NLD suggests that the latter can be seen as an adequate neuropsychological marker of AS. Interestingly, such neuropsychological differences between AS and HFA were captured in the groups' VIQ-PIQ discrepancy, with VIQ being universally higher than PIQ for individuals with AS, whereas no differential was found for individuals with HFA, a finding that is supported by results of the DSM-IV Autism/PDD field trial (Volkmar et al., 1994) and recent neuropsychological research of autism unaccompanied by mental retardation (Minshew, 1992).

The present findings contrast with previous work on the neuropsychology of AS (e.g. Ozonoff et al., 1991; Szatmari et al., 1990). However, the present use of stringent ICD-10 criteria for diagnostic assignment complicates a direct interpretation of differences with previous studies where less systematic and stringent diagnostic assignment was adopted. For example, Szatmari et al.'s study (1990) revealed no significant differences between AS and HFA groups, leading the authors to the conclusion that "it is justified to combine the AS and HFA groups into a more general PDD category (p. 135). However, the adopted inclusionary criteria—(1) isolated behavior; (2) impaired social interaction; (3) one of odd speech, impaired nonverbal communication, or bizarre preoccupations, and (4) onset prior to 6 years of age (p. 131)—defined AS in a much broader fashion than the ICD-10 draft research criteria. The authors' conclusion that AS appears to be "a very mild form of PDD" (p. 136) raises some questions as to the face value of creating the AS grouping apart from the PDD-NOS category, and may account for some of the positive findings (with regard to early history), and the rather broad definition of the syndrome may partly account for the lack of findings in regard to the groups' neurocognitive profiles. Clearly, research findings are dependent upon the nosologic approach adopted. In contrast to Szatmari et al.'s strategy, the present study adopted the ICD-10 approach to AS, which attempts to maximize the differences between HFA and AS in ways compatible with, as yet tentative, clinical research data.

Ozonoff et al.'s study (1991) did use the ICD-10 definition of AS, but modified it by excluding the onset criteria. The exclusion was justified in terms of the current debate regarding the validity of the AS onset criteria (Gillberg & Steffenburg, 1987; Wing, 1988). Although this approach could be well justified, it did make the AS definition broader than the one adopted in the present study. The impact of a given diagnostic system on the assignment of diagnosis is illustrated in Ozonoff et al.'s (1991) finding that 40% of their AS subjects met DSM-III-R (1987) criteria for autism. In many respects, Ozonoff et al.'s (1991) findings were inconsistent with Szatmari et al.'s (1990). For example, in Ozonoff et al.'s (1991) study, the AS and HFA groups did significantly differ in terms of Verbal IQ—Performance IQ differential due to the AS group having significantly higher Verbal IQ.

Clearly, the nosological strategy has a direct impact on findings of studies of AS. Given the current state of affairs, our approach was to select the most phenomenologically prototypical cases of HFA and AS, with a view to maximize differences in developmental history and presentation. Operationally, we decided to adopt the most stringent current definitions of these syndromes. The rationale for this strategy was based on the assumption that if neuropsychological differences could not be found with the extreme cases, then there would be little reason to pursue this line of research. In this effort, we chose to add two additional criteria, which are suggested but not required in ICD-10 and DSM-IV (American Psychiatric Association, 1994), so as to further specify our definition of AS. The two criteria were (a) "delayed motor milestones and presence of motor 'clumsiness'", and (b) "isolated, unusual all-absorbing special skill or activity". This strategy entailed some gains and losses. More stringency was achieved by bringing our defining criteria closer to findings revealed in the Autism/ PDD DSM-IV field trial (Volkmar et al., 1994), according to which it was the case that motor delays and clumsiness, and idiosyncratic/circumscribed interests were very common in AS. However, this approach entailed a modification of the ICD-10 defining criteria, and this should be taken into consideration when interpreting our findings.

For example, the introduction of the motor criterion may have selected a very specific subsample of AS subjects from our original pool of potential participants. This possibility prompted a reanalysis of our data with a view to ascertain whether any additional subjects would have been included in the AS sample had we not made the motor criterion necessary for the diagnosis. From the 33 individuals excluded, only six subjects would have been included in the AS sample using this less restrictive definition; interestingly, however, all these were complex cases which were excluded from further analysis owing to a lack of concordance between clinician-assigned diagnosis and the ICD-10 rating criteria. The inclusion of these six subjects in the AS sample did not significantly alter the results obtained, although the statistical significance level of group comparisons for four neuropsychological items—gross motor skills, visual-motor integration, visual-spatial perception, and visual memory—dropped slightly. There was only one significant alteration of results, and that concerned the group comparison for verbal memory, which became barely significant at the $p < .05$ level. Paradoxically, this was one area for which there was significant differences between the AS and HFA groups in Ozonoff et al.'s (1991) study. This reanalysis notwithstanding, it is still possible that our AS sample represented a specific group of AS individuals whose neuropsychological profile includes motor symptoms.

Another issue relates to the ICD-10 (and our) requirement for "preservation" of language skills early in development, and its possible relationship to later verbal/nonverbal IQ differences as a result of a "downstream" effect. Following this reasoning, the group differences for verbal/performance IQ differential would simply reflect higher verbal skills from the onset. Although this is in fact an empirical issue, it should be clarified that the ICD-10 meaning of "lack of clinically significant delays or deviance in language acquisition" relates to early language, and not language at the time of our examination (as adopted in Ozonoff et. al's (1991) study). As for the possible "downstream" effect, it is indeed possible that later differences may reflect a more basic initial difference in language development. However, the issue of early language acquisition should be seen as rather separate from later language/communication skills. The early preservation of language does not *necessarily* imply that later language skills will be normal; in fact, they often appeared not to be normal, particularly in terms of the suprasegmental, pragmatic, and competence (e.g. nonliteral) aspects of language. That notwithstanding, certain aspects of language functioning (particularly the formal aspects, e.g. vocabulary, grammatical competence) did appear to represent continued areas of strength for individuals with AS.

A final point in regard to the interpretation of our findings concerns the recruitment origin of our sample. In order to ascertain any differences between the Yale group ($N = 24$) and the LDAA group ($N = 16$), we compared the two samples for age, gender, and Full Scale IQ. Although there were no significant differences in terms of age and Full Scale IQ, there were differences in terms of gender, as both female subjects with AS were from the LDAA group.

In summary, the various issues arising from the adoption of different diagnostic approaches in research studies serve to underscore the paramount importance of stringent nosology for the validation and characterization of diagnostic concepts that share several features such as AS and HFA.

The present findings can be seen as a contribution to the validation of AS vis-à-vis HFA, as these two conditions could be distinguished in terms of their neuropsychological characterization. This is a more complex issue, however, given that these two conditions could still share the same etiology or other pathogenetic processes while having phenotypic difference solely accounted for by neuropsychological differences. In this sense, AS and HFA could be seen as the same diagnostic entity expressed differently because of different neuropsychological endowment, similar, to some extent, to the phenomenological differences between lower functioning and higher functioning autism. Whether AS and HFA are truly different diagnostic entities will be clarified only with additional research on the developmental, behavioral genetics, and neuroanatomic aspects of these two conditions. That notwithstanding, the convergence between AS and NLD suggests lines of investigation focused on right-hemisphere abnormalities, or other competing neuroanatomic models [e.g. involving white matter abnormalities (Rourke, 1989)] purported to account for the unique cluster of neuropsychological assets and deficits characterizing NLD. Such research may review mechanisms responsible for disruptions of socialization skills of a different nature than the ones still eluding investigators of autism.

The clarity of results obtained in this study may have been a function of the investigators' decision to include only stringently diagnosed, prototypical cases of AS and HFA. The phenotypic expression of both conditions is probably more heterogenous than evidenced in the present sample (Klin & Volkmar, 1995). However, given the current controversy regarding the validity of AS, our results suggest the importance of utilizing a stringent and operational definition of subjects studied. Conversely, it will be important to explore the possible associations between neuropsychological profiles and varied clinical presentations of this and other syndromes characterized by disabilities of socialization (e.g. the study of individuals with a neuropsychological profile consistent with NLD, but who do not meet criteria for a pervasive developmental disorder).

Finally, regardless of whether or not AS and HFA are truly different diagnostic entities, the significant divergence of neuropsychological profiles suggests that intervention strategies for AS should be of a different nature, directly addressing specific neuropsychological deficits and building on neuropsychological assets, an approach that has been described as very useful with individuals with Nonverbal Learning Disabilities (Klin, 1994; Rourke, 1989).

## REFERENCES

American Psychiatric Association (1994). *Diagnostic and Statistical Manual of Mental Disorders, 4th Edition*. Washington, DC: American Psychiatric Association.

Asperger, H. (1991/1994). Autistic psychopathy in childhood (trans). In U. Frith (Ed.), *Autism and Asperger syndrome* (pp. 37–92). Cambridge: Cambridge University Press.

Asperger, H. (1979). Problems of infantile autism. *Communication, 13*, 45–52.

Bishop, D. (1989). Autism, Asperger's syndrome, and semantic pragmatic disorder: where are the boundaries? *British Journal of Disorders of Communication, 24*, 107–121.

Cicchetti, D. V. & Sparrow, S. S. (1981). Development of criteria for establishing the interrater reliability of specific items in a given inventory: applications to assessment of adaptive behavior. *American Journal of Mental Deficiency, 86,* 127–137.

Dawson, G. (1983). Lateralized brain dysfunction in autism: evidence from the Halstead-Reitan Neuropsychological Battery. *Journal of Autism and Developmental Disorders, 13,* 269–286.

Denckla, M. B. (1983). The neuropsychology of social-emotional learning disabilities. *Archives of Neurology, 40,* 461–462.

Ghaziuddin, M., Tsai, L. Y. & Ghaziuddin, N. (1992a). A comparison of the diagnostic criteria for Asperger syndrome. *Journal of Autism and Developmental Disorders, 22,* 643–649.

Ghaziuddin, M., Tsai, L. Y. & Ghaziuddin, N. (1992b). A reappraisal of clumsiness as a diagnostic feature of Asperger syndrome. *Journal of Autism and Developmental Disorders, 22,* 651–656.

Gillberg, C. (1991). Clinical and neurobiological aspects of Asperger syndrome in six family studies. In U. Frith (Ed.), *Autism and Asperger syndrome* (pp. 122–146). Cambridge: Cambridge University Press.

Gillberg, C. & Steffenburg, S. (1987). Outcome and prognostic factors in infantile autism and similar conditions: a population-based study of 46 cases followed through puberty. *Journal of Autism and Developmental Disorders, 15,* 389–397.

Kanner, L. (1943). Autistic disturbances of affective contact. *Nervous Child, 2,* 217–250.

Klin, A. (1994). Asperger Syndrome. *Child and Adolescent Psychiatric Clinics of North America, 3,* 131–148.

Klin, A. & Volkmar, F. R. (1995). Autism and the pervasive developmental disorders. *Child and Psychiatric Clinics of North America, 4,* 617–630.

Kraemer, H. C. (1988). Assessment of 2 × 2 associations: generalization of signal detection methodology. *American Statistician, 42,* 37–49.

Minshew, N. J. (1992). Neurological localization in autism. In E. Schopler & G. B. Mesibov (Eds). *High-functioning individuals with autism* (pp. 65–90). New York: Plenum Press.

Molina, J. L., Ruata, J. M. & Soler, E. P. (1986). Is there a right-hemisphere dysfunction in Asperger's syndrome? *British Journal of Psychiatry, 148,* 745–746.

Ozonoff, S., Roge, S. J. & Pennington, B. F. (1991). Asperger's syndrome: evidence of an empirical distinction from high-functioning autism. *Journal of Child Psychology and Psychiatry, 32,* 1107–1122.

Rourke, B. (1989). *Nonverbal learning disabilities: the syndrome and the model.* New York: Guilford Press.

Rumsey, J. M. (1992). Neuropsychological studies of high-level autism. In E. Schopler & G. B. Mesibov (Eds), *High-functioning individuals with autism* (pp. 41–64). New York: Plenum Press.

Rutter, M. (1985). Infantile autism and other pervasive developmental disorders. In M. Rutter & L. Hersov (Eds), *Child and Adolescent Psychiatry: Modern Approaches, 2nd ed.* (pp. 545–566). Oxford: Blackwell.

Rutter, M. (1989). Annotation: Child psychiatric disorders in ICD-10. *Journal of Child Psychology and Psychiatry, 30*, 499–513.

Siegel, S & Castellan, N. J. (1988). *Nonparametric statistics for the behavioral sciences, 2nd ed.* New York: McGraw-Hill.

Szatmari, P., Tuff, L., Finlayson, M. A. J. & Bartolucci, G. (1990). Asperger's syndrome and autism neurocognitive aspects. *Journal of the American Academy of Child and Adolescent Psychiatry, 29*, 130–136.

Tantam, D. (1988). Annotation: Asperger's syndrome. *Journal of Child Psychology and Psychiatry, 29*, 245–255.

Tantam, D. (1991). Asperger syndrome in adulthood. In U. Frith (Ed.), *Autism and Asperger syndrome* (pp. 147–183). Cambridge: Cambridge University Press.

Tsai, L. Y. (1992). Diagnostic issues in high-functioning autism. In E. Schopler & G. B. Mesilov (Eds), *High-functioning individuals with autism* (pp. 11–40). New York: Plenum Press.

Voeller, K. K. S. (1986). Right-hemisphere deficit syndrome in children. *American Journal of Psychiatry, 143*, 1004–1009.

Volkmar, F. R. & Cohen, D. J. (1991). Nonautistic pervasive developmental disorders. In R. Michels (Ed.), *Psychiatry (Child Psychiatry, 2*, 1–6). Philadelphia: J. B. Lippincott.

Volkmar, F. R., Klin, A., Siegel, B., Szatmari, P., Lord, C., Campbell, M., Freeman, B. J., Cicchetti, D. V., Rutter, M., Kline, W., Buitelaar, J., Hattab, Y., Fombonne, E., Fuentes, J., Werry, J., Stone, W., Kerbeshian, J., Hoshino, Y., Bregman, J., Loveland, K., Szymanski, L. & Towbin, K. (1994). DSM-IV Autism/Pervasive Developmental Disorder Field Trial. *American Journal of Psychiatry, 151*, 1361–1367.

Volkmar, F. R., Szatmari, P., & Sparrow, S. S. (1993). Sex differences in Pervasive Developmental Disorders. *Journal of Autism and Developmental Disorders, 23*, 579–592.

Weintraub, S. & Mesulam, M. M. (1983). Developmental learning disabilities of the right hemisphere: emotional, interpersonal, and cognitive components. *Archives of Neurology, 40*, 463–468.

Wing, L. (1981). Asperger's syndrome: a clinical account. *Psychological Medicine, 11*, 115–130.

Wing, L. (1988). The continuum of autistic characteristics. In E. Schopler & G. B. Mesibov (Eds), *Diagnosis and assessment in autism* (pp. 91–111). New York: Plenum Press.

Wing, L. (1991). The relationship between Asperger's syndrome and Kanner's autism. In U. Frith (Ed.), *Autism and Asperger syndrome* (pp. 93–121). Cambridge: Cambridge University Press.

Wolff, S. & Chick, J. (1980). Schizoid personality in childhood: a controlled follow-up study. *Psychological Medicine, 10*, 85–100.

World Health Organization (1990). International classification of diseases: Tenth
revision. Chapter V. Mental and behavioral disorders (including disorders of
psychological development). Diagnostic criteria for research (May 1990 draft
for field trials). Geneva, WHO (unpublished), 1990.

# 10

# Self-Competence and Emotional Understanding in High-Functioning Children with Autism

**Lisa Capps and Marian Sigman**
*University of California, Los Angeles*
**Nurit Yirmiya**
*Hebrew University of Jerusalem*

*This study examined the relationships between perceived self-competence, intellectual ability, emotional understanding, and parent report of social adaptation in 18 nonretarded children with autism. Children who perceived themselves as less socially competent demonstrated stronger intellectual capabilities, greater understanding of others' emotional experiences, and were better able to access their own emotional experiences than were those who perceived themselves as more socially competent. According to their parents, children who reported less social competence also displayed more socially adaptive behavior, and expressed more interest and less sadness and fear than did those who reported greater social competence. Discussion focuses on potential effects of this heightened capacity for emotional understanding on self-esteem and implications for intervention with highly intelligent persons with autism.*

Someone says I should have written about the moods I have, but I think I have described fairly well why I think a lot that's hap-

---

Reprinted with permission from *Development and Psychopathology*, 1995, Vol. 7, 137–149. Copyright © 1995 Cambridge University Press.

This research was supported by grants NS25243 from NINDS and HD17662 from NICHD to Marian Sigman. We are grateful to Larry Epstein, Michael Espinosa, B. J. Freeman, and Alma Lopez for their contributions to this research. We also thank the children and families who participated in this project.

pened to me is enough to make anybody moody. Yes, I think anyone normal would find it hard to lead the kind of existence I have. David Miedzianik (1986)

To portray autistic persons' abilities to understand themselves and others it is necessary to adopt a developmental frame—one that brings both chronological and mental age into focus (Macdonald et al., 1989; Prior, Dahlstrom, & Squires, 1990). Older autistic persons, even those who are retarded, manifest abilities not demonstrated by younger autistic persons, suggesting that experience and maturation play a role in the development of emotional understanding. In addition, nonretarded persons with autism display a greater capacity for emotional expressiveness and responsiveness than do retarded autistic persons (Braverman, Fein, Lucci, & Waterhouse, 1989; Ozonoff, Pennington, & Rogers, 1990), and for reading others' mental states (Happe, in press). These findings may suggest that autistic persons apply their mental strengths in ways that help compensate for autistic impairment.

Across the spectrum of abilities and limitations displayed by individuals with autism, the most dramatic discrepancies occur between those who are young and mentally retarded and those who are older and of normal or superior intelligence (Yirmiya & Sigman, 1991). In contrast to young, mentally retarded autistic children, who rarely look up at others' faces to share emotional experiences (Mundy, Sigman, Ungerer, & Sherman, 1986; Sigman, Mundy, Sherman, & Ungerer, 1986) or to make sense of ambiguous and confusing situations (Sigman, Kasari, Kwon, & Yirmiya, 1992), older, nonretarded individuals with autism display a considerable understanding of their own emotions and the emotions of others.

Members of this high-functioning group show an interest in emotional expression. They also demonstrate capacities to discriminate between emotions and to recognize such expressions as a reflection of a person's internal states, similar in many ways to that reported for normally developing children (Harter & Whitesell, 1989; Russell, 1989; Stein & Trabasso, 1989; Stipek, 1983; Thompson, 1989). They are able to talk about their own experiences of simple emotions, such as happiness, sadness, anger, and fear, as well as complex emotions such as pride and embarrassment, which require understanding of cause and consequence (Capps, Yirmiya, & Sigman, 1992). Like normal comparison children (Seidner, Stipek, & Feshbach, 1988), autistic children described feeling proud in relations to events which are the result of purpose and effort, such as "when I won a game," differentiating these from happy circumstances that lie outside their control, such as "getting a new bike." High-functioning individuals with autism have also demonstrated the ability to label complex facial expressions in pictures requiring interpretation of social cues (Capps, Yirmiya, & Sigman, 1992;

see also Van Lacker, Cornelius, & Needleman, 1991). One such picture, for example, depicted a boy exiting a door labeled "Girls."

Although autistic children performed remarkably well, tasks involving complex emotions appeared more taxing for them than for normal controls. The autistic children required more prompting, took more time to respond, and more frequently responded inappropriately. For example, one autistic child described feeling "proud of a dog." Another, when presented with a picture of a boy shaking his fist, said the boy felt "itchy."

In contrast to young, retarded autistic children, who rarely looked up at, much less comforted persons feigning distress (Sigman, Kasari, Kwon, & Yirmiya, 1992), high-functioning autistic persons performed surprisingly well on laboratory measures of empathy (Yirmiya, Sigman, Kasari, & Mundy, 1992). Autistic and normal comparison children were shown videotaped segments depicting scenarios in which a child feels sad, happy, angry, afraid, or proud. Each child viewed the segments on two occasions, at least one week apart. After the first viewing, participants were asked what the child in the scenario was feeling, comprising a measure of their ability to read others' emotions (labeling task). After the second viewing, the children were asked how they felt. Empathy was measured based on the congruence between the emotional state subjects' attributed to the child-protagonist and their own emotional experience.

Although not as adept as normal comparison children, high-functioning autistic individuals were quite accurate in labeling the emotional experience of protagonists. Similarly, although they performed significantly less well than comparison children, the majority of autistic children reported feeling emotions resembling those they attributed to the child-protagonist.

Because participants' faces were videotaped while they watched the vignettes, we were able to code their displays of facial affect, comprising an additional index of empathic responsiveness. Positive, negative, and concentrated facial expressions were coded second by second. In contrast to younger, retarded individuals with autism, who appear to ignore if not avoid affective displays, this high-functioning group was highly attentive and emotionally expressive while observing the tapes (Capps, Kasari, Yirmiya, & Sigman, 1993). In fact, they displayed more positive affect and greater concentration than did comparison children. Furthermore, there was a positive correlation between children's displays of positive affect while viewing the tapes and their performance on the empathy task, suggesting that children who were most expressive while viewing the child-protagonist were most able to share the protagonists' emotional experience.

Rather than simply revising conceptualizations of autism to fit the abilities of these high-functioning individuals, or questioning the appropriateness of the diagnosis in such cases, it is important to consider the development of these emotional strengths. It is very likely that autistic persons of normal or superior intelligence compensate for emotional impairment, such that the abilities they manifest reflect not the absence of deficits, but diligent, often courageous attempts to overcome them.

What are the consequences of what appears to be an alternative, compensatory route to emotional understanding? Although evidence suggests that more highly intelligent autistic persons are better able to identify and share the emotional experiences of others (Yirmiya et al., 1992), we do not know how such persons see themselves. Despite their implications for psychological adjustment and clinical intervention, questions concerning how the ability to read and relate to others' emotions might affect self-concept have not yet been delineated in the literature on autism.

The few studies of self-concept and self-esteem in nonautistic, mentally retarded persons suggests that the incidence of depression is higher among individuals who are mildly retarded than among those who are moderately or severely retarded (Benson & Ivins, 1992; Jacobson, 1982; Reiss, 1985; Reiss & Rojahn, 1993). In the study by Benson and Ivins (1992), mildly retarded adults reported lower self-concept and greater levels of anger than did more severely retarded persons. In addition, subjects' self-reports for depression and self-concept were corroborated by those of informants. There was a lack of concordance between self- and informant-reports of anger, with informants reporting greater degrees of anger than subjects themselves. In discussing the relationship between depression, self concept, and severity of mental retardation, these investigators suggest that individuals functioning in the mild range may be more aware of their limitations and more frustrated by them than are individuals with lesser intellectual capability (Benson & Ivins, 1992; Reiss, 1985; Reiss & Rojahn, 1993).

Given the nature of autistic impairment, the extent to which this line of reasoning can be applied to autism is unclear. The self-reflective and social-comparative processes involved in self-perception are most challenging for autistic persons. This investigation aims to illuminate how autistic persons of average or superior intelligence—persons who seem to apply their intellectual strengths to gain access to social-emotional exchanges—perceive themselves, particularly in social-emotional domains. Although autistic persons' peculiarities and limitations are striking to observers inside and outside of the laboratory, we have little knowledge—and no empirical information—about their own awareness of these shortcomings.[1] Such

---

[1] Although we are not aware of other studies on self-concept in autistic children, autobiographical accounts provide rich information. See Bemporad (1979), Grandin (1984), Grandin and Scariano (1986), Miedzianik (1986) and Williams (1992), as well as analysis by Dewey (1991), Happe (1991), and Volkmar and Cohen (1985).

awareness may be a crucial part of adjustment. As Kanner pointed out in 1973, "[his] most successful autistic patients, unlike most other autistic children, became uneasily aware of their peculiarities, and began to make a conscious effort to do something about them." Kanner did not, however, account for the development of such awareness, nor efforts to alter idiosyncratic characteristics and behaviors.

This study examined the extent to which awareness of peculiarities might be mediated by intelligence and by the ability to read and share the emotions of others. One possibility is that more highly intelligent autistic persons' superior emotional abilities are reflected in their perceived self-competence; that is, because IQ seems to help compensate for social-emotional limitations, children with higher IQ scores may feel more socially competent. Alternatively, those who are most intelligent and best able to read the responses of others may have greater access to appraisals of their quirks and limitations.

A second objective of this study was to investigate the relationships between high-functioning autistic children's perceptions of their own social abilities and their parents' perceptions of the children's social adaptation. On one hand, we thought that parents of autistic children with exceptional cognitive abilities might see their children as better adjusted in general. On the other, it seemed possible that children's cognitive capabilities would engender greater expectations in general, heightening parents' awareness of their children's shortcomings.

A third objective was to examine parents' perceptions of their children's emotional experiences over the course of daily life. We were most interested in whether children's perceived social competence was manifest in their emotional life with others. In particular, we wondered whether children who perceived themselves as less socially competent would more frequently display negative affects such as sadness, fear, and shame.

## METHOD

### Subjects

The sample consisted of 18 children with autism, ranging in age from 9 years, 3 months to 16 years, 10 months ($M = 12$ years, 6 months), and 20 normally developing children, ranging in age from 9 years, 6 months to 14 years, 1 month. Participants had all been followed at University of California, Los Angeles (UCLA) since early childhood and were diagnosed with autism within 2 years prior to initiation of this study by clinicians not affiliated with the project. Because the sample was recruited in 1987–1988, clinicians were using *Diagnostic and Statistical Manual (DSM-III)* diagnostic criteria (American

Psychiatric Association, 1981). To confirm that the children showed symptoms of autism in early childhood, the parents were asked to fill out the Autism Behavior Checklist (ABC; Krug, Arick, & Almond, 1978) using recollections of their children's behaviors at ages 3–5 years. A check of the medical charts for 10 of these children when they were 3–5 years-old showed agreement between the parental recollections of the severity of symptoms and ratings made from clinical descriptions in the charts, $r = .74$ (Yirmiya, Sigman, & Freeman, 1994). The autistic children all had scores over the cut-off score of 68, a reliable indicator of autism (Krug, Arick, & Almond, 1978).

In order to be included in this study, the children were also required to have current Verbal IQ, Performance IQ, and Full-scale IQ scores of 75 or higher (as determined by the Wechsler Intelligence Scale for Children-Revised [WISC-R]) and to be free of additional diagnoses. Full-scale IQ scores ranged from 75 to 136 ($M = 102$).

Children in the comparison group were recruited from private schools and were screened for symptoms of autism by a trained clinical psychologist during administration of intelligence tests. Comparison children were matched with autistic children on gender, Full-scale IQ, and chronological age. The *t*-tests revealed that groups were not statistically different with respect to mental age, Verbal IQ, and Performance IQ. Groups were also matched on ethnicity and socioeconomic status (SES) as determined by the Hollingshead Index (1957). Sample characteristics are presented in Table 1.

TABLE 1
Sample Characteristics

|  | Group | |
|---|---|---|
|  | Autistic<br>($n = 18$) | Normal<br>($n = 20$) |
| Chronological age (years) | 12.4 ± 2.1 | 11.4 ± 2.0 |
| Mental age (years) | 12.3 ± 2.2 | 12.1 ± 2.0 |
| Full-Scale IQ | 101.9 ± 18.6 | 108.4 ± 13.7 |
| Verbal IQ | 98.6 ± 20.5 | 106.9 ± 12.4 |
| Performance IQ | 105.3 ± 19.4 | 105.1 ± 13.9 |
| SES | 3.5 ± 0.9 | 3.7 ± 1.06 |
| Male/Female | 15/3 | 17/3 |
| Caucasian | 11 | 14 |
| Latino | 3 | 2 |
| African-American | 2 | 2 |
| Asian | 2 | 2 |

*Note:* IQ scores are based on the WISC-R. SES was based on a Hollingshead score (1 = lowest to 5 = highest SES). Values are mean ± *SD*.

### Procedures

The children and their parents participated in two 90-min sessions, wherein the children were interviewed individually by a graduate student and parents completed a series of questionnaires. First, the WISC-R was administered to determine the appropriateness of the child as a subject, after which each child received a battery of standardized tests and experimental procedures.

### Measures Administered to Children

**Perceived self-competence.** Children completed the "Perceived Competence Scale for Children" (Harter, 1982), which taps children's sense of competence in four different domains, rather than viewing competence as a unitary concept. The domains include cognitive competence (doing well at school, being smart); social competence (having a lot of friends, being easy to like, an important member of one's class); and physical competence (doing well at sports, learning new games readily, preferring to play rather than watch); and "general self-worth" (being happy with oneself).

The child is presented with a question such as, "Some kids find it hard to make friends, but for other kids it's pretty easy." The child indicates which kind of kid he or she is most like, and then decides whether the description is "sort of true" or "really true." Each item is scored from 1 to 4, 1 indicating low perceived competence and 4 reflecting high perceived competence. Scores are summed and then averaged for each subscale.

**Communication about own emotional experiences.** As reported in Capps, Yirmiya, and Sigman (1992), subjects were given a list of four emotions (sadness, happiness, embarrassment, and pride). Each child was asked to read the list aloud and to tell about a time in which s/he felt each emotion. The order in which different emotional experiences were elicited was randomized. When a child was unable to provide an example, the examiner related a time in which he/she felt the emotion (standard stories) and proceeded through the list before returning to the source of difficulty. Prompting, in the form of repetition, was used when a child did not respond, stated that s/he had never felt the emotion, or could not recall the situation. To measure the difficulty of the task, number of prompts were counted, and latency of response was timed.

**Empathy.** As reported in Yirmiya et al. (1992), participants observed five videotaped vignettes, each of which was 3 min long and involved a child-protagonist experiencing one of the following emotions: happiness, pride, sadness, fear, and anger. Each subject viewed the segments twice, during separate sessions. Both times, after each segment, the participant was given a list of seven emotions. Counterbalancing for condition, on one occasion s/he was asked to circle the emotion being experienced by the protagonist, and on another to report his or her own emotional response.

**Coding.** Each subject received both a labeling score and an empathy score (reflecting the match between the label and the child's own reported feeling) for each of the five segments. Responses were scored as 2 = correct, 1 = incorrect, but appropriate hedonic tone, or 0 = incorrect.

### Measures Administered to Parents

**Vineland adaptive behavior scales.** Parents of autistic children completed the Vineland Adaptive Behavior Scales (VABS; Sparrow, Balla, & Cicchetti, 1984), an interview that provides a measure of children's social and adaptive competencies and yields standardized scores and age equivalents in four domains: Communication, Daily Living Skills, Socialization, and Motor Skills. The VABS has excellent reliability and validity (Cicchetti & Sparrow, 1981; Sparrow, Balla, & Cicchetti, 1984) and has been used extensively with developmentally disabled children (Deckner, Soraci, Deckner, & Blanton, 1981; Loveland & Kelley, 1988; Rodrigue, Morgan, & Geffken, 1991; Volkmar et al., 1987).

**The emotion behavior checklist.** As described in Capps et al. (1993), the Emotion Behavior Checklist (EBC; Izard, Dougherty, Bloxton, & Kotsch, 1974) asks parents to report how often during the past 2 weeks their child showed behaviors that are indicative of the following emotions: interest, joy, sadness, anger, and fear. Each emotion is considered separately and rated in relation to a variety of specific behavioral manifestations of emotion: actions, facial affect, body posture/gait, tone of voice/vocalization, and verbal expression. Ratings are given on a scale of 1–10, with 1 being rarely, 10 very often, and rarely, hardly ever, sometimes, and often falling in between.

## RESULTS

### Child Measures

**Perceived self-competence.** Between-group comparisons of children's overall self-competence ratings were conducted using a Hotellings' $T^2$ test, and results suggested that autistic children perceive themselves to be less competent than comparison children do, $F(3, 36) = -4.59, p < .001$. Subsequent $t$ tests showed that autistic children perceived themselves to be *less* competent than did their nonautistic peers in all but the cognitive domain. Autistic children reported feeling less competent socially, $t = 5.17, df = 36, p < .0001$, and physically, $t = 2.86, df = 36, p < .01$, and reported lower estimates of their overall self-worth, $t = 4.02, df = 36, p < .001$. Results appear in Table 2.

**Correlation with IQ.** Within each group, correlations were computed between the four self-competence scores and Full-scale IQ scores. Within the autistic group, one significant correlation emerged: perceived social competence was *negatively* correlated with Full-scale IQ, $r = .51, p < .04$. That is, autistic children with higher IQ scores appeared to perceive themselves as less socially competent than did autistic children with lower IQ scores. Correlations between perceived self-competence and IQ appear in Table 3.

In the comparison group IQ was positively correlated with children's perceived cognitive competence, $r = .58, p < .01$, but did not correlate with social competence.

TABLE 2
Children's Perceived Self-Competence

|  | Group | |
|---|---|---|
|  | Autistic ($n = 18$) | Normal ($n = 20$) |
| Overall self-competence | 70.9 ± 11.2 | 87.5 ± 11.1 |
| Social competence | 16.8 ± 3.8 | 22.8 ± 3.3* |
| Cognitive competence | 19.5 ± 3.7 | 21.1 ± 3.7 |
| Physical competence | 16.7 ± 4.6 | 20.9 ± 4.4** |
| Global self-worth | 17.9 ± 4.6 | 22.8 ± 2.7*** |

*Note:* Self-competence scores based on the Harter Perceived Self Competence Scales. Values are mean ± *SD*.
*$p < .0001$.
**$p < .01$.
***$p < .001$.

TABLE 3
Correlations Between Autistic Children's IQ
Scores, Perceived Self-Competence,
and Parent's Report of Social Adaptation

| | Full-Scale IQ Autistic Group ($n = 18$) |
| --- | --- |
| Perceived self-competence | |
| Social competence | − 0.51* |
| Cognitive competence | 0.41 |
| Physical competence | − |
| Overall self-worth | − |
| Parent's report of socialization skills | 0.72** |

*$p < .05$.
**$p < .001$.

**Correlations with ability to talk about own emotions and the emotions of others.**  In order to determine whether autistic children's perceived self-competence was related to the ability to describe their own emotions and those of others, social competence scores were correlated with latency to respond, number of prompts, empathy, and labeling scores.

Analyses suggested that autistic children who reported higher social competence manifest greater difficulty talking about their own emotional experiences. Perceived social competence was correlated with latency to respond, $r = .58$, $p < .02$, and with number of prompts, $r = .61$, $p < .01$. There were no significant correlations between perceived self-competence and laboratory measures of the ability to label or to emphathize with others' emotional experiences. However, a trend emerged, suggesting that autistic children who perceive themselves as less socially competent appear better able to label, $r = −.41$, $p = .09$. Correlations between perceived social competence and understanding of emotion in self and others appear in Table 4.

### Parent Measures

**Parents' reports of children's social adaptation.**  Only parents of autistic children completed the Vineland Adaptive Behavior Scale. The mean scores on the three domains were as follows: Communication, 84.4 ($SD = 33.1$), Daily Living Skills, 70.3 ($SD = 23.7$), and Socialization, 64.4 ($SD$

TABLE 4
Correlations Between Autistic Children's IQ
Scores, Perceived Self-Competence,
and Parent's Report of Social Adaptation

|  | Perceived Social Competence Autistic Group ($n = 18$) |
|---|---|
| Ability to talk about own emotions |  |
| Response latency | 0.58* |
| Prompting | 0.61** |
| Labeling others' emotional experiences | − 0.41 |
| Parent's report of children's behavior |  |
| Socialization skills | − 0.48* |
| Display of interest | − 0.63** |

*$p < .05$.
**$p < .01$.

= 22.9). Given that these scores are standardized with a mean normative score of 100 and *SD* of 15, children's reported social and daily living skills are very far below average for their age. Means appear in Table 5.

**Correlations with IQ.** Additional analyses suggested that parents' report of autistic children's social adaptations were highly correlated with children's Full-scale IQ scores, $r = .72$, $p < .001$. Given that children's IQ scores were correlated with parents' report of children's social adaptation

TABLE 5
Parent's Report of Autistic Children's
Socially Adaptive Behavior

|  | Autistic Group ($n = 18$) |
|---|---|
| Socialization domain | 64.4 ± 22.9 |
| Communication domain | 84.4 ± 33.1 |
| Daily living skills | 70.3 ± 23.7 |

*Note:* Scores based on the Vineland Adaptive Behavior Scales; mean standard score for normal children = 100. Values are mean ± *SD*.

and children's own perceptions of their self-competence, the relationship between the latter variables were reanalyzed, partialling out IQ. Results were no longer significant, suggesting that IQ mediates the inverse relationship between children's and parents' perceptions of children's social competence, as well as the positive relationship between children's perceptions of their cognitive competence and parents' perceptions of children's social adjustment. Correlations between parent report of socialization skills and children's IQ scores appear in Table 3.

**Correlations with children's self-perceptions.** Correlations were calculated between the Vineland socialization scores reported by parents of autistic children, and the children's four Harter scores. Results suggested that autistic children's reports about their cognitive competence were positively correlated with parents' perceptions of children's social adjustment, $r = .52, p < .03$. Most strikingly, there was a significant *negative* correlation between children's perceptions of their social competence and parents' reports of their children's social adjustment, $r = -.48, p < .05$. Parents' perceptions of their children's social adaptation were not correlated with children's perceived physical competence, nor with their overall feelings of self-worth. Correlations between children's perceived social competence and parents' perceptions of their children's socialization skills appear in Table 3.

**Correlations with parents' reports of children's emotional experiences.** Analyses of the relationships between parents' reports of their children's displays of five emotions (happiness, interest, sadness, fear, and anger) and children's perceived social competence and overall feelings of self-worth suggested that children who report lower perceived self-worth appear to their parents to show less sadness and fear than children who report higher overall self-worth, $r = .52, p < .05, r = .78, p < .001$, respectively. In addition, parents of children who perceive themselves as having greater social competence report that their children display interest less frequently than do children who perceive themselves as less socially competent, $r = -.63, p < .01$. Correlations between children's perceived social competence and parent report of emotion expression appear in Table 3.

## CONCLUSIONS

This study illuminates the self-perceptions of nonretarded autistic persons. It sheds light on the relationships between perceived self-competence, intellectual capabilities, and emotional understanding, and, in so doing, raises compelling questions for further research.

Results of this study show that perceived social competence is lower among autistic children than typically developing children, and lowest among the most highly intelligent autistic children. These highly intelligent children also have greater access to their own and others' emotional experiences; they are able to talk about their own emotional experiences with greater ease (Capps, Yirmiya, & Sigman, 1992) and are more accurate in labeling the emotions of others (Yirmiya et al., 1992).

One interpretation of these findings is that autistic persons who are more intelligent and better able to read the emotions of others may acquire greater awareness of qualities that differentiate them from normal people. Their cognitive and emotional abilities may yield this knowledge by facilitating their own appraisals of self and others, and by providing access to others' appraisals of their limitations. This particularly high-functioning group may see themselves more accurately, or, in Kanner's terms, they may be "more aware of their peculiarities."

What are the consequences of this awareness? Kanner suggests that for some, awareness of peculiarities leads to "a conscious effort to do something about them." Embedded in questions about consequence are questions about experience. Might such awareness involve depression and hopelessness? The perceived self-competence scale used in this study is not a measure of self-esteem or depression (Harter, 1982). However, many of the items that were highly correlated with autistic children's IQ scores invoke feelings of sadness on the part of researchers, for example, "some kids wish that more people liked them," "some kids find it hard to make friends," "some kids are not very popular," and "some kids wish they were different." The pain one feels in response to visions of the isolated, autistic child is greatly magnified when one imagines the child feels lonely and rejected, rather than detached or unaware. Nevertheless, our responses are not necessarily an accurate index or the way the children feel.

Although we did not assess depression in this sample, parents' perceptions of their children's adjustment and emotional life shed light on the issue. Parents of both young mentally retarded children with autism and these older, nonretarded autistic children report that their children show more negative emotions than did parents of comparison children (Capps et al., 1993). In addition, parents of high-functioning autistic children reported significant deficits in their children's social adaptive behaviors; parents responses to questions on the Vineland Adaptive Behavior Scale place the children 3 $SD$ below the mean for normal children on the Socialization domain, 2 $SD$ below the mean with respect to Daily Living Skills, and 1 $SD$

below the mean in the Communication domain. These scores suggest that even this high-functioning group of autistic persons has extreme difficulty maintaining social relationships and functioning independently.

Given the correlations between IQ scores and adaptive behaviors across domains, it seems that intelligence partially mediates these deficits: the most highly intelligent autistic children are, by parents' report, better able to function in the social world. Yet these same children perceived themselves as less socially competent. That is, within the autistic group, there was an inverse relationship between parents' perceptions of their children and children's self-perceptions; children who report lower social competence are perceived by their parents to be better adjusted socially than are children who report greater social competence.

In keeping with the possibility that the low social-competence ratings represent more accurate self-appraisals, perhaps the heightened awareness of social weaknesses displayed by the most highly intelligent autistic children contributes to socially adaptive behavior reported by their parents. Alternatively, children who rated themselves as less socially competent may focus on their limitations to the exclusion of abilities that are visible to parents, and to a greater degree than autistic persons with less strong intellectual and emotional capabilities. Thus, although illuminating, parent's reports of their children's social adaptation do not resolve questions regarding children's self-esteem.

Information from parents about their children's affective expression may be more relevant. Autistic children who report feeling less competent are perceived by their parents to be more interested, and less often sad and afraid than children who report greater degrees of competence and self-worth. This pattern runs contrary to the notion that autistic children who perceive themselves as less competent are more depressed. It may be that these children do apply their intellectual abilities in ways that facilitates emotional understanding of self and others and highlight qualities that set them apart, but also in ways that such self-appraisals do not lead to depression.

Yet we cannot rule out depression, particularly because the parents of autistic children report more negative affect in the group as a whole, relative to parents of normal children and adolescents. Perhaps the situations that engender positive assessments of autistic children's social functioning by parents have the opposite effect on the children themselves. Given the correlations between IQ and emotional abilities, autistic children who are most capable intellectually are likely to be most inclined to engage in social interactions. For the child, this interaction may highlight limitations and deficits, but to parents, and perhaps to researchers, such attempts index social adjustment. Further, perhaps these children are more often main-streamed. Experiences in mainstreamed environments might make the children more aware of their social limitations, while giving parents the sense that they are better adjusted socially.

These potential consequences of mainstreaming attest to the importance of frames of reference in self-perception and self-esteem. Beginning with the classic work of Festinger (1954), social psychologists have delineated processes of social comparison, through which assessment of abilities, opinions, and overall feelings of self-worth are influenced by how one's attributes compare with those of other people. More recently this research has focused on the effects of social comparison on self-esteem, specifically in terms of whether one is comparing oneself to others who are less fortunate ("downward comparisons") or more fortunate ("upward comparisons") than oneself. Such studies provide strong support for the notion that downward comparisons enhance subjective well-being, because favorable comparisons enable one to feel better about oneself and one's situation (see Wills, 1987, cited in Major, Testa, & Bylsma, 1991).

However, additional studies suggesting that there are circumstances in which upward comparisons are esteem-enhancing (Taylor, Aspinwall, Dakof, & Reardon, 1993; Testa & Major, 1990) led to the identification of two factors that appear to play a crucial role in determining these consequences: relevance of the basis for comparison to self-concept (Major, Testa, & Bylsma, 1991; Tesser, 1988; Tesser & Campbell, 1983), and perceived control over the basis for comparison (Bandura, 1977; Lazarus & Folkman, 1984; Major, Testa, & Bylsma, 1991; Testa & Major, 1990). Laboratory studies suggest that upward social comparisons that are perceived to be relevant to one's self-esteem and unchangeable are particularly likely to lead to negative affect (Weiner, 1986) and social distancing (Salovey & Rodin, 1984).

This social-psychological theory and research is consistent with the aforementioned results of studies finding lower self-concept and higher rates of depression and anger among adults suffering from mild, as opposed to moderate or severe, mental retardation (Benson & Ivins, 1992; Jacobson, 1982; Reiss, 1985; Reiss & Rojahn, 1993). It also has implications for interpreting the findings of this study and for continuing research.

The heightened capacity for emotional understanding displayed by particularly intelligent nonretarded autistic persons, whether they are mainstreamed or not, is likely to expand their frame of reference, thereby increasing the potential for upward social comparison. Furthermore, their superior emotional abilities may not only facilitate social comparison, but also increase the relevance of social dimensions to self-esteem. This question has yet to be addressed, as do questions concerning the extent to which autistic persons perceive their social and emotional limitations as unchangeable. Kanner's (1973) suggestion that his most successful autistic patients became aware of their peculiarities and made a conscious effort to do something about them is promising. So, too, are reports from parents in this study suggesting that autistic children who perceive themselves as less socially competent show less negative emotion at home than do autistic children who perceive themselves as more socially competent—if negative affect is viewed as a manifestation of frustration in the face of unchangeable circumstances.

Nevertheless, the literature on social comparison, coupled with the perceived social competence ratings, and potential risk for depression, among these highly intelligent autistic children has important implications for intervention. Perhaps autistic persons would benefit from the presence of an esteem-enhancing frame of reference. In working with autistic children and their families, it has been our impression that children and parents alike profit from efforts to create a supportive network for the child, composed of people who are aware of the child's history and are familiar with autism. Such networks simultaneously facilitate engagement in social interaction and enable autistic persons' past accomplishments to serve as a basis for evaluation by self and others. It is also noteworthy that in writing about themselves, both Temple Grandin (1984, Grandin & Scariano, 1986) and Donna Williams (1992), two remarkably successful, well-adjusted autistic women, focus on their accomplishments, evaluating themselves in relation to who they were, and to other persons with autism, rather than to normal individuals.

Support groups for high-functioning individuals with autism might also facilitate more positive social comparisons. In addition, given that upward social comparisons that are perceived to be unchangeable are most likely to have depressing effects on self-esteem, it seems critical to work with autistic persons to identify these bases for social comparison and to work toward a plan for self-improvement. This type of intervention would both illuminate the basis for negative self-evaluation and enhance perceived control.

Finally, the results of this study oblige us to be mindful of the frame of reference we use in assessing social functioning, and the possibility that our assessment might diverge from the self-assessments of those we study. When we say an autistic person is "high-functioning" we generally mean relative to other persons with autism. We must work to prevent such labels from eclipsing our view of the subjective experiences of individuals and associated avenues for intervention.

## REFERENCES

American Psychiatric Association (1981). *Diagnostic and statistical manual of mental disorders* (3rd ed.). Washington, DC: Author.

Bandura, A. (1977). Self-efficacy: Toward a unifying theory of behavioral change. *Psychological Review, 89,* 191–215.

Bemporad, J. R. (1979). Adult recollections of a formerly autistic child. *Journal of Autism and Developmental Disorders, 9,* 179–197.

Benson, B. A., & Ivins, J. (1992). Anger, depression, and self-concept in adults with mental retardation. *Journal of Intellectual Disability Research, 36,* 169–175.

Braverman, M., Fein, D., Lucci, D., & Waterhouse, L. (1989). Affect comprehension in children with pervasive developmental disorders. *Journal of Autism and Developmental Disorders, 19,* 301–316.

Capps, L., Kasari, C., Yirmiya, N., & Sigman, M. (1993). Parental perceptions of emotional expressiveness in children with autism. *Journal of Consulting and Clinical Psychology, 61,* 475–484.

Capps, L., Yirmiya, N., & Sigman, M. (1992). Understanding of simple and complex emotions in non-regarded children with autism. *Journal of Child Psychology and Psychiatry, 33,* 1169–1182.

Cicchetti, D. V., & Sparrow, S. S. (1981). Developing criteria for establishing interrater reliability of specific items. Application to assessment of adaptive behavior. *American Journal of Mental Deficiency, 86,* 127–137.

Dewey, M. (1991). Living with Asperger's syndrome. In U. Frith (Ed.), *Autism and Asperger's syndrome* (pp. 184–207). Cambridge: Cambridge University Press.

Deckner, C. W., Soraci, S. A., Deckner, P. O., & Blanton, R. L. (1981). Consistency among commonly used procedures for assessment of abnormal children. *Journal of Clinical Psychology, 37,* 856–862.

Festinger, L. (1954). A theory of social comparison processes. *Human Relations, 7,* 117–140.

Grandin, T. (1984). My experiences as an autistic child and review of selected literature. *Journal of Orthomolecular Psychiatry, 13,* 144–175.

Grandin, T., & Scariano, M. (1986). *Emergence labelled autistic.* Tunbridge Wells, UK: Costello.

Happe, F. (in press). Theory of mind in individuals with autism. *Child Development.*

Happe, F. (1991). The autobiographical writings of three Asperger syndrome adults: problems of interpretation and implications for theory. In U. Frith (Ed.), *Autism and Asperger's syndrome* (pp. 207–242). Cambridge: Cambridge University Press.

Harter, S. (1982). The perceived competence scale for children. *Child Development, 53,* 87–97.

Harter, S., & Whitesell, R. (1989). Developmental changes in children's understanding of single, multiple, and blended emotion concepts. In C. Saarni & P. Harris (Eds.), *Children's understanding of emotion* (pp. 81–116). Cambridge: Cambridge University Press.

Hollingshead, A. B. (1957). *Two factor index of social position.* Unpublished manuscript. Department of Psychology, Yale University, New Haven, CT.

Izard, C. E., Dougherty, F. E., Bloxton, B. M., & Kotsch, W. E. (1974). *The differential emotions scale: A method of measuring the subjective experience of discrete emotions.* Unpublished manuscript. Department of Psychology, University of Delaware, Newark, DE.

Jacobson, J. W. (1982). Problem behavior and psychiatric impairment within a developmentally disabled population. *Applied Research in Mental Retardation, 3*, 121–140.

Kanner, L. (1973). How far can autistic children go in matters of social adaptation? In L. Kanner (Ed.), *Childhood psychosis: initial studies and new insights.* Washington, DC: Winston.

Krug, D. A., Arick, J. R., & Almond, P. J. (1978). *Autism screening instrument for education and planning.* Portland, OR: ASIEP Educational Company.

Lazarus, R. S., & Folkman, S. (1984). *Stress, appraisal, and coping.* New York: Springer.

Loveland, K. A., & Kelley, M. L. (1988). Development of adaptive behavior in adolescents and young adults with autism and Down Syndrome. *American Journal on Mental Retardation, 93*, 84–92.

Macdonald, H., Rutter, M., Howlin, P., Rios, P., Le Couteur, A., Evered, C., & Folstein, S. (1989). Recognition and expression of emotional cues by autistic and normal adults. *Journal Child Psychology and Psychiatry, 30*, 865–877.

Major, B., Testa, M., & Bylsma, W. H. (1991). Responses to upward and downward social comparisons: The impact of esteem-relevance and perceived control. In J. Suls & T. A. Wills (Eds.), *Social comparison: Contemporary theory and research* (pp. 237–260). Hillsdale, NJ: Erlbaum.

Miedzianik, D. C. (1986). *My autobiography.* (Intro, by Elizabeth Newson). Nottingham: Child Development Research Unit, University of Nottingham, UK.

Mundy, P., Sigman, M., Ungerer, J., & Sherman, T. (1986). Defining the social deficits of autism. *Journal of Child Psychology and Psychiatry, 27*, 657–669.

Ozonoff, S., Pennington, B., & Rogers, S. (1989). Are there emotion perceptions deficits in young autistic children? *Journal of Child Psychology and Psychiatry, 51*, 343–361.

Prior, M., Dahlstrom, B., & Squires, T. (1990). Autistic children's knowledge of thinking and feeling states in other people. *Journal of Child Psychology and Psychiatry, 31*, 587–601.

Reiss, S. (1985). Mentally retarded, emotionally disturbed adult. In M. Sigman (Ed.), *Children with emotional disorders and developmental disabilities* (pp. 171–192). Orlando, FL: Grune & Stratton, Inc.

Reiss, S., & Rojahn, J. (1993). Joint occurrence of depression and aggression in children and adults with mental retardation. *Journal of Intellectual Disability Research, 37,* 287–294.

Rodrigue, J. R., Morgan, S. B., & Geffken, G. R. (1991). A comparative evaluation of adaptive behavior in children and adolescents with autism, Down Syndrome, and normal development. *Journal of Autism and Developmental Disabilities, 21,* 187–196.

Russell, J. A. (1989). Culture, scripts, and children's understanding of emotion. In C. Saarni & P. Harris (Eds.), *Children's understanding of emotion* (pp. 293–318). Cambridge: Cambridge University Press.

Salovey, P., & Rodin, J. (1984). Some antecedents and consequences of social comparison jealousy. *Journal of Personality and Social Psychology, 47,* 780–792.

Seidner, L. B., Stipek, D. J., & Feshbach, N. D. (1988). A developmental analysis of elementary school-aged children's concepts of pride and embarrassment. *Child Development, 59,* 367–377.

Sigman, M., Kasari, C., Kwon, J., & Yirmiya, N. (1992). Responses to the negative emotions of others by autistic, mentally retarded, and normal children. *Child Development, 63,* 796–807.

Sigman, M., Mundy, P., Sherman, T., & Ungerer, J. (1986). Social interactions of autistic, mentally retarded, and normal children and their caregivers. *Journal of Child Psychology and Psychiatry, 27,* 647–656.

Sparrow, S. S., Balla, D., & Cicchetti, D. V. (1984). *The Vineland adaptive behavior scales: Interview edition, survey form.* Circle Pines, MN: American Guidance Service.

Stein, N. L., & Trabasso, T. (1989). Children's understanding of changing emotional states. In C. Saarni & P. Harris (Eds.), *Children's understanding of emotion* (pp. 50–80). Cambridge: Cambridge University Press.

Stipek, D. (1983). A developmental analysis of pride and shame. *Human Development, 26,* 42–54.

Taylor, S. E., Aspinwall, L. G., Dakof, G. A., & Reardon, K. K. (1993). Storytelling, social comparison, and social support: Reactions to stories of similar others undergoing stressful events. *Journal of Applied Social Psychology, 23,* 703–733.

Tesser, A. (1988). Toward a self-evaluation maintenance model of social behavior. In L. Berkowitz (Ed.), *Advances in experimental social psychology* (Vol. 21, pp. 181–227). San Diego, CA: Academic Press.

Tesser, A., & Campbell, J. (1983). Self-definition and self-evaluation maintenance. In J. Suls & A. G. Greenwald (Eds.), *Psychological perspectives on the self* (Vol. 2, pp. 1–31). Hillsdale, NJ: Erlbaum.

Testa, M., & Major B. (1990). The impact of social comparison after failure: The moderating effects of perceived control. *Basic and Applied Social Psychology, 11*, 205–218.

Thompson, R. (1989). Causal attributions and children's emotional understanding. In C. Saarni & P. Harris (Eds.), *Children's understanding of emotion* (pp. 117–150). Cambridge: Cambridge University Press.

Van Lacker, D., Cornelius, C., & Needleman, R. (1991). Comprehension of verbal terms for emotions in normal, autistic, and schizophrenic children. *Developmental Neuropsychology, 7*, 1–18.

Volkmar, F. R., & Cohen, D. J. (1985). The experience of infantile autism: A first-person account by Tony W. *Journal of Autism and Developmental Disorders, 15*, 47–54.

Volkmar, F. R., Sparrow, S. S., Goudreau, D., Cicchetti, D. V., Paul, R., & Cohen, D. J. (1987). Social deficits in autism: An operational approach using the Vineland Adaptive Behavior Scales. *Journal of American Academy of Child and Adolescent Psychiatry, 26*, 156–161.

Weiner, B. (1986). Attribution, emotion and action. In R. M. Sorrentino & E. T. Higgins (Eds.), *Handbook of motivation and cognition: Foundations of social behavior* (pp. 281–312). New York: Guilford Press.

Williams, D. (1992). *Nobody nowhere: The remarkable autobiography of an autistic girl*. London: Doubleday.

Yirmiya, N., & Sigman, M. (1991). High-functioning individuals with autism: Diagnosis, empirical findings and theoretical issues. *Clinical Psychology Review, 11*, 669–683.

Yirmiya, N., Sigman, M., & Freeman, B. J. (1994). Comparison between diagnostic instruments for identifying high-functioning children with autism. *Journal of Autism and Developmental Disorders, 24*, 281–292.

Yirmiya, N., Sigman, M., Kasari, C., & Mundy, P. (1992). Empathy and cognition in high-functioning children with autism. *Child Development, 63*, 150–160.

# 11

# The Recognition of Autism in Children with Down Syndrome: Implications for Intervention and Some Speculations About Pathology

**P. Howlin and L. Wing**
*St. George's Hospital Medical School, London*

**J. Gould**
*Centre for Social and Communication Disorders, Kent, U.K.*

*Although autism can occur in conjunction with a range of other conditions, the association with Down syndrome is generally considered to be relatively rare. Four young boys with Down syndrome are described who were also autistic. All children clearly fulfilled the diagnostic criteria for autism required by the ICD-10 or DSM-III-R, but in each case the parents had faced considerable difficulties in obtaining this diagnosis. Instead, the children's problems had been attributed to their cognitive delays, despite the fact that their behaviour and general progress differed from other children with Down syndrome in many important aspects. The implications, for both families and children, of the failure to diagnose autism when it co-occurs with other conditions such as Down syndrome are discussed. Some speculations about possible pathological associations are also presented.*

Although autism is a relatively rare occurrence in people with Down syndrome, there are an increasing number of reports of the two conditions

---

Reprinted with permission from *Developmental Medicine and Child Neurology*, 1995, Vol. 37, 406–414. Copyright © 1995 co-existing. Wing and Gould (1979) carried out an epidemiological study of 35,000 children under the age of 15 years, using the Medical Research Council's Handicaps, Behaviour and Skills (HBS) interview schedule (Wing and Gould 1978). They initially reported one child from a total of 30 fully ambulant children who met two essential criteria for typical autism (Kanner and Eisenberg 1956) and another two children who were severely socially impaired, mute, with no pretend play and marked motor stereo-typies. Although these two were within the autistic spectrum, they were not classified as having Kanner's autism because they showed no adherence to elaborate non-functional routines other than their motor stereotypies. At follow-up, it was clear that one more child with Down syndrome should have been included in the socially impaired but not typically autistic group (Kanner, personal communication). Turk (1992), also using the HBS schedule, reported that 9 per cent of his series of children with Down syndrome met the full ICD-10 criteria for autism (World Health Organization 1993). Ghaziuddin (personal communication) found autism in 10 per cent of his subjects with Downs' syndrome. Gillberg (1986) identified one child with 'classic' autism from a group of 20 children with Down syndrome. Ghaziuddin et al. (1992) found two children who fulfilled DSM-III-R criteria for autism (American Psychiatric Association 1987) from an estimated total of 40 with Down syndrome (based on school-age population figures). Lund (1988), in a Danish epidemiological study of 44 adults with Down syndrome, diagnosed four males and one female as having autism, again using the HBS questionnaire (Wing and Gould 1978).

A number of individual case studies are also reported in the literature. Ghaziuddin et al. (1992) described three cases with Down syndrome who met DSM-III-R criteria for autism and who scored well above the cut-off scores for autism on the Autism Behaviour Checklist (Krug et al. 1980). Two had severe mental impairment and the third was considered to have moderate intellectual impairment. All three had some language, although this was repetitive or non-communicative. Impairments in non-verbal skills, imaginative play, peer relationships and social interactions generally were also noted. Despite the generally low intellectual abilities of the subjects described, the stereotyped and repetitive behaviours they exhibited were not simply those typically associated with severe disability which consist of principally motor mannerisms, stereotypies and self stimulatory behaviours); there was also evidence of the more complex rituals and routines characteristic of autism. These included insistence on repeating the same activities (playing the same records over and over, watching the same television programmes, and lining up and dusting objects), a strong resistance to environmental change, marked attachments to objects, and a tendency to touch or smell people and objects. Bregman and Volkmar (1988) described a 12-year-old girl with Down syndrome and non-verbal abilities in the severely retarded range. She met DSM-III and DSM-III-R criteria for autism and scored within the autistic range on the Childhood Autism Rating Scale (Schopler et al., 1986). Although she did not speak, she had a number of signs and gestures but failed to use these communicatively. Social interactions were markedly impaired and she exhibited many repetitive behaviours and preoccupations with the parts and details of objects. She also tended to smell toys and other objects and to feel them in her mouth.

The seven-year-old Japanese boy described by Wakabayashi (1979) was much more profoundly retarded, and diagnosis in this case is perhaps somewhat less clear-cut (he had, for instance, shown evidence of physical and motor regression at the age of two and a half years, and was now completely dependent on adults for all his needs). However, the author concluded that the boy met both Kanner's (1943) and Rutter's (1965) criteria for autism.

The following case studies describe four boys aged between eight and 11 years, who were seen in early 1993. All had Down syndrome, but in each case the parents had become concerned at their children's failure to make progress and by the realisation that, as they grew older, they clearly differed from their special peer group in many ways, especially in terms of their play and social and communication skills.

## CASE REPORTS

### *Family Background*

Child A, now aged 11 years 5 months, had been adopted at the age of 4 years 9 months by a single mother who had also successfully adopted another child with Down syndrome. Children B and C aged 9 years 11 months and 11 years 8 months, respectively, were being brought up by single divorced parents. Child D, aged eight years, lived with both parents. All children had been born in the UK.

### *Early History*

Down syndrome was diagnosed at birth in all four cases, but whereas the children's additional physical problems were recognised and treated as necessary in the early years, the social, communication and behavioural abnormalities described by the parents seem to have received little attention.

All the children's parents had requested further assessment because they believed these additional problems could not simply be explained by the fact that the child had Down syndrome.

### School Placements

All the children had been placed initially in schools for pupils with severe learning disabilities. Child A had been removed by his mother because she felt the structure was not appropriate to his needs and he had recently been accepted by a school for children with a mixture of communication and behavioural problems. The parents of B and C were also unhappy with the educational provision available, mainly because of the schools' failure to deal adequately with the children's social and communication problems and their ritualistic behaviour. For similar reasons the parents of child D were exploring the possibility of a transfer to a unit specialising in autism.

### Diagnosis

A detailed history of each child's early development was completed in collaboration with the parents. The first three cases were assessed using the HBS (Wing and Gould 1978); the fourth child was assessed using the Autism Diagnostic Interview (ADI) (Le Couteur et al. 1989). The children were also observed individually and formal psychometric assessments were attempted. All clearly fulfilled the diagnostic criteria for autism in terms of their social, play and communication difficulties and the presence of rituals and routines. Case D, for example, scored well above the cut-off levels for autism in all areas assessed on the ADI; thus his score for communication deficits was 13 (cut-off 8), for social impairments 28 (cut-off 11), and for repetitive and stereotyped behaviours 6 (cut-off 3). In all cases abnormalities in development had been noted in the first two to three years of life.

Tables 1 and 2 give details of the research diagnostic criteria for autism specified in the ICD-10 and DSM-III-R classification systems, and show how each of the children met these requirements. Table 3 describes the individual characteristics of the four cases in greater detail.

Because of their chromosomal abnormalities, the difficulties shown by the children had generally been attributed in the past to Down syndrome or their cognitive delays. However, it was evident that they differed in many ways from most other children with this condition. Their social relationships were much less well developed, attachments to adults were delayed; there was little evidence of shared attention, empathy or understanding of

TABLE 1.
Diagnosis According to DSM-III-R Criteria: Autism Present
if There is Impairment in Eight or More Categories (At Least Two from A,
One from B and One from C)

| | Child A | Child B | Child C | Child D |
|---|---|---|---|---|
| A. *Social interaction—impaired in:* | | | | |
| 1. Awareness of others' feelings | + | + | + | + |
| 2. Seeking of comfort | + | + | + | + |
| 3. Imitation | + | + | + | + |
| 4. Social play | + | + | + | + |
| 5. Peer friendships | + | + | + | + |
| B. *Communication—impaired in:* | | | | |
| 1. Verbal or non-verbal communication | − | − | − | − |
| 2. Use of non-verbal communication skills (eye-contact, *etc.*) | + | + | + | + |
| 3. Imagination | + | + | + | + |
| 4. Volume, pitch, intonation *etc.* of speech | NA | NA | NA | NA |
| 5. Content of speech; stereotyped, idiosyncratic, *etc.* | + | + | NA | + |
| 6. Conversational interchange | NA | NA | NA | NA |
| C. *Stereotyped routines* | | | | |
| 1. Motor stereotypies | + | + | + | + |
| 2. Preoccupation with parts of objects | + | + | + | + |
| 3. Distress over trivial changes | + | + | + | + |
| 4. Insistence on routines | + | + | + | + |
| 5. Preoccupation with one narrow interest | + | + | + | + |

+ = impairment present; − = impairment not present; NA = not applicable.

others' feelings, and they failed to use adults for comfort in the usual way. Relationships with other children were particularly poor and often charac- terised by aggression or resistance. Although three of the children had some speech, their language was abnormal, being echolalic or repetitive, and rarely used communicatively. For all children their main mode of com- munication was to take adults by the hand to indicate their needs.

Non-verbal skills such as eye contact and gesture were uniformly poor, and none of the four showed any spontaneous imaginative play. All the children showed stereotyped motor behaviours, which is common in chil- dren with severe learning disabilities. However, they also showed a strik- ing resistance to change and an insistence on routines. Child A spent much

TABLE 2.
Diagnosis According to ICD-10 Criteria: Autism Present if There is Impairment in One or More Symptoms from A and Six or More from B, Including at Least Two from B1, One from B2 and One from B3

|  | Child A | Child B | Child C | Child D |
|---|---|---|---|---|
| *A. Abnormal before 3 years of age in:* | | | | |
| 1. Social communication | + | + | + | + |
| 2. Social attachment and/or interaction | + | + | + | + |
| 3. Functional and/or symbolic play | + | + | + | + |
| *B1. Social interaction—impaired in:* | | | | |
| a. Non-verbal social regulation | + | + | + | + |
| b. Peer relationships | + | + | + | + |
| c. Response to others' emotions; behaviour in social context; integration of social emotional and communicative behaviour | + | + | + | + |
| d. Sharing pleasure with others | + | + | + | + |
| *B2. Communication—impaired in:* | | | | |
| a. Verbal and non-verbal language | + | + | + | + |
| b. Reciprocal conversion | NA | NA | NA | NA |
| c. Meaningful language (*i.e.* language is stereotyped and repetitive) | + | + | NA | + |
| d. Pretend play | + | + | + | + |
| *B3. Stereotyped routines:* | | | | |
| a. Restricted patterns of interest | + | + | + | + |
| b. Adherence to non-functional routines | + | + | + | + |
| c. Motor stereotypies—hand/finger or whole body | + | + | + | + |
| d. Preoccupation with part objects or quantities—feel, smell, *etc.* | + | + | + | + |

+ = impairment present; − = impairment not present; NA = not applicable.

of his time sorting objects into boxes and had very fixed routines, being happiest when sitting by a radiator, and listening to music tapes. He always listened to music before going to sleep, and the last piece heard in the evening had to be the first tune played the next day. Child B was so resistant to change of any kind that his playroom was empty of everything, including floor covering, except for his cassette recorder. If the school bus took a different route he would refuse to get off when it reached his home. Child C always insisted on sitting in specific places, and became very distressed on seeing anyone he knew in an unfamiliar setting; he was very upset when his mother bought a new car or changed the wallpaper, and his

TABLE 3

Characteristics of the Four Children Studied (Age in Parentheses—Years:Months)

| | Child A (11:5) | Child B (9:11) | Child C (11:8) | Child D (8:0) |
|---|---|---|---|---|
| *Original diagnosis* | Down syndrome; infantile spasms | Down syndrome: left hemi-hypertrophy (affecting mainly the leg) | Down syndrome | Down syndrome |
| *Early development* | Miserable; feeding problems | Quiet, unresponsive except to lights | Quiet, unresponsive | Unresponsive |
| *Physical problems* | Walked just before 5 yrs; still has problems walking; nystagmus | Walked at 2 yrs; still has problems walking; odd gait; short-sighted; ambidextrous | Walked at 3 yrs; now runs on toes; heart condition (Fallot's tetralogy). | Walked at 30 mths; possible hearing loss; marked squint |
| *Self-care* | Poor, very dependent toilet-trained at 5 yrs | Limited: not yet dry at night; does not chew food | Toilet-trained at 10; needs help with washing and dressing | Not toilet-trained; needs help with dressing etc. |
| *Communication* | Echoes; takes adults by hand though has Makaton signs and some words | Pulls people by hands; some echolalia; repeats words over and over | No words or consistent signs; pulls adults by hand | Repetitive, noncommunicative use of a few words; takes adults' hands; has signs but does not use |
| *Imagination* | No spontaneous pretend play | No pretend play | No pretend play | No pretend play |

| | | | | |
|---|---|---|---|---|
| *Social development* | Poor eye-contact; ignores or hits children; little show of affection. Does not come for comfort: dislikes physical contact | Poor eye-contact; Aggressive to peers; hugs adults without discrimination; separation anxiety; very disinhibited; no shared attention | Poor eye-contact; pushes other children; dislikes cuddles; shows no greeting behaviour; little affection | Poor eye-contact no greeting or seeking comfort; pushes away other children; no shared attention |
| *Sterotypies* | Jumps, rocks and flaps; hand mannerisms | Flaps and rocks; makes odd noises | Jumps, flaps, spins and rocks | Flaps arms and waves head simultaneously |
| *Special interests* | Audio-tapes; fitting things in boxes; specific videos | Thomas the Tank Engine and Michael Jackson videos | Videos; spinning things; flickering candles | Toilets, taps, switches and doors. Watches Sooty and Sweep videos constantly |
| *Attachment to objects* | Always something in hand | Leaves and sticks | Pink hair brush; other 'twiddlers' | 'Sweep' puppet; piece of hose-pipe |
| *Routines* | Very fixed daily pattern; dislikes new clothes/foods/videos; distressed by change | Distress at change in routes/routines, *etc.* Play room totally empty except for tape-recorder | Hates any change to surroundings/routine. Insists on sitting in fixed places; upset if others in 'wrong' | Obsessional use of toilets, lights, *etc.* Has fixed places for self and objects; drinks only clear liquids |
| *Behaviour* | Aggression, mood swings; resistant to demands/change | Aggressive, destructive; tempers; over-activity | Running away; no sense of danger; throwing objects | Destructive; negativistic; provocative |
| *Psychometry* | No co-operation | Leiter: 4 yrs | No co-operation | No co-operation |
| *Special skills* | 'Amazing memory' | No particular skills | Good memory | None |

life was said to be 'dominated by his repetitive routines and resistance to change'. Child D was obsessed with toilets, light-switches, taps and doors, and although he was not toilet trained, the first thing he would do on entering anyone's house was find and then flush the lavatory. The only videos he watched were old 'Sooty and Sweep' shows, and he carried a Sweep puppet around with him at all times. Cups and chairs had to be placed in fixed positions and he would only drink clear liquids such as mineral water or lemonade. In the garden he had a particular piece of hosepipe that he waved constantly back and forth (and which he always seemed able to find even if his parents hid it). For details of other routines, obsessions and attachments etc., see Table 3.

## IMPLICATIONS OF THE FAILURE TO DIAGNOSE AUTISM

Having first had to come to terms with the fact that their children had Down syndrome, the parents then had to cope with the realisation that their children's development was abnormal even relative to their special peer group. Although the parents had frequently expressed concerns about their children's development, they had tended to be assured that this was all that could be expected. The parents of child D, for instance, had raised the possibility some years earlier that he might be autistic but school records show that staff were 'very reluctant' even to consider this. The professionals in these cases seemed to pay little heed to the fact that, linguistically and socially, the children were falling further and further behind other children with Down syndrome of the same age. Moreover, even if particular problems were acknowledged these were often misinterpreted. For example, although the educational psychologist involved with child B noted that 'it would not do him justice to consider him as just an ordinary Down lad' and remarked on his odd relationships with people and objects in his environment and his need for order and routines, his behaviours seem to have been interpreted by the school as 'naughty' or 'wilful.' Child D's problems were very clearly described by his teachers, but were viewed simply as 'difficult behaviours' and explained away in terms of poor motivation and lack of co-operation. School reports indicated no concern about his social development and gave no indication that he was in any way different from his peers. However, they also noted that his motivation to communicate was 'on his terms only'; that he had 'quite definite likes and dislikes and routine is obviously important to him'; and that his co-operation was poor and he had a tendency to 'opt out' of group activities. He was also observed to place 'objects . . . in very specific places' and was only recently 'becoming more tolerant to touch and physical contact'.

The failure to appreciate the nature of children's learning, behavioural and social difficulties had obvious implications for teaching. For the children described here, there seems to have been a failure to recognise their need for a highly structured environment, involving individualised step-by-step teaching programmes, and in most cases there has been little if any awareness of their lack of social understanding or their need for specialist help to develop communication skills. School reports for child D suggested the need to 'present him with opportunities to enrich the quality of his play activities; to share these with other children and to communicate . . . as often as possible'. Yet no specific strategies for teaching were suggested; nor was his failure to use the limited amount of language he possessed in any communicative way considered significant. However, simply presenting a child with autism with the 'opportunities' to learn is known to be ineffective. Only highly structured teaching specifically geared to the child's particular pattern of skills and deficits is likely to have any significant impact on outcome (Rutter and Baftak 1973, Howlin and Rutter 1987). Psychometric testing proved impossible in three of the four cases reported here (even if the child's own teacher was present) largely because of their lack of co-operation and their stereotyped behaviours. The psychologists involved (P.H. and J.G.) had wide experience of assessing children with autism but were nevertheless unsuccessful in their attempts to carry out formal assessments. If the children's educational needs had been recognised and appropriately catered for at a much earlier stage, such problems might have been avoided.

## SPECULATIONS ABOUT PATHOLOGY

The finding of the co-occurrence of autism or autistic spectrum disorders contrasts with the usual view of people with Down syndrome as being sociable and outgoing. There is no published epidemiological study of the prevalence of autistic spectrum disorders in a large population of children with Down syndrome, but the evidence currently available suggests that it is in the region of 10 per cent for autism. The Camberwell epidemiological study found a total of 13 per cent for the whole spectrum but only 3 per cent for typical autism using the criteria of Kanner and Eisenberg, which tend to give the lowest rates (Wing 1993). The rates from the studies quoted for autistic disorder or autistic spectrum disorders are larger than for the population as a whole, even taking the highest estimate of around one in 200. This includes the rate for autistic spectrum disorders in children with learning disabilities (Wing and Gould 1979) plus the estimate for Asperger syndrome in children mostly with IQ of 70 or above (Ehlers and Gillberg

1993). A more realistic comparison group for the children with Down syndrome comprises those who have moderate, severe or profound learning disabilities (IQ of below 50), among whom the rates for autistic spectrum disorders are much higher than for the general population. In the Camberwell study, among the fully mobile children with IQs of below 50 who did not have Down syndrome there were 16 per cent with Kanner's autism and 57 per cent with other autistic spectrum disorders. Thus children with Down syndrome seem more likely to be autistic or to have other autistic spectrum disorders than would be expected by chance on the basis of total population studies, but are less likely to have these disorders than other children with moderate, severe or profound learning disabilities.

In the present state of knowledge of the causes of autistic conditions, it is possible only to speculate on the aetiological implications of the association of autism and Down syndrome. Given the difference in prevalence rates noted above, it appears at first glance that autistic spectrum disorders in children with Down syndrome cannot be explained away as one of the hazards of having an IQ of below 50. However, in the Camberwell study (Wing and Gould 1979) it was found that 5 per cent of the fully mobile children with profound learning disabilities (IQ of below 20) had Kanner's autism and 90 per cent had other autistic spectrum disorders. If all the children with Down syndrome and autistic spectrum disorders had IQs of below 20, this might explain the association, though not why they had such profound disabilities. In the Camberwell study, three of the children with Down syndrome and an autistic spectrum disorder had profound learning disabilities and one was just above this level, whereas all those with Down syndrome who were sociable were in the severe, moderate or (in one case) mild learning disability ranges. In the present paper, three of the children were untestable and probably had profound learning disabilities, although one was in the moderately disabled range. The levels of ability of the subjects with Down syndrome in the other papers quoted were not given in sufficient detail to allow specific conclusions to be drawn.

Another possibility is that additional medical disorders may be linked with the autism and the very low levels of ability which are not found in most children with Down syndrome. In the Camberwell study, the one child with Down syndrome and Kanner's autism had had infantile spasms and continued to have fits. Of the three with autistic spectrum disorders, all had congenital heart lesions (giving rise to recurrent episodes of cyanosis in at least one child), and two had severe visual impairments (one with myopia, nystagmus and strabismus and the other with cataracts). Among the four cases reported here, two had had serious medical conditions: infantile spasms in one case and a major heart condition (Fallot's tetralogy) in the other; this was repaired but the child remained under constant medical supervision. The other two both had squints and one possibly had hearing loss (Table 3).

Details of associated medical conditions are not available for the other studies quoted, so no definite conclusions can be drawn. However, the possibility that such medical conditions are linked with the autistic spectrum disorders requires careful investigation. The hypothesis would be that Down syndrome itself does not give rise to the brain pathology underlying autism but that the additional medical conditions do affect the relevant parts or functions of the brain.

A further suggestion (Ghaziuddin, personal communication) is that children with Down syndrome and autistic spectrum disorders may be members of families with a high incidence of the latter.

Investigations are needed to establish the nature of the association between the conditions. These ideally should include family and genetic studies and the same types of brain imaging and postmortem examinations of brain pathology, as have been carried out in autism (Bauman and Kemper 1994). Such investigations were not done for the children described in the present paper and no published data are currently available.


## CONCLUSION

The fact that the co-occurrence of autism and Down syndrome is rare seems, unfortunately, to have resulted in the mistaken belief that the two *never* go together. Indeed, the frequency with which the two conditions co-exist may well be greater than previous studies suggest. All the cases described by Ghaziuddin et al. (1992) were seen within the course of a year and the four cases presented above were seen over a period of a few weeks. Nevertheless, even when autistic symptoms are evident in a child with Down syndrome, these tend to be attributed to the associated learning difficulties rather than being adequately assessed in their own right. The diagnosis of autism in other children is usually made well before they reach school age (although of course there are exceptions to this) but diagnosis in Down syndrome tends to be much later. In the present cases the diagnosis of autism was not made until the ages of eight, nine and 11 years; the Wakabayashi (1979) case was seven years old; that of Bregman and Volkmar (1988) 12 years old; in the Ghaziuddin et al. (1992) study, the ages at diagnosis were 17, 14 and 21 years; and in the Lund (1988) study all were adults.

Late diagnosis, or indeed the failure to diagnose at all, may clearly have detrimental and long-term effects on the lives of affected children and their families. The parents of child D, for example, described their increasing dejection as they saw their son 'falling further and further behind', despite help from a private language therapist and a clinical psychologist, and they became convinced that this 'failure' was their own fault. Having access to professional advice from those experienced in the field of autism can be crucial in developing the child's skills, in minimising the impact of routines, obsessions and rituals, and in avoiding the secondary problems that are able to develop if the child's needs are not adequately understood (Wing 1980, Howlin and Rutter 1987). Being put in touch with a local parent support group is also of great benefit to many parents. Above all, appropriate education is essential and although this need not necessarily entail specialist autistic provision, the future of the child's social and communication deficits need to be recognised, understood and adequately catered for.

Finally, for the majority of parents the correct diagnosis, rather than being viewed as an additional burden, comes as a relief, often exonerating them from a sense of guilt that it was they who were the cause of their child's difficulties (Piper and Howlin 1992). Many parents of children with autism already face a battle in obtaining a diagnosis (Smith et al. 1994); it is unacceptable to make the struggle even harder for families who know their child has another life-long disability. Rather than relying on stereotyped and unfounded notions of the sorts of problems that children with Down syndrome may or may not suffer, there is a need for more research into the expected frequency of additional conditions such as autism. Research into the physical problems associated with Down syndrome has resulted in individuals with this condition living much longer and happier lives than was the case 30 years ago (Carr 1994). The recognition of other developmental disorders that may occur (albeit infrequently) with Down syndrome, and the provision of appropriate services, could have an equally beneficial impact on those with a dual disability.

## REFERENCES

American Psychiatric Association (1987) *Diagnostic and Statistical Manual of Mental Disorders, 3rd Edn, Revised (DSM-III-R)*. Washington, DC: American Psychiatric Association.
Bauman, M. L., Kemper, T. L. (Eds.) (1994) *The Neurobiology of Autism*. Baltimore: Johns Hopkins University Press.
Bregman, J. D., Volkmar, F. R. (1988) 'Autistic social dysfunction and Downs' syndrome.' *Journal of the American Academy of Child and Adolescent Psychiatry, 27*, 440–441.

Carr, J. (1994) 'Long term outcome in Downs' syndrome'. *Journal of Child Psychology and Psychiatry. (in press).*

Ehlers, S., Gillberg, C. (1993) 'The epidemiology of Asperger syndrome. A total population study.' *Journal of Child Psychology and Psychiatry 34*, 1327–1350.

Ghaziuddin, M., Tsai, L., Ghaziuddin, N. (1992) 'Autism in Downs' syndrome: presentation and diagnosis.' *Journal of Intellectual Disability Research, 36*, 449–456.

Gillberg, C., Persson, E., Grufman, N., Themner, U. (1986) 'Psychiatric disorders in mildly and severely mentally retarded urban children and adolescents: epidemiological aspects.' *British Journal of Psychiatry, 149*, 68–74.

Howlin, P., Rutter, M. (1987) *Treatment of Autism Children.* Chichester: John Wiley.

Kanner, L. (1943) *'Autistic disturbances of affective contact.' Nervous Child, 2*, 217–250.

—Eisenberg, L. (1956) 'Early infantile autism 1943–1955.' *American Journal of Orthopsychiatry, 26*, 55–65.

Krug, D. A., Arick, J., Almond, P. (1980) 'Behaviour checklist for identifying severely handicapped individuals with high levels of autistic behaviour.' *Journal of Child Psychology and Psychiatry, 21*, 221–229.

le Couteur, A., Rutter, M., Lord, C., Rios, P., Robertson, S., Holdgrafer, M., McLennan, J. D. (1989) 'Autism diagnostic interview: a semi structured interview for parents and carers of autistic persons.' *Journal of Autism and Developmental Disorders, 19*, 363–387.

Lund, J. (1988) 'Psychiatric aspects of Down syndrome.' *Acta Psychiatrica Scandinavica, 78*, 369–374.

Piper, E., Howlin, P. (1992) 'Assessing and diagnosing developmental disorders that are not evident at birth: parental evaluations of intake procedures.' *Child: Care, Health and Development, 18*, 35–55.

Rutter, M. (1965) 'The influence of organic and emotional factors on the origins, nature and outcome of childhood psychosis.' *Developmental Medicine and Child Neurology, 7*, 518–528.

—Bartak, L. (1973) 'Special educational treatment of autistic children: a comparative study. II Follow-up findings and implications for services.' *Journal of Child Psychology and Psychiatry, 14*, 241–270.

Schopler, E., Reichler, R. J., Renner, R. (1986) *The Childhood Autism Rating Scale (CARS) for Diagnostic-Screening and Classification of Autism.* New York: Irving.

Smith, B., Chung, M. C., Vostanis, P. (1994) 'The path to care in autism; is it better now?' *Journal of Autism and Developmental Disorders (in press).*

Turk, J. (1992) 'Children with Down's syndrome and Fragile X syndrome: a comparison study.' *Society for Study of Behavioural Phenotypes: 2nd Symposium Abstracts.* Oxford: SSBP.

Wakabayashi, S. (1979) 'A case of infantile autism associated with Down syndrome.' *Journal of Autism and Developmental Disorders, 9*, 31–36.

Wing, L. (1980) Autistic Children: *A Guide for Parents*. London: Constable.

—(1993) 'The definition and prevalence of autism: a review.' *European Journal of Child and Adolescent Psychiatry, 2*, 61–74.

—Gould, J. (1978) 'Systematic recording of behaviours and skills of retarded and psychotic children.' *Journal of Autism and Childhood Schizophrenia, 8*, 79–97.

—(1979) 'Severe impairment of social interaction and associated abnormalities in children: epidemiology and classification' *Journal of Autism and Developmental Disorders, 9*, 11–29.

World Health Organization (1993) *The ICD-10 Classification of Mental and Behavioural Disorders: Diagnostic Criteria for Research*. Geneva: WHO.

# 12

# Use of Methylphenidate in the Treatment of Children with Autistic Disorder

**Humberto Quintana and Boris Birmaher**
*Western Psychiatric Institute and Clinic, Pittsburgh*

**Deborah Stedge, Susan Lennon, and Jane Freed**
*New York State Psychiatric Institute*

**Jeffrey Bridge**
*Western Psychiatric Institute and Clinic, Pittsburgh*

**Larry Greenhill**
*New York State Psychiatric Institute*

*The use of psychostimulants in autistic disorder has not received extensive evaluation. Furthermore, their use for the symptomatic control of autistic disorder has been felt to be contraindicated. This study investigates the use of methylphenidate (MPH) for the treatment of selected symptoms of autistic disorder. Ten children, ages 7–11, with a DSM-III-R diagnosis of autistic disorder participated in a double-blind crossover study using placebo and two MPH doses (10 mg or 20 mg bid). Subjects showed modest but statistically significant improvement on MPH over placebo. No significant side effects including worsening stereotypic movements occurred on either dose. Improvement in hyperactivity and lack of adverse effects suggest that MPH may be useful in the treatment of hyperactive autistic children.*

Autistic disorder is manifested by pervasive impairments in communicative, cognitive, and social development. In addition, some autistic patients show other associated features such as stereotypic and repetitive

Reprinted with permission from the *Journal of Autism and Developmental Disorders*, 1995, Vol. 25, No. 3, 283–294. Copyright © 1995 Plenum Publishing Corporation.

movements, lability of mood, impulsiveness, short attention span, and hyperactive behavior (Campbell & Green, 1985; Geller, Guttmacher, & Bleeg, 1981). Few medications such as naltrexone, clomipramine, and haloperidol have been shown to improve some of the above associated features (Anderson et al., 1989; Campbell et al., 1990; Campbell, Anderson, Small, Adams, Gonzalez, & Ernst, 1993; Gordon et al., 1993; McDougle et al., 1992). Among these medications, however, haloperidol has been the most extensively studied (Sloman, 1991) and has been found to be among the most useful for the symptomatic treatment of these patients (Campbell et al., 1978; Campbell, Gonzalez, Ernst, et al., 1993; Campbell, Geller, & Cohen, 1977; Vitriol & Farber, 1981). For example, Anderson et al. (1984) in a double-blind, placebo-controlled study on 45 autistic children (mean age 4.5) of whom 42 were mildly mentally retarded, reported that haloperidol was associated with decreases in hyperactivity, temper tantrums, withdrawal, stereotypies, and an increase in social relatedness. Treatment with haloperidol, however, may cause numerous significant short-term and long-term, possibly irreversible side effects. For instance, over a period of 5 years, 20% of children taking neuroleptics developed signs of tardive dyskinesia and other extrapyramidal effects (Campbell, Adams, Perry, Spencer, & Overall, 1988; Gualtieri et al., 1980, 1984). Also, it seems that acute dystonias occur much more frequently in children (10 to 19 years old) than adults (Keepers, Clappison, & Casey, 1983). Therefore, in view of these various complications and potential dangers inherent in the use of neuroleptics (Gualtieri et al., 1984; Perry, Campbell, Green, Small, & Trill, 1985; Sloman, 1991), alternate medications should be considered. Among the medications to be considered, the stimulants may play a role in the symptomatic control of the impulsivity, short attention span, and hyperactivity found in some autistic patients. As reviewed by Birmaher, Quintana, and Greenhill (1988), there are few reports on the use of stimulants with children with autistic disorder. Earlier studies showed that stimulants increased the irritability and stereotypic movements in autistic children (Campbell et al., 1978). These studies included a heterogeneous sample of children with diverse psychiatric disorders such as schizophrenia, autism, and organic disorders. It is important, however, to note that DSM-II (American Psychiatric Association [APA], 1968) did not include autism as a diagnostic category; only in DSM-III (APA, 1980) was this diagnostic category included. Moreover, most of these patients were taking neuroleptics and the stimulants were given without a washout period from the neuroleptics. Hence, withdrawal dyskinesias may have been confused with increased stereotypic movements induced by the stimulants.

Some studies have reappraised the use of stimulants for the treatment of autistic children and have yielded more positive effects. Hoshino, Kumashiro, Kanero, and Takahashi (1977) in an uncontrolled study, administered methylphenidate (MPH; 10 to 15 mg) to children with autism. The MPH was given for a period from 2 weeks up to 14 months. The children were rated by a nonblind psychiatrist and by nonblind parents. Of the 12 children who followed the protocol, 7 improved in the ratings for hyperactivity, impulsivity, and concentration. The main side effects were anorexia, irritability, insomnia, and aggressive behavior, all of which responded to dose reduction. Geller et al. (1981) administered 5 to 10 mg of dextroamphetamine to two autistic children aged 9 and 12 years old. These children showed improvement in their hyperactivity, attention span, and aggressive behavior without the development of side effects. Vitriol and Farber (1981) reported similar results after treating a 1-year-old autistic child with MPH 10 mg/day. Strayhorn, Rapp, Donina, and Strain (1988), in a blind randomized (ABA) trial of MPH in an autistic child, found significant improvement in attention and activity, destructive behavior, and stereotypic movements. Birmaher et al. (1988) in an open study administered MPH to 9 autistic children in doses ranging from 10 to 50 mg/day. Eight children showed improvement in hyperactivity, impulsivity, and attention span. There were no major side effects or worsening of stereotypic movements suggesting that stimulants may be used for the symptomatic control of autistic patients.

This article is the first reported double-blind crossover study that evaluates MPH efficacy and side effects in the treatment of children with autistic disorder.

## METHOD

### *Subjects*

Subjects were recruited from the New York State Psychiatric Institute outpatient clinic. Inclusion criteria included DSM-III-R (APA, 1987) criteria for autistic disorder, and a Childhood Autism Rating Scale (CARS, Schopler, Reichler, & Renner, 1988); a score of 15–29 is given as nonautistic by Schopler, Reichler, and Renner (1985). In addition, children were accepted if they had been off neuroleptics for a period of at least 1 month or if their parents would agree to have them off neuroleptics for 1 month prior to the start of the study. Subjects were excluded if they had been on MPH at any time before entry into the study and if they had a history of seizure disorder or other major neurological or medical illness.

Ten children referred to our clinic over a 6-month period met study criteria. Subjects' ages ranged from 7–11 ($M = 8.5 \pm 1.3$); there were 6 boys and 4 girls; the mean Developmental Quotient was $64.3 \pm 9.9$. Developmental Quotient is a numerical measure of mental capability determined by dividing mental age score achieved in our patients by Stanford-Binet Test by the patient's chronological age and multiplying by 100 (50–55 to 70 = mild intellectual impairment; 35–40 to 50–55 = moderate intellectual impairment) (APA, 1987; Gelfand, 1980). The mean CARS score was $41.6 \pm 10.6$. Subjects received MPH in the range of 0.37 to 0.74 mg/kg per day. Table 1 depicts subject demographics and MPH doses in mg/kg.

All of the children included in the study had been on neuroleptic medication (haloperidol, chlorpromazine, etc.) at some point over the course of their lives but had not been previously treated with MPH or with any other medications. In this study, the 10 subjects demonstrated a wide range of baseline behaviors including withdrawn, isolative, passive, aggressive (including temper tantrums), and agitated behaviors. Five of the subjects (1, 3, 5, 9, & 10) were on neuroleptic medication prior to entry into the study. With parental consent, they were weaned off the neuroleptic and

TABLE 1
Demographics, Disorder Severity, and MPH Dose

| Subject | Age | Sex | Developmental Quotient | Total CARS[a] | MPH (g/dose, 10 mg/kg) | MPH (g/dose, 20 mg/kg) |
|---|---|---|---|---|---|---|
| 1[b,c] | 8 | M | 58 | 51.5 | 0.31 | 0.61 |
| 2 | 9 | M | 84 | 30.0 | 0.21 | 0.42 |
| 3[b,c] | 11 | F | 50 | 54.0 | 0.20 | 0.40 |
| 4 | 7 | F | 75 | 34.0 | 0.33 | 0.68 |
| 5[b,c] | 8 | M | 65 | 36.0 | 0.29 | 0.58 |
| 6 | 9 | M | 72 | 30.0 | 0.25 | 0.48 |
| 7 | 10 | F | 58 | 36.5 | 0.27 | 0.54 |
| 8 | 7 | F | 70 | 30.5 | 0.32 | 0.65 |
| 9[b,c] | 9 | M | 60 | 59.5 | 0.17 | 0.34 |
| 10[b] | 7 | M | 65 | 36.5 | 0.29 | 0.58 |
| | | | Mean MPH dose | | 0.26 | 0.53 |

[a] Childhood Autistic Rating Scale.
[b] Subject had been on neuroleptics prior to study.
[c] Decided to remain on methylphenidate (followed for 1 year).

were off medications for at least 1 month prior to entry into the study. None of these subjects developed withdrawal dyskinesias during the weaning period. During the study the patients received only MPH.

## *Design*

The study took place in the Children's Day Hospital at the New York State Psychiatric Institute. Admission procedures included a history, physical examination, and routine laboratory tests completed by the pediatrician (J.F.).

The study design was a crossover MPH versus placebo with each limb divided into a low- versus high-dose trial. After a 2-week medication-free period (baseline period), the children were randomly assigned to be treated with MPH or placebo as follows: 10 mg am and noon doses every day for 1 week, and 20 mg am and noon doses every day for the 2nd week. Thereafter, subjects underwent a crossover to MPH or placebo for another 2-week trial as described above. The subjects were observed and rated on the last day of each week for 3 hours in a simulated structured classroom situation in which mental age-related classroom tasks were presented and during free play. The study was completed in 6 weeks which included 2 weeks baseline, 2 weeks of methylphenidate or placebo 10 mg bid, and 2 weeks of methylphenidate or placebo 20 mg bid.

The dosage of methylphenidate (10 mg bid, 20 mg bid) was selected based on our (B.B., H.Q.) previous clinical experience and our open study (Birmaher et al., 1988), where 50% of subjects responded to MPH 10 mg bid dose and 50% had responded to MPH 20 mg bid dose.

Except for the observation day at the day hospital when our nurses (D.S., S.L.) administered the am dose of MPH/placebo, the subjects' parents administered the MPH or placebo am dose at home during the week, and a school nurse administered the noon dose. Observation of the children's behavior began 30 min after the MPH or placebo dose and lasted for 3 hours. The CARS, the Aberrant Behavior Checklist (Aman & Singh, 1985), and the Conners Teacher Questionnaire (CTQ) were done independently by two psychiatrists (H.Q., B.B.), and the pediatrician (J.F.) completed the Abnormal Involuntary Movements Scale (Guy, 1976) and the Side-effects Checklist for stimulant medication. These investigators, the children, and the parents were blind to drug and drug dose. The Conners Parent Questionnaires (Conners, 1973) were completed by the children's parents, who based their answers on observations of at-home behavior for the week prior to assessment at the partial hospital.

## Measures

The following measures were used in this study: Childhood Autism Rating Scale—a total score of 15–29 equals nonautistic, mildly to moderately autistic is 30–36.5, and severely autistic is 37–60 (Schopler et al., 1985, 1988); the 10-item Conners Abbreviated Parent Questionnaire (maximum score 30 points); the hyperactivity factor of the CTQ (a score equal to or greater than 1.8 is considered 2 *SD* above the mean for normal children) (Conners, 1973; Goyette, Conners, & Sulrick, 1978); and the Aberrant Behavior Checklist (total score 174) (behavior is a slight problem 1–58; moderate behavior problem is equal to 59–116; severe behavior problem is equal to 117–174) (Aman & Singh, 1985). The Aberrant Behavior Checklist includes Subscale I—irritability factor (maximum score 45), Subscale III—stereotypies (maximum score 21), and Subscale IV—hyperactivity factor (maximum score 48) (Aman & Singh, 1985).

Side effects were measured by the Side Effects Checklist for Stimulant Medication, which included irritability, headache, stomache aches, tics, lack of appetite, weight loss, insomnia, and hallucinations (Campbell et al., 1972); the Abnormal Involuntary Movements Scale (AIMS) (total score 42); the Aberrant Behavior Checklist, Subscale III for stereotypies (maximum score 21) (Aman & Singh, 1985). The two psychiatrists, Quintana and Birmaher, independently completed the CTQ, and Aberrant Behavior Rating scales and the pediatrician (J.F.) completed the Side-effects Checklist. Rating forms were completed at the end of the 3-hour observation period, except for the Conners Parent Questionnaire which was completed at home by the parents.

## Data Analysis

The data were normally distributed, thus parametric statistics were used for the analysis. Intraclass correlation coefficients (ICC) for rating scales administered by the psychiatrists were above .85, thus only average scores for each rating scale are presented. Analysis of variance (ANOVA) showed no medication order effects, therefore, the data for placebo and MPH were collapsed. Since there were no statistically significant differences between the two placebo and the two MPH doses, the mean placebo and MPH scores were used for the statistical analysis. Two-tailed paired *t* tests were used to compare differences between groups. Analysis of covariance (ANCOVA) was used to examine the effects of age, developmental quotient, dose, and baseline scores.

## RESULTS

### Clinical Ratings

As shown in Table 2, subjects on MPH showed a statistically significant improvement over placebo on their hyperactivity as measured by the CTQ (1.3 ± 0.7 vs. 1.5 ± 0.3, $t = 2.69$, $p = .02$), the Aberrant Behavior Checklist-total (42.0 ± 18.3 vs. 52.4 ± 22.5, $t = 2.43$, $p = .04$), Aberrant Behavior Checklist-irritability factor (4.0 ± 3.8 vs. 7.2 ± 6.3, $t = 3.23$, $p = .01$), and Aberrant Behavior Checklist-hyperactivity factor (12.1 ± 9.4 vs. 19.8 ± 17.9, $t = 2.82$, $p = .02$). Controlling for baseline scores yielded similarly significant results. There were no age, dose, or developmental quotient effects. Also, compared to their respective baseline scores both MPH and placebo showed statistically significant reductions on the Aberrant Behavior Checklist, total score, irritability factor, hyperactivity factor, and CTQ scores (Table 2).

### Side Effects

As shown in Table 2, there were no statistically significant side effects between MPH and placebo. The percentage occurrence of side effects while patients were on the high dose of methylphenidate (20 mg) was irritability, 4%; headache 1%; stomache ache 3%; tics, 0%: lack of appetite, 20%; weight loss, 0%; insomnia, 5%, and hallucinations, 0%. In addition, there were no statistically significant differences between MPH and placebo in the AIMS, and the Aberrant Behavior Checklist-stereotypic movements subscale. There were no age, developmental quotient, and dose effects.

## DISCUSSION

In this study we found MPH associated with a modest but statistically significant improvement in hyperactivity over placebo with no significant side effects including worsening of behavior (irritability, tantrums, or withdrawal) or worsening in stereotypic movements. Whereas both clinical experience and some published reports have reported a worsening in behavior such as irritability, temper tantrums, and stereotypic movements in autistic patients treated with psychostimulants, hyperactivity has been reported to have improved (Anderson et al., 1989). In this study, although our 10 subjects demonstrated a wide range of baseline behaviors including withdrawal, isolation, passivity, aggression, and agitation, there were no

TABLE 2
Comparison Between Baseline, Placebo, and MPH Treatment in Autistic Children ($n = 10$)[a]

| Variable | Baseline | Placebo | Methylphenidate | Statistics | | |
|---|---|---|---|---|---|---|
| | | | | Comparison | $t$ | $p$ |
| Aberrant Behavior Checklist-total | 70.2 ± 34.3 | 52.4 ± 22.5 | 42.0 ± 18.3 | MPH vs. Pb<br>MPH vs. B<br>Pb vs. B | 2.43<br>4.08<br>3.16 | .04<br>.003<br>.01 |
| Aberrant Behavior Checklist-Irritability | 11.8 ± 11.2 | 7.2 ± 6.3 | 4.0 ± 3.8 | MPH vs. Pb<br>MPH vs. B<br>Pb vs. B | 3.23<br>2.80<br>2.12 | .01<br>.02<br>.06 |
| Aberrant Behavior Checklist-Stereotypies | 7.0 ± 4.2 | 5.4 ± 2.5 | 4.5 ± 3.6 | ns | | |
| Aberrant Behavior Checklist-Hyperactivity | 25.5 ± 15.3 | 19.8 ± 12.9 | 12.1 ± 9.4 | MPH vs. Pb<br>MPH vs. B<br>Pb vs. B | 2.82<br>4.61<br>2.63 | .02<br>.001<br>.03 |
| Conners Teacher Questionnaire | 1.8 ± 0.5 | 1.5 ± 0.3 | 1.3 ± 0.3 | MPH vs. Pb<br>MPH vs. B<br>Pb vs. B | 2.69<br>3.63<br>2.36 | .02<br>.006<br>.04 |
| Conners Parent Questionnaire | 28.1 ± 7.8 | 26.2 ± 8.3 | 24.9 ± 6.6 | ns | | |
| Abnormal Involuntary Movements Scale | 15.0 ± 7.0 | 11.7 ± 7.8 | 13.0 ± 7.8 | ns | | |
| Side-effects Checklist | 8.1 ± 5.8 | 6.9 ± 4.1 | 6.1 ± 4.5 | ns | | |

[a] Key: B: Baseline, Pb: placebo, and ns = Not significant. Aberrant Behavior Checklist-total; slight problem = 1–58, moderate = 59–116, severe = 117–174; Irritability (maximum 45); Stereotypies (maximum 21); Hyperactivity (maximum 48); CTQ-range 0–30; Conners Parent Questionnaire; 0–40 range. Abnormal Involuntary Movements Scale; range 0–48; Side-effects checklist for stimulants medication, range 0–48.

significant differences or worsening in behaviors as measured by the Aberrant Behavior Scales and parents' reports between these baseline behaviors and the behaviors of subjects during MPH treatment. Furthermore, although there were no significant differences between MPH and placebo with respect to hyperactivity on the Conners Parent Questionnaire ratings, this lack of significant difference may be due to the fact that the Conners Parent Questionnaires were done by the parents at home on different days and times than the ratings done by the psychiatrists. Another interpretation could be that the Conners Parent Questionnaire results indicate that the medication treatment seemed to produce effects in the partial hospital/ clinic setting but that comparable levels of improvement were not noted at home. However, it is interesting that despite the apparent lack of response on the Conners Parent Questionnaire, five parents opted to keep their children on MPH.

Although there was a statistical improvement while on MPH, as measured by CTQ Scales and Aberrant Behavior Scales-hyperactivity subscale, some behavioral problems prevailed. For example, at the end of the study, in addition to MPH, two subjects (1 and 9) were restarted on haloperidol at bedtime. Both of these patients had preexisting sleeping problems, severe impulsivity, intermittent aggressive and self-injurious behavior. Therefore, based on this study, it is our recommendation that MPH be tried first for *hyperactive* autistic children, and that later, a neuroleptic could be added if needed. We are suggesting this for consideration since in our experience certain baseline behavioral problems such as intermittent aggressivity and injurious behavior may require the short use of a more potent agent such as a neuroleptic. Therefore it is possible that MPH is most effective in children who are mildly to moderately ill and not severely ill. However, in these cases, the dose and use of a neuroleptic may be minimized if combined with MPH or in some cases the use of MPH may allow the use of a neuroleptic to be avoided.

It is interesting to note that autistic children on placebo showed a decrease in the hyperactivity scores when compared with their respective baseline scores. This may be due to the fact that autistic patients tend to show a delayed adaptation to new experimental environments such as the partial hospital environment where this study was carried out (Campbell et al., 1977). Therefore, 1 day a week for 2 weeks of baseline may not be enough time to allow for an adequate adaptation when doing a pharmacological study with children with autistic disorder.

Another variable to consider when looking at the response of children with developmental disorders to stimulants is the developmental quotient. In this domain, Aman (1988) found that in contrast to mentally retarded children with developmental quotients above 48, those with developmental quotients below 48 did not respond to MPH. We did not find any relationship between developmental quotient and response to MPH. However, our sample was small and all our subjects had developmental quotients above 48.

It was not clear why there were no statistical differences between the two doses of MPH; however, similar results have been reported in the treatment of attention deficit hyperactivity disorder (ADHD). For example, Barkley, DuPaul, & McMurray (1991), reported that three doses of MPH (5, 10, and 15 mg. twice daily) were equally effective for the treatment of ADHD in children.

Although our results show the usefulness of MPH in a group of children with autism, there are some shortcomings in the interpretation of the results. First, the study was limited to the treatment of a small sample of children. Second, the children in our study were observed intensively only during a 3-hour period one time per week. Therefore, this intense but time-limited observation period may not be sufficient when evaluating children with autistic disorder, especially since children with autism may respond adversely to environmental changes and may have clinical pictures that wax and wane in severity over time. Third, no specific measures of cognition were used in this study; therefore, no comments could be made with respect to medication effects on cognition.

An additional limitation was the use of the Conners Teacher and Parent Questionnaire in this study, since they have not been standardized for children with autism. We chose these scales because of their proven sensitivity in assessing stimulant response in children with ADHD. In fact, the CTQ scores significantly correlated with other scales used in this study and in autistic children. For example, the correlation of the Conners Teacher's Questionnaire with the Aberrant Behavior Checklist-hyperactivity subscale was $.95, p = .0005$.

In conclusion, the improvement in hyperactivity without the development of side effects seen in our previous methylphenidate open study (Birmaher et al., 1988) and in this double-blind crossover study suggests that methylphenidate may have a role in the treatment of a group of hyperactive children with autistic disorder. Further studies with larger samples are warranted.

## REFERENCES

Aman, M. (1988). The use of methylphenidate in autism [Letter to the editor]. *Journal of the American Academy of Child and Adolescent Psychiatry, 27*, 821–822.

Aman, M., & Singh, N. N. (1985). The Aberrant Behavior Checklist. *Psychopharmacological Bulletin, 21*, 845–850.

American Psychiatric Association. (1968). *Diagnostic and statistical manual of mental disorders (2nd ed.)*. Washington, DC: Author.

American Psychiatric Association. (1980). *Diagnostic and statistical manual of mental disorders (3rd ed.)*. Washington, DC: Author.

American Psychiatric Association (1987). *Diagnostic and statistical manual of mental disorders (3rd ed., rev)*. Washington, DC: author.

Anderson, L., Campbell, M., Grega, D., et al. (1984). Haloperidol in the treatment of infantile autism: Effects on learning and behavioral symptoms. *American Journal of Psychiatry, 141*, 1195–1202.

Anderson, L. T., Campbell, M., Adams, P., Small, A. M., Perry, R., & Small, J. (1989). The effects of haloperidol on discrimination learning and behavioral symptoms in autistic children. *Journal of Autism and Developmental Disorders, 19*, 227–239.

Barkley, R. A., DuPaul, G. J., & McMurray, M. B. (1991). Attention deficit disorder with and without hyperactivity: Clinical response to 3 dose levels of methylphenidate. *Pediatrics, 87*, 519–531.

Birmaher, B., Quintana, H., & Greenhill, L. (1988). Methylphenidate treatment of hyperactive autistic children. *Journal of the American Academy of Child and Adolescent Psychiatry, 27*, 248–251.

Campbell, M., Adams, P., Perry, R., Spencer, E. K., & Overall, J. E. (1988). Tardive and withdrawal dyskinesia in autistic children: A prospective study. *Psychopharmacology Bulletin, 24*, 251–255.

Campbell, M., Anderson, L. T., Meier, M., Cohen, I. L., Small, A. M., & Green, W. H. (1978). A comparison of haloperidol, behavior therapy, and their interactions in autistic children. *Journal of the American Academy of Child Psychiatry, 17*, 640–655.

Campbell, M., Anderson, L., Small, A., Adams, P., Gonzalez, N., & Ernst, M. (1993). Naltrexone in autistic children: Behavioral Symptoms and Attentional Learning. *Journal of the American Academy of Child and Adolescent Psychiatry, 32*, 1283–1291.

Campbell, M., Anderson, L., Small, A., et al. (1990). Naltrexone in autistic children: A double-blind and placebo controlled study. *Psychopharmacological Bulletin, 26*, 130–135.

Campbell, M., Fish, B., David, R., Shapiro, T., Collins, P., & Koch, C. (1972). Response to triiodothyronine and dextroamphetamine: A study of preschool, schizophrenic children. *Journal of Autism and Childhood Schizophrenia, 2*, 343–358.

Campbell, M., Geller, B., & Cohen, I. L. (1977). Current status of drug research and treatment in autistic children. *Journal of Pediatric Psychology, 2*, 153–161.

Campbell, M., Gonzalez, N. M., Ernst, M., et al. (1993). Neuroleptics. In J. S. Werry & M. G. Aman (Eds.), *Practitioners guide to psychoactive drugs for children and adolescents* (pp. 269–296). New York: Plenum Press.

Campbell, M., & Green, W. H. (1985). Pervasive developmental disorders of child-hood. In H. I. Kaplan & B. J. Sadock (Eds.), *Comprehensive textbook of psychiatry* (Vol. 4, 4th ed., pp. 1672–1683).

Conners, C. K. (1973). Rating scales for use in drug studies with children. [Special issue] *Psychopharmacological Bulletin, 9*, 24–42.

Gelfand, R. (1980). Glossary. In H. I. Kaplan, A. M. Freedman, & B. Sadock (Eds.), *Comprehensive textbook of psychiatry* (Vol. 3, 3rd ed., p. 3334). Baltimore: Williams & Wilkins.

Geller, B., Guttmacher, L., & Bleeg, M. (1981). Coexistence of childhood onset pervasive developmental disorder and attention deficit disorder with hyperactivity. *American Journal of Psychiatry, 138*, 388–389.

Gordon, C. T., State, R. C., Nelson, J. E. et al. (1993). A double-blind comparison of clomipramine, desipramine, and placebo in the treatment of autistic disorder. *Archives of General Psychiatry, 50*, 441–447.

Goyette, C., Conners C. K., & Sulrick, R. F. (1978). Normative data on revised Conners parent and teacher ratings scales. *Journal of Abnormal Child Psychology, 6*, 221–230.

Gualtieri, C. T., Barnhill, J., McGinsey, J., et al. (1980). Tardive dyskinesia and other movement disorders in children treated with psychotropic drugs. *Journal of the American Academy of Child Psychiatry, 19*, 491–510.

Gualtieri, C. T., Quade, D., Hicks, R. D., et al. (1984). Tardive dyskinesia and other clinical consequences of neuroleptic treatment in children and adolescents. *American Journal of Psychiatry, 141*, 20–23.

Guy, W. (1976). *ECDEU assessment manual of psychopharmacology*. Rockville, MD: NIMH Psychopharmacology Research Branch.

Hoshino, Y., Kumashiro, H., Kanero, M., & Takahashi, Y. (1977). The effects of methylphenidate in early infantile autism and its relation to serum serotonin levels. *Folia Psyciatrica et Neurologica Japonica, 31*, 605–614.

Keepers, G. A., Clappison, V. J., & Casey, D. E. (1983). Initial anticholinergic prophylaxis for neuroleptic-induced extrapyramidal syndromes. *Archives of General Psychiatry, 40*, 1113–1117.

McDougle, C. L., Price, L. H., Volkmar, F. R. et al. (1992). Clomipramine in autism: Preliminary evidence of efficacy. *Journal of Academy of Child and Adolescent Psychiatry, 31*, 746–750.

Perry, R., Campbell, M., Adams, P., et al. (1989). A multidimensional long term efficacy of haloperidol in autistic children: Continuous versus discontinuous drug administration. *Journal of American Academy of Child and Adolescent Psychiatry, 28*, 87–92.

Perry, R., Campbell, M., Green, W., Small, A., & Trill, M. (1985). Neuroleptic related dyskinesias in autistic children: A prospective study. *Psychopharmacology Bulletin, 21*, 140–143.

Schopler, E., Reichler, R. J., & Renner, B. (1985). Childhood Autism Rating Scale (CARS). *Psychopharmacology Bulletin, 21*, 1052–1053.

Schopler, E., Reichler, R. J., & Renner, B. (1988). *Childhood Autism Rating Scale (CARS)*. Los Angeles: Western Psychological Services.

Sloman, L. (1991). Use of medications in pervasive developmental disorders. *Psychiatric Clinics of North America, 14*, 165–182.

Strayhorn, J. M., Rapp, N., Donina, W., & Strain, P. S. (1988). Randomized trial of methylphenidate for an autistic child. *Journal of the American Academy of Child and Adolescent Psychiatry, 27*, 244–247.

Vitriol, C., & Farber, B. (1981). Stimulant medication in certain childhood disorders. *American Journal of Psychiatry, 138*, 1517–1518.

# Part IV

# CLINICAL ISSUES

The first paper in this section alerts clinicians to the possibility that some cases of childhood onset Obsessive-Compulsive Disorder (OCD) and Tourette's syndrome (TS) may be precipitated or exacerbated by an infection-triggered autoimmune response. Allen, Leonard, and Swedo present the cases of four participants in an open treatment study. All were boys between the ages of 12 and 13 years of age, who displayed abrupt, severe onset or worsening of Obsessive-Compulsive Disorder or tics in association with either a recent group A beta-hemolytic streptococcus (GABHS) or viral infection and whose symptoms improved following immunomodulatory treatments including plasmapheresis, intravenous immunoglobulin, or immunosuppressive doses of prednisone.

This innovative approach to treatment derives from the integration of informed clinical observation and systematic review of previously published information. In brief, the episodic, gradual waxing and waning of symptoms typical of many cases of OCD and TS is strikingly similar to the course of movements in Sydenham's chorea, a variant of rheumatic fever. In addition, many Sydenham's patients also display obsessive-compulsive symptoms and/or tic-like adventitial movements. These observations led the authors to hypothesize that similar mechanisms might underlie symptom expression in all three conditions. Via a process analogous to Sydenham's chorea, infections with group A beta-hemolytic streptococci, and possibly other agents as well, could trigger autoimmune responses that could cause or exacerbate some cases of childhood onset OCD or tic disorders. Therefore in at least some instances, immunomodulatory treatments should result in decreased symptoms, and the improvement described in the case reports, summarized in the present paper, is consistent with this expectation.

Although preliminary, these results raise the possibility of more effective treatments for some individuals whose OCD and/or tic disorder may have an autoimmune etiology. The authors specify criteria for the diagnosis of pediatric, infection-triggered, autoimmune neuropsychiatric disorders (PITANDs) and invite referral of patients for enrollment in a treatment protocol with a double-blind placebo-controlled component, currently underway at NIMH. In addition, the authors advise inquiring about recent illnesses, obtaining a throat culture and streptococcal serologic studies on initial presentation, and monitoring throat cultures for asymptomatic GABHS at intervals thereafter. As early treatment of streptococcal infections could theoretically limit the immune response and potentially blunt increases in obsessions, compulsions, or tics, all clinicians should be aware of these simple and straightforward recommendations.

Although prevailing clinical wisdom has long held to the rarity of child-hood onset mania, a spate of recent case reports have challenged this belief. In the second paper in this section, Wozniak, Biederman, Kiely, Ablon, Farone, Mundy, and Mennin examine the prevalence, characteristics, and correlates of "manic-like" symptoms in children under the age of 12, evaluated at a pediatric psychopharmacology clinic.

The study sample was drawn from a pool of 262 consecutive referrals to the clinic. All children were evaluated using the Schedule for Affective Disorders and Schizophrenia for School-Age Children—Epidemiologic Version (K-SADS-E) administered to the mother by carefully trained and supervised raters. Two groups of clinically referred children were identified: 42 who met full criteria for a DSM-III-R diagnosis of mania and 164 who met criteria for ADHD without mania. An additional group of 84 similarly assessed participants in family genetic studies of ADHD, who were without either mania or ADHD, constituted a third comparison group. The clinical picture was fully compatible with the DSM-III-R diagnosis of mania in 16 percent (N = 43) of referred children. Of these, the vast majority (84 percent) had a chronic course, and all but one also met criteria for ADHD.

To help clarify the issue of overlap between ADHD and mania, the authors reanalyzed the data after removal of symptoms common to both disorders: distractibility, motoric hyperactivity, and talkativeness. Seventy-six percent (N = 32) of the 42 children meeting criteria for mania and ADHD continued to meet full or subthreshold criteria for mania, and all ADHD diagnoses retained either full or subthreshold diagnostic status after subtraction of the three overlapping symptoms. Compared with ADHD children without mania, manic children had significantly higher rates of major depression, psychosis, multiple anxiety disorders, conduct disorder, and oppositional defiant disorder. Psychosocial functioning was significantly more impaired and almost a quarter of children who met criteria for a diagnosis of mania had had at least one psychiatric hospitalization.

While the data of the present study strongly suggest that mania, comorbid with ADHD, may be relatively common among psychiatrically referred children, particularly among those who are seriously disturbed, the authors underscore that these results should be interpreted with caution, a caution clearly reflected in the title of the paper "Mania-Like Symptoms Suggestive of Childhood-Onset Bipolar Disorder in Clinically Referred Children." Further studies using a broader sampling frame that includes a greater number of females, in which data is obtained directly from children as well as parents, are clearly needed. Nevertheless, the results of this study underscore that children with ADHD who also "meet criteria for mania" have a severe clinical picture that leads to considerable psychiatric and psychosocial disability beyond that conferred by ADHD, and clinicians should be alert to the possibility of concomitant Bipolar Disorder.

While, "what is beautiful is good" is a powerful stereotype, as Sheerin, MacLeod, and Kusumakar point out in the third paper in this section, "Psychosocial Adjustment in Children with Port-Wine Stains and Prominent Ears," much of the available information on psychological sequelae of facial disfigurement is anecdotal. These authors utilize standardized instruments to evaluate the psychosocial adjustment of two groups of children with facial disfigurements. Children with port-wine stains (PWS) and prominent ears (PE) were chosen for study because as groups they provide a measure of disfigurement that is not confounded by other illness, disability, or intervention variables. Forty-two children with PWS and 32 children with PE, who were between the ages of 7 and 16, completed the Harter Self-Perception Profile, the Revised Children's Manifest Anxiety Scale, the Children's Depression Inventory, the Disfigurement Perception Scale, while the parents completed the Child Behavior Checklist.

Responses were compared with normative data for the local population or with a control group of 32 nondisfigured children matched to the PWS group for age, sex, skin color, and social class. While there was no correlation between degree of disfigurement and level of psychosocial adjustment, children with PE had poorer self-perception, were more anxious, had more other internalizing as well as externalizing symptoms, and had more social problems than children with PWS. While children with PWS functioned as well as or better than nondisfigured peers on measures of psychosocial adjustment, children with PE scored lower than nondisfigured peers on measures of self-perception and parent-rated social and attentional problems.

The authors interpret the differences in results between the two groups as suggesting that "disfigurement" is an umbrella term encompassing a heterogenous group of children whose problems may have subtle but significant different influences on psychosocial adjustment. While the generalizability of the results is to some extent limited by the relatively small sample size, unbalanced sex distribution, as well as the fact that all subjects had sought or been referred for corrective plastic surgery, the authors thoughtful discussion of the findings, together with a critical assessment of the relevant literature, provides clinicians with a general framework for conceptualizing the difficulties experienced by individual children with facial disfigurements, which further informs decision making regarding both the desirability and timing of surgical intervention.

The final paper in this section "Psychological Science and the Use of Anatomically Detailed Dolls in Child Sexual-Abuse Assessments" is the report of a working group, commissioned by the American Psychological Association to prepare a comprehensive review of the scientific and clinical knowledge base on anatomically detailed (AD) dolls. AD dolls are often used in sexual-abuse evaluation and treatment with children, but their use is controversial. Some unresolved questions include the following: Do AD dolls assist children in reporting or communicating about sexual experiences? Are AD dolls intrinsically suggestive of sexual acts? Are they suggestive only in the context of leading questioning or only with young children? Are there children for whom AD dolls elicit false reports, regardless of the questioning context? Do examiners misinterpret children's innocent behavior with AD dolls as indicative of abuse?

Koocher, Goodman, White, Friedrich, Sivan, and Reynolds acknowledge that there are no simple answers and that it is difficult to avoid dichotomous thinking about AD doll use. Nevertheless, their examination of the history of the use of AD dolls in clinical inquiry and summary of relevant bodies of research including that on sexual behaviors in children, the normative use of AD dolls in nonreferred children, play behavior, and emotional reactions to AD dolls, as well as memory and suggestibility issues relating to AD doll use, make an important clarifying contribution and delineates areas for future research.

Koocher, Goodman, White, Friedrich, Sivan, and Reynolds conclude that while AD dolls can provide a useful communication tool in the hands of a trained professional interviewer, there are pitfalls inherent in their use. In particular, clinicians must recognize that AD dolls are not a psychological test with predictive validity per se and that definitive statements about child sexual abuse cannot be made on the basis of spontaneous or guided "doll play" alone. In addition, particular caution is called for when interpreting the reports of children ages four years and under, most particularly when affirmations to leading questions about "being touched" are concerned and when repeated misleading questioning has been used. Special recognition of normative differences between children of different racial and socioeconomic groups needs to be part of training professionals who use AD dolls in clinical inquiry. On the basis of their assessment of current knowledge, Koocher et al. further recommend that the American Psychological Association consider revising those elements of the Statement on the Use of Anatomically Detailed Dolls in Forensic Evaluations, issued in 1991, which attest to the existence of valid "doll-centered assessment" techniques which may provide the best available practical solution to the pressing clinical problem of investigating the possible presence of sexual abuse of a child.

# 13

# Case Study: A New Infection-Triggered, Autoimmune Subtype of Pediatric OCD and Tourette's Syndrome

**Albert J. Allen, Henrietta L. Leonard, and Susan E. Swedo**
*National Institute of Mental Health, Bethesda, Maryland*

*A review of clinical observations and literature reports leads to the hypothesis that, via a process analogous to Sydenham's chorea, infections with group A β-hemolytic streptococci, among others, may trigger autoimmune responses that cause or exacerbate some cases of childhood-onset obsessive-compulsive disorder (OCD) or tic disorders (including Tourette's syndrome). If this hypothesis is correct, then immunological treatments should lead to decreased symptoms in some cases. Four cases with abrupt, severe onset or worsening of OCD or tics are presented from an open treatment study. All were boys aged 10 to 14 years. One had OCD, one had Tourette's syndrome, and two had both OCD and Tourette's syndrome. Clinically and on standardized rating scales, their symptoms were in the moderate to very severe range. Two had evidence of recent group A β-hemolytic streptococci infections, and the others had histories of recent viral illnesses. Two were treated with plasmapheresis, one with intravenous immunoglobulin, and one with immunosuppressive doses of prednisone. All had a clinically significant response immediately after treatment. Diagnostic*

Reprinted with permission from the *Journal of the American Academy of Child and Adolescent Psychiatry*, 1995, Vol. 34, No. 3, 307–311. Copyright © 1995 by the American Academy of Child and Adolescent Psychiatry.

The authors acknowledge the invaluable contributions of Xavier Castellanos, M.D. Ms. Sara Dow, Susan Leitman, M.D., Gary Mosher, M.D., Collette Parker, M.D., Mr. Daniel Richter, Kenneth Rickler, M.D., Norman Rosenthal, M.D., Mark Schapiro, M.D., Gregory J. Swedo, M.D.

*criteria are provided that describe these cases of pediatric, infection-triggered, autoimmune neuropsychiatric disorders (PITANDs). Suggestions are made regarding the evaluation and management of patients who may have this condition.*

An episodic, gradual waxing and waning of symptoms is typical of many cases of obsessive-compulsive disorder (OCD), and a similar symptom course has been associated with Tourette's syndrome (TS) and other tic disorders (American Psychiatric Association, 1994). In pediatric patients with OCD, we have noted a subgroup whose waxing and waning of symptoms is distinguished by a sudden, dramatic onset of clinically significant symptoms followed by a slow waning over a period of months. This pattern is strikingly reminiscent of the course of movements in Sydenham's chorea, a variant of rheumatic fever (Swedo, 1994). Indeed, patients with Sydenham's chorea frequently reported a concomitant onset of obsessions and compulsions with their movements (Swedo et al., 1989). In one case series, we subsequently found that about three quarters of the patients had obsessive-compulsive symptoms and one third had frank OCD (Swedo et al., 1993). The obsessive-compulsive symptoms appeared shortly before the onset of choreic movements, and they waxed and waned in severity concomitant with the chorea. It is interesting that approximately one third of children with OCD in one National Institute of Mental Health (NIMH) study had mild choreiform movements (Denckla, 1989). We therefore speculated that Sydenham's chorea might serve as a medical model for OCD (Swedo, 1994). There also appears to be an association between Sydenham's chorea and tic disorders. In addition to the choreic movements, many Sydenham's patients have tic-like, adventitial movements, an observation that was originally made by Osler (1894) and was recently extended by Kiessling et al. (1993) in their report of patients with increased tics after a community outbreak of streptococcal pharyngitis.

The above observations led us to propose that, in pediatric patients, streptococcal infections ("strep throats" and other infections caused by group A β-hemolytic streptococci, GABHS) could trigger the sudden onset or episodic worsening of OCD and/or tic disorders (including TS) via an autoimmune process analogous to Sydenham's chorea (Swedo, 1994; Swedo et al., 1994). This hypothesis suggests that treatments that alter immune function might benefit some children experiencing acute, severe exacerbations of OCD and TS (Swedo, 1994). Furthermore, if this is true, then identifying such children becomes important from both a clinical and research perspective as a different approach assessment and treatment would be indicated. Four cases treated in an open NIMH trial are presented below; pertinent data and ratings are summarized in Table 1.

## CASE 1

B.J. was a 14-year-old with a 1.5-year history of OCD and mild tics, which had been stable for several months while he was taking a combination of clomipramine and fluoxetine. Then, during a summer soccer camp, his OCD symptoms suddenly worsened dramatically. On his return home, his psychiatrist consulted one of us (S.E.S.), who suggested a throat culture be done. The culture was positive and GABHS pharyngitis was diagnosed, although B.J.'s last sore throat had resolved a month earlier. Two weeks later, he came to the NIMH for evaluation. His obsessions included a fear for his own and his father's safety, a need for symmetry, and perfectionistic concerns. His predominate compulsions were checking behaviors and exercises (e.g., fingertip pushups) that had to be performed perfectly or repeated until he was unable to continue. At that time, more than 90% of his waking hours were occupied by obsessions and compulsions. Neurological examination revealed motoric hyperactivity and mild choreiform movements.

Because of the severity of B.J.'s OCD, his suspicious movements, and his sudden worsening during a streptococcal infection, he was treated with a series of six plasma exchanges over a period of 2 weeks. During this time there was a marked decline in his OCD symptoms (Table 1). Subjectively, the patient and his family reported he was "80% better." A magnetic resonance imaging scan done after four plasma exchanges showed a 25% decrease in the size of the head of the caudate compared to a scan done before treatment (Swedo et al., 1994). After plasmapheresis he began a regimen of penicillin as prophylaxis against GABHS infections. He continued to do well at follow-up several months later.

## CASE 2

T.J. was a 10-year-old who had no history of psychiatric or neurological problems. The weekend after several family members had the "flu," he had sudden onset of severe obsessions about viruses and chemicals, and he began compulsive hand-washing. After a month of continuous illness, psychiatric treatment was sought and he started sertraline therapy, with only partial symptom relief of his OCD after 2 months. He was then evaluated at the NIMH (3 months after the onset of his illness). At that time his fore-

TABLE 1
Demographic, Clinical, and Treatment Data

| | Case 1 (B.J.) | Case 2 (T.J.) | Case 3 (S.J.) | Case 4 (J.J.) |
|---|---|---|---|---|
| Sex, age (years) | Male, 14 | Male, 10 | Male, 13 | Male, 13 |
| Diagnosis (including predominate obsessions and compulsions) | Mild motor and vocal tics, OCD (exercise, need for perfection) | OCD (contamination) | TS | ADHD, TS, OCD (contamination, rereading, need for perfection) |
| Prodromal symptoms or prior episodes | Yes | No | Yes | Yes |
| Suspected infectious trigger for treatment episode | GABHS pharyngitis (positive culture) | Viral, possibly influenza | Viral, possible influenza | GABHS pharyngitis (positive culture) |
| Duration of episode before treatment | 2 weeks | 3 months | 5 months | 1 month |
| Laboratory results before treatment | ASO = 340 Anti-DNAse B = 1:340 ANA negative | ASO, ANA negative | ASO = 240 ANA positive, 1:320, speckled | ASO, ANA negative |
| Pretreatment ratings[a] | C-YBOCS = 40 (maximum possible score) | C-YBOCS = 25 | Ex MTR = 13 Ex VTR = 2 Hx MTR = 18 Hx VTR = 5 | C-YBOCS = 28 Ex MTR = 9 Ex VTR = 12 Hx MTR = 16 Hx VTR = 19 |

| Treatment Posttreatment ratings[b] (% change from pretreatment) | | |
|---|---|---|
| Plasmapheresis C-YBOCS = 19.5 (−51%) | Plasmapheresis C-YBOCS = 10 (−60%) | Prednisone Ex MTR = 8 (−38%) |
| | | Ex VTR = 2 (0%) |
| | | Hx MTR = 10 (−44%) |
| | | Hx VTR = 0 (−100%) |
| | | IVIG C-YBOCS = 26 (−7%) |
| | | Ex MTR = 4 (−56%) |
| | | Ex VTR = 4 (−67%) |
| | | Hx MTR = 6 (−62%) |
| | | Hx VTR = 12 (−37%) |

*Note:* OCD = obsessive-compulsive disorder; TS = Tourette's syndrome; ADHD = attention-deficit hyperactivity disorder; GABHS = group A β-hemolytic streptococci; ASO = anti-streptolysin O; Anti-DNAse B = anti-streptococcal DNAse B; ANA = antinuclear antibodies; C-YBOCS = Children's Yale-Brown Obsessive Compulsive Scale (Goodman and Price, 1992) (a score of 20 reflects OCD symptoms of moderate severity; scores range from 0 to 40); Ex MTR = examiner's motor tic ratings on the Shapiro tic rating scale (Shapiro et al., 1978) (a score of 12 reflects tics of moderate severity; scores range from 0 to 20); Ex VTR = examiner's vocal tic ratings on the Shapiro tic rating scale (Shapiro et al., 1978); Hx MTR = historical (from parent/child) motor tic ratings on the Shapiro tic rating scale (Shapiro et al., 1978) (a score of 15 reflects tics of moderate severity; scores range from 0 to 25); Hx VTR = historical (from parent/child) vocal tic ratings on the Shapiro tic rating scale (Shapiro et al., 1978); IVIG = intravenous immunoglobulin.

[a] All ratings shown are the means from two physicians with training in mental health research.
[b] Posttreatment ratings are within a month of completing treatment.

arms and hands were chapped and red, and contamination fears prevented him from fully opening his mouth so that he was unable to eat in the hospital or have a throat culture.

Because of the abrupt onset of his symptoms and their severity, T.J. was treated with six plasma exchanges over a period of 2 weeks. Penicillin prophylaxis was not prescribed because his episode of OCD appeared to have been virally triggered. His symptoms declined noticeably during plasmapheresis—after the fourth exchange he could eat at the hospital and permitted a throat culture. His symptoms were so improved 1 month after plasmapheresis that his sertraline dosage was being tapered, with only subclinical obsessions and compulsions remaining (Table 1). He was reported to be doing well several months later.

## CASE 3

In 1987, when S.J. was 7 years old, painful ulcers developed on his mouth and lips, and he was noted to have a positive antinuclear antibody titer with speckled pattern. Shortly after this, he had the first of many GABHS infections, which continued until 1989 when he had a tonsillectomy. After the surgery he began to experience motor tics (craning of his neck, eye-blinking, shoulder-shrugging) and vocal tics ("clicking" sounds), which were eventually diagnosed as TS. His tics declined after he began to take a low dose of fluphenazine and were stable for approximately 18 months. Shortly after a bout of the "flu," his tics escalated dramatically. Of particular concern were new, violent tics of his head and neck that were so extreme that S.J. had physical discomfort. Now 13 years old, he was referred to the NIMH for evaluation. He was found to have an antinuclear antibody titer of 1:320 (speckled pattern), and subsequently a transient rash developed. A rheumatologist concluded he did not have lupus, however.

Six months after his viral illness, S.J. was treated with immunosuppressive doses of prednisone. A clinically significant improvement in his tics was evident 2 weeks later (Table 1), although residual movements remained. His tics again worsened suddenly a few weeks later, after a viral respiratory infection and an allergic reaction to an influenza immunization. A retrial of prednisone at that time was unsuccessful (no change in tic ratings, data not shown).

## CASE 4

J.J. was a 13-year-old with a long history of asthma, hyperactivity, TS, and OCD. He had previously been enrolled in several protocols at the National

Institutes of Health (NIH) for these illnesses. His neuropsychiatric symptoms were believed to be episodic but had been relatively well controlled for about 6 months while he was taking a combination of methylphenidate and clomipramine. After a documented case of GABHS pharyngitis, he experienced rapid, severe worsening of both his TS and OCD. This occurred during a family trip to Thailand and Arizona, during which the family had to alter their travel plans because of J.J.'s obsessive fears that the plane would crash. J.J. also had severe vocal tics (spitting and nearly continuous screaming) during the trans-Pacific flights, and he was unable to finish any reading material because he felt the need to reread every sentence many times.

Approximately 2.5 months after his infection and a month after his symptoms increased, he was treated with intravenous immunoglobulin (1 mg/kg per day for 2 days). His parents reported that his tics began to improve within a week of the intravenous immunoglobulin treatment. At 1 month follow-up (Table 1), there was a clinically significant improvement in his tics, but his OCD was essentially unchanged. His parents reported that J.J. was doing well several months later, at which time he entered a protocol (NIH protocol 93-M-0122) comparing penicillin with placebo as prophylaxis against neuropsychiatric episodes triggered by GABHS infections.

## DISCUSSION

We report these cases because our preliminary evidence suggests that immunomodulatory treatments may improve symptoms for some OCD and TS patients with severe illness due to a postulated autoimmune etiology. Further research is needed to establish the efficacy of these interventions as the novelty of this approach, the economic costs, and the potential medical risks demand scientific proof rather than anecdotal evidence. A treatment protocol with a double-blind, placebo-controlled component has been approved by the NIMH institutional review board and is under way. (To refer patients, contact the authors.) Although our preliminary results promise great treatment benefit to some individuals with this subtype of pediatric OCD and/or tic disorders, ultimately such research may be more important because of information it provides about the etiology of some OCD and TS cases. In turn, this may lead to the development of new, more specific treatment and prevention regimens.

The essential features of these cases are summarized by the phrase: pediatric, infection-triggered, autoimmune neuropsychiatric disorders (PITANDs). Some of these cases may be triggered by viruses rather than GABHS, as in cases 2 and 3 presented here. At this time, no laboratory measure appears to be both sensitive and specific for PITAND cases. Thus, identification of cases currently depends on the patients' clinical histories. The following criteria appear to accurately identify this subgroup of patients:

1. Pediatric onset: symptoms of the disorder first become evident between 3 years of age and the beginning of puberty.
2. At some time in his or her life, the patient must have met diagnostic criteria for OCD and/or tic disorder.
3. The onset of clinically significant symptoms must be sudden (with or without a subclinical prodrome) and/or there must be a pattern of sudden, recurrent clinically significant symptom exacerbations and remissions. Onset of a specific episode typically can be assigned to a particular day or week, at which time symptoms seemed to "explode" in severity.
4. Increased symptoms should not occur exclusively during stress or illness, should be pervasive, should be of sufficient severity to suggest the need for treatment modifications, and (if untreated) should last at least 4 weeks before improvement is noted.
5. During OCD and/or tic exacerbations, the major of patients will have an abnormal neurological examination, frequently with adventitious movement (e.g., mild chorea).
6. There must be evidence of an antecedent or concomitant infection. Such evidence might include a positive throat culture, positive streptococcal serological findings (e.g., anti-streptolysin O or anti-streptococcal DNAse B), or a history of illness (e.g., pharyngitis, sinusitis, or flu-like symptoms).
7. Patients may or may not continue to have clinically significant symptoms between episodes of their OCD and/or tic disorder.

By design, these criteria permit patients with both very severe and relatively mild symptoms to be diagnosed with PITANDs. This is important because infectious and autoimmune processes may be amenable to preventive interventions, and thus recognition of early, less affected cases may be desirable.

At present, identification of PITAND cases may be important for two reasons. First, patients with this syndrome may be candidates for experimental treatment protocols that could directly benefit the patient and increase our knowledge about this condition. Second, it is our clinical impression that some of these patients may benefit from careful monitoring by physicians for GABHS infections. This is based, in part, on the fact that, before the onset of routine penicillin prophylaxis, rheumatic fever episodes were reduced merely by surveillance throat cultures and aggressive treatment of GABHS (for review, see Foggo, 1985). Early treatment of streptococcal infections could theoretically limit the immune response (Berrios et al., 1985) and potentially blunt increases in obsessions, compulsions, or tics. Thus, on initial presentation, we would suggest inquiring about recent illnesses and obtaining a throat culture and streptococcal serological studies (anti-streptolysin O and/or anti-streptococcal DNAse B). Subsequent preventive care might include periodic throat cultures for asymptomatic GABHS infections (as was found in case 1) and treatment of positive cultures. As research in this area proceeds, these patients may also benefit from new diagnostic tests, treatments, or prophylactic measures. Indeed, we are currently engaged in a double-blind, placebo-controlled trial of penicillin for the prevention of OCD disorder exacerbations.

## REFERENCES

American Psychiatric Association (1994), *Diagnostic and Statistical Manual of Mental Disorders, 4th edition (DSM-IV)*. Washington, DC: American Psychiatric Association

Berrios X, Quesney F, Morales A, Blazquez J, Bisno AL (1985), Are all recurrences of pure Sydenham chorea true recurrences of acute rheumatic fever? *J Pediatr* 107:867–872

Denckla MB (1989), Neurological examination. In: *Obsessive-Compulsive Disorder in Children and Adolescents*, Rapoport JL, ed. Washington, DC: American Psychiatric Press, pp 107–118

Foggo BA (1985), Sore throat, antibiotics and rheumatic fever. *Fam Pract* 2: 101–107

Goodman WK, Price LH (1992), Assessment of severity and change in obsessive compulsive disorder. *Psychiatry Clin North Am* 15:861–869

Kiessling LS, Marcotte AC, Culpepper L (1993), Antineuronal antibodies in movement disorders. *Pediatrics* 92:39–43

Osler W (1894), *On Chorea and Choreiform Affections*. Philadelphia: HK Lewis

Shapiro AK, Shapiro ES, Bruun RD, Sweet RD (1978), *Gilles de la Tourette Syndrome*. New York: Raven Press

Swedo SE (1994), Sydenham's chorea: a model for childhood autoimmune neuropsychiatric disorders. *JAMA* 272:1788–1791

Swedo SE, Leonard HL, Kiessling LS (1994), Speculations on antineuronal antibody-mediated neuropsychiatric disorders of childhood. *Pediatrics* 93: 323–326

Swedo SE, Leonard HL, Schapiro MB et al. (1993), Sydenham's chorea: physical and psychological symptoms of St Vitus dance. *Pediatrics* 91:706–713

Swedo SE, Rapoport JL, Cheslow DL et al. (1989), High prevalence of obsessive-compulsive symptoms in patients with Sydenham's chorea. *Am J Psychiatry* 146:246–249

PART IV: CLINICAL ISSUES

# 14

# Mania-Like Symptoms Suggestive of Childhood-Onset Bipolar Disorder in Clinically Referred Children

**Janet Wozniak and Joseph Biederman**

*Massachusetts General Hospital and Harvard Medical School, Boston*

**Kathleen Kiely and J. Stuart Ablon**

*Massachusetts General Hospital, Boston*

**Stephen V. Faraone**

*Massachusetts General Hospital and Harvard Medical School, Boston*

**Elizabeth Mundy and Douglas Mennin**

*Massachusetts General Hospital, Boston*

**Objective:** *To examine the prevalence, characteristics, and correlates of mania among referred children aged 12 or younger. Many case reports challenge the widely accepted belief that childhood-onset mania is rare. Sources of diagnostic confusion include the variable developmental expression of mania and its symptomatic overlap with attention-deficit hyperactivity disorder (ADHD).* **Method:** *The authors compared 43 children aged 12 years or younger who satisfied criteria for mania, 164 ADHD children without mania, and 84 non-ADHD control children.* **Results:** *The clinical picture was fully compatible with the DSM-III-R diagnosis of mania in 16% (n = 43) of referred chil-*

Reprinted with permission from the *Journal of the American Academy of Child and Adolescent Psychiatry*, 1995, Vol. 34, No. 7, 867–876. Copyright © 1995 by the American Academy of Child and Adolescent Psychiatry.

This work was supported in part by the National Alliance for Research on Schizophrenia and Depression, by the Eli Lilly Pilot Research Award through the American Academy of Child and Adolescent Psychiatry (Dr. Wozniak), and by grants RO1 MH41314-07 and RO1 MH50657-02 from the National Institute of Mental Health (Dr. Biederman).

*dren. All but one of the children meeting criteria for mania also met criteria for ADHD. Compared with ADHD children without mania, manic children had significantly higher rates of major depression, psychosis, multiple anxiety disorders, conduct disorder, and oppositional defiant disorder as well as evidence of significantly more impaired psychosocial functioning. In addition, 21% (n = 9) of manic children had had at least one previous psychiatric hospitalization.* **Conclusions:** *Mania may be relatively common among psychiatrically referred children. The clinical picture of childhood-onset mania is very severe and frequently comorbid with ADHD and other psychiatric disorders. Because of the high comorbidity with ADHD, more work is needed to clarify whether these children have ADHD, bipolar disorder, or both.*

As far back as the 1920s, Kraepelin (1921) documented that 4 (0.4%) of 903 manic-depressive patients had onset of symptoms before the age of 10 years. Loranger and Levine (1978) retrospectively evaluated 200 adult bipolar patients and found that first symptoms had occurred between the ages of 5 and 9 years in 1 (0.5%) of these patients. Goodwin and Jamison (1990, pp. 186–209) conducted a similar study, reviewing 898 cases from 1977 to 1985. They found that 3 (0.3%) had onset before age 10 years. While this literature supported the existence of childhood-onset mania, it also indicated that it may be rare. A literature review by Anthony and Scott (1960) suggested that childhood mania was indeed uncommon. In reviewing 28 papers published between 1884 and 1954, Anthony and Scott (1960) reported that only 3 (5%) of the 60 cases of purported childhood mania actually met their criteria for bipolar disorder. While their pioneering work was the first attempt to operationalize the diagnosis of childhood mania, Anthony and Scott's criteria stressed the presence of classic Kraepelinian symptoms plus clinical features that do not resemble *DSM-III, DSM-III-R,* or *DSM-IV* criteria. Thus, Anthony and Scott's criteria may have led unintentionally to the underdiagnosis of childhood-onset cases and an underestimation of the prevalence of bipolar disorder in children.

In recent years, however, the view that childhood-onset mania is rare has been challenged by a plethora of case reports and case series (Campbell, 1952; Coll and Bland, 1979; Davis, 1979; Feinstein and Wolpert, 1973; Frommer, 1968; Geller et al., 1994; Kasanin, 1931; McHarg, 1954; McKnew et al., 1974; Potter, 1983; Poznanski et al., 1984; Sylvester et al., 1984; Tomasson and Kuperman, 1990; Varanka et al., 1988; Varsamis and MacDonald, 1972; Weinberg and Brumback, 1976). Weller et al. (1986)

searched the literature of case reports describing children with severe psychiatric symptomatology (excluding developmental disorders and attention-deficit hyperactivity disorder [ADHD]). Of 157 such cases, 19 (12%) were diagnosed as manic in the original reports and another 19 (12%) of cases previously diagnosed as psychotic or schizophrenic were rediagnosed by the authors as manic according to *DSM-III* criteria. This review suggested that juvenile mania may be common among referred children with severe psychopathology but that it may be difficult to diagnose. In a recent follow-up study of 79 children with major depression, Geller et al. (1994) reported that bipolarity developed in 25 (32%).

While developmental variations have been accepted in *DSM-III, DSM-III-R*, and *DSM-IV* for major depression, no similar accommodations have been made for mania (Cantwell and Carlson, 1983). Unlike adult bipolar patients, manic children are seldom characterized by euphoric mood (Carlson, 1983). Rather, the most common mood disturbance in manic children may be better characterized as irritable, with "affective storms" or prolonged and aggressive temper outbursts (Davis, 1979). For example, one literature review (Carlson, 1983) found that bipolar children under the age of 9 years had more irritability, crying, and psychomotor agitation than older bipolar children, who were more likely to be "classically manic" with euphoria and grandiosity. In addition, it has been suggested that the course of childhood-onset bipolar disorder tends to be chronic and continuous rather than episodic and acute, as is characteristic of the adult disorder (Carlson, 1983; Carlson, 1984; Feinstein and Wolpert, 1973; McGlashan, 1988). Thus, examination of the clinical phenomenology and course of manic children could help clarify diagnostic uncertainties of childhood bipolar disorder.

Another potential source of diagnostic confusion in childhood-onset mania is its symptomatic overlap with ADHD. Noting that distractibility, impulsivity, hyperactivity, and emotional lability are characteristic of both ADHD and bipolar disorder, Carlson (1984) concluded that the relationship between these two disorders required further clarification. Most of the available case reports of manic children commented on the overlap of symptoms between these two disorders (Potter, 1983; Poznanski et al., 1984).

This report examines the prevalence, characteristics, and correlates of mania among referred children aged 12 years or younger. Based on the available literature, we hypothesized that (1) mania would be identifiable in referred children; (2) the clinical picture of childhood-onset mania would be irritable and mixed, and the course would be chronic; (3) children satisfying criteria for mania would frequently also meet criteria for ADHD;

and (4) children with both mania, and ADHD would have the clinical features of both disorders.

## METHOD

The sample consisted of all children, 12 years or younger, who had been consecutively referred to a pediatric psychopharmacology clinic since 1991. Each had been evaluated comprehensively with a structured diagnostic interview ($n = 262$). From this pool of clinic subjects we identified those meeting full criteria for a *DSM-III-R* diagnosis of mania ($n = 43$). This clinic sample is *unselected* in that children were referred for a pediatric psychopharmacology evaluation but not for evaluation of any specific disorder. For comparison, we used information from ADHD children without mania referred to the same clinical center during the same period of time ($n = 164$). For additional comparison we used information from a pool of non-ADHD control children of both genders without mania participating in family genetic studies of ADHD ($n = 84$) (Biederman et al., 1992). For simplicity of exposition, children satisfying criteria for mania are referred to as "manic," children satisfying criteria for ADHD without mania are referred to as "ADHD," and those without mania or ADHD as "non-ADHD controls."

All children were evaluated using the Schedule for Affective Disorders and Schizophrenia for School-Age Children-Epidemiologic Version (K-SADS-E) (Orvaschel and Puig-Antich, 1987) administered to the mother by raters who had been trained and supervised by the senior investigator (J.B.). For the clinic sample, raters were blind to the clinical diagnosis apart from their knowledge that the child had been referred to a pediatric psychopharmacology clinic. The clinic children and the non-ADHD control children were evaluated using identical methodology and by the same pool of raters. These non-ADHD control children had been evaluated by raters who were blind to diagnostic status in a family study of boys and girls with ADHD (Biederman et al., 1992). The approach taken by the K-SADS-E to evaluate these criteria is similar to that taken by the original SADS. First, a period of time characterized by the features in section A is established; then each of the criteria in B are addressed. For example, to assess B1 the interviewer would ask the parent: During this period did [child's name] feel especially self-confident? Like he/she could do anything? Was special? In what way? Special powers? Stronger? Smarter?

For every diagnosis, information was gathered regarding the ages at onset and offset of symptoms, number of episodes, and treatment history. All diagnoses were reviewed by a diagnostic sign-off committee chaired by the service chief (J.B.), who reviewed both the items endorsed during the interview along with detailed notes taken by the interviewer. Moreover, for this study, a second board-certified child and adolescent psychiatrist (J.W.) reviewed all case material, including the audiotape of the structured interview, to confirm that all diagnoses of mania were clinically meaningful. Since the anxiety disorders comprise many syndromes with a wide range of severity, we use two or more anxiety disorders to indicate the presence of a clinically meaningful anxiety syndrome and refer to this as "multiple anxiety disorders" as we have elsewhere (Biederman et al., 1990).

Diagnoses presented for review were considered positive only if a consensus was achieved that criteria were met to a degree that would be considered clinically meaningful. By "clinically meaningful" we mean that the data collected from the structured interview indicated that the diagnosis should be a clinical concern because of the nature of the symptoms, the associated impairment, and the coherence of the clinical picture. A key point is that these diagnoses were made as part of the clinical assessment procedures for our clinic; they were not simply research diagnoses computed by counting symptoms endorsed and applying an algorithm. We consider these diagnoses "clinically meaningful" because they are routinely used in planning the treatment of children in our clinic.

We computed κ coefficients of agreement between the trained raters and three experienced, board-certified child and adult psychiatrists who reviewed the audiotaped interviews. Based on 115 interviews, all disorders achieved κ values higher than .82. The mean κ was 90. We attained a κ of 1.0 for ADHD and .91 for mania.

To be given the lifetime diagnosis of mania, the child had to meet full *DSM-III-R* criteria for a manic episode with associated impairment. Thus, a child must have met criterion A for a period of *extreme* and persistently elevated, expansive, or irritable mood; plus criterion B, manifested by three (four if the mood is irritable only) of seven symptoms during the period of mood disturbance; plus criterion C, associated impairment.

We examined the extent of symptom overlap between mania and ADHD in children with both disorders. Of seven criteria for a manic episode, three are shared with the criteria for ADHD: distractibility, motoric hyperactivity, and talkativeness. Thus, to avoid counting symptoms twice toward the diagnosis of both ADHD and mania, we reassessed each individual after subtracting the three overlapping symptoms and applying the same criteria required in *DSM-III-R* for diagnosis.

We also obtained information regarding cognitive functioning using subtests from the WISC-R, the Wide Range Achievement Test, and the Gilmore Oral Reading test. To evaluate school functioning, we assessed—

on the basis of parent reports—three straightforward indices of school failure: placement in special classes, in-school tutoring, and repeated grades. Psychosocial functioning was assessed using the *DSM-III-R* Global Assessment of Functioning (GAF) (0 = worst to 90 = best).

Data are expressed as means ± standard deviations. Continuous data were analyzed by analysis of variance and categorical data by $\chi^2$ analyses. Significant overall analyses of variance were followed by pairwise tests with corrections for multiple comparisons using Fisher's Protected Least Significant Difference tests. All analyses were two-tailed; statistical significance was set at the 1% level ($p \leq .01$).

## RESULTS

From the pool of 262 consecutive referrals of children 12 years of age and younger, 79% ($n = 207$) met criteria for either mania or ADHD (Table 1). Sixteen percent ($n = 43$) of the 262 referrals met criteria for mania and 79% ($n = 206$) met criteria for ADHD. Of the 206 ADHD patients, 80% ($n = 164$) did not meet criteria for mania. The overlap between mania and ADHD was asymmetrical: the 42 patients with both ADHD and mania were 98% of the 43 manic children but only 20% of the 206 ADHD children. There were no meaningful differences between the manic, ADHD, and control children in sociodemographic characteristics such as age, socioeconomic status, grade placement, or gender distribution (Table 1).

Seventy percent of manic children ($n = 30$) had onset of mania-like symptoms at age 5 or younger. For 23% ($n = 10$) of the manic children, symptoms of mania were reported as "always present," and an exact age of onset could not be established. In these cases, the age at onset was coded as 1 year. Among manic children, the duration of illness represented on average 38% of the child's life for mania and 68% for ADHD. Although the age at onset of ADHD or duration of ADHD did not differ between manic and ADHD children, manic children had significantly more ADHD symptoms than did ADHD children (12.6 versus 11.2, $p \leq .001$) (Table 1).

Significant differences were also observed in treatment histories. Manic children had a significantly higher rate of prior need for combined medication and psychotherapy treatment than did ADHD children (51% [$n = 22$] versus 24% [$n = 40$], $p < .001$). In addition, manic children also had a significantly higher rate of previous psychiatric hospitalization than did ADHD children (21% [$n = 9$] versus 2% [$n = 4$], $p \leq .001$) (Table 1).

Of the 43 children who met criteria for mania, 77% ($n = 33$) did so because of extreme and persistent irritability, 9% ($n = 4$) because of both eu-

TABLE 1
Sociodemographic and Clinical Characteristics of Sample

| Clinical Variables | Manic Children (n = 43) | | ADHD Children (n = 164) | Non-ADHD Control (n = 84) | Significance: p Value |
|---|---|---|---|---|---|
| **Demographic** | | | | | |
| Socioeconomic status: mean ± SD | 2.3 ± 1.3 | | 1.9 ± 1.2 | 1.9 ± 1.1 | NS |
| Age (yr): mean ± SD | 7.9 ± 2.6 | | 8.8 ± 2.2 | 9.0 ± 2.1 | NS |
| Grade placement: mean ± SD | 2.5 ± 2.4 | | 3.3 ± 2.1 | 3.6 ± 2.3 | NS |
| Males: No. (%) | 36 (84) | | 141 (85) | 71 (85) | NS |
| **Treatment history: No. (%)** | | | | | |
| Psychotherapy only | 21 (49)[b] | | 55 (34)[b] | 1 (1) | <.001 |
| Medication only | 6 (14)[b] | | 43 (26)[b] | 0 (0) | <.001 |
| Therapy and medication | 22 (51)[a,b] | | 40 (24)[b] | 0 (0) | <.001 |
| Hospitalization | 9 (21)[a,b] | | 4 (2) | 0 (0) | <.001 |
| | Mania (n = 43) | ADHD (n = 42) | | | |
| **Illness history: mean ± SD** | | | | | |
| Age of onset (yr) | 4.4 ± 3.1[c] | 2.5 ± 1.9 | 3.0 ± 2.1 | | NS |
| Duration of illness (yr) | 3.0 ± 2.1 | 5.4 ± 2.5 | 5.7 ± 2.8 | | NS |
| No. of symptoms | 5.2 ± 1.1 | 12.6 ± 1.7[a] | 11.2 ± 1.9 | | NA |

*Note:* ADHD = attention-deficit hyperactivity disorder; NS = not significant; NA = not applicable; PLSD = Protected Least Significant Difference.

[a] p ≤ .001 versus ADHD children by $\chi^2$ analysis, t test, or Fisher's PSLD.
[b] p ≤ .001 versus non-ADHD control by $\chi^2$ analysis, t test, or Fisher's PSLD.
[c] p ≤ .001 versus ADHD in manic children by $\chi^2$ analysis, t test, or Fisher's PSLD.

phoria and irritability, and 5% ($n = 2$) because of euphoria. The remaining 9% ($n = 4$) of children met criteria for mania because they were described as being full of energy or having many thoughts. Eighty-four percent ($n = 36$) had a chronic course and 16% ($n = 7$) had episodic difficulties (that is, more than one episode of mania was reported). Among the manic children 14% ($n = 6$) had mania only, 84% ($n = 36$) had a mixed presentation in which both symptoms of mania and major depression co-occurred, and 2% ($n = 1$) of the manic children had a biphasic presentation characterized by nonoverlapping episodes of mania and major depression. Of the manic children with major depression, the onset of the major depression preceded the onset of mania in 43% ($n = 16$), postceded it in 19% ($n = 7$), and was simultaneous in 38% ($n = 14$).

To help clarify the overlap between ADHD and mania, we examined the extent of symptom overlap in the two disorders after removal of the overlapping symptoms (distractibility, motoric hyperactivity, and talkativeness). Seventy-six percent ($n = 32$) of the 42 children meeting criteria for mania and ADHD continued to meet full (50%, $n = 21$) or subthreshold (26%, $n = 11$) criteria for mania after the three overlapping symptoms were removed. Subthreshold was defined as meeting more than half of the symptoms required for full diagnosis. Similarly, in this group, all ADHD diagnoses retained either full (95%, $n = 30$) or subthreshold (5%, $n = 2$) diagnostic status after subtraction of the three overlapping symptoms.

Table 2 shows the prevalence of comorbid psychiatric disorders in manic and ADHD children. With the exception of simple phobia, significant differences were detected between the groups in *all* assessed psychiatric disorders (all $p$ values $\leq .01$, Table 2). Although the rates of these disorders were significantly higher in both manic and ADHD children than in controls, they were much higher in manic than in ADHD children, reaching statistical significance for comparisons between manic and ADHD children for major depression, psychosis, conduct disorder, oppositional defiant disorder, multiple anxiety disorders, overanxious disorder, separation anxiety disorder, agoraphobia, and panic disorder (all $p$ values $\leq .01$) (Table 2).

Both manic and ADHD children showed more impaired scores than controls on most cognitive measurements (Table 3). Manic children had significantly more impaired scores than non-ADHD controls on the WISC-R Vocabulary and Digit Span subscales and on the WISC-R estimated Verbal IQ, and ADHD children had significantly more impaired scores than non-ADHD controls on the WISC-R Digit Symbol subscale (all $p$ values $\leq .01$) (Table 3).

Both manic and ADHD children had significantly higher rates of learning disabilities than non-ADHD controls. In addition, the rate of reading

TABLE 2
Rates of Additional Psychiatric Diagnoses

| Psychiatric Diagnoses | Manic Children (n = 43) | | ADHD Children (n = 164) | | Non-ADHD Control (n = 84) | | Significance* (df = 2): p Value |
|---|---|---|---|---|---|---|---|
| | No. | % | No. | % | No. | % | |
| Major depression | 37 | 86[a,b] | 63 | 38[b] | 3 | 4 | <.001 |
| Psychosis | 7 | 16[a] | 3 | 2 | NA | 0 | <.001 |
| Conduct disorder | 16 | 37[a,b] | 24 | 15[b] | 0 | 0 | <.001 |
| Oppositional defiant disorder | 38 | 88[a,b] | 78 | 48[b] | 3 | 4 | <.001 |
| Multiple anxiety disorders (≥2) | 24 | 56[a,b] | 43 | 26[b] | 1 | 1 | <.001 |
| Overanxious disorder | 21 | 49[a,b] | 39 | 24[b] | 2 | 2 | <.001 |
| Separation anxiety disorder | 19 | 44[a,b] | 36 | 22[b] | 4 | 5 | <.001 |
| Agoraphobia | 14 | 33[a,b] | 24 | 15[b] | 1 | 1 | <.001 |
| Panic disorder | 4 | 9[a,b] | 1 | 0.6 | 0 | 0 | <.001 |
| Social phobia | 10 | 23[b] | 26 | 16[b] | 1 | 1 | <.001 |
| Simple phobia | 8 | 19 | 28 | 17 | 7 | 8 | .138 |
| Obsessive-compulsive disorder | 5 | 12[b] | 7 | 4 | 0 | 0 | .008 |
| Tic disorders | 11 | 26[b] | 49 | 30[b] | 5 | 6 | <.001 |

*Note:* ADHD = attention-deficit hyperactivity disorder; PLSD = Protected Least Significant Difference; NA = not applicable.

* Overall comparisons between manic, ADHD, and non-ADHD control by $\chi^2$ analyses or by analysis of variance.

[a] $p \leq .01$ versus ADHD by $\chi^2$ analysis or by Fisher's PLSD.

[b] $p \leq .01$ versus non-ADHD control by $\chi^2$ analysis or by Fisher's PLSD.

TABLE 3
Rates of Cognitive, Social and School Functioning

| | Manic Children (n = 43) | ADHD Children (n = 164) | Non-ADHD Control (n = 84) | Significance* (df = 2): p Value |
|---|---|---|---|---|
| Cognitive Functioning: mean ± SD | | | | |
| WISC-R subscale percentiles | | | | |
| Vocabulary | 54.2 ± 29.7[b] | 65.1 ± 29.8 | 75.0 ± 21.5 | .002 |
| Block Design | 61.6 ± 29.6[b] | 69.5 ± 27.9[b] | 86.4 ± 18.2 | <.001 |
| Oral Arithmetic | 45.8 ± 30.3[b] | 56.1 ± 28.9[b] | 70.0 ± 26.3 | <.001 |
| Digit Span | 36.0 ± 24.9[b] | 45.9 ± 28.8 | 55.9 ± 26.3 | .004 |
| Digit Symbol | 51.6 ± 27.3 | 48.2 ± 31.9[b] | 66.1 ± 23.7 | <.001 |
| Estimated IQ scores | | | | |
| Verbal IQ | 102.4 ± 14.9[b] | 108.6 ± 16.0 | 113.5 ± 12.7 | .005 |
| Performance IQ | 105.9 ± 16.0[b] | 111.4 ± 15.9[b] | 121.3 ± 12.4 | <.001 |
| Full Scale IQ | 103.5 ± 11.5[b] | 110.0 ± 13.3[b] | 117.4 ± 10.4 | <.001 |
| Freedom from Distractibility | 44.8 ± 26.7[b] | 50.3 ± 29.6[b] | 69.1 ± 23.0 | <.001 |
| Academic achievement | | | | |
| Achievement tests: mean ± SD | | | | |
| WRAT Arithmetic percentiles | 30.9 ± 28.0[b] | 45.6 ± 32.7[b] | 69.8 ± 27.2 | <.001 |
| WRAT/Gilmore Reading standard scores | 90.5 ± 20.8 | 100.9 ± 17.8 | 102.9 ± 13.2 | .012 |
| Learning disabilities: No. (%) | | | | |
| Arithmetic | 6 (30)[b] | 22 (24)[b] | 5 (6) | .003 |
| Reading | 8 (42)[a,b] | 13 (14) | 4 (5) | .001 |
| Psychosocial functioning: mean ± SD | | | | |
| Global Assessment of Functioning | 43.0 ± 7.3[a,b] | 50.0 ± 5.1[b] | 72.0 ± 8.2 | <.001 |
| School Functioning: No. (%) | | | | |
| Repeated grade | 8 (19) | 30 (18) | 4 (5) | .011 |
| Tutoring | 19 (45)[b] | 85 (52)[b] | 18 (21) | <.001 |
| Placement in a special class | 14 (33)[b] | 52 (32)[b] | 2 (2) | <.001 |

*Note:* ADHD = attention-deficit hyperactivity disorder; WRAT = Wide Range Achievement Test; PLSD = Protected Least Significant Difference.

* Overall comparisons between manic, ADHD, and non-ADHD control by $\chi^2$ analyses or by analysis of variance.
[a] $p \leq .01$ versus ADHD by $\chi^2$ analysis or by Fisher's PLSD.
[b] $p \leq .01$ versus non-ADHD control by $\chi^2$ analysis or by Fisher's PLSD.

disability was significantly higher in manic than in ADHD children (Table 3). Similarly, both manic and ADHD children had significantly more impaired GAF scores than did non-ADHD controls (43 versus 50 versus 72, $p$ values $\leq .01$), and manic children had significantly more impaired GAF scores than did ADHD children ($p \leq .01$) (Table 3). Both manic and ADHD children compared with controls had significantly higher rates of school dysfunction (Table 3).

## DISCUSSION

Our systematic evaluation of structured interview-derived data from a sample of clinically referred children showed that (1) a clinical picture compatible with the diagnosis of mania was identified in 16% of psychiatrically referred children; (2) the clinical picture in these children was predominantly irritable and mixed, and the course was chronic; (3) children meeting criteria for mania frequently met criteria for ADHD; and (4) children with mania-like symptoms often met structured interview-derived diagnostic criteria for major depression and psychosis, had higher rates of psychiatric hospitalization, and showed evidence of severely impaired psychosocial functioning. Although preliminary, these cross-sectional findings suggest that children with mania-like clinical features may suffer from an early form of bipolar disorder.

The 16% rate of mania-like symptoms in our pool of psychiatrically referred children challenges the commonly held notion that mania is rare or nonexistent in children. This rate is consistent with the findings of Weller et al. (1986), who estimated a rate of mania of 22% among severely disturbed children.

Our findings indicate that mania can begin in very early childhood. The majority (70%) of cases began at or before age 5 years, and in 23% the parents reported that symptoms of mania had been "always present" and were unable to establish an exact age at onset. Even when parents were able to pin down an age at onset, most reported a very early onset. This suggests that the onset of juvenile mania may be insidious, manifesting itself in some children at the beginning of life. This aspect coupled with its chronicity may make identification difficult. The finding that childhood mania may have an insidious onset is consistent with other findings of insidious onset reported in nonbipolar depression (Kovacs et al., 1984a,b) and in early-onset bipolar disorder (Akiskal et al., 1985).

We found that the predominant mood in the children meeting criteria for mania was that of severe irritability rather than euphoria. This is consistent with other work documenting that manic episodes in young children are seldom characterized by euphoric mood (Carlson, 1983, 1984). Of course, irritability is a common symptom in childhood psychopathology, and tantrums are common among children with ADHD. However, the type of irritability observed in our children with mania-like symptoms was very severe and often associated with violence. For example, several children when irritable used knives to threaten others, to stab the furniture or floor, or to cut off a cat's tail. Most of the children were described as assaultive when irritable. One child attempted to smother his mother with a pillow. Other children were described in the medical charts as "completely wild," "explosive," "extremely aggressive," or "creating a war zone." The irritability in these children rapidly became violent, resulting in throwing and breaking things, kicking down doors, and destroying property. This type of severe irritability and "affective storms," associated with prolonged and nonpredatory aggressive outbursts (Davis, 1979), is precisely the one identified in the literature dealing with childhood-onset mania. In our sample, the severe irritability was the most common reason for these children to be psychiatrically hospitalized. Despite the fact that irritability is an accepted component of criterion A for mania in *DSM-III, DSM-III-R,* and *DSM-IV* and a common feature of adult bipolar disorder (Goodwin and Jamison, 1990, pp. 186–209), its presence may have contributed to the underidentification of mania in children. In the absence of euphoria, clinicians may attribute irritability in a child to psychosocial factors or conduct disorder rather than to mania.

Our results also indicated that childhood-onset mania is commonly mixed, with symptoms of depression and mania occurring simultaneously. This finding is consistent with a body of literature suggesting that the earlier the onset of bipolar disorder, the greater the frequency of mixed states (Ryan and Puig-Antich, 1986). Mixed manic states have been described as the most likely presentation of mania in juveniles (Goodwin and Jamison, 1990, pp. 186–209; Ryan and Puig-Antich, 1986). In a recent literature review, McElroy et al. (1992) estimated that 30% of bipolar adults present with a mixed bipolar state, associated with younger age of onset, suicidality, longer duration of illness, poorer outcome, and more neuropsychiatric abnormalities, representing a most severe form of the illness and among the most difficult to manage clinically. Given the possible continuity of bipolar disorder from childhood to adulthood, it is conceivable that childhood-onset mania increases the risk for a mixed disorder throughout the life cycle with its attendant complex course and poor therapeutic responsivity.

Our findings document that childhood-onset mania is commonly chronic rather than episodic. Although information about the course of juvenile bipolar disorder is sparse, Carlson (1983) notes that discrete episodes are difficult to delineate in younger children. A chronic course may make mania difficult to identify if clinicians are expecting to observe specific episodes or mood swings (Feinstein and Wolpert, 1973; Poznanski et al., 1984). A chronic course, however, has been well documented in studies of manic adults (Tsuang et al., 1979). For example, epidemiological studies indicate that as many as 22% of bipolar subjects have a chronic course (Goodwin and Jamison, 1990, pp. 127–156). It remains to be determined whether chronic childhood mania leads to a chronic course in adulthood.

Our finding of a high overlap between mania and ADHD is consistent with previous studies of juvenile mania (Potter, 1983; Poznanski et al., 1984), studies of childhood histories of bipolar adults (Sachs et al., 1993; Winokur et al., 1993), and high-risk studies of children of bipolar parents (Grigoroiu-Serbanescu et al., 1989; Kestenbaum, 1979). Most case reports of childhood-onset mania note symptoms of hyperactivity preceding or occurring simultaneously with those of mania. In a recent article, Winokur et al. (1993) showed that bipolar adults and their adult bipolar relatives were more likely to have had a childhood history of hyperactivity than were unipolar subjects and their relatives. Sachs et al. (1993) found comorbid ADHD exclusively among early-onset (before age 18) bipolar adults.

The overlap between mania and ADHD may have led to confusion as to whether these children have ADHD, mania, or both. Our data show that children fulfilling diagnostic criteria for both ADHD and mania have correlates of both disorders, thus supporting the notion that both conditions may be present. The patterns of psychiatric comorbidity, cognitive impairment (learning disability), and school failure identified in youngsters with mania plus ADHD in our series are consistent with findings in ADHD children without mania in this study as well as with findings reported in referred samples of ADHD children (Faraone et al., 1993; Semrud-Clikeman et al., 1992). Moreover, the clinical picture of ADHD in the manic children was extremely severe, as characterized by a significantly higher number of ADHD symptoms, by the significantly higher rate of reading disability, and by a greater need for aggressive treatments than that reported for other ADHD children (Tables 1 and 3). In addition, the significantly elevated rates of major depression, psychosis, and psychiatric hospitalization in manic children compared with ADHD children support the diagnosis of mania in these children (Gershon, 1990), supporting our contention that both disorders may be present.

Since ADHD and mania individually are associated with high morbidity and disability, their co-occurrence may herald a most severe clinical picture of high morbidity and perhaps mortality. For example, a study of adolescent suicide found that adolescents who completed suicide had significantly higher rates of bipolar disorder, especially mixed subtype, and a higher rate of comorbid ADHD than those who attempted suicide (Brent et al., 1988). Because ADHD can compound the impulsivity of a severe mixed manic state, the combination of ADHD and mania can be potentially lethal.

Although children meeting diagnostic criteria for mania also frequently met criteria for ADHD, ADHD children less frequently met criteria for mania: the rate of ADHD in children with mania was 98%, while the rate of mania in children with ADHD was only 20%. This asymmetrical overlap between mania and ADHD suggests divergent validity: it shows that a manic clinical picture is not a common correlate of ADHD. This finding is consistent with a study by Fristad et al. (1992). These authors found that children with mania and children with ADHD received similar scores on the Conners ADHD rating scale, while manic children scored significantly higher than ADHD children on the Mania Rating Scale.

Our data on symptom expression for ADHD and mania show that in the manic children with ADHD in our sample, the ADHD and mania diagnoses could not be accounted for by the symptoms shared by the two disorders (distractibility, motoric hyperactivity, and talkativeness). The ability to retain diagnostic status for both mania and ADHD after removing overlapping symptoms supports the assertion that each diagnosis was made robustly, with more than the minimum criteria met.

Our findings indicating that psychosis is more common among children meeting criteria for mania than among children with ADHD without mania are consistent with a large body of literature suggesting that bipolar disorder frequently presents with psychosis (Goodwin and Jamison, 1990, pp. 15–55), especially in juveniles (Ballenger et al., 1982; McGlashan, 1988). It is for this reason that juvenile mania may frequently be misdiagnosed as schizophrenia. Given the literature on psychosis and mania, psychosis could be considered another correlate of bipolar disorder.

In addition to comorbidity with ADHD, bipolar children also had a high degree of comorbidity with anxiety disorders. This finding is consistent with previous, usually incidental, reports in the literature. Carlson and Kashani (1988) found that nonreferred adolescents with manic symptoms were more likely than controls to meet criteria for anxiety disorders. Bashir et al. (1987) noted that anxiety disorders were present in 53% of 30 adolescents with diagnosed mania or hypomania. Similarly, Zahn-Waxler et al. (1988) and Sachs et al. (1993) both reported an increased risk for anxiety in high-risk children of bipolar parents. Clearly, more work is needed to understand further the overlap between anxiety and mania. However, our findings suggest that the presence of anxiety disorders may be characteristic of juvenile-onset mania.

Although our data provide evidence for the validity of childhood-onset mania, they should be interpreted with caution. We have used the terms "mania-like symptoms" and "children who meet criteria for mania" to underscore the developmental complexities of making bipolar diagnoses in young children, especially in the context of comorbid ADHD. We have shown here, and in a different sample (S. Milberger, J. Biederman, S.V. Faraone, J. Murphy, M.T. Tsuang, unpublished), that these shared criteria cannot account for the observed comorbidity. However, the phenomenology of both disorders includes impulsivity and overactivity, poor judgment and irritability. Also, although the chronic course of manic symptomatology in our sample is more similar to ADHD than it is to "classic" bipolar disorder, some forms of mania also can take a chronic course. Furthermore, the presence of chronicity and mixed symptoms with major depression make this clinical picture of bipolar disorder in children "atypical" by adult standards and contributes to the difficulty in distinguishing these children from those with ADHD.

Thus, our work raises several nosological questions. Are "children who meet criteria for mania" severe cases of ADHD with affective dysregulation? If so, do they fall on a continuum of severity with other ADHD cases or do they constitute an etiologically or pathophysiologically distinct subtype? Alternatively, are these children truly cases of bipolar disorder? If so, are they nosologically distinct from classic bipolar disorder or do their atypical symptoms and course indicate a varying developmental expression of bipolar disorder? Treatment, family, and follow-up studies are needed to clarify the nosological status of "children who meet criteria for mania." However, these nosological questions should not obscure a key clinical point: "children who meet criteria for mania" have a severe clinical picture that leads to considerable psychiatric and psychosocial disability beyond that conferred by ADHD. Since ADHD will often be diagnosed in such children, clinicians should be alert to the potential of concomitant bipolar disorder.

Although it would be premature to establish diagnostic rules for childhood mania, our work and that of others suggests some initial approaches. Qualitative aspects of symptomatology may be helpful in assessing bipolarity that is concomitant with ADHD (Casat, 1982). For example, in bipolar disorder overactivity may be expressed during goal-directed activity, whereas in ADHD the overactivity may be more pervasive. Also, the impulsivity characteristic of manic episodes may involve the pursuit of pleasurable activities having a high potential for adverse consequences while, in contrast, the impulsivity of the ADHD child is manifest as a pervasive failure of inhibition not limited to pleasurable activities. Weinberg and Brumback (1976) noted that in contrast to the relatively chronic hyperactivity of the ADHD child, the overactivity of the manic child may emerge quickly and could show a change from prior behavior. Also, the grandiose symptoms of bipolar disorder are not part of ADHD. Another notable distinction highlighted by Bowring and Kovacs (1992) is that irritability, rather than euphoria, is the essential disruption-of-mood characteristic of childhood mania. The labile and irritable mood of the manic child is associated with levels of agitation and belligerence that are not common features of ADHD.

In addition to the questions raised by these differential diagnostic issues, our findings should be evaluated in light of specific methodological limitations. Although acceptable reliability data for the mood disorder modules of the K-SADS-E have been documented (Chambers et al., 1985), less is known about the validity of the modules. However, structured diagnostic interview techniques can minimize informant and clinician bias and may represent an improvement over the standard clinical assessment (Robins, 1985). Given a reluctance to diagnose bipolar disorder in young subjects, structured interviews provide a means of identifying cases that might otherwise have been misattributed. Moreover, in our series, structured interview data were always reviewed by an experienced, board-certified child and adolescent psychiatrist (J.B.) before final diagnostic assignment, enhancing the credibility of the findings.

In this study, all structured interviews about the child were done with a parent, usually the mother. Although children are not always good reporters of their lifetime psychopathology, future studies would benefit from direct interview of the child in addition to the parent.

Data regarding age at onset and offset of symptoms were obtained by retrospective recollection by the child's mother. A possible recollection bias makes this method imprecise. Moreover, many of the ages at onset of disorders of interest could not be precisely reported. Instead, the mother indicated that the child had had the disorder "always" or "since birth." We coded this as age 1 year. Although these data generate intriguing hypotheses about early onset for childhood mania, more work is needed to precisely estimate the age at onset. Clearly, identification of these children at an earlier age would aid in characterizing further their course and presentation.

Inasmuch as 98% of the children with mania-like symptoms also had ADHD, our results may not generalize to manic children who do not have ADHD. More generally, because we studied children referred to a pediatric psychopharmacology clinic, our findings should generalize to similar clinics treating severely disturbed children, but they may not generalize to other psychiatric sampling frames or to community samples. It is possible that our clinic has become well known for the treatment of ADHD children or the management of difficult, comorbid cases. This might explain the high rate of ADHD seen in our sample of referred manic children. However, our clinic is not a specialty clinic: no specific diagnosis is required for referral or acceptance. Thus, the rates of mania and comorbid ADHD are "naturalistic" rates not biased by preselection by the investigator on either clinical or research grounds. Clearly, more work is needed to further address this issue with large and diagnostically representative samples of general clinic referrals as well as epidemiological samples.

Also, as most of our subjects were male, additional work with females is needed to determine whether our results would generalize to females. However, these findings should be of use to the many child psychiatrists who work in clinics treating clinically referred children. To our knowledge, possibly as a result of diagnostic prejudices, no epidemiological study to date has assessed bipolar disorder among children in a community sample.

Despite these limitations, our findings indicate that a clinical picture compatible with the diagnosis of childhood mania can be identified in children by using systematic assessment methodology. Our data also suggest that juvenile mania may be more common than previously recognized. This clinical picture compatible with the diagnosis of mania is characterized by severe irritability, a mixed presentation with symptoms of depression and mania, and a chronic course. Although mania and ADHD have overlapping symptoms, our work suggests that both conditions may coexist. More work needs to be done to evaluate further the overlap between ADHD and mania in children to determine the implications of the comorbid condition for clinical and research work.

## REFERENCES

Akiskal HS, Downs J, Jordan P (1985), Affective disorders in referred children and younger siblings of manic-depressives: mode of onset and prospective course. *Arch Gen Psychiatry* 42:996–1003.

Anthony J, Scott P (1960), Manic-depressive psychosis in childhood. *J Child Psychol Psychiatry* 1:53–72.

Ballenger JC, Reus VI, Post RM (1982), The "atypical" picture of adolescent mania. *Am J Psychiatry* 139:602–606.

Bashir M, Russell J, Johnson G (1987), Bipolar affective disorder in adolescence: a 10-year study *Aust N Z J Psychiatry* 21:36–43.

Biederman J, Faraone SV, Keenan K et al. (1992), Further evidence for family-genetic risk factors in attention deficit hyperactivity disorder (ADHD): patterns of comorbidity in probands and relatives in psychiatrically and pediatrically referred samples. *Arch Gen Psychiatry* 49:728–738.

Biederman J, Rosenbaum JF, Hirshfeld DR et al. (1990), Psychiatric correlates of behavioral inhibition in young children of parents with and without psychiatric disorders. *Arch Gen Psychiatry* 47:21–26.

Bowring MA, Kovacs M (1992), Difficulties in diagnosing manic disorders among children and adolescents. *J Am Acad Child Adolesc Psychiatry* 31:611–614.

Brent DA, Perper JA, Goldstein CE et al. (1988), Risk factors for adolescent suicide: a comparison of adolescent suicide victims with suicidal inpatients. *Arch Gen Psychiatry* 45:581–588.

Campbell J (1952), Manic depressive psychosis in children, report of 18 cases. *J Nerv Ment Dis* 116:424–439.

Cantwell DP, Carlson GA, eds (1983), *Affective Disorders in Childhood and Adolescence. An Update*. Child Behavior and Development Series. New York: Spectrum.

Carlson GA (1983), Bipolar affective disorders in childhood and adolescence. In, *Affective Disorders in Childhood and Adolescence: An Update*, Cantwell DP, Carlson GA, eds. New York. Spectrum, pp 61–83.

Carlson GA (1984), Classification issues of bipolar disorders in childhood. *Psychiatr Dev* 2:273–285.

Carlson GA, Kashani JH (1988), Manic symptoms in a non-referred adolescent population. *J Affect Disord* 15:219–226.

Casat CD (1982), The under- and over-diagnosis of mania in children and adolescents. *Compr Psychiatry* 23:552–559.

Chambers W, Puig-Antich J, Hirsch M et al. (1985), The assessment of affective disorders in children and adolescents by semistructured interview. *Arch Gen Psychiatry* 42:696–702.

Coll PG, Bland R (1979), Manic depressive illness in adolescence and childhood: review and case report. *Can J Psychiatry* 24:255–263.

Davis RE (1979), Manic-depressive variant syndrome of childhood: a preliminary report. *Am J Psychiatry* 136:702–706.

Faraone SV, Biederman J, Krifcher Lehman B et al. (1993), Intellectual performance and school failure in children with attention deficit hyperactivity disorder and in their siblings. *J Abnorm Psychol* 102:616–623.

Feinstein SC, Wolpert EA (1973), Juvenile manic-depressive illness, clinical and therapeutic considerations. *J Am Acad Child Psychiatry* 12:123–136.

Fristad MA, Weller EB, Weller RA (1992), The Mania Rating Scale: can it be used in children? A preliminary report. *J Am Acad Child Adolesc Psychiatry* 31:252–257.

Frommer E (1968), Recent developments in affective disorders. *Br J Psychiatry* 2:117–136.

Geller B, Fox L, Clark K (1994), Rate and predictors of prepubertal bipolarity during follow-up of 6- to 12-year-old depressed children. *J Am Acad Child Adolesc Psychiatry* 33:461–468.

Gershon ES (1990), Genetics. In *Manic-Depressive Illness*, Goodwin F, Redfield Jamison K, eds. New York: Oxford University Press, pp 373–401.

Goodwin F, Jamison K (1990), *Manic-Depressive Illness.* New York: Oxford University Press.

Grigoroiu-Serbanescu M, Christodorescu D, Jipescu I, Totoescu A, Marinescu E, Ardeleau V (1989), Psychopathology in children aged 10–17 of bipolar parents' psychopathology rate and correlates of the severity of the psychopathology *J Affect Disord* 16:167–179.

Kasanin J (1931), The affective psychoses in children. *Am J Psychiatry* 10: 897–926.

Kestenbaum CJ (1979), Children at risk for manic-depressive illness: possible predictors *Am J Psychiatry* 136: 1206–1208.

Kovacs M, Feinberg T, Crouse-Novak M, Paulauskas S, Pollock M, Finkelstein R (1984a), Depressive disorders in childhood: II. A longitudinal study of the risk for a subsequent major depression. *Arch Gen Psychiatry* 41:643–649.

Kovacs M, Feinberg TL, Crouse-Novak M, Paulauskas SL, Finkelstein R (1984b), Depressive disorders in childhood: I. A longitudinal prospective study of characteristics and recovery. *Arch Gen Psychiatry* 41:229–237.

Kraepelin E (1921), *Manic-Depressive Insanity and Paranoia.* Edinburgh: Livingstone.

Loranger A, Levine P (1978), Age at onset of bipolar affective illness. *Arch Gen Psychiatry* 35:1345–1348.

McElroy SL, Keck PE, Pope HG, Hudson JI, Faedda G, Swann AC (1992), Clinical and research implications of the diagnosis of dysphoric or mixed mania or hypomania. *Am J Psychiatry* 149:1633–1644.

McGlashan T (1988), Adolescent versus adult onset of mania. *Am J Psychiatry* 145:221–223.

McHarg JF (1954), Mania in childhood. *Arch Neurol Psychiatry* 72:531–539.

McKnew D, Cytryn L, White I (1974), Clinical and biochemical correlates of hypomania in a child. *J Am Acad Psychiatry* 13:576–584.

Orvaschel H, Puig-Antich J (1987), *Schedule for Affective Disorders and Schizophrenia for School-Age Children-Epidemiologic Version.* Ft Lauderdale, FL. Nova University, Center for Psychological Study.

Potter RL (1983), Manic-depressive variant syndrome of childhood. Diagnostic and therapeutic considerations. *Clin Pediatr (Phila)* 22:495–499.

Poznanski E, Israel M, Grossman J (1984), Hypomania in a four-year-old. *J Am Acad Child Psychiatry* 23:105–110.

Robins LN (1985), Epidemiology: reflections on resting the validity of psychiatric interviewing. *Arch Gen Psychiatry* 42:918–924.

Ryan ND, Puig-Antich J (1986), Affective illness in adolescence In: *American Psychiatric Association Annual Review*, Frances AJ, Hales RE, eds Washington, DC, American Psychiatric Press, pp 420–450.

Sachs GS, Conklin A, Lafer B, Thibault AB, Rosenbaum JF, Biederman J (1993), Psychopathology in children of late vs early onset bipolar probands. *Proceedings of the Annual Meeting of the American Academy of Child and Adolescent Psychiatry.*

Semrud-Clikeman MS, Biederman J, Sprich S, Krifcher B, Norman D, Faraone S (1992), Comorbidity between ADHD and learning disability: a review and report in a clinically referred sample. *J Am Acad Child Adolesc Psychiatry* 31:439–448.

Sylvester CE, Burke PM, McCauley EA, Clark CJ (1984), Manic psychosis in childhood. Report of two cases. *J Nerv Ment Dis* 172:12–15.

Tomasson K, Kuperman S (1990), Bipolar disorder in a prepubescent child: case study. *J Am Acad Child Adolesc Psychiatry* 29:308–310.

Tsuang MT, Woolson R, Fleming JA (1979), Long-term outcome of major psychoses: I. Schizophrenia and affective disorders compared with psychiatrically symptom-free surgical conditions. *Arch Gen Psychiatry* 36:1295–1301.

Varanka TM, Weller RA, Weller EB, Fristad MA (1988), Lithium treatment of manic episodes with psychotic features in prepubertal children. *Am J Psychiatry* 145:1557–1559.

Varsamis J, MacDonald SM (1972), Manic depressive disease in childhood. *Can J Psychiatry* 24:279–281.

Weinberg WA, Brumback RA (1976), Mania in childhood. *Am J Dis Child* 130: 380–385.

Weller RA, Weller EB, Tucker SG, Fristad MA (1986), Mania in prepubertal children: has it been underdiagnosed? *J Affect Disord* 11:151–154.

Winokur G, Coryell W, Endicott J, Akiskal H (1993), Further distinctions between manic-depressive illness (bipolar disorder) and primary depressive disorder (unipolar depression). *Am J Psychiatry* 150:1176–1181.

Zahn-Waxler C, Mayfield A, Radke-Yarrow M, McKnew D, Cytryn L, Davenport Y (1988), A follow-up investigation of offspring of parents with bipolar disorder. *Am J Psychiatry* 145:506–509.

# 15

# Psychosocial Adjustment in Children with Port-Wine Stains and Prominent Ears

**Declan Sheerin**
*Regional Child and Family Centre, Drogheda, Ireland*
**Morag MacLeod**
*Mental Welfare Commission, Edinburgh, Scotland*
**Vivek Kusumakar**
*Dalhousie University, Halifax, Nova Scotia*

**Objective:** *To evaluate psychosocial adjustment in children with port-wine stain (PWS) and children with prominent ears (PE).* **Method:** *Thirty-two children aged 7 to 16 years with facial PWS and 42 children with PE were evaluated using the Harter Self-Perception Profile, the Revised Children's Manifest Anxiety Scale, the Children's Depression Inventory, the Disfigurement Perception Scale, and the Child Behavior Checklist. Results were compared with normative data for the local population or with a control group. Profile scores were correlated with severity of the PWS or prominence of the ears.* **Results:** *Children with PE had poorer self-perception, higher concentration anxiety, and more internalizing and externalizing symptoms, and they were more withdrawn and had more social problems than children with PWS. The children with PWS functioned as well as or better than nondisfigured peers on measurements of psychosocial adjustment, while children with PE scored lower than nondisfigured peers on measures of self-perception and parent-rated social and attention problems. There was no correlation*

Reprinted with permission from the *Journal of the American Academy of Child and Adolescent Psychiatry*, 1995, Vol. 34, No. 12, 1637–1647. Copyright © 1995 by the American Academy of Child and Adolescent Psychiatry.

*between degree of disfigurement and level of psychosocial adjustment.* **Conclusions:** *Psychosocial adjustment varied according to the nature of the disfigurement or deformity and was unrelated to the severity of the disfigurement.*

Children born with facial vascular malformations are said to suffer severe psychological and emotional difficulties (Diwan, 1990). These disfigurements lead to a significant degree of social stigmatization, often commencing when the child enters school (Lanigan and Cotterill, 1989). The discomfort caused by being marked with a port-wine stain (PWS) has led many individuals to use cosmetics to conceal their PWS (Kalick et al., 1981).

The influence of the patient's birthmark on his or her emotional life is dependent on location, type, size, and contour in addition to parental and societal attitudes (Harrison, 1988). Facial birthmarks usually have the more devastating effect. The size and contour of the vascular anomaly is important, not just because of the proportionate impact of the birthmark on physical appearance but also because the more severe the disfigurement, the more vigorous the employment of psychological defenses, particularly the primitive defenses of denial and avoidance, to protect the person from the pain of having the defect (Harrison, 1988).

Sociological studies support the view that appearance and disfigurement are associated with psychosocial morbidity (Bull and Stevens, 1981; Dion and Berscheid, 1974; Langlois and Downs, 1979). A child or adolescent with an unattractive appearance will be disadvantaged in a variety of areas. Attractive individuals are judged to be more socially desirable than unattractive individuals and are expected to have better prospects for happier social and professional lives (Dion et al., 1972).

"What is beautiful is good" is a powerful internally consistent stereotype in social life which affects the youth of society as well as unattractive children (Kalick, 1978). Its influence may extend to preschool children and infants (Clifford and Walster, 1973; Dion, 1972; Dion and Berscheid, 1974). Corter et al. (1978) have shown that nurses in charge of premature infants give a better intellectual prognosis to the children they perceive to be more physically attractive. Unattractive children appear to be significantly disadvantaged in society; the facially disfigured may suffer even more. In support of this, McCabe and Marwit (1993) reported that negative evaluation of personal attractiveness in children aged 8 to 14 years was associated with dysphoria.

Research on PWS and other disfigurements goes back four decades. Access to disfigured children has invariably been through plastic surgery clinics and had originally focused on craniofacial deformities and cleft lips and palates; more recently, with progress in operative and laser techniques, PWS and prominent ears (PE) have been targeted for research. Harper and Richman (1978) state that the type of disability has differential effects on adolescent personality characteristics. When disfigurement involves the face, the complexity and intensity of feelings appear most pronounced (Nordlicht, 1979). Disfigurement of the face should be distinguished from that affecting other parts of the body.

Young but not older children with PE have been shown to report significantly more teasing than their nondisfigured peers; however, family members do not appear to relate to each other and to the outside world any differently from control families (Bradbury et al., 1992). In a study of 21 children with PE, self-esteem, trait anxiety, and depression were not significantly different from normative scores, though the trend was for lower scores (J. Doe, personal communication, 1992). Anomalies of the ears (for example, adherent ear lobes or malformed, asymmetrical, or soft and pliable ears) but not PE have been associated with other dysmorphic features and with hyperactive behavior in boys (Pomeroy et al., 1988; Waldrop and Halverson, 1971).

Many studies quoted as evidence for the psychological and emotional sequelae of being disfigured are anecdotal (Bull, 1990; Lansdown et al., 1991); failed to use reliable measurements; used self-reports, where statements are questionable indices of stigmatization (Lanigan and Cotterill, 1989); or did not use control groups or locally based normative data. Cleft and craniofacial deformity studies that looked at the impact of disfigurement on psychosocial adjustment have been confounded by the associated sufferings of these children—hearing, speech, and early feeding problems; hospital admissions; and operative interventions (Bradbury, 1993). No studies have comprehensively assessed psychosocial functioning in children with PWS or PE. As groups they provide a measure of disfigurement that is not confounded by other illness, disability, or intervention variables.

The aim of this study was to evaluate the psychosocial adjustment of two groups of children with congenital facial deformity—those with PWS and those with PE—and to address the following questions:

1. Is psychosocial adjustment in children with congenital facial disfigurement lower than that of nondisfigured children?
2. Does severity of disfigurement correlate with self-concept or psychosocial adjustment?
3. Is facial disfigurement a risk factor for later psychosocial maladjustment and if so, does this inform treatment strategies?

Although psychological disturbance per se is not an indication for plastic surgery, it is often justified upon the assumption that disfigurement is a risk factor for the development of psychosocial maladjustment. Self-perception is but one indicator of psychosocial adjustment. The wide age range of children in this study may reveal effects of disfigurement upon self-perception as the children grow older. Such a finding would suggest the need for early intervention and therefore inform treatment strategies.

## METHOD

### Description of Samples

**PWS group.** Between 1991 and 1992 an assessment was made of the psychosocial adjustment of 32 children (aged 7 to 16 years) with facial PWS referred to the Laser Clinic in Edinburgh, Scotland. When families received their appointments they were informed about this study and consent was requested. All consecutive referrals aged between 7 and 16 years were invited to participate and all agreed. All assessments were carried out before the children were seen by the plastic surgeon or received any laser treatment.

**PE group.** Over the same time frame 47 children (aged 7 to 14 years) with PE admitted to the plastic surgery ward in Edinburgh for corrective surgery were assessed by a child psychiatrist at the time of admission, using the same instruments. Consent was requested at the time of admission to the ward, and all consecutive admissions but one agreed to participate.

**Control group.** Thirty-two nondisfigured children, matched to the PWS group for age, sex, skin color, and social class, were recruited through two Edinburgh schools following approval by the Education Department Research Committee. The children were randomly selected and matched from the schools' registers and parental consent was sought. This group was assessed at the beginning of term or midterm when no examinations were current or pending. They were administered the Children's Depression Inventory (CDI) and the Revised Children's Manifest Anxiety Scale (RCMAS). The Harter Self-Perception Profile was not administered as local normative data were available.

**Demographics.** As this study was part of a descriptive account of children referred for plastic surgery, the original samples of PWS (n = 32) and PE groups ($n = 47$) differ significantly in demographic characteristics (Table 1). There were twice as many girls in the PWS group and twice as many boys in the PE group. Ages ranged from 7 to 16 years, though the PE group were younger. For these reasons, only certain descriptive comparisons of the two groups could be made. Social class was defined according to the classification of the Office of Population Census and Surveys (1980). The distribution of both groups across the social classes is similar. Because of the age and sex differences in the PWS and PE subjects, two subgroups of 21 children matched for age, sex, skin color, and social class were isolated for further comparative analyses.

## *Measures*

**Severity of disfigurement.** PWSs have a number of visible components that may influence overall appearance—size, position, type of stain, color, and local gigantism. These parameters were assessed and recorded by a plastic surgeon. Size was measured in square centimeters for the area of the PWS that covered the face or neck. Size was further grouped into four categories: small ($<10$ cm), medium (10 to 25 cm), large (25 to 50 cm) and extra-large ($>50$ cm). In addition, a composite score was formulated on the basis of the model proposed by Quaba (1989). The components of this score were size (small, medium, large, or extra-large); position (peripheral-hidden, peripheral-visible, central—not involving the eyes or mouth, or central—involving the eyes or mouth); color (pink, red, or purple); stain (confluent, confluent with satellites, or patchy); and presence of local gigantism (yes or no). The composite score was heavily weighted to reflect the importance of position and size to severity.

PE were assessed by a lay panel of three judges (a child, an adolescent, and an adult) who viewed standardized color photographs of the children with facial features obscured so that only prominence was rated. Degree of prominence was rated on a 5-point Likert scale. Interrater reliability results indicated agreements ranging from 0.37 to 0.63 and 0.57 among sets of judges. Results were analyzed for the three separate judges' ratings, rather than constructing a composite score.

**Self-perception profile for children.** The Self-Perception Profile for Children (Harter, 1985) is based on a multidimensional, developmental perspective of the self in which several domains of self-conceptions exist at successive portions of the life span (McGuire, 1994 Lerner and Jovanovic, 1990). The scale is a 36-item, self-completed questionnaire that

TABLE 1
Demographic Characteristics of the Samples

| | Port-Wine Stain ($n = 32$) | Prominent Ears ($n = 47$) | Age- & Sex-Matched Group ($n = 21$) |
|---|---|---|---|
| Sex | | | |
| Male | 7 | 31 | 7 |
| Female | 25 | 16 | 15 |
| Age | | | |
| Mean (yr) | 11.0 | 9.1 | 10.4 |
| Range | (7–15) | (7–13) | (7–13) |
| Social class, No. (%)[a] | | | |
| I | 3 (6) | 2 (6) | 1 (5) |
| II | 7 (15) | 4 (12) | 2 (8) |
| III | 21 (45) | 12 (38) | 10 (45) |
| IV | 6 (12) | 5 (16) | 3 (14) |
| V | 1 (2) | 1 (3) | 1 (5) |
| Unemployed | 6 (12) | 5 (16) | 5 (23) |
| Unknown | 3 (6) | 3 (9) | |

[a] Approximate percentages.

measures six subscales of self-perception: Global Self-Esteem, Scholastic Performance, Social Acceptance, Athletic Competence, Physical Appearance, and Behavior. Internal consistency reliability scores of .73 to .85 and convergent validity scores of .47 and .64 have been quoted (McGuire, 1994).

Hoare et al. (1993) administered this questionnaire to 5,000 children in the Edinburgh region (5% of the school population). Their study has provided recent normative figures from the local population. Among Hoare and colleagues' findings was that the Physical Appearance subscale was highly correlated with global self-worth. This supports Harter's claim that self-perceptions about physical appearance invariably account for the major proportion of the variance in feelings of general self-worth or self-esteem (Lerner and Jovanovic, 1990).

**Disfigurement perception scale.** The Disfigurement Perception Scale (DPS) is a 10-item questionnaire devised for the study and based on the literature concerning the problems that children with birthmarks have and on a pilot study of the questionnaire, conducted with 10 children with PWS. It measured the following: the degree to which the child is upset by the birthmark, the social consequences of having a birthmark, the effects of the birthmark on self-image and social image, and the use of camouflage and the desire for treatment. Each item was scored on a 0- to 2-point scale and was structured in the format of the CDI, where the child chooses between three statements, i.e.: "I rarely feel upset by my birthmark" (0); "I often feel upset by my birthmark" (1); "I always feel upset by my birthmark" (2). A test-retest reliability study ($n = 12$) conducted on each item of the DPS revealed $\kappa$ scores ranging from .40 to 85, with seven items having $\kappa$ scores greater than .60.

**Revised children's manifest anxiety scale.** This 37-item self-administered questionnaire measures different aspects of trait anxiety. Besides an overall anxiety score, it also yields three subscale scores: Physiological Anxiety, Worry and Oversensitivity, and Concentration Anxiety (Castaneda et al., 1956; Reynolds and Richman, 1978).

**Children's depression inventory.** The CDI, one of the most commonly used self-report questionnaires designed to measure childhood depression, has been validated and standardized in several studies (M. Kovacs, unpublished).

**Child behavior checklist.** The Child Behavior Checklist (CBCL) was completed by the parents of each child. It is usually referenced in the research literature to the normative data supplied by Achenbach (1991). It consists of 118 behavioral problem items, each scored on a 3-point scale. This gives a total behavior problem score and two broad-band subscale scores, Externalizing and Internalizing. Eight narrow-band syndromes are also derived: Withdrawn, Somatic Complaints, Anxious/Depressed, Social Problems, Thought Problems, Attention Problems, Delinquent Behavior, and Aggressive Behavior. Various forms of reliability and validity (including cross-cultural validity) studies have been documented and have supported the usefulness of the instrument.

### Statistical Analysis

Continuous variables such as self-perception and DPS scores are presented as means and standard deviations. For each of the two groups, means were compared by two-tailed $t$ tests to assess significant differences Relationships between severity of disfigurement and self-perception scores were determined using Spearman correlation coefficients. Statistical significance was set at $p < .05$. All data were analyzed using the Statistical Package for the Social Sciences (SPSS) (Norusis, 1991).

Although 47 children with PE and 32 children with PWS were included in the study, the numbers vary throughout this article for three reasons: (1) there was variable applicability of questionnaires to age ranges; (2) a subgroup of age- and sex-matched children from both groups was isolated for further analysis; and (3) a control group of 32 children was matched to the PWS group.

### RESULTS

### Self-Perception Scores

Self-perception results were compared to normative data (Hoare et al., 1993) drawn from the same population area as the PWS, PE, and control groups. Table 2 presents the self-perception results for both groups as standardized $z$ scores (i.e., where the normal population mean $= 0$ and its standard deviation $= 1$). Children with PWS scored significantly better on Scholastic Performance and Global Self-Esteem ($p < .01$) than the normal population. They also rated themselves as having higher Social Acceptance ($p < .001$). They did not rate their Physical Appearance lower than normal children rated theirs. In contrast, children with PE rated themselves lower than did normal children on athletic ($p < .05$) and physical subscales ($p < .01$).

TABLE 2

Port-Wine Stain and Prominent Ears Groups: Standardized $z$ Scores for Self-Perception
Compared to Normative Data

| Harter Subscale | Port-Wine Stain ($n = 32$) | | | Prominent Ears ($n = 41$) | | |
|---|---|---|---|---|---|---|
| | Mean | SD | $p$ Value | Mean | SD | $p$ Value |
| Scholastic | 0.54 | 0.91 | <.01 | 0.31 | 0.88 | <.05 |
| Social | 0.55 | 0.70 | <.001 | −0.03 | 0.96 | NS |
| Athletic | 0.36 | 1.02 | NS | −0.36 | 0.97 | <.05 |
| Physical | 0.26 | 0.97 | NS | −0.48 | 0.95 | <.01 |
| Behavioral | 0.28 | 1.02 | NS | 0.12 | 0.88 | NS |
| Global | 0.53 | 0.89 | <.01 | −0.07 | 0.86 | NS |

*Note:* NS = not significant.

As the PWS and PE groups were not matched for age and sex, we cannot compare them because any differences could be explained by either variable itself. Therefore, a subgroup of 21 children matched for age, sex, skin color, and social class was extracted from each group and comparisons were again made using a paired $t$ test. Table 3 shows that the PE group, compared with the PWS group, rated themselves significantly lower on Athletic Competence ($p < .05$) and lower on Physical Appearance (approaching significance), and there was a trend to rate themselves lower on Global Self-Esteem.

## Correlations

Figure 1 shows that there was no correlation between the size of the birthmark and Global Self-Esteem (each point on the graph represents an individual case). Nor was there any correlation between the size of the birthmark and Physical Appearance self-perception, the composite score and Global Self-Esteem, or the composite score and Physical Appearance.

There were no significant correlations ($p < .01$) between the position, size, or composite score for the birthmark and anxiety or depression ratings using the RCMAS and the CDI or parent ratings using the CBCL.

For the PE group, CDI and RCMAS scores did not correlate with the degree of prominence assessed by any of the three judges. Nor did CBCL scores correlate with severity, with the exception of Thought Problems ($p < .01$ for one rater but not the other two). Also, there were no correlations between the prominence of the ears and Harter self-perception scores.

## Perceptions of Disfigurement and Psychosocial Adjustment

The two age- and sex-matched groups were compared on the disfigurement variables of the DPS. The children with PE reported that friends make fun of them more than did children with PWS ($p < .01$). They reported that they dislike looking at their faces in the mirror more ($p < .05$) and reported more overall upset by their disfigurement ($p = .06$). Children with PWS were more likely to report that others like their appearance ($p < .05$).

Total scores for the DPS for both groups of children were correlated with the Harter scores (Table 4). Children who were more negative about their PE scored significantly lower on Physical Appearance than did children who were more positive ($p < .05$). Children who were more negative about their PWS scored worse on Behavior ($p < .01$) and on Global Self-Esteem ($p < .001$) than did children who were more positive. In other words, there was a correlation between being negative about one's birthmark and being

TABLE 3

Harter Self-Perception Scores: Comparison of Age- and Sex-Matched
Port-Wine Stain and Prominent Ears Groups

| Harter Subscale | Port-Wine Stain ($n = 21$) | | Prominent Ears ($n = 21$) | | $t$ Value | $p$ Value |
|---|---|---|---|---|---|---|
| | Mean | SD | Mean | SD | | |
| Scholastic | 3.10 | 0.59 | 3.02 | 0.52 | 0.51 | NS |
| Social | 3.28 | 0.51 | 3.06 | 0.57 | 1.60 | NS |
| Athletic | 3.12 | 0.70 | 2.61 | 0.62 | 2.82 | <.05 |
| Physical | 2.93 | 0.71 | 2.56 | 0.58 | 3.26 | .05 |
| Behavioral | 2.98 | 0.58 | 2.91 | 0.56 | 0.72 | NS |
| Global | 3.37 | 0.49 | 3.11 | 0.50 | 2.93 | .08 |

*Note:* NS = not significant.

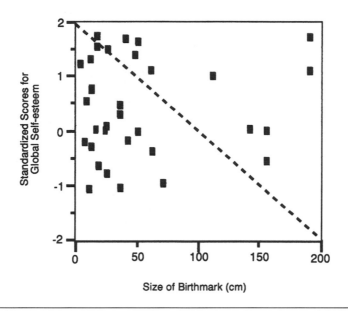

**Figure 1.** Correlation between Global Self-Esteem subscale and size of birthmark.

more globally negative about oneself. Figure 2 shows more graphically the decline in Global Self-Esteem as children become more negative about their birthmarks.

Children who were more upset by their birthmark (Q1 of the DPS) scored higher for Thought Problems ($p < .05$), Attention Problems ($p < .05$), and Aggressive Behavior ($p < .05$) on the CBCL. In addition, the PWS group's overall score on the DPS correlated significantly with the total CDI score ($p < .5$), total anxiety score ($p < .01$), Worry and Oversensitivity ($p < .001$), and Concentration Anxiety ($p < .001$). Against parent-rated CBCLs, the total DPS score correlated with the Total Problem score ($p < .01$), Externalizing score ($p < .05$), Attention Problems ($p < .05$), and Aggressive Behavior ($p < .01$).

The total DPS score for children with PE was related to the total CDI score ($p < .001$), Concentration Anxiety ($p < .05$), and parent-rated Social Problems ($p < .05$).

## Age Trends in Self-Perception

Although children with PWS appear to function well with regard to self-perception, it is important to look at how scores vary as children get older

TABLE 4

Correlations Between Disfigurement Perception Scale and Harter Self-Perception Scale for Both Groups

| | SC | SO | AT | PH | BE | GL |
|---|---|---|---|---|---|---|
| DPS (PWS) | −.35 | −.29 | −.34 | −.31 | −.59** | −.63*** |
| DPS (PE) | −.21 | −.27 | −.15 | −.34 | −.28 | −.21 |
| DPS¹ (PWS) | −.34 | −.19 | −.26 | −.18 | −.27 | −.38* |

*Note:* SC = Scholastic subscale of Harter Self-Perception Scale; SO = Social; AT = Athletic; PH = Physical; BE = Behavioral; GL = Global; DPS (PWS) = Disfigurement Perception Scale for port-wine stain group; PE = prominent ears group; DPS¹ (PWS) = the first question of the DPS.

* $p < .05$; ** $p < .01$; *** $p < .001$.

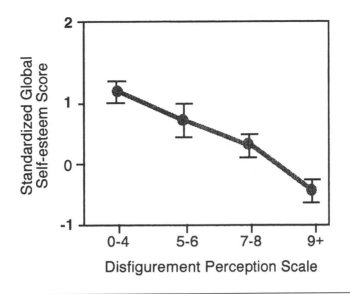

**Figure 2.** Relationship between Global Self-Esteem for children with port-wine stains and the Disfigurement Perception Scale (DPS). DPS scores are grouped by approximate quartiles. Global Self-Esteem scores are presented as means and standard errors.

and how they compare to normal children at different ages. For most of the subscales of self-perception, there was no difference in the age trend of scores for children with PWS compared with those of normal children, with one exception—Physical Appearance. For normal girls there was a decline in perceived physical appearance in late childhood and adolescence (Figure 3). But for the girls with PWS, whose Physical Appearance scores in early childhood were much higher than those of normal children, there was a plummeting in physical appearance self-perception from late childhood to midadolescence. The rate of decline or the angle of descent, compared with that of nondisfigured girls, is significant ($p < .01$). The numbers in each age bracket are, however, too small for anything other than tentative inferences to be made. There were no significant age trends for children with PE.

### Behavior, Depression, and Anxiety Scores

To compare CBCL scores for both groups with the published norms, standardized scores were calculated from the $T$ scores by subtracting the mean

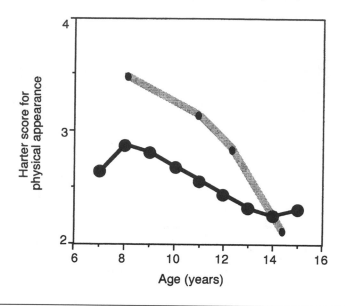

**Figure 3.** Age trends for girls' perception of their physical appearance. *Circles with light shading* represent the port-wine stain group. *Large circles with boldface line* represent norms Physical Appearance scores for girls with port-wine stains are grouped by approximate quartiles.

and dividing by the standard deviation of the published norms. Parents of children with PE ($n = 47$) and parents of children with PWS ($n = 32$) rated their children little differently from those of nondisfigured children of the same sex and age, with some exceptions. The narrow-band syndromes of Social Problems and Attention Problems were significantly higher for the PE group than for normal children ($p < .05$). Children with PWS scored significantly lower than the norm for Social Problems ($p < .05$).

Table 5 shows that children with PE had significantly more problems than children with PWS on the following scores: Total Problem score ($p < .01$); Internalizing score ($p < .01$) and Externalizing score ($p < .05$). In addition, they were considered more withdrawn ($p < .05$), had more social problems ($p < .05$), were more anxious/depressed ($p = .05$), and tended to be more aggressive ($p = .06$).

CDI and RCMAS scores for children with PWS ($n = 32$) were compared with those of an age- and sex-matched control group. There were few differences. Children with PWS had less self-rated Concentration Anxiety than did matched controls ($p < .05$). There were no significant differences

TABLE 5

Comparison of Child Behavior Checklist, Anxiety and Depression Rating Scales
for Age- and Sex-Matched Port-Wine Stain and Prominent Ear Subgroups

| | Port-Wine Stain (n = 21) | | Prominent Ears (n = 21) | | t Value | p Value |
|---|---|---|---|---|---|---|
| | Mean | SD | Mean | SD | | |
| **CBCL** | | | | | | |
| Total score | 46.7 | 12.6 | 57.4 | 10.9 | −2.9 | <.01 |
| Internalizing score | 47.6 | 9.9 | 57.3 | 10.3 | −3.3 | <.01 |
| Externalizing score | 47.4 | 11.3 | 54.7 | 10.5 | −2.1 | <.05 |
| Withdrawn | 53.4 | 5.3 | 58.1 | 6.5 | −2.4 | <.05 |
| Somatic Complaints | 53.3 | 5.5 | 57.2 | 12.2 | −1.6 | NS |
| Anxious/Depressed | 52.7 | 5.4 | 57.7 | 10.1 | −2.1 | .05 |
| Social Problems | 53.0 | 5.5 | 60.2 | 10.8 | −2.6 | <.05 |
| Thought Problems | 53.7 | 6.3 | 54.0 | 7.3 | −0.2 | NS |
| Attention Problems | 56.0 | 7.3 | 58.9 | 9.4 | −1.1 | NS |
| Delinquent Behavior | 55.2 | 7.0 | 55.8 | 7.2 | −0.2 | NS |
| Aggressive Behavior | 53.0 | 5.6 | 57.2 | 8.6 | −1.9 | .06 |
| CDI total | 7.3 | 5.1 | 8.4 | 6.7 | −0.83 | NS |
| **RCMAS** | | | | | | |
| Physiological Anxiety | 2.9 | 2.4 | 2.8 | 2.6 | 0.14 | NS |
| Worry and Oversensitivity | 2.8 | 2.7 | 3.3 | 2.8 | −1.10 | NS |
| Concentration Anxiety | 0.9 | 1.1 | 1.9 | 1.8 | −3.00 | <.01 |
| RCMAS total | 6.1 | 5.3 | 8.0 | 6.6 | −1.22 | NS |

*Note:* CBCL = Child Behavior Checklist; CDI = Children's Depression Inventory; RCMAS = Revised Children's Manifest Anxiety Scale; NS = not significant.

between the CDI and RCMAS scores for the subgroup of children with PE ($n = 21$) compared with a matched group of controls.

In comparisons of depression and anxiety scores for the PWS and PE subgroups (Table 5), the only significant difference found was that children with PE had higher levels of Concentration Anxiety ($p < .01$).

CBCL scores were correlated against self-perception scores using Spearman correlation coefficients. For the children with PWS, self-rated behavior problems were significantly correlated with externalizing symptoms ($p < .01$) and Aggressive Behavior ($p < .05$), while poor scholastic self-perception was correlated with Attention Problems ($p < .05$) and the Anxious/Depressed subscale ($p < .05$). For the PE group, lower self-rated Physical Appearance correlated with both externalizing problems ($p < .05$) and Delinquent Behavior ($p < .05$). In addition, self-rated behavior problems correlated with Total Problem score, Internalizing score, Externalizing score, Thought Problems, and the Aggressive Behavior subscale (all at $p < .05$).

## DISCUSSION

The literature on the psychosocial impact of disfigurement or deformity is controversial (Bernstein, 1976; Corah and Corah, 1963; Spriestersbach, 1973; Watson, 1964). Although adults with PWS are said to have high levels of psychological morbidity due to stigmatization, the results of standard psychological screening tests for psychiatric illness, depression, or anxiety were found to be similar to those for controls (Lanigan and Cotterill, 1989). Adults with PWS reported that as children they were acutely aware of the reaction of others to their birthmark (Malm and Carlberg, 1988). They were teased at school and asked intrusive questions by strangers. The term "psychological morbidity" mentioned in many plastic surgery studies is misleading, referring more to disfigurement-related stresses or social discomforts than to its standard meaning in mental health.

Although the results of cleft, craniofacial, hemangioma and PE studies (Bradbury et al., 1992; Brantley and Clifford, 1979; Dieterich-Miller et al., 1992; Doe, personal communication, 1992; Goodstein, 1968; Harper and Richman, 1978; Kapp, 1979; McWilliams, 1982; Pertschuk and Whitaker, 1982) suggest that children with facial deformity do not have serious psychosocial problems, there is some indication, if only anecdotal, that deformity has a more diffuse influence on feelings and the way the problems of living are approached. Deformity does "arouse social responses that influence life patterns in subtle ways" (McWilliams, 1982). Studies that have utilized less structured approaches to evaluation—for instance, psychiatric and behavioral observations—have found the facially disfigured to be overly conscious of negative reactions in others and unhappy as a result (Macgregor, 1951). Studies that have used checklists and standardized questionnaires may have failed to unearth more subtle and more "deeply personal anxieties" (McWilliams, 1982) such as these. Harper and Richman's work on social inhibition may reflect the subtle manifestations of distress for disfigured children (Harper and Richman, 1978).

The findings in this study reveal that children with PE have social, attention, and self-perception difficulties (athletic and physical), that is, the more "subtle" behavioral manifestations of distress. This supports the findings from studies of children with craniofacial deformities and cleft lip/palate which consistently demonstrate that these children have problems in social relationships. Thus, social acceptance is reported to be a problem for some children with cleft lip/palate (Goodstein, 1968); the more craniofacially deformed adolescent boys have problems with socialization (Pertschuk and Whitaker, 1982); and adolescents with cleft lip/palate experience more anxiety, ruminative self-doubt, and discomfort in interpersonal relationships (Harper and Richman, 1978) and less "global happiness and satisfaction" than their peers (Kapp, 1979). All these studies have methodological problems, yet the themes of diffuse unhappiness and problems in socialization recur.

Sociological studies emphasize the influence of the stereotype "what is beautiful is good" in shaping public views of the disfigured. However, it is not without its critics. Dermer and Thiel (1975) noted a dark side to the stereotype: "what is beautiful is self-centred" or egotistical or dishonest. In a meta-analytic review of research on the stereotype, Eagly et al. (1991) conclude that in large part the stereotype "what is beautiful is good" is correct but is highly variable, dependent crucially on the type of inference the perceiver is asked to make. Good looks induce strong inferences about social competence and less strong inferences about adjustment and intellectual competence, and they have little impact on beliefs about integrity and concern for others.

Nevertheless, sociological studies do suggest that unattractive children are disadvantaged in society, the facially disfigured even more so. Care, however, must be taken in coupling disadvantage with psychological morbidity. It is not the same thing to say that the facially disfigured who suffer social disadvantage suffer psychological distress. There is insufficient robust research to link the social disadvantages of disfigurement with psychological morbidity. Even were such a link to be proven, it would not of itself provide evidence for continuity but rather point to linkage, the nature of which may be direct or indirect. For instance, family competencies in coping with the birth and early upbringing of a disfigured child may provide a healthy environment for ego-functioning and self-image as well as a protective shell of family functioning within which the child may prosper. Although initial negative maternal reactions have been noted following the birth of a craniofacially deformed child (Clifford, 1979), long-term acceptance of these children in their families is the norm (Marsh, 1980). If familial rejection is occurring, then it is subtle and well hidden. Adolescent and adult craniofacial patients uniformly denied mistreatment by parents, though they noted some rejection by peers (Pertschuk and Whitaker, 1982). Compensatory parental coping may in large measure redress the deficits of disfigurement, at least for the younger child. Disfigurement is clearly a complex construct where many factors interrelate. Thus, it is not surprising that the research presented here reveals no correlation between severity of disfigurement and the degree of psychosocial distress measured on any of the scales used.

In addition, the results of sociological studies on attractiveness and unattractiveness should not be confused with the problems faced by children with PWS or PE. The equation "PWS child = unattractive child" is clearly mistaken. Some PWS and PE children are attractive, and "what is beautiful is good" may not be relevant to them.

The strong relationships found in this study between disfigurement-related stresses (measured by the DPS) and self-perception, parent-rated psychological and behavioral functioning, and child-rated anxiety and depressive feelings point to the complex interplay of psychosocial adjustment and the personal emotional management of disfigured appearance. The results do not, however, indicate the nature of the interplay of these forces or whether there is a common yet covert third factor. They do, on the other hand, indicate that clinically the child who answers affirmatively to the simple question "does your birthmark upset you a lot?" is less likely to be coping well than the child who answers "no."

The differences in results between the two groups in this study suggest that "disfigurement" is an umbrella term that covers a heterogeneous group whose problems may have subtle but significantly different influences on psychosocial adjustment. It may be that being "disfigured" (i.e., having a PWS) is different from being "deformed" (i.e., Crouzon's syndrome) and that having a PWS (clearly abnormal) is different from having PE (an exaggeration of the normal). It is possible that children with clearly abnormal disfigurements are more likely to receive uniformity of opinion about their disfigurement and uniformity of support from their immediate family than are children with deformities that are exaggerations of the normal. This may in part explain the higher morbidity in the PE group.

The close correlations revealed in this study between the DPS scores and Harter, CBCL, CDI, and RCMAS scores lend some support to the construct validity of the DPS.

There are a number of limitations in this study. A control group was used only for the measurement of anxiety and depressive symptoms while normative data were used in analyzing CBCL and Harter results. The evaluation of ear prominence must be questioned given the poor interrater reliability for one set of judges, though acceptable interrater reliability was achieved for the other two sets. A further limitation is that the numbers in the groups are small. PWSs occur in an estimated 1 in 3,000 births, so that getting larger numbers for research is problematic. The sex difference of the two groups represents a bias in referral as the incidence of PWS and PE is identical in both sexes. Hypothetically, this bias could indicate that PE are more of a problem for boys who, for instance, cannot so easily hide their ears behind their hair. The inherent problems of comparing outpatient and inpatient samples need to be stated. The groups may differ in motivation and severity. Furthermore, the population of children in this study is a select population. They have sought or been referred to plastic surgeons and may well differ from those children with PWS or PE who have not attended a clinic. Also, two different yet mutually exclusive dynamic routes for referral of disfigured children to plastic surgery can be conceptualized (Figure 4), making analysis and discussion of the findings more complex. Is there a difference in parental coping and resources between referred and nonreferred families? At present, there is no firm answer to this question. Only 1 family in 80 refused to participate in the study, suggesting selection bias toward the motivated, involved family.

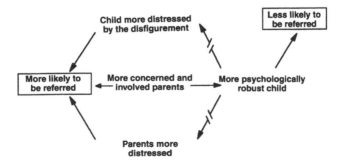

**Figure 4.** Possible characteristics of referred and nonreferred children with port-wine stains. *Solid arrows* connote positive influence. *Broken arrows* connote inhibitory influence.

Disfigurement is perhaps best understood in terms of risk and protective factors. A risk factor "is an element which, if present, increases the likelihood of developing emotional or behavioral disorders in children" (Grizenko and Fisher, 1992, p. 711). Risk factors can be defined as factors that increase a child's vulnerability in situations of stress. Protective factors, elements that modify, ameliorate, or alter a person's responses to stress act in counterbalance to risk factors. It could be that having good social skills and a significant adult figure in the life of a child with a PWS are protective factors. Understanding the complex interaction of risk and protective factors is beyond the scope of this study; however, a greater insight into the problems of disfigured children will doubtless require careful investigation of the interplay of disfigurement as a risk factor and family, socioenvironmental, and temperamental variables as protective factors.

In conclusion, children with PE do have problems with self-esteem. Their parents rated them as having significantly more social and attention problems than normal children and higher Externalizing, Internalizing, and Total Problem scores than children with PWS. They were also more distressed by their disfigurement and its effect on their lives than were children with PWS, who appeared to function at normal or above-normal levels, particularly in areas where decompensation could be expected. For instance, PWS children saw themselves, and their parents rated them, as being more socially competent than normal children. Do their high self-perception scores, low parent ratings of social problems, and normal scores on other indices of psychosocial adjustment represent an overcompensation process, where mental defenses or resources are channeled into vulnerable areas that can be bolstered throughout childhood in the safe protection of the family, only to be demolished in adolescence? Is there overcompensation or overcoping in these children and their families which does not survive the rigors of adolescence? Two threads appear to play a part. On the one hand, the ambiguity of support for children with deformities that represent exaggerations of the normal may impair the formation of a "stable, coherent self-concept," an ambiguity that children with PWS are largely spared (Kalick et al., 1981). On the other, appearance does seem to be a less salient issue for younger children—children regard their PWSs as less noticeable and less unattractive than do adults (Lanigan, 1991)—in contrast to the expanding world of adolescents, where they are neither known, supported, nor automatically accepted (Pertschuk and Whitaker, 1982).

The decline in self-rated physical appearance in girls with PWS from childhood to adolescence suggests that such a process may be the case for at least one aspect of psychological functioning. Remembering that the perception of physical appearance is most closely correlated with global self-esteem, then the consequences of such a precipitous decline in physical appearance for these children are obvious. Nevertheless, it must be remembered that this was not the case for any of the other parameters of self-perception.

To treat or not to treat? Children with PE referred for corrective surgery are likely to be having difficulties in some areas of their psychological functioning. However, the linkage may not be direct and the indication for surgical intervention would need to be based on, among other things, longitudinal studies that demonstrate postsurgery benefits to psychosocial functioning in the short, medium, and long term. Such studies with adequate methodology do not exist. What about facial PWS? There may well be "a medical necessity" to treat PWS. But is there a psychological one? If the trends toward a decline in physical appearance are replicated in a larger study, then intervention at an early age and before the disruptions of laser treatment upon school attendance intervene, could be justified but only if supported by longitudinal studies. Current results, however, do suggest that children with PWS referred to a plastic surgeon are not psychosocially maladjusted or in any psychological sense noticeably different from nondisfigured children. This does not, however, vitiate the suspicion that as adolescents and adults, people with PWS have subtle interpersonal difficulties and problems with psychosocial adjustment. It remains to be seen whether future research utilizing more sensitive measures for capturing "subtle" interpersonal difficulties can unearth the long-suspected difficulties of disfigured children and the adults they become.

## REFERENCES

Achenbach TM (1991), *Manual for the Child Behavior Checklist14–18 and 1991 Profile*. Burlington: University of Vermont Department of Psychiatry

Bernstein NR (1976), *Emotional Care of the Facially Burned and Disfigured*. Boston: Little Brown

Bradbury E (1993), Psychological approaches to children and adolescents with disfigurement, a review of the literature. *ACPP Rev Newsl* 15:1–6

Bradbury E, Hewison J, Timmons MJ (1992), Psychological and social outcome of prominent ear correction in children. *Br J Plast Surg* 45:97–100

Brantley H, Clifford E (1979), Cognitive, self-concept and body image measures of normal, cleft palate and obese adolescents. *Cleft Palate J* 16:177–182

Bull R, Stevens J (1981), The effects of facial disfigurement on helping behaviour. *Ital J Psychol* 8:25–31

Bull RH (1990), Society's reactions to facial disfigurement. *Dental Update* pp 202–205

Castaneda A, McCandless BR, Palermo DS (1956), The children's forms of the Manifest Anxiety Scale. *Child Dev* 27:317–326

Clifford E (1979), Psychological aspects of the craniofacial experience. In *Symposium on Diagnosis and Treatment of Craniofacial Anomalies*. Converse JM, ed. St Louis, Mosby

Clifford MM, Walster E (1973), The effect of physical attractiveness on teacher expectations. *Sociol Educ* 46:248–258

Corah NL, Corah PL (1963), Study of body image in children with cleft palates and cleft lips. *J Genet Psychol* 103:133–137

Corter C, Trehub S, Boukvdis C, Ford L, Clehoffer L, Minde K (1978), Nurses judgements of the attractiveness of premature infants. *Infant Behav Dev* 1: 373–380

Dermer M, Thiel DL (1975), When beauty may fail. *J Pers Soc Psychol* 31: 1168–1176

Dieterich-Miller CA, Cohen BA, Liggert J (1992), Behavioral adjustment and self-concept of young children with hemangiomas. *Pediatr Dermatol* 9:241–245

Dion K (1972), Physical attractiveness and evaluations of children's transgressions. *J Pers Soc Psychol* 24:207–213

Dion K, Berscheid E (1974), Physical attractiveness and peer perception among children. *Sociometry* 37:1–12

Dion K, Berscheid E, Walster E (1972), What is beautiful is good. *J Pers Soc Psychol* 24:285–290

Diwan R (1990), Laser therapy in the treatment of congenital vascular abnormalities. *Md Med J* 39:343–347

Eagly AH, Ashmore RD, Makhijani MG, Longo LC (1991), What is beautiful is good, but . . . : a meta-analytic review of research on the physical attractiveness stereotype. *Psychol Bull* 110:109–128

Goodstein LD (1968), Psychosocial aspects of cleft palate. In *Cleft Palate and Communication*, Spriestersbach DC, Sherman D, eds. New York: Academic Press

Grizenko N, Fisher C (1992), Review of studies of risk and protective factors for psychopathology in children. *Can J Psychiatry* 37:711–721

Harper DC, Richman LC (1978), Personality profiles of physically impaired adolescents. *J Clin Psychol* 34:636–642

Harrison A (1988), The emotional impact of a vascular birthmark. In: *Vascular Birthmarks: Haemangiomas and Malformations*. Mulliken JB, Young AE, eds. Philadelphia: Saunders

Harter S (1985), *Manual for the Self-Perception Profile for Children* Denver: University of Denver

Hoare P, Elton R, Greer A, Kerley S (1993), The standardisation of the Harter Questionnaire with Scottish schoolchildren. *Eur Child Adolesc Psychiatry* 2:19–33

Kalick SM (1978), Towards an interdisciplinary psychology of appearances. *Psychiatry* 41:243–253

Kalick SM, Goldwyn RM, Noe JM (1981), Social issues and body image concerns of port wine stain patients undergoing laser therapy. *Lasers Surg Med* 1:205–213

Kapp K (1979), Self-concept of the cleft lip and/or palate child. *Cleft Palate J* 16:171–176

Langlois JH, Downs AC (1979), Peer relations as a function of physical attractiveness the eye of the beholder or behavioral reality? *Child Dev* 50:409–418

Lanigan S (1991), The stigma of port-wine stains. *Br J Hosp Med* 45:274–276

Lanigan SW, Cotterill JA (1989), Psychological disabilities amongst patients with port-wine stains. *Br J Dermatol* 121:209–215

Lansdown R, Lloyd J, Hunter J (1991), Facial deformity in childhood: severity and psychological adjustment. *Child Care Health Dev* 17:165–171

Lerner RM, Jovanovic J (1990), The role of body image in psychosocial development across the life span: a developmental contextual perspective. In *Body Images, Development, Deviance and Change*. Cash TF, Pruzinsky T, eds. New York: Guilford Press

Macgregor FC (1951), Some psycho-social problems associated with facial deformities. *Am Sociol Rev* 16:629–638

Malm M, Carlberg M (1988), Port-wine stain: a surgical and psychological problem. *Ann Plast Surg* 20:513–516

Marsh JL (1980), Comprehensive care of craniofacial anomalies. *Curr Probl Pediatr* 10:1

McCabe M, Marwit SJ (1993), Depressive symptomatology, perceptions of attractiveness, and body image in children. *J Child Psychol Psychiatry* 34:1117–1124

McGuire S (1994), Measuring self-concept in children. *ACPP Rev Newsl* 16:83–87

McWilliams BJ (1982), Social and psychological problems associated with cleft palate. *Clin Plast Surg* 9:317–326

Nordlicht S (1979), Facial disfigurement and psychiatric sequelae. *NY State J Med* 1382–1384

Norusis MJ (1991), *The SPSS Guide to Data Analysis for SPSS/PC?+*. Chicago: SPSS Inc

Office of Population Census and Surveys (1980), *Classification of Occupations* London: HMSO

Pertschuk MJ, Whitaker LA (1982), Social and psychological effects of craniofacial deformity and surgical reconstruction. *Clin Plast Surg* 9:297–306

Pomeroy JC, Sprafkin J, Gadow KD (1988), Minor physical anomalies as a biological marker for behavior disorders. *J Am Acad Child Adolesc Psychiatry* 27:466–473

Quaba A (1989), Results of argon laser treatment for port-wine stains: a method of assessment. *Br J Plast Surg* 42:125–132

Reynolds CR, Richmond BO (1978), What I think and feel, a revised measure of children's manifest anxiety. *J Abnorm Child Psychol* 6:271–280

Spriestersbach DC (1973), *Psychosocial Aspects of the Cleft Palate Problem*. Vol 1. Iowa City: University of Iowa Press

Waldrop MF, Halverson CF (1971), Minor physical anomalies and hyperactive behavior in young children. In *The Exceptional Infant*. Hellmuth J, ed. New York: Brunner/Mazel

Watson CG (1964), Personality adjustment in boys with cleft lip and palate. *Cleft Palate J* 1:130–138

# 16

# Psychological Science and the Use of Anatomically Detailed Dolls in Child Sexual-Abuse Assessments

**Gerald P. Koocher**
*Harvard Medical School, Boston*

**Gail S. Goodman**
*University of California, Davis*

**C. Sue White**
*Case Western Reserve University School of Medicine, Cleveland*

**William N. Friedrich**
*Mayo Clinic, Rochester, Minnesota*

**Abigail B. Sivan**
*Rush-Presbyterian–St. Luke's Medical Center, Chicago*

**Cecil R. Reynolds**
*Texas A&M University College Station*

*Many devices are used in child assessment and treatment as communication aids, projective tools, and symbolic means of interaction. None are as hotly debated in their application among mental health professionals as dolls with genital details.*

Reprinted with permission from *Psychological Bulletin*, 1995, Vol. 118, No. 2, 199–222. Copyright © 1995 by the American Psychological Association, Inc.

This article is the work of the Anatomical Doll Working Group functioning with financial support from the American Psychological Association and consisting of William N. Friedrich, Gail S. Goodman, Gerald P. Koocher (Chair), Abigail B. Sivan, C. Sue White, and Cecil R. Reynolds. The content of this article is solely our work and does not necessarily represent the policy of the American Psychological Association.

We appreciate the detailed constructive critique provided by Barbara Boat and David Faust in response to earlier versions of this article and the sharing of ideas and works in progress by Maggie Bruck, Steve Ceci, and Paul Meehl.

*Anatomically detailed (AD) dolls are often used in sexual-abuse evaluation and treatment with children, but such applications are controversial. This article is the product of a working group formed to review AD doll research and practice. This article reviews historical use of dolls in clinical inquiry and research on sexual behaviors in children, normative use of AD dolls in nonreferred children, differences in children's play behavior and emotional reactions to AD dolls, and memory and suggestibility issues relating to AD-doll use. Recommendations for future research are provided.*

On February 8, 1991, the American Psychology Association's (APA) Council of Representatives formally adopted the following *Statement on the Use of Anatomically Detailed Dolls in Forensic Evaluations*:

Anatomically detailed dolls are widely used in conducting assessments in cases of alleged child sexual abuse. In general, such dolls may be useful in helping children to communicate when their language skills or emotional concerns preclude direct verbal responses. These dolls may also be useful communication props to help older children who may have difficulty expressing themselves verbally on sexual topics.

These dolls are available from a variety of vendors and are readily sold to anyone who wishes to purchase them. The design, detail, and nature of the dolls vary considerably across manufacturers. Neither the dolls, nor their use, are standardized or accompanied by normative data. There are currently no uniform standards for conducting interviews with the dolls.

We urge continued research in quest of more and better data regarding the stimulus properties of such dolls and normative behavior of abused and nonabused children. Nevertheless, doll-centered assessment of children when used as part of a psychological evaluation and interpreted by experienced and competent examiners, may be the best available practical solution for a pressing and frequent clinical problem (i.e., investigation of the possible presence of sexual abuse of a child).

Therefore, in conformity with the *Ethical Principles of Psychologists*, psychologists who undertake the doll-centered assessment of sexual abuse should be competent to use these techniques. We recommend that psychologists document by video-tape (whenever possible), audiotape, or in writing the procedures they use for each administration. Psychologists should be prepared to provide clinical and empirical rationale (i.e., published studies, clinical experience, etc.) for procedures employed and for interpretation of results derived from using anatomically detailed dolls (American Psychological Association, 1991).

This statement was the end result of a 4-year process and considerable compromise among competing political entities within APA. The goal of the proponents was to place on the record for the forensic community a statement confirming that anatomically detailed (AD) dolls can play an important and valid role in the clinical assessment of child sexual abuse. The statement also lists a number of caveats, professional cautions, and contextual concerns. Some members of the council opposed the statement as potentially restricting professional discretion or as creating standards that might lead to litigation against some practitioners. During the debate on the resolution, it became clear to many council members that there was no comprehensive review of the scientific and clinical knowledge base on AD-doll use in the scholarly literature. The council then approved funding for a group of scholars to prepare such a review. This article is the product of the working group.

It is well-known that young children's reports of events are often less complete than those of older children and adults. It is also well-known that cues and reenactment can at times result in elicitation of more complete information from children (e.g., Flavell, 1985; Kail, 1990; Piaget & Inhelder, 1973; Price & Goodman, 1990; Ratner, Smith, & Padgett, 1990). Moreover, there is little doubt that children's ability to express themselves in language improves with age. If AD dolls provide memory cues and a means for event reenactment, thus aiding the communication process, one might expect such dolls to be beneficial for obtaining information from children. Professionals who use AD dolls in child-abuse investigations emphasize these possible benefits (e.g., Conerly, 1986; Everson & Boat, 1994; Yates & Terr, 1988a, 1988b). Alternatively, there are others who view children as prone to sexual fantasy and highly suggestible. These people express concern that AD dolls may be suggestive per se and may stimulate sexual and other fantasy (e.g., Ceci & Bruck, 1994; Gardner, 1991; King & Yuille, 1987; R. J. Levy, 1989; Yates & Terr, 1988a, 1988b). These opposing views underlie much of the controversy regarding AD-doll use.

Other core issues in the AD-doll controversy concern interviewers' possible contamination of child interviews and their potential misinterpretation of children's responses to AD dolls. Interviewers who are not properly trained and victim sensitive may contaminate the validity of interview data whether they use AD dolls or not (H. Levy, Kalinowski, Markovic, Pittman, & Ahart, 1991). Similarly, clinicians who are unfamiliar with appropriate validity standards in the behavioral sciences may also be prone to justify a forensic determination of child sexual abuse on the basis of doll play alone where it may not be warranted (Wolfner, Faust, & Dawes, 1993). Because AD dolls are easily purchased and used with forensic diagnostic intent by individuals with little or no behavioral science or forensic training, considerable vigilance in interpreting data collected from using AD dolls is warranted. However, even if considerable vigilance is expended, psychologists must determine whether AD doll-aided professionals reach valid conclusions.

Differing perspectives on the benefits and dangers of using AD dolls in sexual-abuse assessments have resulted in a lively debate, and a number of pressing questions have emerged: Do AD dolls assist children in reporting or communicating about sexual experiences? Are AD dolls intrinsically suggestive of sexual acts? Are they suggestive only in the context of leading questioning? Are they suggestive only with young children? Are children so suggestible and prone to sexual fantasy that AD dolls elicit false reports regardless of questioning context? Is there a subset of children for whom AD dolls elicit false reports? Do adults misinterpret children's innocent behavior with AD dolls (e.g., exploration of the AD doll's orifices) as indicative of abuse? Are objections raised by some adults to the use of AD dolls on the basis of valid scientific principles? Are some adults so resistant to believing children's reports of sexual abuse that they focus on the potential for misinterpretation of AD-doll play as a way of dismissing children's disclosures?

The answers to these questions are not simple. Although it is difficult to avoid dichotomous thinking about AD-doll use, clearly there are both potential benefits and problems associated with it. In this article, we explore the historical use of dolls in clinical inquiry, followed by an overview of what is known about sexual behaviors in childhood. Next, we review studies on nonreferred and referred children's reactions to AD dolls and examine research on children's memory and suggestibility in relation to AD-doll interviews. Finally, we suggest productive arenas for future investigation.

## USE OF DOLLS IN CLINICAL INQUIRY

The use of dolls as tools in clinical inquiry with children has been documented since the 1920s (Group for the Advancement of Psychiatry, 1982).

Dolls and doll play have been regarded as integral tools and valued modes of interaction between mental health professionals and children since the beginning of the child-study and play-therapy movements. As early as 1928, Anna Freud acknowledged that work with children required "certain modifications and alterations" (p. 2) when compared to work with adults.

Although Anna Freud (1928) and Melanie Klein (1932) differed in their interpretation of the play situation, both agreed that the "play technic [sic] worked out by Mrs. Klein has the greatest value for the observation of the child" (Freud, 1928, p. 30).

> Instead of losing time and energy keeping track of the child in its domestic environment, we transplant at one stroke its entire known world to the room of the analyst without any interference for the time being. We thus have an opportunity to become familiar with its various reactions, the strength of its aggressive inclinations, its capacity for sympathy, as well as its attitude toward different objects and persons which are represented by the dolls." (Freud, 1928, p. 30)

Dolls are routinely included among the essential equipment for a playroom in which to interact with young children, and their use is consistent with any theory of psychotherapy (Edington, 1985). In the therapeutic context, dolls afford the opportunity to "recreate self, family, and day-to-day events" (Wright, Everett, & Roisman, 1986, p. 93). Dolls are an "expedient" by which the child "is given the opportunity to reproduce the exact mental mechanisms which are disturbing him [or her]" (Solomon, 1938, p. 492).

In the 1930s, researchers explored the use of other stimuli, such as drawings and photos, through which children could project their feelings and express their developing sense of self (Horowitz, 1939). However, in their assessments of the racial identification of African American children during the 1940s and 1950s, the Clarks (1958) returned to the use of dolls rather than more abstract representations. They used a simple paradigm in which children were asked to choose which one of four Black or White dolls most closely fit a series of questions designed to elicit preferences and identifications. The findings from these interviews were highly influential (Kluger, 1975) and, in fact, were ultimately heard in the United States Supreme Court in the celebrated case of *Brown v. Board of Education* (1954) to illustrate the damage created by segregation. Moreover, the Clarks's doll technique continues to be a popular means to study the racial preferences of young children as illustrated by research on the effectiveness of interventions designed to reduce negative racial stereotypes (Powell-Hopson & Hopson, 1988).

The collective experience of generations of clinicians as well as that of researchers in child development suggests that child's play is often a reflection of the reality of his or her experience (Sivan, 1991). In several contexts, dolls may offer children a means of expressing themselves when words are not available either because of limited vocabulary or warnings not to speak about a given topic, as is often the case in circumstances of sexual abuse (Sinason, 1988).

## EVOLUTION OF THE USE OF SEXUALLY AD DOLLS

Although there is no record of the precise date on which AD dolls made their appearance in clinical work, the best guess is that the first dolls specifically manufactured with genital representations appeared in the mid-1970s. Prior to that time, some clinicians may have used AD dolls that were individually modified for purposes other than sexual-abuse investigations. Although precise documentation is elusive, two historically separate events illustrate how use of AD dolls evolved.

The first occurred in Eugene, Oregon in the mid-1970s when Virginia Friedemann, a police detective, and Marcia Morgan, the director of a rape victim assistance program, recognized the need "to establish more clear communication between interviewers and children" (Friedemann & Morgan, 1985, p. iv) in cases of alleged sexual abuse. As a result, "natural dolls" were developed, and subsequently Friedemann and Morgan formed the first company to produce such dolls on a large scale. Other companies then followed suit.

The second historical line of AD-doll development was more serendipitous. In the late 1970s and early 1980s, Cleveland (Ohio) Metropolitan General Hospital (CMGH) was unofficially designated as the county's receiving hospital for the majority of sexual-abuse cases involving young children. Because there were no guidelines or specific graduate-level mental health training for evaluating allegations of sexual abuse, front-line clinicians were forced to create ad hoc methods of evaluation for significant numbers of young children. In struggling with this problem, it was noted that homemade dolls with anatomical details were used in some hospital locations as teaching tools to prepare children for impending medical procedures (e.g., catheterizations). A set of such dolls was secured for use in abuse evaluations by a group at CMGH. By 1983, AD dolls were a regular part of abuse evaluations with young children at CMGH, and data obtained in these assessments were routinely presented in court as indicators of sexual abuse.

Despite the early clinical enthusiasm, caution soon took hold. There were no scientific bases on which to reach conclusions using AD-doll data. The clinical sample was small, and there were no normative data on nonabused children. As a result, a study that became one of the first research articles published on AD dolls was initiated (White, Strom, Santilli, & Halpin, 1986), and a structured interview protocol was developed. There are undoubtedly more stories of how AD dolls became a part of local interviewing practices in cases of suspected child sexual abuse, but these two anecdotes reflect the evolution of clinical guidelines developed on an ad hoc basis out of urgent forensic and clinical need (White, Strom, & Santilli, 1985).

In the strictest sense, this evolutionary pattern highlights a significant ethical problem: how to develop new assessment strategies predicted on urgent clinical necessity while maintaining adequate scientific rigor. Because of the forensic events that routinely issue from disclosure of alleged sexual abuse, testimony and data on the basis of unvalidated and nonstandardized AD-doll assessments quickly made their way into the legal system. Some scholars have argued that application should "follow knowledge gained from research, rather than precede it" (Wolfner et al., 1993, p. 9). Although we agree in principle, practitioners on the front line of child sexual-abuse work were often in the position of choosing between urgent clinical need and ideal standards for development and validation of assessment techniques. In addition, as discussed later in this article, conducting normative research presents its own set of ethical and methodological problems. The significant ethical difficulty arrived when persons without scientific training or appropriate caution (i.e., police, child welfare workers, and others including, alas, some psychologists and psychiatrists) began using AD dolls as though almost anything done with them yielded data of intrinsic validity for evaluation of sexual abuse (e.g., see *In re Amber B.*, 1987).

In any case, by the mid-1980s, with increased reporting and investigation of child sexual-abuse allegations, the use of AD dolls became widespread. During this time, the issue arose as to whether AD dolls constitute a "psychological test" for sexual abuse.

## ARE AD DOLLS A "PSYCHOLOGICAL TEST"?

Over the years, one significant problem has been the assumption on the part of some that AD dolls constitute some form of psychological test with demonstrated potential for detecting child sexual abuse or for stating with a degree of certainty that sexual abuse occurred. Such assumptions are unfounded and dangerous for a variety of reasons.

To elevate AD dolls to the status of a psychological test grants implications of utility and benefit that are undeserved and without basic foundation. The National Research Council, APA, the American Educational Research Association, and the National Council on Measurement in Education have all endorsed the position that, properly used, psychological tests provide a better basis for making certain decisions than would otherwise be available (Committee to Develop Standards for Educational and Psychological Testing, 1985). *Psychological tests* are tools of measurement based on psychological science. Measurement is a set of rules for assigning numbers to objects or events such as behavior, responses to questions, and the like. A psychological test provides a set of standardized procedures for the presentation of common (i.e., standardized) stimuli with rules for recording responses to the stimuli and rules for then assigning quantitative features (i.e., a score) to the elicited responses. Clearly, AD dolls do not meet any of these requirements as yet (Skinner & Berry, 1993), although one can imagine developing a test that includes a standardized set of AD dolls. At present, AD dolls are not standardized as stimulus materials; they appear in many shapes, sizes, colors, and even have varying genital and related characteristics that may affect a child's perceptions and responses to AD dolls. The questions used to elicit responses, the question sequencing, and the positioning of an AD doll-aided interview in the forensic process have not been standardized, and no quantifiable means of evaluating responses has been proffered.

Although some suggested protocols for use of AD dolls have been published (see, for example, American Professional Society on the Abuse of Children's *Guidelines*, 1990; Boat & Everson, 1986; Friedemann & Morgan, 1985; H. Levy et al., 1991; White et al., 1986), there is no uniform acceptance of such suggestions. In addition, there is no documentation of validity of AD dolls or of these suggested protocols for forensic purposes. No one knows if different AD dolls lead to different responses by children, how varying the questions or their sequence causes children to alter their responses, or how these variables may interact with each other or the timing of using AD dolls in interviews during what may be months (or even a year or more) of investigative procedures.

Some may assume AD dolls are appropriately labeled if called a projective test or instrument. However, even projective techniques have a standard set of stimulus materials and specific rules of inquiry, and most have a set of scoring criteria. AD dolls have none of these attributes and cannot be said accurately to have been derived from or fit properly even on a post hoc basis the projective hypothesis (e.g., see Chandler, 1990).

In summary, the requisite information is simply unavailable and not known to be forthcoming to allow AD dolls to be used as a test (see Committee to Develop Standards for Educational and Psychological Testing's *Standards for Educational and Psychological Testing*, 1985, especially Part II, sections 6 and 7). Consistent with this conclusion, Everson and Boat (1994) found that none of the 16 published guidelines or the 4 unpublished but widely disseminated protocols endorsed use of AD dolls as a "diagnostic test."

If not a test, what are AD dolls? As Everson and Boat (1994) pointed out, AD dolls can serve a variety of functions, including (a) a comforter (e.g., to create a more relaxed atmosphere during a sexual-abuse interview), (b) an icebreaker (e.g., to introduce in a nonleading way the topic of sexuality and to convey that the interviewer is comfortable talking about sex), (c) an anatomical model (e.g., a model for body-part naming), (d) a demonstration aid (e.g., props to show and tell what happened), (e) a memory stimulus (e.g., to trigger memory of sexual experiences), and (f) a diagnostic screen (e.g., to provide an opportunity for children to spontaneously reveal sexual knowledge but with major reliance on children's verbal statements rather than their behavioral interactions with AD dolls).

In general, AD dolls might be considered a diverse set of stimuli that can function as communication and memory aids to children and other individuals who have immature language, cognitive, or emotional development or impaired communication skills. AD dolls are simply intended to assist in the communication process allowing children and others to demonstrate acts for which they have limited verbal descriptions and limited familiarity in life or about which they are too embarrassed to speak. How well they serve these functions and their effects on the accuracy and completeness of a child's recounting of sexually related events are the topics of other sections of this article concerning research on AD dolls.

## AD-DOLL INTERVIEWS: SURVEY FINDINGS ON USE AND PROFESSIONAL TRAINING

Given that AD dolls do not constitute a test for child sexual abuse and that no standardization exists, how then are AD dolls used in actual practice? How much training do professionals have in using AD dolls to interview children? What are the characteristics or features of the AD dolls used? In addition, what do professionals say they take as evidence of sexual abuse when children interact with AD dolls? For example, if a child inserts a finger into one of the doll's body openings, do professionals interpret such actions as a sign of sexual victimization? Fortunately, these important questions have been the topic of research.

In a survey of professionals in North Carolina undertaken in 1985, Boat and Everson (1988b) attempted to evaluate (a) who was using AD dolls, (b) what kind of training these individuals had received, (c) what AD dolls were being used, (d) how AD dolls were used, and (e) what criteria interviewers used to make judgments about children's responses to AD dolls. Out of 600 requests, they received replies from 295 professionals in the area of child investigation; child protection workers ($N = 92$), law enforcement officers ($N = 46$), mental health practitioners ($N = 60$), and physicians ($N = 97$). Of these, one third had used AD dolls for more than 1 year. Child protection workers were the most active users (68%), law enforcement next (35%), followed by mental health professionals (28%) and physicians (13%). Although respondents in all four groups indicated they intended to increase their use of AD dolls, the child protection workers and mental health practitioners were the most zealous advocates of escalating their usage.

When Boat and Everson (1988b) examined respondents' levels of training with regard to AD dolls, the authors' response categories ranged from "formal workshops" to simple "discussions with a supervisor or colleague." Even with this broad definition, however, fewer than 50% of each type of respondent, except mental health practitioners, had any training. Put in perspective, however, there were fewer mental health practitioners using AD dolls (only 28% of those surveyed). One also suspects that most of the reported training involved "discussions with a supervisor or colleague" or reading books on interviewing (Harnest & Chavern, 1985) as professional workshop training on AD-doll usage did not begin to appear until 1985 (White, 1985a, 1985b) and was not widely offered until the late 1980s. Those who had adopted some kind of formal assessment guidelines did not exceed 20% of the Boat and Everson sample, but the precise nature of the guidelines is unknown because the first published set came with Friedemann and Morgan's (1985) AD dolls.

The results of a more recent study by Kendall-Tackett and Watson (1992) of changes in professionals' training and AD-doll use can be contrasted with the results of Boat and Everson (1988b). In 1989, Kendall-Tackett and Watson contacted by phone 201 mental health and law enforcement professionals in the Boston area, achieving a 99% compliance rate for the interview. Seventy-three percent used AD dolls, and mental health professionals were more likely to use them than law enforcement professionals. Whereas Boat and Everson found that only 47% of professionals received training in AD-doll use, Kendall-Tackett and Watson reported that 97% of their interviewees had received training, often from more than one source (e.g., professional workshops and supervisors). Furthermore, 78% followed a standardized protocol. Several possible explanations for differences in their results compared with Boat and Everson's results include differences in response rate, cities, training opportunities, and the 3-year period separating data collection across the two studies. However, regarding the latter possibility, Kendall-Tackett and Watson noted that 59% of the Boston-area professionals used AD dolls for 4 years or more, indicating that timing between the two surveys cannot completely explain the discrepancies.

## Variable Procedures in Interviews

**Number of sessions and number of dolls.** At the time of the Boat and Everson (1988b) survey, single investigatory sessions with AD dolls were the norm, although frequency varied by profession (e.g., mental health professionals used a single interview 86% of the time; but for child protective workers and law enforcement officers, the figures were 48% and 40% of the time, respectively). By the mid- to late 1980s, however, many evaluators were recommending more than one session for investigating sexual-abuse allegations (e.g., Boat & Everson, 1986; White, 1986). Consistent with such advise, Kendall-Tackett and Watson (1992) found that 44% of Boston-area professionals present AD dolls for two or three sessions and 34% always have AD dolls present.

When AD dolls were first introduced, most practitioners recommended using a family cluster of dolls consisting of father, mother, brother, and sister figures (Boat & Everson, 1986; Friedemann & Morgan, 1985; White, Strom, & Santilli, 1983) to represent the nuclear American family. By the end of the 1980s, however, some were advocating for a larger set of dolls that would also reflect the living circumstances of the nontraditional family. For example, in their third protocol revision, White and colleagues (1987) recommended a set of eight dolls. Current practices vary widely, but our discussions with front-line workers suggest that most continue to use four AD dolls, primarily because of ease of availability (i.e., most manufacturers sell basic sets consisting of four dolls), convenience (i.e., storing and transporting) and cost (i.e., the average cost is $250 to $300 for a set of four).

**Matching race with victim.** Do evaluators match AD dolls racial characteristics with that of the alleged victim? In the 1985 survey by Boat and Everson (1988b), mental health practitioners reportedly did so 81% of the time, physicians 63%, child protection workers 60%, and law enforcement officers 43%. Throughout the 1980s, recommendations about race matching evolved from specific matching advice (Boat & Everson, 1986; Friedemann & Morgan, 1985; White, Strom, Santilli, & Quinn, 1987) to recommendations of at least having different races available (Boat & Everson, 1986; White et al., 1987), to actually presenting a cross-section of races representative of the child's community (MacFarlane & Krebs, 1986). However, Kendall-Tackett and Watson (1992) reported that 74% of their respondents still matched the complexion of the AD dolls with the race of the child.

Although there are no data to indicate what is typical practice nationwide, racial matching should be carefully thought out prior to the selection of AD dolls. First, one should recognize that AD dolls are manufactured in a variety of complexion colors and features, which are marketed as Caucasian, Black/African American, Asian, and Hispanic. When one considers that there are no validity studies to assess children's perceptions of such presumed representations for each manufacturer's product, trying to match the racial characteristics of an AD doll and alleged victim has no documented scientific or clinical basis with respect to a child's actual behavior. Second, the child evaluated may not have a single racial identity in his or her heritage or may be exposed to potential perpetrators of more than one race, or both. Thus, matching the child's and AD dolls' racial characteristics may wrongly imply that the alleged perpetrator is of a particular race. Third, there are no data to support the conclusion that children use the cue of race to represent the alleged perpetrator. If there is a mental representation or linking between the AD doll and alleged perpetrator at all (e.g., if abuse has actually occurred), the scientific community has yet to produce the data describing which children use what cues as representative. The implications of race matching are sufficiently complex that extreme caution is warranted. For example, one should not conclude that the use of any given doll from a multi-colored array constitutes valid or reliable racial identification of an alleged perpetrator per se.

**Body-part survey.** A body-part survey involves assessing the child's knowledge of body-part name and function. The first body-part survey known to have been incorporated into a set of guidelines was in 1983 by White, Strom, and Santilli. By the end of the 1980s, most guidelines (Boat & Everson, 1986; Friedemann & Morgan, 1985; White et al., 1987) recommended body-part surveys as integral components of an abuse evaluation, so the interviewer would know the child's preferred names for the parts which might be discussed in subsequent abuse disclosure and would have an initial assessment of the child's level of knowledge of sexual anatomy. Indeed, Kendall-Tackett and Watson (1992) found that the naming of body parts was indicated by professionals as the most frequent use of AD dolls compared with having children act out what happened or observing children in free play with AD dolls and that all of these uses were particularly likely with young children (e.g., children under 6 years) compared with children 6 years and above.

**Dressed or undressed presentation.** Whether AD dolls should be presented dressed or undressed has been a controversial issue since such dolls were first introduced. Friedemann and Morgan (1985) have continued to assert that presentation can be done either way without harm to the child's emotional development or to the investigation of the case. Others have argued for systematic undressing of the AD dolls (Boat & Everson, 1986; White et al., 1987) or having the AD dolls prearranged in various stages of undress. Boat and Everson's (1988a, 1988b) data as well as Kendall-Tackett and Watson's (1992) data indicate that most evaluators present AD dolls clothed. In the latter study, of the professionals who used AD dolls, 99% presented clothed AD dolls to children and 73% had children undress the AD dolls.

**Background knowledge or blind interview** .Should interviewers be blind to background information about the alleged abuse before interviewing children with AD dolls? Some professionals prefer to know almost nothing about a case except the child's name and age, believing (probably correctly) that the legal system will then be more willing to accept the information obtained (White, 1986). Other professionals feel that it is important to know something about the alleged abuse (e.g., Boat & Everson, 1986). Research specifically testing the value of blind versus informed AD-doll interviews has not been conducted.

### *Doll Features*

With the increasing reports of allegations of child sexual abuse, the demand for AD dolls grew significantly as the 1980s progressed. Not all who use AD dolls for investigative work use dolls that were specifically manufactured for this purpose. Of those in Boat and Everson's (1988b) survey who actually used AD dolls ($N = 119$), only about half were using a set specifically manufactured as AD dolls. Others used Cabbage Patch Dolls with genitalia sewn on, modified versions of Barbie, or some other readily available doll.

**Nonsexual.** A wide variety of features is available on specifically manufactured AD dolls. *Digitated fingers*: Some AD dolls are manufactured with totally gloved hands or thumbgloved hands such that there are no individual fingers. Others have distinct fingers created with internal wires such that the digits can be separated or individually bent into specific positions, or both. *Facial expressions*: AD dolls come with a variety of facial expressions; such as smiling, straight lipped, or a turned-down mouth; some have eyes gazing forward, others seem to glance to the side. *Facial parts*: Some AD dolls have all of their facial features designed in detail, and some are even accentuated by cloth design. Others have all the features painted on. Still others omit some features of the normal head (e.g., many omit ears).

**Sexual.** The presentation of sexual anatomy is the primary reason for the use of AD dolls. How these body parts are accentuated varies across manufacturers. Some are stuffed, some are given different colors from the rest of the doll, and some are drawn on the AD doll's body in two dimensions. Some have large body openings (e.g., mouth, anus, and vagina); others have no openings at all. Some of the openings are large enough to accommodate a child's finger but not an adult's finger. Some have secondary sexual characteristics, such as pubic hair and breasts. Although critics have charged that the sexual parts on AD dolls are exaggerated (Berliner, 1988; Freeman & Estrada-Mullaney, 1988), Bays (1990), the only study to evaluate the proportion of such parts, reported that the AD dolls had genitalia of proportional size to the human figure.

### Professionals' Interpretations of Children's Responses

**"Very convincing" evidence.** As part of their survey, Boat and Everson (1988b) asked their participants what they would accept as very convincing evidence of sexual abuse in 3- to 5-year-old children. All of the physicians reported that children who made verbal statements would be believed. Still, a substantial 88% of child protection workers and mental health practitioners would regard the child's verbal statement as very convincing evidence. Law enforcement officers were more skeptical; only 69% reported a willingness to accept verbal report unquestionably. If a child demonstrated sexual activities with AD dolls but made no accompanying verbal statement, children under 3 years were believed by only 25% of law officers and between 57% and 69% of the other professionals surveyed. AD doll demonstration with verbal description increased the perceived credibility to 56% (law enforcement) and as much as 76–92% for other professionals. The most convincing evidence with AD dolls was ascribed to 6- to 12-year-old children's reports that included verbal description. Whether the same data would be found were the survey undertaken today is questionable because of increasing challenges to children's statements in some sectors.

Interestingly, in a more recent survey, Conte, Sorenson, Fogarty, and Rosa (1991) reported that professionals rated AD dolls as the assessment tool most often used by them for evaluating child sexual abuse and rated children's responses to AD dolls as important in substantiating reports of child sexual abuse. However, these professionals also indicated that the latter responses were not nearly as important as other signs such as physical indicators of sexual abuse and age-inappropriate sexual knowledge.

**What is considered normal behavior?** Boat and Everson's (1988b) survey also produced data that described what professionals considered children's "normal" behaviors with the AD dolls. Almost everyone agreed that a child's undressing AD dolls and touching the doll's genitals were within normal limits. When, however, the child touched the AD doll's breasts or anal area, law officers were less likely to consider this normal, whereas most other professionals did. If the child placed the AD dolls on top of each other, 50% of the protective service workers considered this normal behavior, as did 39% of the physicians and 29% of the mental health providers. Only 6% of the law enforcement officers considered this juxtapositioning within normal limits. If vaginal penetration was demonstrated on the dolls, less than 15% of any professional group considered it normal behavior. Notably, there were individuals in all professional groups who thought that for 2- to 5-year-olds, the demonstration of sexual intercourse, oral-genital contact, and anal penetration were all normal behaviors. The accuracy of such beliefs may be contrasted with normative data obtained from children with no known history of sexual abuse, discussed later in this article.

So far, this review concentrates on survey data concerning AD doll use in actual practice. We now turn to the scientific research base relevant to AD dolls. However, before discussing such research, ethical and methodological considerations must be highlighted because these considerations mold and constrain scientists' efforts to understand the impact of AD dolls on children's play behavior and reports of sexual abuse.

## ETHICAL AND METHODOLOGICAL CONSIDERATIONS

Realistic scientific research is needed to answer important questions about the use of AD dolls in the clinical and forensic context. However, a number of ethical and methodological issues influence the definitiveness of such research. For example, investigators studying the normative behavior of children with AD dolls often hope to exclude from their studies children with a history of sexual victimization. Obviously, if a researcher wants to study nonabused children's reactions to AD dolls, it is important to have a nonabused sample. Although researchers can ask parents whether their children have been abused, it is impossible to know for certain whether abused children have inadvertently slipped into a sample. Parents may not know whether the child was abused or may not define certain actions as abusive. Moreover, the very act of asking poses ethical issues. If the family admits to sexual abuse, the researcher may be obligated to report it to government authorities. One way around this problem is to ask parents whether any one of a number of eligibility requirements, presented as a group, describes the child (e.g., Is the child mentally retarded? Is the child a fluent speaker of English? Does the child have emotional problems? Is the child a victim of sexual abuse?) without asking them to point out which question applied. Parents can also be forewarned during recruitment that they will be asked to sign a statement that their child is not to their knowledge a victim of sexual abuse and that suspicions of abuse must be reported to authorities under law.

In contrast, some investigators may want to study child victims' use of AD dolls (e.g., to investigate how abused children react to AD dolls). Again, the researcher is faced with the dilemma of knowing with certainty a child's abuse history. The researcher interested in child victims' AD doll use may also face a perplexing situation in determining who should provide consent for a child's participation in research. If the child is in state custody, must the child welfare authorities provide consent, or is it sufficient to obtain consent from a foster parent? Should the children's actual parents be contacted, even if they may have been involved in the abuse? Such decisions are typically negotiated between researchers and institutional review boards, university attorneys, and other various agencies involved.

Methodological and ethical concerns also affect the types of situations studied. There are increasing demands for research to be ecologically valid in relation to the context of child sexual-abuse investigations. For example, studies of children's memory and suggestibility have often involved artificial laboratory situations in which children are asked to recall words or pictures, thus limiting ecological validity (Goodman, Rudy, Bottoms, &

Aman, 1990). However, ethical limitations clearly exist with respect to the ecological validity of AD-doll research. For example, investigators cannot contrive a totally realistic forensic atmosphere in which parents believe their children have been abused. They cannot randomly assign children to abused and nonabused groups. Researchers must often walk a tightrope in trying to ensure that their studies are ecologically valid and that they respect participants' welfare and rights. There are dangers on both sides. On the one hand, if researchers put child participants in compromising situations, the children's welfare could be harmed. On the other hand, when studies do not sufficiently mimic actual forensic situations and their results are consequently misleading, reliance on such studies for determining forensic practice, influencing court decisions, and setting social policy could lead to grave injustices for actual child victims and innocent defendants. Some argue that it is impossible to generalize from studies of AD dolls to actual child sexual-abuse interviews because of the dramatic differences in context (e.g., Ceci & Bruck, 1993, 1994); this has not stopped some of these same investigators from applying their findings on AD dolls to legal cases (Bruck & Ceci, 1993). Although the issue of ecological validity is critically important, it should be kept in mind that there is not just one context inherent in child sexual-abuse interviews (Brigham, 1991). A range exists, and current studies may generalize about some situations but not about others.

With these considerations in mind, we now turn to a brief review of empirical studies that have explored children's normative sexual behaviors generally and then their normative behavior with AD dolls specifically.

## CHILDREN'S SEXUAL BEHAVIORS

A child's behavior with anatomical dolls is presumably related to a variety of factors, one of which is the extent and nature of sexual behavior exhibited by the child. Sexual behavior is influenced by the family context and the child's experience, normative or traumatic, with sexuality.

The family context is central to an understanding of sexual behavior in children. Mrazek and Mrazek (1981) discuss a continuum of acceptable sexuality in families, ranging between the extremes of complete permissiveness on the one hand and complete repression on the other. Families establish a "psychosexual equilibrium" derived from (a) the parent's sexual adjustment, (b) the child's developing sexuality, (c) the impact of the child's sexual development on parental sexual adjustment, and (d) the interaction triggered as the child's sexual development causes parents to reexperience memories and feelings related to their own sexual development.

Psychosexual development begins at birth, although there are few major changes in physical sexual development prior to puberty. Rutter (1971) reported that during the 2- to 5-year-old period, both sexes show increased genital interest and genital play. He also reported findings of sexual play or genital handling by male and female preschoolers, with male children exhibiting significantly more masturbatory activity. Interestingly, sexual anatomy content responses to the Rorschach inkblots are most frequent in childhood among 5- to 7-year-olds (Ames, Learned, Metraux, & Walker, 1974), perhaps reflecting the increased developmental curiosity noted by Rutter.

Other research suggests that some occasional sexual behavior directed at adults is common in young children. A recent study based on interviews with parents of 576 children, aged 2 to 10 years, found that a child's touching a parent's genitals was "not uncommon on an incidental basis" (Rosenfeld, Bailey, Siegel, & Bailey, 1986). Rosenfeld and colleagues undertook the data collection to provide a basis for testimony in a case of alleged sexual abuse and concluded that such touching could be a response to normal curiosity in a child.

In a random sample of 880 children aged 2 to 12 years, screened for the absence of sexual abuse, touching a mother's breasts at least once in the previous 6 months was reported for 31% of the children, ranging from a high of 48% and 44% of the 2- to 6-year-old girls and boys, respectively, to a low of 9% and 12% of the 7- to 12-year-old girls and boys, respectively (Friedrich, Grambach, Broughton, Kuiper, & Beilke, 1991). These findings are even more interesting given other data from the same study that established a positive link between sexual behavior in the home (e.g., family nudity, available pornography, opportunities to witness intercourse, etc.) and the child's overall level of sexual behavior as measured by a sexual behavior rating scale completed by parents.

Sexual games are a relatively common occurrence in childhood. Lamb and Coakley (1993) studied female college students' recollections of childhood sexual play. A total of 85% of the women studied remembered a childhood sexual game. The data also suggest a broad range of behavior, with six of the nine categories of play described as normal. These games included "playing doctor," exposure, experiments in stimulation (usually of the genitals), kissing, and fantasy sexual play. Normal play included slight persuasion or coercion. Gordon and her colleagues (1990a, 1990b) studied another aspect of sexual behavior (i.e., sexual knowledge) that is also critical for understanding normative sexuality, especially because clinicians have contended that precocious sexual knowledge may be a clinical marker for sexual abuse. Gordon's research with 130 children between the ages of 2 and 7 years revealed significant age and social class differences. A number of areas of sexual knowledge were studied (i.e., gender, sexual and nonsexual body parts and functions, sexual behavior, pregnancy, and abuse prevention). Although none of the children demonstrated much knowledge of adult sexual behavior, younger children generally knew less than older ones. Lower socioeconomic status (SES) children had less knowledge than children in middle and upper SES groups with respect to sexual body parts, pregnancy, and abuse prevention. This may have been because of more restrictive attitudes toward sexuality evident among lower SES parents.

Sexual knowledge includes knowing names for genitalia. Many families teach children idiosyncratic names for body parts. For example, Fraley and her colleagues (1991) studied genital naming among mothers of *nonreferred* children (that is, children with no known history of sexual abuse) under age 4 and found that only 30% of boys and 21% of girls had been taught to use the words *penis* and *vagina*, respectively. Fully one third of the girls and nearly a fifth of the boys they studied had been given no name for their genitals. A study that used AD dolls to evaluate children's knowledge of sexual body parts reported that among 2- to 6-year-old nonreferred children, names for the breast, buttocks, and penis were reported more accurately than for anus or scrotum (Schor & Sivan, 1989). Clearly, some objective basis for clarifying meaning would be needed in interviewing such children no matter how accurate their memories.

Overall, these findings suggest that, in normative samples, children will engage in exploration of genitals (e.g., playing doctor) and certain sexually related acts (e.g., kissing). It follows that children might also display such behaviors with AD dolls. The studies provide no evidence that children 7 years old or younger usually know about such adult sexual acts as intercourse, oral sex, or anal sex, which might make demonstrations of such actions with AD dolls more suspect. However, it is unclear when children start hiding their knowledge from adults. Furthermore, studies of children's interactions with AD dolls, reviewed later, indicate that some groups of nonreferred children may know more than the previous studies would suggest.

The studies previously mentioned indicate that a continuum exists of acceptable sexuality in families and of sexual behavior and knowledge in children. Sexual abuse would be expected to affect the continuum point on which a child's sexual behavior and knowledge falls. *Sexual abuse* is an event or series of events with psychological effects that vary along several dimensions or factors (for reviews, see Browne & Finkelhor, 1986; Kendall-Tackett, Williams, & Finkelhor, 1992), including traumatic sexualization, which involves the stress inherent in a precocious introduction to sexual behavior. Finkelhor and Browne (1985) identified several psycho-logical sequelae of traumatic sexualization (e.g., confusion of sex with love, increased salience of sexual issues, and behavioral manifestations such as sexual preoccupation, sexual aggression, and the inappropriate sex-ualization of parenting). In children, the sexualized behaviors that can fol-low traumatic sexualization include excessive masturbation or preoccupa-tion with one's own or others' genitalia; developmentally inappropriate sexual behavior with peers, younger children, or animals; sexual promis-cuity; and prostitution. In the most current and comprehensive review of the effects of child sexual abuse, Kendall-Tackett et al. concluded that sex-ualized behavior was reported more often in sexually abused than in non-sexually abused children, even when comparisons involved nonabused but clinical samples of children. Posttraumatic stress disorder-like behavior was the only other behavior to share this distinction. Although these be-haviors should not be used by themselves as confirmation of sexual abuse, they are important clinical indicators.

Consistent with Browne and Finkelhor's (1986) and Kendall-Tackett et al.'s (1992) conclusions, Gil and Johnson (1993) reported a study that was based on evaluations of children referred because of their sexual behav-ior. The children were grouped into four categories: normal sexual explo-ration, sexually reactive, extensive mutual sexual behaviors, and molest-ing behaviors. The large majority of children in the latter three groups had been sexually abused or exposed to high degrees of family sexuality or violence, or both. Particularly relevant to the AD-doll controversy, Browne and Finkelhor contended that inappropriate sexualized, aggres-sive play is the most reliable behavioral consequence of childhood sexual abuse. Presumably such play could be directed at dolls as well as peers and adults.

Does child sexual abuse result in increased sexual knowledge? Although an increase might be expected, one of the few studies to examine this issue did not uncover a significant difference in referred and nonreferred chil-dren's sexual knowledge (Gordon, Schroeder, & Abrams, 1990b). However, children who had experienced sexual abuse were more emotionally reactive than nonabused children to pictures depicting ambiguous sexual acts.

These studies are not without their faults. For example, empirical liter-ature regarding increased sexual behavior among sexually abused children has relied primarily on parent reports (e.g., Friedrich et al., 1992; White, Halprin, Strom, & Santilli, 1988). However, the empirical assessment of sexual behavior through direct observation of behavior in interview or play settings that include AD dolls is an even more controversial topic and is the focus of the next discussion.

## NORMATIVE BEHAVIOR WITH AD DOLLS

Research examining children's reactions to AD dolls has focused on a variety of sexually related and emotional behaviors exhibited by children when interacting with these special props (e.g., the touching of AD dolls' genitals, digital penetration, intercourse, and emotional reactions such as avoidance of the AD dolls). Table 1 presents an outline of these studies. In some studies, relatively large samples of nonabused children were observed under a number of different conditions, and their behaviors were

TABLE 1

Summary of Research Samples and Activities for Studies of Nonreferred and Referred Children's Interactions with Anatomically Detailed Dolls

| Study | Nonabused (*N*) | Abused (*N*) | Age | Gender F | Gender M | Type of observation |
|---|---|---|---|---|---|---|
| Gabriel (1985) | 16 | — | 2–5 | 8 | 8 | Free play Interview |
| White et al. (1986) | 25 | 25 | 2–6 | 29 | 21 | Interview |
| Jampole & Weber (1987) | 10 | 10 | 3–8 | 16 | 4 | Free play Interview |
| Sivan et al. (1988) | 144 | — | 3–8 | 72 | 72 | Free play Interview |
| August & Forman (1989) | 16 | 16 | 5–8 | 32 | | Directed play Story telling |
| Glaser & Collins (1989) | 86 | — | 2–6 | 46 | 40 | Free play with and without peers Interview in small groups |
| Everson & Boat (1990) | 209 | — | 2–5 | 103 | 106 | Interview Free play |
| Realmuto et al. (1990) | 9 | 6 | 4–8 | 13 | 2 | Interview |
| Cohn (1991) | 35 | 35 | 2–6 | 46 | 24 | Free play Interview |
| Kenyon-Jump et al. (1991) | 9 | 9 | 3–5 | 10 | 8 | Free play |
| Rudy (1991) | 10 | 10 | 4–6 | 20 | 0 | Interview Story telling Free play |
| Dawson et al. (1992) | 20 | — | 3–8 | 10 | 10 | Interview Free play |

*Note.* F = female; M = male.

categorized for the presence or absence of explicit sexual activity. In other studies, the frequencies of various interactions with AD dolls including sexual behaviors were compared in relatively small samples of suspected or confirmed sexual abuse victims and in matched control groups of non-victims (i.e., children with no known history of sexual abuse).

### Nonreferred Samples

How do nonabused children react to AD dolls? That is, what is the nature of children's normative behavior with these special props? This is a critical question because if nonabused children show evidence of sexual behaviors with AD dolls, such behaviors could be misinterpreted as evidence of sexual abuse. In an earlier article, Gabriel (1985) described observations of 16 nonreferred children, 2 to 5 years old, in free-play interactions with AD dolls. Gabriel noted that many of the children showed behaviors with AD dolls that might be considered "suggestive" of abuse (e.g., touching and commenting on the AD dolls' genitals and inserting fingers into the AD dolls' orifices); however, none of his examples are of children clearly depicting sexual acts (e.g., intercourse). Some of the ambiguous behavior evidenced by the children could conceivably be misinterpreted as signs of abuse (e.g., a 2.5-year-old child who said "choo-choo-ing" when asked what a penis is for and a girl who put a boy AD doll under her skirt). The author concluded that such behavior, combined with the "thought processes" of the young child, made evidence collected from interviews with AD dolls highly suspicious. However, for the study the observer "made a number of inquiries" about the AD dolls, but the inquiries were unspecified. This same observer coded the children's responses, but it is unclear whether the observer was blind to the hypotheses. Operationally defined coding categories were not presented in the article (although examples are given), and reliability of coding is not indicated. Furthermore, Gabriel's conclusion contains an untested assumption that some of the children's behaviors would be misinterpreted as signs of abuse. Thus, although the study provides interesting descriptive data and was the first of its kind, methodological problems limit the conclusions that can be reasonably drawn from it.

Sivan, Schor, Koeppl, and Noble (1988) examined the behaviors of a relatively large sample ($N = 144$) of nonreferred children with AD dolls in three within-subject conditions: (a) with an adult present, (b) without an adult present, and (c) without an adult present but with the AD dolls having been undressed during an interview in which body-part names had been reviewed. In general, the 3- to 8-year-old children found the AD dolls no more attractive than other toys provided; no instances of role-playing explicit sexual behavior and very few instances of aggressive behavior with the AD dolls were observed. The presence of a female as opposed to a male interviewer increased the likelihood that the children would interact with the dolls. Undressing the dolls also increased the likelihood of interaction, particularly of dressing the dolls, perhaps suggesting that the nonreferred children were less comfortable when the dolls were undressed. However, Sivan et al. did not provide details about such activities as touching the dolls' genitals or about other ambiguous behavior that could conceivably be mistaken by some for signs of sexual abuse. In addition, the sample group consisted of middle-class children only and, as acknowledged by Sivan et al., the conditions of the study did not mimic those of a child-abuse investigation. Nevertheless, the Sivan et al. study provided support for the claim that AD dolls in and of themselves do not lead to sexualized activity in nonreferred children.

Glaser and Collins (1989) observed a sample of 86 nonreferred preschool children in a play situation that included focusing the children on the novelty of the AD dolls and inviting the children to play with the dolls during several intervals of free play, undressing the dolls, naming body parts and their functions, and redressing the dolls. Although the two scorers were not naive to the hypotheses, independent coding by two scorers of the children's behavior, including touching of genitalia and so forth, was obtained. Results indicated that three fourths of the 2- to 6-year-old children spontaneously undressed the AD dolls, and 71% eventually touched the male doll's penis, whereas only 4% touched the vaginal opening. There was considerable variation in the children's responses to the genitalia (e.g., matter-of-fact noticing, avoidance, and excitement). None of the children inserted their fingers into the vaginal or anal opening.

In total, five children's play actions with the AD dolls showed sexualized qualities. Specifically, two of the 3-year-old female participants demonstrated an intercourse position (but not intercourse itself). One of these children also demonstrated hitting the adult female doll around the breasts. It was learned later that this child had been made to watch pornography at home, that her name appeared on a child-abuse registry, and that she had witnessed domestic violence against her mother. A third girl joined the adult dolls' genitalia and demonstrated kissing. The source of this 4-year-old's sexual knowledge remained unknown. A fourth girl, also 4 years of age, demonstrated "rocking in intercourse motion" (Glaser & Collins, 1989) with her own body when squeezing the AD doll. Glaser and Collins later discovered that the child had observed sexual activity between her brother and her friend. Finally, the most troubling case was a 4-year-old girl who, when asked about the function of the penis, proceeded to suck it. She later commented, regarding penises, that they smell and "they say open your mouth." When the child's parents were appraised of this behavior, the father admitted to having found his daughter examining his pornographic literature. (The family was referred to local social services.) These examples suggest that, for at least some children, AD dolls may elicit reenactment of sexual or aggressive experiences and observations.

Glaser and Collins (1989) concluded that although AD dolls cannot be regarded as a "clinically reliable screening test for sexual abuse" (p. 559), it was unlikely that explicit sexual play with AD dolls arises from innate factors or that the dolls lead the children to sexual play. Thus, they suggested that interviewers further explore the sources of learning that contribute to a given child's demonstrating explicit sexual acts.

Similarly, Everson and Boat (1990; Boat & Everson, 1994a) examined the behaviors of 209 nonreferred children, ages 2 to 5 years old, who were screened for possible sexual abuse under free-play and directed-play conditions. The latter included the prompt "show me what the dolls can do together." The authors found that 6% (12 children) "demonstrated behavior clearly depicting sexual intercourse" (Everson & Boat, 1990, p. 741) across free- and directed-play conditions. None of the 2-year-olds demonstrated clear intercourse positioning. However, 18% of the 5-year-olds showed suggestive intercourse positioning when the interviewer was present, and 12% of the 5-year-olds showed clear intercourse positioning when alone. Notably, as age increased, there was a greater likelihood that the child when left alone would demonstrate intercourse positioning. Genital intercourse positioning was more likely to occur than either oral or anal intercourse positioning. African American children with low SES backgrounds were more likely than both their middle-class African American peers and Caucasian peers to demonstrate clear intercourse positioning. Male children were equally likely to demonstrate clear intercourse positioning whether the interviewer was present or not, whereas female children were only seen to do so when left alone with the AD dolls.

Boat and Everson (1994a) concluded that there was little support for the idea that exposure to the AD dolls induced sexually naive children to fantasize about sex or to act in sexually explicit ways. However, they did suggest that AD dolls "do provide sexually knowledgeable children with at least implicit permission and perhaps, encouragement to reveal their knowledge of sexuality in play" (Everson & Boat, 1990, p. 741). These authors, like Glaser and Collins (1989), were able to identify "relatively benign" sources for the sexual behaviors demonstrated (e.g., exposure to pornography and observation of sexual behavior among teenage relatives).

In addition, Boat and Everson observed that explicit sexual play varied with the child's age and family characteristics, leading the authors to suggest that there may be a need for differential norms to interpret AD-doll play of children from different backgrounds (Everson & Boat, 1990, p. 742).

Boat and Everson (1989) conducted follow-up evaluations with 10 *demonstrators*, 10 *avoiders*, and 20 controls from the original 209 individuals. Sixteen months later, all three groups still exhibited similar behaviors. None of the children were avoidant of the AD dolls; about 25% of the controls and 20% of the demonstrators showed explicit sexual positioning. None of the avoiders showed the dolls in sexualized positions. Questions were also asked to ascertain the sources of the children's knowledge of genital intercourse. Avoiders had less explicit sexual knowledge than did the other groups, an observation confirmed by their parents, who reported never having given their children descriptions of sexual intercourse.

Finally, Dawson, Vaughan, and Wagner (1992) examined 20 nonreferred, middle-class Caucasian children's interactions with AD dolls. The children named body parts on the AD dolls, demonstrated with dressed and then undressed AD dolls such activities as what the child and the child's father do alone together, and engaged in free play. There were no instances of children reenacting sexual intercourse, oral sex, or fondling. Low levels of sexual aggression (e.g., hitting the dolls' genitals) were observed; high levels of sexual exploratory play and nonsexual aggression were reported, especially when the AD dolls were undressed. This small sample study again shows low levels of explicit sexual demonstration with AD dolls in middle-class, Caucasian preschool children whose families agreed to participation in such research projects.

In summary, normative studies of children's interactions with AD dolls have focused on spontaneous and directed play in nonreferred children, analyzing the children's behavior for evidence of sexualized or aggressive play. Virtually all of these studies found that many of the children inspected and touched sexual body parts. However, play demonstrating explicit sexual activity such as intercourse or oral-genital contact was rare in these nonreferred samples. The exception was a study in which the children were primed with the prompt "show me what these dolls can do together." In the study, a group of low SES African-American male 5-year-olds displayed clear sexual intercourse positioning at rates higher than their more socially advantaged peers.

In drawing conclusions from extant research, one must keep in mind that most studies have not varied such background factors as SES and ethnicity, which Everson and Boat's (1990) results indicate may be significant influences on children's behavior. In future research, it will be important for investigators to include a diverse, representative sample of nonabused children and specify clearly the refusal rate or to target certain groups of children who are likely to become involved in child sexual-abuse investigations. Studies of children's normative behavior with AD dolls have not attempted to mimic the context created by actual child-abuse investigations and have not systematically varied the extent of children's exposure to AD dolls. Non-abused children's behavior with these dolls may be affected by such factors.

### Referred Versus Nonreferred Groups

A related area of research focuses on comparing referred and nonreferred children's behavior with AD dolls. The main goal of such research is to determine whether abused and nonabused children interact differently with AD dolls. White et al. (1986) conducted the first systematic study comparing the behavior of children suspected of being sexually abused (*referred*) with the behavior of children with no known history of sexual abuse (*nonreferred*). The researchers used a structured AD-doll interview and compared the responses of twenty-five 2- to 6-year-old children referred for abuse evaluations with the responses of 25 nonreferred children of the same ages. Using a 5-point scale with indicators ranging from *no suspicion* to *very high suspicion*, the authors reported that the nonreferred group had a significantly lower rating of suspected abuse as indicated by sexually explicit behaviors demonstrated with AD dolls. The 3-year-olds were the most reactive to sexual features on the dolls.

Jampole and Weber (1987), with a small sample of 10 referred and 10 nonreferred children between the ages of 3 and 8 years, introduced the children to the AD dolls and asked them to name body parts. The children were then left to play with the dolls for 15 min without an adult present; after the 15 min, the researcher returned to the playroom, and the child was allowed to continue playing for 1 hr from the beginning of the session. Ninety percent of sexually abused children demonstrated sexual behaviors with the AD dolls, whereas only 20% of the nonreferred children ($N = 2$) showed these behaviors. Increased sexual behavior with the dolls was noted when the researcher was out of the room. The sample in this study raises questions of ascertainment bias because the nonabused children were either the sons or daughters of social service agency employees or were in legal custody of social services for reasons other than sexual abuse. Not only was the sample of nonreferred children unrepresentative of such children generally but also the sampling raises questions about whether the nonreferred children in state custody who demonstrated sexual acts were in fact undetected victims of sexual abuse or had been prematurely exposed to sexual behavior in other ways.

August and Forman (1989) conducted another comparative study of referred and nonreferred children. Two groups, each with 16 girls between the ages of 5 and 8 years, were presented with a set of AD dolls and an extra set of clothes. The children were asked to change the clothes on the dolls when the examiner left the room; on the examiner's return, the children were asked to tell a story about the family of AD dolls. Results indicated that when left alone, the referred children played less with the dolls but were more aggressive and investigated the genital parts more than the nonreferred children. The authors concluded that children referred for evaluation of suspected sexual abuse respond differently than nonreferred children to AD dolls, particularly when left alone with the dolls. Furthermore, they suggested that there may be a subgroup of sexually abused children who respond with high levels of aggression and another subgroup that is avoidant of interaction with AD dolls. The small sample size, as well as the lack of delineation of the participants' characteristics, was a significant limitation to the conclusive statements on the basis of this study, as was the use of parametric statistics in a study with category data.

Rudy (1991) also compared referred and nonreferred children's behavior with AD dolls in a study that included twenty 4- to 6-year-old girls matched in age, race, SES, and receptive vocabulary. Children's behavior with AD dolls was observed during a three-phase session, consisting of AD-doll introduction and body-part naming, the child telling a story with the AD dolls, and the child being left alone with the AD dolls. Children's behavior with AD dolls was coded by raters naive to the children's abuse status and to the study's hypotheses. Referred children displayed significantly more sexualized behavior with AD dolls than did nonreferred children during the introductory and body-part naming phase but not during the other two phases. Moreover, referred children engaged in sexual behavior for longer periods of time than did nonreferred children, and they also engaged in more and longer aggressive behavior toward the AD dolls than did nonreferred children. The two groups of children did not significantly differ in exploration of the AD dolls' sexual parts. Thus, despite the small sample size (10 children in each group) and despite the limited amount of time referred children spent engaging in sexualized and aggressive behaviors (i.e., $M = 3.5$ and 1 s, respectively), significant differences in sexual and aggressive behaviors were obtained. Rudy concluded that referred children exhibit different behaviors with AD dolls than do nonreferred children.

Although significant differences in referred and nonreferred children's behavior with AD dolls were detected in the previous studies, such differences are not always found. For example, Cohn (1991) compared the behaviors of 36 children referred for suspected abuse with 36 nonreferred children matched on age and gender. No statistically significant differences were reported between the groups; however, similar to Everson and Boat's (1990) results, trends in the data and demographic differences lead Cohn to suggest further studies of the linkage between sexuality in the home and AD-doll interactions of young children.

Kenyon-Jump, Burnette, and Robertson (1991) compared the behaviors of nine sexually abused preschoolers with nine control children matched on age, gender, race, family status, and SES. Like Cohn (1991), Kenyon-Jump and colleagues found no statistically significant difference in explicit sexual behavior. Suspicious behaviors such as putting one's hands between one's legs when combined with explicit sexual behavior did yield a statistically significant difference between the groups, despite the small sample size; this finding was not explained by the authors.

Finally, a lack of difference in AD-doll interaction was also noted between two small samples of emotionally disturbed preschoolers: one group of children who had been sexually abused and another who had not (Allen, Jones, & Nash, 1989). Allen et al. suggested that pathogenic family histories may mask the differences seen with samples not matched on degree of family disturbance.

An important question related to the one previously addressed concerns professionals' ability to reliably categorize a child as abused or nonabused on the basis of the child's behavior with AD dolls. Realmuto and his colleagues (Realmuto, Jensen, & Wescoe, 1990; Realmuto & Wescoe, 1992) studied a small group of 15 children under the age of 7 years, including 6 children with a documented history of sexual abuse and 9 without a known history, with the purpose of examining the reliability of professional decision making when using AD dolls as "a sole test of sexual abuse." The children were interviewed with a standardized protocol that avoided direct questioning about abuse incidents. Instead, Realmuto and colleagues analyzed the children's spontaneous remarks and the behaviors elicited in 15-min interactions with AD dolls. The interviewer was blind to the abuse status of the child and rated the child's interview according to the criteria provided by White et al. (1986). Proper classification was obtained for 53% of the sample. When 14 professionals rated the interview, there was little agreement in their determinations ($\kappa = .355$), a finding that lead the authors (Realmuto & Wescoe, 1992) to conclude that discrepancies in training and experience may be contributing to the variance. The authors made several useful suggestions about the direction of research on clinical decision making and determinations of child sexual abuse, but because of experimental constraints (e.g., no abuse-oriented questions and brief interviews), care should be taken regarding generalized application of these results.

Two studies provide information regarding front-line clinical use of AD dolls when suspicions of abuse arise. Although these studies do not technically compare referred with nonreferred children, they may have included both groups because abuse was not yet verified. Regardless, the studies provide important information concerning the amount of information obtained from children in sexual-abuse assessments conducted with and without AD dolls. Leventhal, Hamilton, Rekedal, Tebano-Micci, and Eyster (1989) examined records of interviews with young children (under 7 years old) who had been seen for sexual-abuse evaluations. The children had been interviewed first without and then with AD dolls. Unfortunately, the confounding of order-of-interview format and AD-doll use makes it difficult to distinguish AD-doll versus reinterviewing effects. In any case, without the dolls, 13% gave detailed descriptions of the alleged abusive behavior. In contrast, 48% of these children reported details of the alleged abuse when interviewed with the dolls. In the no AD-doll condition, the alleged perpetrator was named 32% of the time, whereas 67% of those in the AD-doll condition named the alleged abuser. If the adult who accompanied the child strongly suspected abuse, the child was more likely to provide a detailed description with AD dolls; this result could reflect either a suggestibility effect on the child's part or a valid suspicion of abuse and greater parental support on the adult's part (Lawson & Chaffin, 1992).

Unfortunately, the authors did not present information about whether the adults' suspicions of abuse correlated with objective indicators of abuse, such as physical findings; detailed description and demonstration of abuse were unrelated to the presence of physical evidence. Children were more likely to be rated as definitely abused when the AD-doll information was included in the assessment than when it was excluded, and of the children considered to have been definitely abused, 38% did not provide evidence of abuse except during the AD-doll interview. These results led the investigators to conclude that the use of the AD dolls gave the children the freedom to provide more details of their experiences. The authors did note, however, that children younger than 3 years old were generally unable to provide detailed verbal descriptions about the alleged abuse experience under either condition, although a number of these young children demonstrated what had allegedly happened when provided with AD dolls.

However, in a study conducted by Britton and O'Keefe (1991), 2- to 10-year-old children were interviewed with either AD dolls or nondetailed dolls (e.g., regular Ken and Barbie or Cabbage Patch). In general, there was no difference between the AD dolls and other dolls in eliciting information; two thirds of each group were able to give detailed accounts. Girls tended to use AD dolls as props to report their allegations, whereas boys were more likely to describe their experiences using nondetailed dolls (66% vs. 44%).

In summary, although a number of studies have uncovered significant differences between referred and nonreferred children's interactions with AD dolls, the findings are mixed. The diversity of findings across studies of referred and nonreferred children's displays of sexual behaviors with AD dolls are not surprising. The studies differ widely in the size and composition of their samples and the methodology used. One would not expect all sexually abused children to display increased sexual behavior with AD dolls. Likewise, one might expect that certain groups of nonabused children will show evidence of more sexualized behavior than other nonabused groups. Interestingly, in a number of studies in which no difference was found, the data point to the possible importance of family circumstances or psychological disturbance in nonabused samples as contributing to a lack of difference between referred and nonreferred children's display of sexual behavior with AD dolls.

The studies are also in general agreement in several respects. First, clearly using AD dolls in evaluations does not inherently distress or overstimulate children. Second, using the dolls can clearly assist in identifying children's preferred or idiosyncratic names for body parts. Third, using AD dolls often results in increased verbal productions during standardized research interviews. Regarding the important question of whether more or less accurate determinations of child sexual abuse are made when children are interviewed with AD dolls, the studies by Leventhal et al. (1989) provide relevant information but not conclusive answers. The clear message is consistent with a key point in the statement adopted by the APA Council and presented at the beginning of this article: "Such dolls may be useful in helping children to communicate when their language skills or emotional concerns preclude direct verbal responses. These dolls may also be useful communication props" (American Psychological Association, 1991, p. 722).

## MEMORY AND SUGGESTIBILITY CONCERNS

A central concern about the role of AD dolls in forensic interviews is that children's memory may be contaminated and their suggestibility increased when AD dolls are introduced to the interview context. What does research indicate about the impact of AD dolls on children's memory and suggestibility? As an important backdrop for answering this question, we first consider certain legal issues and interviewing practices that influence the research questions asked and the procedures used. We then discuss several critical issues concerning children's cognitive development, memory, and suggestibility as they relate to children's use of AD dolls. Finally, we review studies that specifically investigated effects of AD dolls on children's memory reports and suggestibility.

### Legal Issues and Interviewing Considerations Relevant to Children

Concerns about children's memory and suggestibility play a prominent role in investigations and trials of child sexual abuse, whether AD dolls are involved or not. However, these concerns may be exacerbated when AD dolls are used. Prosecutors report that when child sexual-abuse cases go to trial, defense attorneys "almost always" or "frequently" challenge the accuracy of a child victim—witness's testimony by asserting, for example, that the child's memory is inaccurate or that the child was led or coached into making a false allegation, is confused (e.g., confused a sexual dream with reality), or is identifying the wrong person (see Goodman, 1993). Moreover, although prosecutors report that AD dolls are useful in reducing children's trauma when testifying, they also report that such use is a source of defense challenges.

Although a number of legal issues are relevant to a general discussion of children's memory and suggestibility when AD dolls are used in interviews, such discussion would lead too far afield. The issues of leading questions and coercive interviewing require mention, however. There is substantial concern that *leading questions* may be necessary to facilitate disclosure of abuse by some children in formal legal settings (e.g., Keary & Fitzpatrick, 1994), but such leading questions may also result in false reports by nonabused children, especially when AD dolls are used (Raskin & Yuille, 1989). Thus, it is important to understand what constitutes a leading question from a legal perspective. Although a precise definition remains elusive, questions that introduce or imply information not already offered by a witness are typically considered leading. Under this nebulous definition, if a child were asked "What happened?" (an open-ended question) and then "What else happened?" (which might seem innocuous enough), the latter question can technically be defined as leading. A question that included specific reference to a person and an act (e.g., "Did Uncle Henry touch your bottom?") would be a relatively clear case of a leading question. Because so many questions qualify as leading, interviewers face a challenging task in questioning children. In any case, when leading questions are combined with AD dolls in an interview, the child's credibility as a witness may be especially likely to come under forensic attack.

Legal and psychological debate also revolves around what constitutes a coercive or contaminated interview versus a supportive or sufficiently probing interview (e.g., White & Quinn, 1988). In actual cases, *coercive-interviewing* techniques have been used in conjunction with AD dolls (e.g., *State of New Jersey v. Michaels*, 1993). Many would agree that when interviewers pressure children (e.g., "Tell me about the time he kissed you and then you can go home") or badger children with overly repeated questions about the abuse but not taking no for an answer, such techniques add to the leading nature of an interview (Quinn, White, & Santilli, 1989; White & Quinn, 1988); how often such techniques are actually used with AD dolls and how often they result in false reports of abuse is a related but distinct issue, however. Ironically, the same techniques that some consider coercive and that may result in inaccuracies from nonabused children might be successful in obtaining accurate and complete information from frightened, embarrassed, or guilt-ridden children (Goodman & Clarke-Stewart, 1991). Research empirically validating what constitutes coercive versus sufficiently probing techniques concerning sexual experiences is surprisingly sparse. Keep in mind, however, that the relevant concern for research on AD dolls is whether AD dolls add to error rates above the use of leading questions and coercive-interviewing techniques. Ideally, appropriate comparisons should be included within studies (e.g., examination of effects of leading questions with vs. without AD dolls); unfortunately, they too seldom are.

Willingness to use leading questions, AD dolls, and even coercive techniques in an interview may be influenced by concern about how to balance risks of false reports versus risks of continued abuse. Professionals and laypersons differ in how they weigh these two risks. Some appear more willing to err on the side of child protection, whereas others appear more willing to err on the side of protecting the rights of defendants (e.g., Bottoms, 1993; Finlayson & Koocher, 1991). Members of the former group might be less opposed to using leading questions, a certain degree of coaxing, and AD dolls, whereas members of the latter group might be more troubled by using leading questions, pressuring, and AD dolls.

The previous interviewing considerations affect professionals' use of AD dolls. For fear that a child's accuracy or credibility (or both) will be damaged, many interviewers try to avoid leading questions and leading approaches to AD-doll use. Some professionals avoid AD dolls altogether. The previous issues also affect research on memory and suggestibility when children are confronted with AD dolls and the conclusions that different researchers are willing to reach.

## Developmental Issues

The use of AD dolls with children is, at its core, a developmental issue. Therefore, it is important to include a brief discussion of cognitive development and its interaction with memory and suggestibility as they relate to AD-doll use.

Research confirms that complex interactions involving many factors (e.g., developmental level, task, and context) influence children's performance on cognitive tasks (e.g., Fischer & Bullock, 1984; Melton & Thompson, 1987). It follows that complex interactions also affect children's behavior with AD dolls. Within this framework, memory, suggestibility, and AD-doll use have multiple determinants, developmental level being an important but not the sole influence. Consistent with this view, when a task is simplified, when appropriate cues are available, and when the socioemotional context is supportive, young children typically provide more complete and accurate memory reports than when a task is complex requiring coordination of multiple higher level representations, when appropriate cues are unavailable, and when the socioemotional context is nonsupportive (e.g., Donaldson, 1979; Fischer & Bullock, 1984; Goodman, Bottoms, Schwartz-Kenney, & Rudy, 1991; Kail, 1990; Price & Goodman, 1990). For example, memory performance may falter when inaccurate or irrelevant cues in the form of toy props are introduced (Pipe, Gee, & Wilson, 1993; Saywitz, Goodman, Nicholas, & Moan, 1991; i.e., in some situations, AD dolls could constitute misleading or irrelevant cues), when the language used in an interview is unfamiliar and abstract (Brennan & Brennan, 1988; Carter, 1991; Perry et al., 1993), and when the emotional context is intimidating (Goodman et al., 1991; Hill & Hill, 1987; Saywitz & Nathanson, in press).

Some very young children may not yet have the representational skills to appreciate the full symbolic nature of props, such as AD dolls (DeLoache, 1990, in press). Although task difficulty can affect a child's ability to activate emerging representational skills (DeLoache, Kolstad, & Anderson, 1991), developmental level may place important limits on children's ability to recount an event using AD dolls. Fischer and Lazerson (1984) describe a sequence of children's pretend play involving props that may also apply to AD-doll use. According to this sequence, in the transition from sensorimotor to preoperational intelligence, children can act out familiar actions with their own body (e.g., to use their own body to pretend to go to sleep). Once the child is capable of mentally coordinating single representations (often by about 2 years of age), the child can act out a single action and then later (by around 3 years of age) act out a series of related actions with a prop. As the child's cognitive development advances further, the child of about 4 years of age is able to use a prop to relate one social category (e.g., mother or father) to another social category (e.g., daughter or son). It would be of considerable interest to test whether this developmental sequence applies to children's use of AD dolls to report experienced events from memory.

Although studies of adults' use of AD dolls to reenact experienced events are lacking, note that task and context affect adults' memory performance as well (e.g., Chi, 1978; Loftus, 1979; Tulving, 1983). Moreover, individual differences within any age group can be striking; when recounting an event, some children are more accurate than others, and some children are more accurate than some adults (Leippe, Manion, & Romanczyk, 1993). Still, the optimal level of performance a young child can reach is unlikely to match that of an older child or adult (Fischer, 1980). For example, older children and adults, on average, can be expected to reenact complex events with dolls and props with greater completeness and accuracy than can younger children.

**Memory.** If young children were incapable of remembering their experiences, using AD dolls to elicit memory reports would be futile. However, even infants show evidence of preverbal memory (e.g., Rovee-Collier, 1989), and 2- and 3-year-olds can verbalize memories for events that occurred at least 6 months earlier (Fivush, Gray, & Fromhoff, 1987). Behavioral indexes, such as interactions with toy props, reveal that 2-year-olds have traces of nonverbal memories for experiences that occurred in infancy (Myers, Clifton, & Clarkson, 1987). However, for young children (e.g., 2-year-olds), parental discussion of events may be important for retention of specific experiences; without such discussion, an enduring, consciously accessible episodic memory of a specific experience in early childhood may not form (Nelson, 1993).

When compared with older children and adults, preschool children tend to recall significantly less information in free recall and make more errors in answering questions (e.g., Goodman & Reed, 1986; Poole & Lindsay, 1994), including questions that deal with abuse-related information (e.g., being kissed and having one's bottom touched). Nevertheless, by the age of about 4 years, children can show surprising accuracy in answering questions about abuse-related actions (e.g., Rudy & Goodman, 1991; Tobey & Goodman, 1992), although accuracy is not guaranteed (e.g., Lepore & Sesco, 1994). As studies reviewed later in this article indicate, to date the presence versus absence of AD dolls has not been proven to significantly increase children's commission errors to such questions.

Some of children's memory deficits reflect a limited knowledge base compared with that of adults (Chi, 1978). Children who have experienced sexual abuse would be expected to have relevant knowledge of the experience, a knowledge that might be reflected in their AD-doll reenactment. Although repeated experience with an event generally strengthens memory, it can also result in confusions across similar instances, especially for young children (e.g., Farrar & Goodman, 1992), in part because their semantic knowledge tends to intrude into their episodic reports of a specific experience (Mandler, 1984). As a result, in some situations a young child might reenact general knowledge with an AD doll rather than a specific experience. When semantic-based AD-doll reenactment reflects age-inappropriate sexual knowledge, suspicion of premature exposure to sexuality or sexual abuse might reasonably be raised. Alternatively, when reenactment is based on inaccurate stereotypes or inaccurate interpretations of events, errors may result (e.g., Clarke-Stewart, Thompson, & Lepore, 1989; Leichtman & Ceci, 1995).

Although young children's memories may be more fragile and fade more quickly than adults' memories (Brainerd, Renya, Howe, & Kingma, 1991; Flin, Boon, Knox, & Bull, 1992; Howe, 1991), traumatic and stressful events can be retained over significant periods of time by young children (e.g., Goodman, Hirschman, Hepps, & Rudy, 1991; Steward, 1993; Terr, 1988), and it is well documented that central features of traumatic events may be reenacted by children in their doll play (e.g., Terr, 1988). Thus, even if a young child cannot be brought to articulate a traumatic memory in words or has difficulty using AD dolls to reenact an event in response to an interviewer's command, a child's posttraumatic play with AD dolls may reflect a child's experiences.

For both neutral and traumatic events, because children typically retain more information than they report in free recall (Kail, 1990), scientists and professionals who work with children have long relied on specific questioning and use of props such as dolls, to help elicit more complete memory reports from children. Children's limited memory-retrieval abilities may lag behind their abilities to reenact simple events (Piaget & Inhelder, 1973; Price & Goodman, 1990). Although props at times provide communication and memory interference (e.g., distraction and misleading cues), a number of studies also indicate facilitative effects of props on memory (Pipe et al., 1993; Price & Goodman, 1990).

**Suggestibility.** Of particular concern in the AD-doll debate is children's suggestibility. Young children, on average, tend to be more suggestible than older children or adults (for reviews, see Ceci & Bruck, 1993; Saywitz & Goodman, in press). To the extent that children's compared to adults' memories possess less *memory strength*, there is an increased possibility of suggestibility and incorporation of misleading postevent information (Loftus, 1979; Schwartz-Kenney & Goodman, 1991). However, when forgetting rates are controlled, age differences in some forms of suggestibility may disappear (Howe, 1991). Thus, for salient features of an event to which children attend, consider important, and thus encode well, children may at times be no more susceptible to forgetting, memory impairment, and suggestibility effects than adults. A number of factors influence memory strength and resistance to suggestion, such as the centrality and salience of event information (e.g., Loftus, 1979; Schwartz-Kenney & Goodman, 1991), delay (Goodman, Hirschman, et al., 1991; Loftus, 1979), participation in an event (Baker-Ward, Hess, & Flannagan, 1990; Lindberg, McComas, Jones, & Thomas, 1993; Rudy & Goodman, 1991; Tobey & Goodman, 1992), expectations and discrepancy (Baker-Ward, Gordon, Ornstein, Larus, & Clubb, 1993; List, 1986; Pezdek, 1994), repeated interviewing (Leichtman & Ceci, 1995; Warren, Hagood, & Snider, 1993), and rehearsal (Brainerd & Ornstein, 1991). Moreover, although memory strength may be linked to suggestibility, it is as yet unclear whether it is a singularly determining factor or whether social factors (e.g., demand characteristics; Zaragoza, 1991) or personality factors (e.g., attachment status and temperament; Goodman, Batterman-Faunce, Quas, Riddlesberger, & Kuhn, 1993; Gordon et al., 1993) are even more controlling. These same factors can be expected to affect children's suggestibility in response to questions asked in interviews that contain AD dolls.

In actual cases, forensic interviewers have at times combined repeated abuse suggestions, an accusatory context, and biased interviewing with the use of AD dolls (e.g., *State of New Jersey v. Michaels*, 1993), a combination that could enhance the chances of obtaining a false report of sexual abuse. There is growing research that when an interviewer repeatedly communicates accusation or intimidation, increased memory distortion and suggestibility can result, at least in young children (Clark-Stewart et al., 1989; Goodman, Bottoms, et al., 1991; Leichtman & Ceci, 1995; Tobey & Goodman, 1992). However, the influence of intimidation, accusatory context, and repetition of misleading questions has not been put to scientific test specifically in relation to interviews that include AD dolls. Moreover, it is unknown whether similar interviewing techniques are successful, or even necessary, in obtaining disclosures of actual abuse from frightened or embarrassed children and how best to balance the risk of obtaining a false report with the need to detect actual abuse.

**Distinguishing fantasy from reality.** Children's accuracy of reports when interviewed with AD dolls is not related to memory alone; it may also be influenced by children's ability to distinguish fantasy (i.e., play, imagination, and cognition) from reality. Such influences are of particular concern when children are interviewed with AD dolls because of the fear that toys such as dolls may be associated in children's minds with fantasy play. Differentiation between fantasy and reality has a developmental course, but children nevertheless evidence a basic understanding of "pretend" at young ages (DiLalla & Watson, 1988; Wellman & Estes, 1986). Research on "reality monitoring" also indicates that younger children may have more difficulty than older children differentiating their own thoughts from reality (e.g., Johnson & Foley, 1984), but literature focuses chiefly on mundane events rather than those of personal significance to children. To the extent that children might confuse fantasy with reality, and to the extent that certain props such as AD dolls might promote such confusion, caution in interpreting children's reports from AD-doll interviews is warranted. However, there is little solid research evidence indicating that young children have spontaneous sexual fantasies (e.g., of copulation) that they then confuse with reality, which is an issue of greater forensic concern in many situations in which AD dolls are used.

**Communication and language.** Use of age-inappropriate language by an interviewer can lead to confusion and increased error (Carter, 1991; Goodman & Aman, 1991; Perry et al., 1993), which could affect an interview that includes AD dolls. Moreover, some young children provide incoherent narratives or recall a different event than the one in question, without communicating the difference to the interviewer. Young children will often expect adults to know and understand what they mean when communicating. Such children, usually under the age of 7 years, may not sense or comprehend incompleteness or ambiguity of their communication and may not indicate that they do not understand an interviewer's question (Saywitz & Snyder, 1993). Confusions resulting from such language and communication problems in interviews that include AD dolls may enhance errors of false reports as well as false denial. In some studies, including ones that involved AD dolls, language was implicated as one of the main causes of children's errors in answering questions about an experienced event (e.g., Goodman & Aman, 1991; Saywitz et al., 1991).

**Recounting sexually related events.** One rationale for AD-doll use is that children may be hesitant to discuss sexual matters outright. Most studies of children's cognitive and memory development have not focused on sexually related information, and thus it is unclear how the findings of such studies apply to children's disclosure of sexual abuse. Although most young children have quite limited sexual knowledge (Gordon, Schroeder, & Abrams, 1990a, 1990b; but see Boat & Everson, 1988a; Everson & Boat, 1990), with development, children gain awareness that sexually related activity is taboo, not generally talked about, embarrassing, and best kept a secret (Goldman & Goldman, 1982). Older children's reports of genital touch in particular may thus be inhibited relative to their reporting of other types of information. In support of this assertion, Saywitz et al. (1991) found that 7-year-olds were less likely than 5-year-olds to report genital touch. Again consistent with the idea that older children may be inhibited when reporting sexually related information, 9- to 10-year-olds in Edwards and Forman's (1989) study tended to avoid AD-doll reenactment of information concerning intrafamilial sexual abuse. Although older children's advanced cognitive skills often make them better able than younger children to recount events completely and accurately, beliefs and feelings about the appropriateness of sexual activity and about discussion of sexual matters may inhibit children's reports of sexual abuse. AD dolls might make it easier for such children to report sexual events (e.g., by permitting them to reenact rather than verbalize events or by providing social cues that discussion of genitally related information is acceptable).

**Summary.** Children do show cognitive and memory deficits compared with adults, and these deficits are likely to affect children's performance in interviews that include AD dolls. Some of these deficits are due to limits in cognitive and language development; others may be due to a more limited knowledge base concerning a particular domain. However, factors related to task complexity, cues, and socioemotional context can potentially reduce age differences in memory. Age differences in children's willingness to report sexually related information may also affect typical developmental patterns, with older children not necessarily providing more complete and accurate reports. Still, under a variety of interviewing contexts, young children—especially preschoolers—can be expected to provide less complete reports, to make more errors, and to be more suggestible on average compared with older children and adults. Age differences may be exacerbated by language and communication difficulties, intimidation, and an accusatory context. Children's cognitive limitations may at times adversely affect interviews that include AD dolls; however, such deficits also underlie why AD dolls can, at other times, lead to more complete and accurate reports from children.

## Studies Concerning Memory and Suggestibility

Only a handful of studies have directly investigated the effects of AD dolls on nonabused children's memory and suggestibility. In one of the first studies to explore this issue (Goodman & Aman, 1991; Goodman et al., 1990), eighty 3- and 5-year-old middle-class children participated individually in games such as Simon Says with a male confederate. A week later, children were individually interviewed in one of four conditions: (a) no dolls (AD or regular) present, (b) AD dolls in view but out of reach, (c) regular dolls present for acting out the event, and (d) AD dolls present for acting out the event. During the interview, children were first asked to describe the earlier play session using free recall; those children in the two doll reenactment conditions were asked to demonstrate as well as tell what happened as part of their free recall. All children were then asked a set of specific and misleading questions, including some questions that might be of particular interest in abuse investigations such as "Did he touch your private parts?" and "Did he spank you like this?" (with the researcher demonstrating the act with the AD doll).

When verbal responses in free recall were considered, a significant age difference but not a significant doll-condition difference emerged. When behavioral responses in the two doll conditions were contrasted, again only a significant age effect was uncovered. However, further analyses indicated that the amount of accurate information provided by older children in free recall was increased by reenactment with regular and AD dolls compared with the no-doll conditions, whereas the amount of accurate information provided by younger children was increased primarily by regular rather than AD dolls (see Goodman et al., 1990). Importantly, there were no significant differences in the amount of incorrect recall as a function of doll condition. In response to the specific and misleading questioning, although few 3-year-olds made commission errors to abuse-related questions, they did so more often than 5-year-olds (e.g., 3-year-olds were more likely to falsely affirm the question "He took your clothes off, didn't he?"). Commission errors were particularly likely when the children did not understand the terms used (e.g., .,"private parts"). In any case, this error rate did not significantly differ as a function of doll condition.

Goodman and Aman (1991) observed that some of the 3-year-olds did not seem to understand that the dolls were supposed to be used to symbolically represent themselves. For example, when asked to act out the event with AD dolls or regular dolls, some young children made statements such as "but I'm not a doll." DeLoache and Marzolf (1994) explored this finding further in a study of 2.5- to 4-year-olds' use of AD dolls (see also De-Loache, in press). Seventy-two middle-class children interacted with a male confederate by engaging in play activities, some of which involved touching and placing stickers on the child. In an immediate interview, children were asked to place stickers on the AD doll in the same place where the stickers had been placed on them. The children were then asked to answer questions about where they were touched (e.g., "Where did Don touch you?") and then to indicate these places on the AD doll (e.g., "Show me on the doll where Don touched you").

Four-year-old children were very accurate in sticker placement on the AD doll (92% correct), but 2.5-year-olds were not (41% correct). Many 2.5-year-olds did not constrain sticker placement by their own experiences and instead placed stickers incorrectly on the AD doll. Importantly, response accuracy to questions about touch was higher when children were asked to describe where they had been touched than when they had to show the same thing on the AD doll, a pattern that was especially true for 2.5-year-olds. Interestingly, when asked misleading questions about where they were touched, both 2.5- and 4-year-olds were more accurate in their verbal responses than 3-year-olds. These findings indicate that some young children may not understand the dolls' symbolic function in terms of serving as a model to indicate an experienced event (see also Gordon et al., 1993). However, because the AD dolls remained clothed throughout the DeLoache and Marzolf (1994) study, their experiment is arguably more about children's use of dolls than about children's use of AD dolls. Possible effects of the AD dolls' genital features (e.g., greater avoidance of or greater interest in the dolls) remain unknown on the basis of this otherwise informative research.

It should be kept in mind that the children in the Goodman and Aman (1991) and DeLoache and Marzolf (1995) studies were not interviewed about an event involving genital touch; AD dolls would be expected to be of particular benefit precisely for such events. For example, the Goodman and Aman study concerned whether children who did not experience genital contact would be more likely to falsely report genital touch and abuse-related actions when interviewed with AD dolls than without such dolls. The results indicated that AD dolls did not intrinsically heighten the chances of obtaining a false report of sexual abuse, although some young children may have difficulty understanding the AD doll's symbolic function.

Children's use of AD dolls to accurately report an event involving genital touch was first investigated by Saywitz et al. (1991). The Saywitz et al. study also explored the reports of children who had not experienced genital contact. Seventy-two 5- and 7-year-old girls were given a complete medical checkup by a pediatrician at a university-affiliated hospital. Standard medical checkups of girls by the pediatrician at the hospital typically involved a vaginal and anal examination (i.e., visually inspecting and touching the labia and checking for an anal reflex). For purposes of the study, this part of the checkup was omitted for half of the children at each age. The advantage of this design is that for the children who had the vaginal and anal examination, the researcher could explore the children's reports, including AD doll-aided reports, of actual genital touch, whereas for children who did not have vaginal or anal touch, the researchers could explore children's tendency to make false reports of genital contact.

After either 1 week or 1 month, the children were interviewed about the checkup; the interview involved free recall, AD-doll reenactment, and directive questioning. The directive questioning included two AD doll-aided leading questions about the checkup that were of special interest. Specifically, the interviewer held up a naked AD doll and asked "Did the doctor touch you here?" (pointing to the AD doll's vaginal area) and "Did the doctor touch you here?" (pointing to the AD doll's anal area). Note that the comparisons across interview format (e.g., free recall and AD doll) were within subject. There was not a "no AD doll" group, and therefore no leading question effects comparisons were possible.

Of most concern to this article is the children's reports of genital touch. To the free-recall question "What happened last time you went to the doctor's office?", only 8 of the 36 children who had the vaginal and anal examination reported vaginal touch, and only 4 of the children reported anal touch. When asked to demonstrate what happened using AD dolls, only 6 of the 36 children reported vaginal touch, and only 4 reported anal touch. It was only when asked the specific (leading) questions during which the AD doll was used that most of the children reported genital contact; at that point, 31 children affirmed the vaginal touch, and 25 children affirmed the anal touch.

Of the 36 children who did not have vaginal or anal touch as part of the checkup, none of the children falsely reported genital contact in free recall or AD-doll reenactment, but 3 children falsely affirmed genital touch when the leading questions using the AD doll were asked. Only 1 of the 3 children provided false detail, claiming that the doctor had used a stick to conduct the anal examination and that it tickled.

The Saywitz et al. (1991) study identifies advantages and disadvantages to using AD doll-aided leading questions with children. On the one hand, it was only when the AD doll-aided leading questions were asked that the majority of the children revealed the genital touch they actually experienced. The omission error rate without use of the AD doll-aided leading questions was substantial at about 60%. Reenactment with AD dolls was not particularly facilitative of disclosure of genital touch, but then again these were not children who had been sexually violated or traumatized. On the other hand, for children who did not experience genital touch, there was a relatively small risk of a false report when the AD doll-aided leading questions were asked; specifically, 8% of the children falsely affirmed genital touch, with only 3% (one child) providing false detail. None of the children falsely indicated genital touch when asked to reenact the event with AD dolls. This study thus indicates that AD doll-aided leading questions can help elicit accurate reports of genital touch from children who have experienced such touch, but that at the same time such questioning may lead to an increase in false reports by children who have not experienced genital contact.

A study that was recently completed on forty 3-year-old children underscores the need for caution in interpreting some young children's behavior with AD dolls as indicative of abuse (Bruck, Ceci, & Francoeur, 1994). Borrowing the methodology developed by Saywitz et al. (1991), Bruck and colleagues also examined children's use of AD dolls to recount medical examinations that involved or did not involve genital touch. All of the children were nonreferred and had no history or suspicion of sexual abuse. The 3-year-olds were examined by their regular pediatrician with their mothers present. For half of the children, the examination included inspection and touching of the child's buttocks and genitals. During this portion of the examination, the pediatrician never inserted anything into the genital opening. Immediately following the examination, the children were interviewed by a research assistant using an AD doll of the same gender as the child. The interviewer asked the child to name all body parts, including anus and genitalia. During this part of the inquiry, the child was asked a leading yes-no question, "Did the doctor touch you here?" Each child was also offered an AD doll and some other props and asked to demonstrate how the doctor touched the child's "genitals" (e.g., "Show me on the doll how Dr. Francoeur touched your penis"), an even more strongly leading question and misleading for children in the non-genital-exam condition. Finally, children who experienced the genital and anal examination were asked to demonstrate on their own bodies parts of the examination. (Those children who had not had their buttocks and genitals checked were not asked to demonstrate on their own bodies the examination of these areas.)

When the experimenter pointed to the AD doll's buttocks and genital area and asked, "Did the doctor touch you here?", 45% of the children who had been touched in those areas accurately answered yes. Fifty percent of those who had not been examined on the buttocks or genital area answered correctly with a no, but the remaining 50% incorrectly affirmed such touch in response to the leading question, a potentially dangerous error were suspicions of criminal behavior involved.

During the second phase of the interview, which involved children using the AD doll and props to show what happened under force of more highly leading questioning, about half (55%) of the children who did not receive the genital examination were accurate by not showing such touch, but the remaining 45% erred. For the children who actually experienced the genital examination, the error rate reached as high as 75% when the researchers included omission errors and incorrect insertions of the children's fingers into anal or genital cavities in demonstrating the touch actually experienced. The children's accuracy did not significantly differ when demonstrations with the AD doll and demonstrations with the children's own bodies were compared.

These data indicate that under certain conditions of testing, a significant number of 3-year-olds can be lead to make false reports of genital touch in interviews when AD dolls are used and that a similar number who actually experienced noninvasive genital touch do not report it when questioned with AD dolls. However, in this study it cannot be determined whether the children who did not experience genital touch would have provided as many false affirmations to leading questions had the AD dolls not been present. The children's scores may reflect children's general suggestibility or younger children's lack of understanding of the task (e.g., the children's response rate tended to hover around chance levels) as opposed to heightened suggestibility because of the presence of AD dolls. That they provided about as many errors to leading questions when demonstrating on their own bodies as with AD dolls also indicates that the AD dolls did not significantly add to the children's error rates. Moreover, because the children were examined by their regular physician, there may have been confusion on the children's part about former examinations by him or her.

The Bruck et al. (1994) study also raises questions about how children's responses should be scored. It may be very difficult for children (and adults, for that matter) to tell if they were touched externally or if slight penetration occurred when lying in a prone position that makes visual observation difficult. Documenting that such differentiation is not always made by children is of interest, but at what point should such responses be scored as errors? Furthermore, combining across different types of errors that have very different legal implications is potentially misleading. Decisions about what constitutes an error and how to report one's data can affect conclusions reached.

Although the Saywitz et al. (1991) and Bruck et al. (1994) studies concern children's reports of genital touch, the children in those studies did not experience painful, invasive touch or actual genital penetration. A recent study (Goodman, 1994) examined children's use of AD dolls to report invasive, painful urethral penetration. In the study, approximately 46 children were interviewed after experiencing a radiological test that was conducted on a physician's order for medical purposes in a hospital. The interview, which took place 1 to 3 weeks after the medical procedure, consisted of free-recall questions and prompts (e.g., "Tell me everything that happened when you got that medical test" and "What else happened?") followed by a request for a reenactment of what happened using an AD doll and props. Findings revealed that older children provided, on average, more correct information than younger children regardless of the type of interview (free recall vs. AD-doll reenactment). Additionally, younger children overall tended to make more errors than older children.

Specifically, 3- to 4-year-olds provided somewhat more correct information when using AD dolls than in free recall, but they also provided more incorrect information. The younger children's errors were especially associated with the distractor props provided (e.g., a tongue depressor). In contrast, AD dolls aided older children (5- to 10-year-olds) in providing additional correct information without a significant increase in error. Although this study did not include a comparison group of non-genitally touched children, thus failing to address the issue of false reports of genital touch, it is relevant to the important question of whether AD dolls aid children who have experienced invasive genital contact report such experiences. The findings suggest that AD dolls may result in additional correct information from older children, but the increase in correct information for younger children may be offset by an increase in error. However, Goodman and colleagues (Goodman, 1994) noted that the additional correct information provided by even the young children was often helpful in specifying more exactly how the child's urethra was penetrated.

Only a few other studies have appeared in the literature in which investigators who have an objective record of an event have collected data relevant to children's suggestibility with AD dolls. Two such studies compare use of AD dolls with other interviewing techniques. Steward and Steward (1989) were interested in 3- to 6-year-old children's reports of bodily touch when children were interviewed with a verbal interview versus with AD dolls, drawings, or a computer-interviewing protocol. They found that all three "stimulus supported" interviews were superior in eliciting information from children compared with a purely verbal interview. Edwards and Forman (1989) invited forty-five 9- to 10-year-old girls to watch a 12 min videotape that provided information on sexual abuse and its prevention. After a delay of between 4 to 6 hr, the children were interviewed about the videotape in one of three conditions; verbal, AD doll, and drawing. For the verbal condition, the children were asked to recall everything they could about the videotape. The children in the AD-doll condition were also asked to show and tell what happened in the videotape. The children in the drawing condition were asked to draw pictures of what happened in the videotape as well as to recall everything about it. Although the children who used the AD dolls or who produced drawings recalled somewhat more than the children in the verbal condition, the differences were not statistically significant. On average, the children provided little incorrect information regardless of interview condition, although one child produced much more inaccurate information than the other children tested.

In summary, research to date mainly supports use of AD dolls as a communication or memory aid for children 5 years or older, albeit with a certain risk of contributing to some children's errors if misleading questions are used. Interestingly, it seems that many children beyond the preschool years are unlikely to make commission errors to abuse inquiries, at least under the conditions examined in the previous studies. Greater caution is needed when preschool children are interviewed with AD dolls because of these younger children's greater tendency toward suggestibility and difficulties with symbolic representation. Further research that includes preschool children will provide important clues about interviewing children ages 4 years and under with AD dolls. Although findings to date indicate that young preschoolers are more prone than older children to falsely report in a leading AD doll-aided interview, these results do not rule out AD dolls' potential usefulness in forensic investigations involving young children. For example, if a young child evidenced inappropriate sexual knowledge by spontaneously acting out a sexual event with AD dolls, such behavior might still aid the interviewer to accurately infer what happened even if the child had difficulty forming a symbolic representation of her- or himself in relation to an AD doll when directed to do so by an interviewer. If a child provides a verbal disclosure of abuse, use of AD dolls after the disclosure as a communication aid for clarifying what occurred may be helpful. In any case, because AD dolls are particularly likely to be used with young children (Kendall-Tackett & Watson, 1992), further research with preschool populations is clearly warranted, as is particular caution in interpreting young children's responses to AD dolls.

It could be legitimately argued, however, that extant research has not included interviews that are as suggestive as some actual forensic investigations, that the forensic context of the interviews was not realistic (e.g., the children did not think anyone was in trouble, nor were they subjected to repeated interrogations), and that the events studied did not approximate closely enough the events about which children might show confusion and thus greater error. Extant studies have also not examined cumulative effects of AD-doll exposure. On the one hand, because any tool or technique can be misused, there may be situations in actual practice in which AD dolls are associated with false reports of abuse or with interviewers forming incorrect conclusions of abuse regardless of a child's age. On the other hand, the current research examining children's memory and suggestibility in interviews that include AD dolls does not address situations in which children attempt to recount actual abusive events and is just beginning to study painful or repeated genital touch or both, factors that also might affect children's performance. Further research may inform interviewers about how to optimize children's disclosures of actual abuse and at the same time minimize children's false reports of abuse, whether AD dolls are used or not.

### A Final Dilemma

The nature of clinical cases involving allegations of child sexual abuse often demand binary categorization (i.e., the abuse did or did not occur). Unlike medicine, where one might use a bacterial culture to document a streptococcal infection, whether the infection is minor or life-threatening, there is no "gold standard" criterion or litmus test of whether alleged abuse took place. In some instances, clinicians may disagree about whether acts acknowledged to have taken place were abusive. In a rare case of alleged child sexual abuse, a gold standard may be approached (e.g., when an articulate child makes an unambiguous report, corroborated by both physical findings and adult witnesses). However, for the most part, clinicians are stuck with contradictory assertions and fallible indicators on which experienced practitioners tend to disagree vociferously. In the words of Paul Meehl (personal communication, April 6, 1993), "clinical experience simply has not sufficed to produce convergence of expert opinion" on this issue. Meehl suggests the application of a taxometric approach to address this problem in a boot-strapping manner (see, e.g., Meehl, 1992). Although such an application is desirable in the long run, methodological barriers abound.

In the face of these observations, one must consider whether the incremental validity provided by using AD dolls in an interview "adds to the predictive accuracy of existing methods" (Wolfner et al., 1993, p. 8). One must also consider the cognitive capability of human beings. Clinicians often claim to base their judgments on configural analysis and integration of many arrays of data; however, research suggests that such subjective beliefs are largely illusory (Faust, 1989). Reviewing clinicians' ability to integrate complex data interactions, Wedding and Faust (1989) found that problems involving the integration of "even two to three variables may outstrip human cognitive capacities" (p. 246). Such cognitive research indicates that clinical judgments that are purportedly based on the integration of many variables can generally be duplicated by merely adding the variables together (Faust, 1989; Wedding & Faust, 1989).

Much human "data processing" is automatic, subject to habit, or otherwise occurs outside of conscious awareness, thus limiting insight about potential biases. The arena of child sexual abuse is one in which many of the performers have strong affective beliefs or attitudes, which may influence them outside of a conscious-rational process. Are the data to be gleaned in interviews featuring AD dolls of sufficient validity in this context that they ought to be among the few given weighty consideration in arriving at clinical conclusions? Are such data significant enough to warrant incorporation as incremental data in an actuarial prediction model? In the context of the studies reviewed here, it does not seem unreasonable to draw on AD-doll data in the cautious and thoughtful manner proposed by the APA council's resolution. Perhaps the concerns advanced by Faust and his colleagues (1989) on the matter of data integration do apply in the context of clinical judgments using AD-doll data in child sexual-abuse cases much as they do in neuropsychology (Wedding & Faust, 1989). Research focused on answering that question seems the best solution.

### Future Research Directions

Many pressing questions about the impact of AD dolls on children's memory and suggestibility remain to be explored or have received insufficient research attention. A number of issues that require further research were mentioned; additional important issues are addressed here. Research is needed on optimal techniques for AD-doll use (e.g., number of AD dolls to use, similarity of props to offenders and events, types of questions to ask, inclusion of other props, and duration of exposure to AD dolls); use of AD dolls to recount repeated versus single events; use of AD dolls to reenact traumatic versus neutral events; further exploration of the basis for developmental differences in AD-doll use; effects of repeated suggestions, repeated exposure to AD dolls, naming of body parts at the start of interviews, and accusatory context on children's AD-doll reports; effects of AD dolls on person identification (e.g., of culprits and other children); effectiveness of AD-doll use in developmentally disabled or language-impaired children; effects of prior sexual knowledge and disorganized family life; and cultural differences that might affect children's recounting of events with AD dolls. In regard to referred children's use of AD dolls, research is needed that takes not only age but also severity and type of sexual abuse into account, in case degree and type of traumatization affect the likelihood of AD-doll reenactment. In general, research should examine separately, when possible, the various functions of AD dolls articulated by Boat and Everson (1994b).

Moreover, psychologists need to know more about the use of AD dolls in actual practice. An ongoing study by Boat and Everson (1994a) on the use of AD dolls by social service professionals should shed important light on the actual practices of interviewers when AD dolls are used in child sexual-abuse investigations, a study that may confirm or shatter some currently held beliefs about actual practice with AD dolls. Perhaps of most concern, there is a nearly complete void in the research literature concerning the process of decision making by professionals and lay people and their abilities to reach the truth on the basis of children's use of AD dolls. Even if young children have difficulty using AD dolls optimally, in the end, it is the fact finder's (e.g., interviewer's and juror's) assessment that matters most.

It goes without saying that assessments of children who report abuse or who are alleged to have been abused are complex. However, this complexity is often ignored by critics of the use of AD dolls who focus on the incidence of false positives that result if one uses interactions with AD dolls as a single indicator or criterion for the evaluation of sexual abuse (Realmuto et al., 1990; Wolfner et al., 1993). In daily practice, professionals, especially mental health professionals, use a wide variety of techniques when evaluating suspected child victims (Kendall-Tackett, 1992). Most of these professionals do so in an effort to achieve responsible clinical decision making. Reviews (Mann, 1991; White, 1991) of current practice attest to this goal. In this context, we disagree with the conclusion of Wolfner et al., (1993) that the APA council resolution at the beginning of this article has "no merit" (p. 9). The data summarized here illustrate both merits and pitfalls inherent in AD-doll use. We agree that the data on AD dolls may be equivocal when claims for diagnostic discrimination are made (Ceci & Bruck, 1993). We agree with the APA resolution that AD dolls can still provide a useful communication tool in the hands of a trained professional interviewer with the following caveats:

1. AD dolls are not a psychological test with predictive (or postdictive) validity per se.

2. Definitive statements about child sexual abuse cannot be made on the basis of spontaneous or guided "doll *play*" alone. A clinical interview by a skilled clinician is not play.

3. Particular caution is called for when interpreting the reports of children ages 4 years and under, at least so far as when affirmations to leading questions about "being touched" are concerned and when repeated misleading questioning has been used.

4. In light of current knowledge, we recommend that APA reconsider whether valid "doll-centered assessment" techniques exist and whether they still "may be the best available practical solution" (APA, 1991, p. 722) for the pressing and frequent problem of investigation of child sexual abuse.

5. Special recognition of normative differences between children of different racial groups and socioeconomic strata should be a part of training professionals who use AD dolls in clinical inquiry.

## REFERENCES

Allen, M. E., Jones, P. D., & Nash, M. R. (1989, August). *Detection of sexual abuse among emotionally disturbed preschoolers: Unique effects of sexual abuse as observed on doll play and other standard assessment procedures.* Paper presented at the Annual Convention of the American Psychological Association, New Orleans, LA.

American Professional Society on the Abuse of Children. (1990). *Guidelines for psychosocial evaluation of suspected sexual abuse in young children.* Unpublished manuscript, Chicago, IL.

American Psychological Association. (1991). Minutes of the Council of Representatives. *American Psychologist, 46*, 722.

Ames, L. B., Learned, J., Metraux, R. W., & Walker, R. N. (1974). *Child Rorschach responses: Developmental trends from two to ten years.* New York: Bruner/Mazel.

August, R. I., & Forman, B. D. (1989). A comparison of sexually abused and non-sexually abused children's behavioral responses to anatomically correct dolls. *Child Psychiatry and Human Development, 6*, 39–47.

Baker-Ward, L., Gordon, B., Ornstein, P., Larus, N., & Clubb, P. (1993). Young children's long-term retention of a pediatric examination. *Child Development, 64*, 1519–1533.

Baker-Ward, L., Hess, T. M., & Flannagan, D. A. (1990). The effects of involvement on children's memory for events. *Cognitive Development, 5*, 55–69.

Bays, J. (1990). Are the genitalia of anatomical dolls distorted? *Child Abuse and Neglect, 14*, 171–175.

Berliner, L. (1988). Anatomical dolls. *Journal of Interpersonal Violence, 3*, 468–470.

Boat, B. W., & Everson, M. D. (1986). *Using anatomical dolls: Guidelines for interviewing young children in sexual abuse investigations.* Chapel Hill: University of North Carolina.

Boat, B. W., & Everson, M. D. (1988a). Research and issues in using anatomical dolls. *Annals of Sex Research, 1,* 191–204.

Boat, B. W., & Everson, M. D. (1988b). Use of anatomical dolls among professionals in sexual abuse evaluations. *Child Abuse and Neglect, 12,* 171–179.

Boat, B. W., & Everson, M. D. (1989, August). *Anatomical doll play among young children. A follow-up of sexual demonstrators and doll avoiders.* Paper presented at the 97th Annual Convention of the American Psychological Association, New Orleans, LA.

Boat, B. W., & Everson, M. D. (1994a). Exploration of anatomical dolls by nonreferred preschool-aged children: Comparisons by age, gender, race and socioeconomic status. *Child Abuse and Neglect, 18,* 139–154.

Boat, B. W., & Everson, M. D. (1994b). Functional uses of anatomical dolls in child sexual abuse investigations. *Profiles of research grants funded by NCCAN.* National Clearinghouse on Child Abuse and Neglect Information, Washington, DC.

Bottoms, B. L. (1993). Individual differences in perceptions of child sexual assault victims. In G. S. Goodman & B. L. Bottoms (Eds.), *Child victims, child witnesses* (pp. 235–247). New York: Guilford Press.

Brainerd, C., & Ornstein, P. A. (1991). Children's memory for witnessed events: The developmental backdrop. In J. Doris (Ed.), *The suggestibility of children's recollections* (pp. 10–20). Washington, DC: American Psychological Association.

Brainerd, C., Renya, V., Howe, M., & Kingma, J. (1991). The development of forgetting and reminiscence. *Monographs of the Society for Research in Child Development, 55* (3–4, Serial No. 222).

Brennan, M., & Brennan, R. (1988). *Strange language: Child victims under cross examination.* Riverina, Australia: Charles Stuart University.

Brigham, J. (1991). Issues in the empirical study of the sexual abuse of children. In J. Doris (Ed.), *The suggestibility of children's recollections* (pp. 110–114). Washington, DC: American Psychological Association.

Britton, H. L., & O'Keefe, M. A. (1991). Use of nonanatomical dolls in the sexual abuse interview. *Child Abuse and Neglect, 15,* 567–573.

Brown v. Board of Educ., 347 U.S. 483 (1954).

Browne, A., & Finkelhor, D. (1986). Impact of child sexual abuse: A review of the research. *Psychological Bulletin, 99,* 66–77.

Bruck, M., & Ceci, S. J. (1993). *Amicus brief on behalf of Kelly Michaels.* Unpublished manuscript, McGill University, Montreal, Canada.

Bruck, M., Ceci, S. J., & Francoeur, E. (1994). *Anatomically detailed dolls do not facilitate preschoolers' reports of touching.* Paper presented at the annual meeting of the Canadian Pediatric Society, St. John's, Newfoundland, Canada.

Carter, C. (1991). *Influences of language and emotional support on children's testimony.* Unpublished dissertation, State University of New York-Buffalo.

Ceci, S. J., & Bruck, M. (1993). Suggestibility of the child witness: A historical review and synthesis. *Psychological Bulletin, 113*, 403–439.

Ceci, S. J., & Bruck, M. (1994). Translating research into policy. *Society for Research in Child Development Social Policy Report, 7*(3), 1–29.

Chandler, L. A. (1990). The projective hypothesis and the development of projective techniques for children. In C. R. Reynolds & R. W. Kamphaus (Eds.), *Handbook of psychological and educational assessment of children. Vol. 2. Personality, behavior, and context.* New York: Guilford Press.

Chi, M. T. H. (1978). Knowledge structures and memory development. In R. Siegler (Ed.), *Children's thinking: What develops?* Hillsdale, NJ: Erlbaum.

Clark, K. B., & Clark, M. P. (1958). Racial identification and preference in negro children. In E. Maccoby, J. Newcomb, & H. Hartley, (Eds.), *Readings in social psychology.* New York: Holt.

Clarke-Stewart, A., Thompson, L., & Lepore, S. (1989, March). Manipulating children's interpretations through interrogation. In G. S. Goodman (Chair), *Can children provide accurate testimony?* Symposium presented at the Society for Research in Child Development Meetings, Kansas City, MO.

Cohn, D. S. (1991). Anatomical doll play of preschoolers referred for sexual abuse and those not referred. *Child Abuse and Neglect, 15*, 455–466.

Committee to Develop Standards for Educational and Psychological Testing. (1985). *Standards for educational and psychological testing.* Washington, DC: American Psychological Association.

Conerly, S. (1986). Assessment of suspected child sexual abuse. In K. MacFarlane & J. Waterman (Eds.), *Sexual abuse of young children* (pp. 30–51). New York: Guilford Press.

Conte, J., Sorenson, M. A., Fogarty, L., & Rosa, J. D. (1991). Evaluating children's reports of sexual abuse: Results from a survey of professionals. *American Journal of Othropsychiatry, 61*, 428–437.

Dawson, B., Vaughan, A. R., & Wagner, W. G. (1992). Normal responses to sexually anatomically detailed dolls. *Journal of Family Violence, 7*, 135–152.

DeLoache, J. (1990). Young children's understanding of models. In R. Fivush & J. Hudson (Eds.), *Knowing and remembering in young children* (pp. 94–126). Cambridge, England: Cambridge University Press.

DeLoache, J. (in press). The use of dolls in interviewing young children. In M. Zaragoza, J. Graham, & G. Hall (Eds.), *Memory and testimony in the child witness.* Newbury Park, CA: Sage.

DeLoache, J., Kolstad, V., & Anderson, K. N. (1991). Physical similarity and young children's understanding of scale models. *Child Development, 62*, 111–126.

DeLoache, J., & Marzolf, D. (1994). *The use of dolls to interview young children: Issues of symbolic representation.* Manuscript submitted for publication, University of Illinois, Champaign-Urbana.

DiLalla, L. F., & Watson, M. W. (1988). Differentiation of fantasy and reality: Preschoolers' reactions to interruptions in their play. *Developmental Psychology, 24,* 286–291.

Donaldson, M. (1979). *Children's minds.* New York: Norton.

Edington, G. (1985). Hand puppets and dolls in psychotherapy with children. *Perceptual and Motor Skills, 61,* 691–696.

Edwards, C. A., & Forman, B. D. (1989). Effects of child interview method on accuracy and completeness of sexual abuse information recall. *Social Behavior and Personality, 17,* 237–247.

Everson, M. D., & Boat, B. W. (1990). Sexualized doll play among young children: Implications for the use of anatomical dolls in sexual abuse evaluations. *Journal of the American Academy of Child and Adolescent Psychiatry, 29,* 736–742.

Everson, M. D., & Boat, B. W. (1994). Putting the anatomical doll controversy in perspective: An examination of the major uses and criticisms of the dolls in child sexual abuse evaluations. *Child Abuse and Neglect, 18,* 113–130.

Farrar, M. J., & Goodman, G. S. (1992). Developmental differences in event memory. *Child Development, 63,* 173–187.

Faust, D. (1989). Data integration in legal evaluations: Can clinicians deliver on their premises? *Behavioral Sciences and the Law, 7,* 469–483.

Finkelhor, D., & Browne, A. (1985). The traumatic impact of child sexual abuse: A conceptualization. *American Journal of Orthopsychiatry, 55,* 530–541.

Finlayson, L., & Koocher, G. P. (1991). Professional judgment and reporting in child sexual abuse cases. *Professional Psychology: Research and Practice, 22,* 464–472.

Fischer, K. W. (1980). A theory of cognitive development: The control and construction of hierarchies of skills. *Psychological Review, 87,* 477–531.

Fischer, K. W., & Bullock, D. (1984). Cognitive development in school-age children: Conclusions and new directions. In W. Collins (Ed.), *Development during middle childhood: The years from six to twelve* (pp. 70–146). Washington, DC: National Academy Press.

Fischer, K. W., & Lazerson, A. (1984). *Human development.* New York: Freeman.

Fivush, R., Gray, J. T., & Fromhoff, F. A. (1987). Two year olds talk about the past. *Cognitive Development, 2,* 393–410.

Flavell, J. H. (1985). *Cognitive development.* Englewood Cliffs, NJ: Prentice-Hall.

Flin, R., Boon, J., Knox, A., & Bull, R. (1992). The effects of a five-month delay on children's and adults' eyewitness memory. *British Journal of Psychology, 83,* 323–330.

Fraley, M. C., Nelson, E. C., Wolf, A. W., & Lozoff, B. (1991). Early genital naming. *Developmental and Behavioral Pediatrics, 12,* 301–304.

Freeman, K. R., & Estrada-Mullaney, T. (1988). Using dolls to interview child victims: Legal concerns and interview procedures. *National Institute of Justice Reports, 107,* 1–6.

Freud, A. (1928). *Introduction to the technique of child analysis.* New York: Nervous and Mental Disease Publishing.

Friedemann, V., & Morgan, M. (1985). *Interviewing sexual abuse victims using anatomical dolls. The professional's guidebook.* Eugene, OR: Shamrock Press.

Friedrich, W. N., Grambach, P., Broughton, D., Kuiper, J., & Beilke, R. L. (1991). Normative sexual behavior in children. *Pediatrics, 88,* 456–464.

Friedrich, W. N., Grambach, P., Damon, L., Hewitt, S. K., Koverola, C., Lang, R. A., Wolfe, V., & Broughton, D. (1992). Child Sexual Behavior Inventory: Normative and clinical comparisons. *Psychological Assessment, 4,* 303–311.

Gabriel, R. M. (1985). Anatomically correct dolls in the diagnosis of sexual abuse of children. *The Journal of the Melanie Klein Society, 3,* 40–51.

Gardner, R. (1991). *Sex abuse hysteria: Salem witch trials revisited.* Cresskill, NJ: Creative Therapeutics.

Gil, E., & Johnson, T. C. (1993). *Sexualized children.* New York: Launch Press.

Glaser, D., & Collins, C. (1989). The response of young, non-sexually abused children to anatomically correct dolls. *Journal of Child Psychology and Psychiatry, 30,* 547–560.

Goldman, R., & Goldman, J. (1982). *Show me yours.* Victoria, Australia: Penguin.

Goodman, G. S. (1993, August). *Child victims, child witnesses.* Invited address presented at the Annual Meeting of the American Psychological Association, Toronto, Canada.

Goodman, G. S. (1994, August). *Update on developmental research on child sexual abuse.* Session presented at the Annual Convention of the American Psychological Association, Los Angeles, CA.

Goodman, G. S., & Aman, C. J. (1991). Children's use of anatomically detailed dolls to recount an event. *Child Development, 61,* 1859–1871.

Goodman, G. S., Batterman-Faunce, J. M., Quas, J., Riddlesberger, M., & Kuhn, J. (1993, March). Children's memory for stressful events: Theoretical and developmental considerations. In N. Stein (Chair), *Emotional events and memory.* Symposium presented at annual meeting of the Society for Research in Child Development, New Orleans, LA.

Goodman, G. S., Bottoms, B. L., Schwartz-Kenney, B., & Rudy, L. A. (1991). Children's memory for a stressful event: Improving children's reports. *Journal of Narrative and Life History, 1,* 69–99.

Goodman, G. S., & Clarke-Stewart, A. (1991). Suggestibility in children's testimony: Implications for child sexual abuse investigations. In J. L. Doris (Ed.), *The suggestibility of children's recollections* (pp. 92–105). Washington, DC: American Psychological Association.

Goodman, G. S., Hirschman, J. E., Hepps, D., & Rudy, L. A. (1991). Children's memory for stressful events. *Merrill Palmer Quarterly, 37,* 109–158.

Goodman, G. S., & Reed, R. S. (1986). Age differences in eyewitness testimony. *Law and Human Behavior, 10*, 317–322.

Goodman, G. S., Rudy, L. A., Bottoms, B. L., & Aman, C. (1990). Children's concerns and memory: Issues of ecological validity in the study of children's eyewitness testimony. In R. Fivush & J. Hudson (Eds.), *Knowing and remembering in young children* (pp. 249–284). New York: Cambridge University Press.

Gordon, B. N., Ornstein, P. A., Nida. R. L., Follmer, A., Crenshaw, M. C., & Albert, G. (1993). Does the use of dolls facilitate children's memory of visits to the doctor? *Applied Cognitive Psychology, 7*, 459–474.

Gordon, B. N., Schroeder, C. S., & Abrams, J. M. (1990a). Age and social-class differences in children's knowledge of sexuality. *Journal of Clinical Child Psychology, 19*, 33–43.

Gordon, B. N., Schroeder, C. S., & Abrams, J. M. (1990b). Children's knowledge of sexuality: A comparison of sexually abused and non-abused children. *American Journal of Orthopsychiatry, 60*, 250–257.

Group for the Advancement of Psychiatry. (1982). *The process of child therapy.* New York: Brunner/Mazel.

Harnest, J., & Chavern, H. E. (1985). *A survey of the use of anatomically correct dolls in sex education, investigation, therapy, and courtroom testimony.* Paper presented at the Seventh World Congress of Sexology, New Delhi, India.

Hill, P., & Hill, S. (1987). Videotaping children's testimony: An empirical view. *Michigan Law Review, 85*, 809–833.

Horowitz, R. E. (1939). Racial aspects of self-identification in nursery school children. *Journal of Psychology, 7*, 91–99.

Howe, M. (1991). Misleading children's story recall: Forgetting and reminiscence of the facts. *Developmental Psychology, 27*, 746–762.

In re Amber B. et al., 91 *Cal. Rptr.* 3d 682 (Calif. Ct. App. 1987).

Jampole, L., & Weber, M. K. (1987). An assessment of the behavior of sexually abused and nonabused children with anatomically correct dolls. *Child Abuse and Neglect, 11*, 187–192.

Johnson, M., & Foley, M. (1984). Differentiating fact from fantasy. *Journal of Social Issues, 40*, 33–50.

Kail, R. (1990). *The development of memory in children* (3rd ed.). New York: Freeman.

Keary, K., & Fitzpatrick, C. (1994). Children's disclosure of sexual abuse during formal investigation. *Child Abuse and Neglect, 18*, 543–548.

Kendall-Tackett, K. A. (1992). Beyond anatomical dolls: Professionals' use of other play therapy techniques. *Child Abuse and Neglect, 16*, 139–142.

Kendall-Tackett, K. A., & Watson, M. W. (1992). Use of anatomical dolls by Boston-area professionals. *Child Abuse and Neglect, 16*, 423–428.

Kendall-Tackett, K. A., Williams, L., & Finkelhor, D. (1992). Impact of sexual abuse on children: A review and synthesis of recent empirical findings. *Psychological Bulletin, 113*, 164–180.

Kenyon-Jump, R., Burnette, M. M., & Robertson, M. (1991). Comparison of behaviors of suspected sexually abused and nonsexually abused preschool children using anatomical dolls. *Journal of Psychopathology and Behavioral Assessment, 13*, 225–240.

King, M. A., & Yuille, J. (1987). Suggestibility and the child witness. In S. J. Ceci, M. P. Toglia, & D. F. Ross (Eds.), *Children's eyewitness memory* (pp. 24–35). New York: Springer-Verlag.

Klein, M. (1932). *The psychoanalysis of children*. London: Hogarth Press.

Kluger, R. (1975). *Simple justice*. New York: Knopf.

Lamb, S., & Coakley, M. (1993). "Normal" childhood sexual play and games: Differentiating play from abuse. *Child Abuse and Neglect, 17*, 515–526.

Lawson, L., & Chaffin, M. (1992). False negatives in sexual abuse disclosure interviews. *Journal of Interpersonal Violence, 7*, 532–542.

Leichtman, M. D., & Ceci, S. J. (1995). The effects of repeated questions and stereotypes on preschoolers' reports. *Developmental Psychology, 31*, 568–578.

Leippe, M. R., Manion, A., & Romanczyk, A. (1993). Discernability or discrimination? Understanding jurors' reactions to accurate and inaccurate child and adult eyewitnesses. In G. Goodman & B. Bottoms (Eds.), *Child victims, child witnesses: Understanding and improving testimony* (pp. 169–202). New York: Guilford Press.

Lepore, S. J., & Sesco, B. (1994). Distorting children's reports and interpretations of events through suggestion. *Journal of Applied Psychology, 79*, 108–120.

Leventhal, J. M., Hamilton, J., Rekedal, S., Tebano-Micci, A., & Eyster, C. (1989). Anatomically correct dolls used in interviews of young children suspected of having been sexually abused. *Pediatrics, 84*, 900–906.

Levy, H., Kalinowski, N., Markovic, J., Pittman, M., & Ahart, S. (1991). *Victim-sensitive interviewing in child sexual abuse. A developmental approach to interviewing and consideration of the use of anatomically detailed dolls.* Chicago: Department of Pediatrics, Mount Sinai Hospital Medical Center.

Levy, R. J. (1989). Using "scientific" testimony to prove child sexual abuse. *Family Law Quarterly, 23*, 383–409.

Lindberg, M., McComas, L., Jones, S., & Thomas, S. (1993, March). *Similarities and differences in eyewitness testimonies for children who directly versus vicariously experience stress.* Paper presented at the annual meeting of the Society for Research in Child Development, New Orleans, LA.

List, J. A. (1986). Age and schematic differences in the reliability of eyewitness testimony. *Developmental Psychology, 22*, 50–57.

Loftus, E. F. (1979). *Eyewitness testimony*. Cambridge, MA: Harvard University Press.

MacFarlane, K., & Krebs, S. (1986). Techniques of interviewing and evidence gathering. In K. MacFarlane & J. Waterman (Eds.), *Sexual abuse of young children: Evaluation and treatment* (pp. 67–100). New York: Guilford Press.

Mandler, J. (1984). *Stories, scripts, and scenes: Aspects of schema theory.* Hillsdale, NJ: Erlbaum.

Mann, T. (1991). Assessment of sexually abused children with anatomically detailed dolls: A critical review. *Behavioral Sciences and the Law, 9*, 43–51.

Meehl, P. E. (1992). Factors and taxa, traits and types, differences of degree and differences in kind. *Journal of Personality, 60*, 117–174.

Melton, G. B., & Thompson, R. (1987). Getting out of a rut: Detours to less traveled paths in child-witness research. In S. Ceci, M. J. Toglia, & D. Ross (Eds.), *Children's eyewitness memory* (pp. 209–229). New York: Springer-Verlag.

Mrazek, D. A., & Mrazek, P. B. (1981). Psychosexual development within the family. In P. B. Mrazek & C. H. Kempe (Eds.), *Sexually abused children and their families* (pp. 17–32). New York: Pergamon.

Myers, N. A., Clifton, R. K., & Clarkson, M. G. (1987). When they were very young: Almost threes remember two years ago. *Infant Behavior and Development, 10*, 123–132.

Nelson, K. (1993). The psychological and social origins of autobiographical memory. *Psychological Science, 4*, 7–14.

Perry, N., Claycomb, L., Dostal, C., Flanagan, C., McAuliff, B., & Tam, P. (1993, March). *When lawyers question children: Is justice served?* Paper presented at the annual meeting of the Society for Research in Child Development, New Orleans, LA.

Pezdek, K. (1994). *Children's suggestibility and resistance to suggestion.* Paper presented at the Conference on Applied Cognitive Psychology, Claremont Graduate School, Claremont, CA.

Piaget, J., & Inhelder, B. (1973). *Memory and intelligence.* New York: Basic Books.

Pipe, M. E., Gee, S., & Wilson, C. (1993). Cues, props, and context: Do they facilitate children's reports. In G. S. Goodman & B. L. Bottoms (Eds.), *Child victims, child witnesses* (pp. 25–46). New York: Guilford Press.

Poole, D., & Lindsay, D. S. (1994, April). *Interviewing preschoolers' Effects of nonsuggestive techniques, parental coaching, and leading questions on reports of nonexperienced events.* Paper presented at the American Psychology and Law Society Meetings, Santa Fe, NM.

Powell-Hopson, D., & Hopson, D. S. (1988). Implications of doll color preferences among Black preschool children and White preschool children. *Journal of Black Psychology, 14*(2), 57–63.

Price, D. W. W., & Goodman, G. S. (1990). Visiting the wizard: Children's memory for a recurring event. *Child Development, 61*, 664–680.

Quinn, K. M., White, S., & Santilli, G. (1989). Influences of an interviewer's behaviors in child sexual abuse investigations. *Bulletin of the American Academy of Psychiatry and the Law, 17*, 45–52.

Raskin, D., & Yuille, J. (1989). Problems in evaluating interviews of children in sexual abuse cases. In S. J. Ceci, D. Ross, & M. Toglia (Eds.), *Perspectives on children's testimony* (pp. 184–207). New York: Springer-Verlag.

Ratner, H. H., Smith, B., & Padgett, R. J. (1990). Children's organization of events and event memories. In R. Fivush & J. Hudson (Ed.), *Knowing and remembering in young children* (pp. 65–93). New York: Cambridge University Press.

Realmuto, G. M., Jensen, J. B., & Wescoe, S. (1990). Specificity and sensitivity of sexually anatomically correct dolls in substantiating abuse: A pilot study. *Journal of the American Academy of Child and Adolescent Psychiatry, 29*, 743–746.

Realmuto, G. M., & Wescoe, S. (1992). Agreement among professionals about child's sexual abuse status: Interviews with sexually anatomically correct dolls as indicators of abuse. *Child Abuse and Neglect, 16*, 719–725.

Rosenfeld, A. A., Bailey, R. R., Siegel, B., & Bailey, G. (1986). Determining incestuous contact between parent and child: Frequency of children touching parent's genitals in a nonclinical population. *Journal of the American Academy of Child and Adolescent Psychiatry, 25*, 481–484.

Rovee-Collier, C. (1989). The joy of kicking: Memories, motives, and mobiles. In P. R. Solomon, G. R. Goethals, C. M. Kelley, & B. R. Stephens (Eds.), *Memory: Interdisciplinary approaches*. New York: Springer-Verlag.

Rudy, L. A. (1991). *Interactions of sexually abused and nonabused children with anatomically correct dolls*. Unpublished master's thesis, Ohio State University, Columbus.

Rudy, L. A., & Goodman, G. S. (1991). Effects of participation on children's reports: Implications for children's testimony. *Developmental Psychology, 27*, 1–26.

Rutter, M. (1971). Normal psychosexual development. *Journal of Child Psychology and Psychiatry, 11*, 259–283.

Saywitz, K., & Goodman, G. S. (in press). Interviewing children in and out of court: Current research and practical implications. In L. Berliner, J. Bulkley, J. Briere, & T. Reid (Eds.), *Handbook of child sexual abuse*. Newbury Park, CA: Sage.

Saywitz, K., Goodman, G. S., Nicholas, E., & Moan, S. (1991). Children's memories of physical examinations involving genital touch: Implications for reports of child sexual abuse. *Journal of Consulting and Clinical Psychology, 59*, 682–691.

Saywitz, K., & Nathanson, R. (in press). Children's testimony and their perceptions of stress in and out of the courtroom. *Child Abuse and Neglect*.

Saywitz, K., & Snyder, L. (1993). Improving children's testimony through preparation. In G. S. Goodman & B. L. Bottoms (Eds.), *Child victims, child witnesses* (pp. 117–146). New York: Guilford Press.

Schor, D. P., & Sivan, A. B. (1989). Interpreting children's labels for sex-related body parts of anatomically explicit dolls. *Child Abuse and Neglect, 13*, 523–531.

Schwartz-Kenney, B., & Goodman, G. S. (1991, April). *Memory impairment in children*. Paper presented at the meetings of the Society for Research in Child Development, Seattle, WA.

Sinason, V. (1988). Dolls and bears: From symbolic equation to symbol: The significance of different play material for sexually abused children and others. *British Journal of Psychotherapy, 4*, 349–363.

Sivan, A. B. (1991). Preschool child development: Implications for investigation of child abuse allegations. *Child Abuse and Neglect, 15*, 485–493.

Sivan, A. B., Schor, D. P., Koeppl, G. K., & Noble, L. D. (1988). Interaction of normal children with anatomical dolls. *Child Abuse and Neglect, 12*, 295–304.

Skinner, L., & Berry, K. (1993). Anatomically detailed dolls and the evaluation of child sexual abuse allegations: Psychometric considerations. *Law and Human Behavior, 17*, 399–422.

Solomon, J. (1938). Active play therapy. *American Journal of Orthopsychiatry, 8*, 479–498.

State of New Jersey v. Kelly Michaels, 2 NJ Super., 593 (1993).

Steward, M. (1993). Understanding children's memories of medical procedures: "He didn't touch me and it didn't hurt." In C. A. Nelson (Ed.), *Minnesota Symposium on Child Psychology: Memory and affect in development* (pp. 171–225). Hillsdale, NJ: Erlbaum.

Steward, M., & Steward, J. (1989). *The development of a model interview for young child victims of sexual abuse: Comparing the effectiveness of anatomical dolls, drawings, and videographics.* Final Report to the National Center on Child Abuse and Neglect, Washington, DC.

Terr, L. (1988). What happens to early memories of trauma? A study of 20 children under age 5 at the time of the documented traumatic events. *Journal of the American Academy of Child and Adolescent Psychiatry, 27*, 96–104.

Tobey, A. E., & Goodman, G. S. (1992). Children's eyewitness memory: Effects of participation and forensic context. *Child Abuse and Neglect, 16*, 779–796.

Tulving, E. (1983). *Elements of episodic memory.* Oxford, England: Oxford University Press.

Warren, A., Hagood, P. L., & Snider, C. (1993, March). *Repeatedly questioning children: Does practice make perfect?* Paper presented at the annual meeting of the Society for Research in Child Development, New Orleans, LA.

Wedding, D., & Faust, D. (1989). Clinical judgment and decision making in neuropsychology. *Archives of Clinical Neuropsychology, 4*, 233–265.

Wellman, H. M., & Estes, D. (1986). Early understanding of mental entities: A reexamination of childhood realism. *Child Development, 57*, 910–923.

White, S. (1985a, October). *Objective data collection using anatomically correct dolls in the assessment of sexual abuse in very young children.* Workshop presented at the American Academy of Child and Adolescent Psychiatry, San Antonio, TX.

White, S. (1985b, October). *The use of anatomical dolls in child sexual abuse evaluations.* Presented at the National Summit Conference on Diagnosing Child Sexual Abuse, Los Angeles, CA.

White, S. (1986). Uses and abuses of anatomically correct dolls. *Children, Youth, and Families Newsletter, 9*, 3.

White, S. (1991). Using anatomically detailed dolls in interviewing preschoolers. In C. E. Schaefer, K. Gitlin, & A. Sandgrund (Eds.), *Play, diagnosis and assessment*. New York: Wiley.

White, S., Halpin, B. M., Strom, G. A., & Santilli, G. (1988). Behavioral comparisons of young sexually abused, neglected, and non-referred children. *Journal of Clinical Child Psychiatry, 17*, 53–61.

White, S., & Quinn, K. M. (1988). Investigatory independence in child sexual abuse evaluations: Conceptual considerations. *Bulletin of the American Academy of Psychiatry and the Law, 17*, 269–278.

White, S., Strom, G., & Santilli, G. (1983). *Research guidelines for interviewing young children with anatomically correct dolls*. Unpublished manuscript, Case Western Reserve University School of Medicine, Cleveland, OH.

White, S., Strom, G., & Santilli, G. (1985). *A protocol for interviewing preschoolers with the sexually anatomically correct dolls*. Unpublished manuscript, Case Western Reserve University School of Medicine, Cleveland, OH.

White, S., Strom, G., Santilli, G., & Halpin, B. M. (1986). Interviewing young sexual abuse victims with anatomically correct dolls. *Child Abuse and Neglect, 10*, 519–529.

White, S., Strom, G., Santilli, G., & Quinn, K. M. (1987). *Clinical guidelines for interviewing young children with anatomically correct dolls*. Unpublished manuscript, Case Western Reserve University School of Medicine, Cleveland, OH.

Wolfner, G., Faust, D., & Dawes, R. M. (1993). The use of anatomically detailed dolls in sexual abuse evaluations: The state of the science. *Applied & Preventive Psychology, 2*, 1–11.

Wright, L., Everett, F., & Roisman, L. (1986). *Experiential psychotherapy with children*. Baltimore: Johns Hopkins University Press.

Yates, A., & Terr, L. (1988a). Anatomically correct dolls: Should they be used as the basis for expert testimony? *Journal of the American Academy of Child and Adolescent Psychiatry, 27*, 254–257.

Yates, A., & Terr, L. (1988b). Issue continued: Anatomically correct dolls: Should they be used as the basis for expert testimony? *Journal of the American Academy of Child and Adolescent Psychiatry, 27*, 387–388.

Zaragoza, M. (1991). Preschool children's susceptibility to memory impairment. In J. Doris (Ed.), *The suggestibility of children's memory* (pp. 27–39). Washington, DC: American Psychological Association.

# Part V

# ISSUES IN TREATMENT

The four papers in this section address issues important in the treatment of children and adolescents with psychiatric disorders. In the first Allen, Leonard, and Swedo review *Current Knowledge of Medications for the Treatment of Childhood Anxiety Disorders*. Information derives from a *Medline*-assisted review of the literature. Particular attention was given to reports of dosage, response, and side effects of medications. Wherever possible, primary references included reports of blinded controlled medication trials in children with anxiety disorders diagnosed by structured criteria. Only 13 controlled studies, 5 for obsessive-compulsive disorder (OCD), 4 for school refusal/separation anxiety disorder, and 4 for avoidant/overanxious disorder or mixed diagnostic groups were located. This is in stark contrast to the fact that studies of children and adolescents have reported rates of anxiety disorders as between 8 and 9% in community samples. Because the number of controlled studies is so low, the authors also have considered critically information which derives from open trials, case reports and controlled trials in adults.

There is good evidence that clomipramine is effective for OCD and some additional evidence supports the efficacy of fluoxetine. Results of investigations of the pharmacologic treatment of separation anxiety and school phobia have been mixed, but suggest that imipramine and the benzodiazepines may be helpful. Less is known about the pharmacotherapy of other childhood anxiety disorders. Open trials with buspirone have suggested efficacy for overanxious disorder. However, a controlled trial with alprazolam did not. Panic disorder is just beginning to receive attention in children and anecdotal reports with imipramine and alprazolam are encouraging. While the SSRI's are promising in terms of a better tolerated side effect profile and evidence of efficacy for a variety of disorders in adults, their application in children is yet to be systematically investigated.

The authors conclude that research on pharmacological treatments for childhood anxiety disorders is in its infancy, with few trials using placebo controls, double-blind design, adequate medication doses, and/or well-defined, homogeneous patient populations. Consequently, in the absence of systematic treatment guidelines, clinicians must carefully consider the relative risk-to-benefit ratio when medicating children with anxiety disorders. The information provided in this review provides a sound basis for the making of informed choices.

In the second paper in this section, Dow, Sonies, Scheib, Moss, and Leonard present a comprehensive overview of the assessment and treatment of children with selective mutism in the light of a recent shift in views regarding etiology. Psychodynamic factors, long considered as etiologically preeminent are currently deemphasized. Instead, it has been proposed that selective mutism is better conceptualized as a childhood anxiety disorder. The failure of affected children to speak in specific social situations, although speaking in other settings, may well be a manifestation of a shy, inhibited temperament, likely modulated by psychodynamic and psychosocial issues, and in some cases associated with other developmental delays, speech and language disorder, or difficulty in processing social cues. Although the diagnostic criteria for selective mutism are straightforward, the differential diagnosis can be more complex. Speech inhibition can be a secondary symptom of many other psychiatric disorders including pervasive developmental disorder, schizophrenia and severe mental retardation. Moreover, speech and language problems can also be comorbid with selective mutism. Consequently any child for whom the diagnosis is considered should have a comprehensive evaluation to rule out other explanations for the mutism and to assess comorbid factors.

Assessment is based on information obtained from parents and direct examination of the child. Dow et al. emphasize that every child referred for selective mutism requires a comprehensive evaluation that addresses neurological, psychiatric, audiological, social, academic, and speech and language concerns. A helpful table summarizes these essential components. In the past, many selectively mute children did not receive complete assessments, either because clinicians believed they were untestable due to lack of verbal response or because they were thought to be unnecessary. These authors underscore that not only is it possible to fully evaluate children who are selectively mute, but that such evaluations are a critical first step in identifying primary and comorbid issues and in developing an appropriately individualized treatment plan. Cognitive-behavioral techniques, psychodynamic psychotherapy, medication and speech and language therapy can all be integrated to decrease anxiety and to foster speech and social interaction. While further research is required to evaluate the comparative effectiveness of these different approaches, this summary provides a most useful guide to clinicians called upon to evaluate and treat a selectively mute child.

The third paper in this section *Pemoline Effects on Children with ADHD*, serves to acquaint readers with an alternative psychopharmacological treatment for Attention-Deficit Hyperactivity Disorder (ADHD). Used in only 2% of children who receive stimulant medication for the treatment of

ADHD, pemoline has been much less extensively studied than the much more frequently administered methylphenidate (MPH). Moreover, as Pellham, Swanson, Furman and Schwindt point out, anecdotal reports of practitioners in clinic settings suggest that pemoline is not as effective as MPH.

The present study was designed to examine the effects of different doses of pemoline administered to children with ADHD in a laboratory classroom setting. Subjects were 28 children who ranged in age from 5 to 12 years, who met DSM-III criteria for ADD. After a two-week baseline, a double-blind crossover design was used to compare placebo, 18.75 mg, 37.5 mg, 75 mg, and 112.5 mg of pemoline, q.a.m., with each dose administered for one week. Medication was given at 9:00 AM and performance was measured immediately and again at 2, 4, and 6 hours after ingestion. Dependent measures included number of math problems completed correctly in a 15 minute period, teacher-recorded rates of on-task behavior and noncompliance, and teacher ratings on an Abbreviated Conners Teacher Rating Scale.

The results indicated that pemoline has clear beneficial effects on measures of classroom behavior and academic performance, comparable to those reported in studies of MPH. Pemoline becomes effective within 2 hours postingestion when it has been given for between 2 and 5 consecutive days. It's effects in the dose range from 18.75 and 112.5 are linear, although effectiveness is minimal at the lowest dose. Side effects were also minimal and not associated with increasing dose. These findings serve to disconfirm the widespread belief that pemoline has a delayed onset of 3 or more weeks and is not as efficacious for children with ADHD as MPH. Moreover because pemoline's effects last for at least 7 hours, it can provide all-day coverage of school behavior and performance as well as coverage of at least some after-school activity and homework time. As many middle school children and adolescents with ADHD are reluctant to take medications in school, pemoline becomes an important alternative long-acting preparation for the treatment of ADHD.

The final paper in this section examines another aspect of the treatment of children with ADHD; the efficacy of methylphenidate in children with comorbid ADHD and tic disorder. As Gadow, Sverd, Sprafkin, Nolan, and Ezor point out, information deriving from case reports and patient questionnaire surveys have been interpreted as indicating that administration of stimulants is ill-advised in the treatment of ADHD in children with tic disorder. The present report presents data from study of 34 prepubertal children with ADHD and tic disorder. Subjects, who were between 6 and 11 years of age received placebo and three dosages of methylphenidate (0.1, 0.3, and 0.5 mg/kg) twice daily for two weeks each, under double-blind conditions. Once the medication evaluation began, each child and at least one parent came to the clinic at two-week intervals for a clinical evaluation which included several standardized tic rating scales. In addition, children attended a simulated classroom where they were videotaped. Parents and teachers also completed tic rating scales. Methylphenidate was found to be effective in suppressing hyperactive, disruptive, and aggressive behavior. There was no evidence that methylphenidate altered the severity of tic disorder, but a small, neither clinically nor statistically significant effect on the frequency of motor (increase) and vocal (decrease) tics was observed.

While the authors conclude that methylphenidate appears to be a safe and effective treatment for children with ADHD and comorbid tic disorder, they do caution in a thoughtful discussion that the findings not be interpreted as indicating that methylphenidate is universally benign with regard to tic exacerbation. The possibility that it can have an adverse effect on tics in specific children cannot be entirely ruled out. All psychotherapeutic medications are capable of inducing or exacerbating comorbid conditions. In addition, this eight-week study does not address the possibility that tic exacerbations might result from longer-term drug exposure. The findings of a study of maintenance therapy, currently in progress, are eagerly awaited.

# 17

# Current Knowledge of Medications for the Treatment of Childhood Anxiety Disorders

**Albert John Allen, Henrietta L. Leonard and Susan E. Swedo**
*National Institute of Mental Health, Bethesda, Maryland*

**Objective:** *This report will review the costs, risks, and benefits of potentially useful medications for the treatment of children and adolescents with anxiety disorders and will identify areas where data are limited and additional research is needed.* **Method:** *A* Medline-*assisted review of the literature was performed. Attention was given to dosage, response, and side effects of medications. Wherever possible, blinded, controlled medication trials in children with anxiety disorders (diagnosed by structured criteria) were targeted for use as the primary references. Relatively few systematic studies were found, so information from open trials and case reports also was included, as were controlled trials in adult populations.* **Results:** *The largest body of work supporting the use of medications for childhood anxiety came from studies of obsessive-compulsive disorder, where clomipramine and fluoxetine have been found effective in systematic studies. In other childhood anxiety disorders, there are conflicting data about the efficacy of medications, such as tricyclic antidepressants, benzodiazepines, serotonin reuptake inhibitors, β-blockers, and monoamine oxidase inhibitors.* **Conclusions:** *This review of the systematic pharmacological trials for childhood anxiety disorders revealed only 13 controlled*

*studies: 5 for obsessive-compulsive disorder, 4 for school refusal/
separation anxiety disorder, and 4 for avoidant/overanxious
disorder or mixed diagnostic groups. Medications appear to be
helpful for childhood anxiety disorders, although definitive
pharmacotherapeutic data are lacking for many conditions. A
systematic study of these medications is required to establish
safety and efficacy in the pediatric age group. Evolving diagnostic criteria and terminology, the presence of comorbid diagnoses (especially affective disorders), and inadequate medication dosages may be factors hindering research in this field.
Until additional research is done, clinicians must carefully consider the relative risk-to-benefit ratio when prescribing these
medications.*

Anxiety is defined as apprehension, tension, or uneasiness from anticipation of danger, the source of which is largely unknown or unrecognized. It is
regarded as pathological when it interferes with achievement of desired goals,
quality of life, or emotional comfort (Hales and Yudofsky, 1987). Clinicians
have long recognized the importance of treating the symptom of anxiety
in children and adolescents. As early as 1959, Rodriguez et al. reported a
follow-up study of a group of children with school phobia, a condition often
including prominent anxiety features (Rodriguez et al., 1959); and in an open
trial, D'Amaro (1962) found chlordiazepoxide superior to psychosocial treatments for school refusal. Yet, despite these early reports and continued attention given to pediatric anxiety disorders, much uncertainty remains concerning the appropriate diagnosis and treatment of these conditions.

This review provides a broad overview of the pharmacological treatment
of childhood anxiety disorders and addresses the issues of changing diagnostic criteria and availability of new medications. It differs from previous
reviews (Allen et al., 1993; Leonard and Rapoport, 1989) in that its primary
focus is the consideration of evidence for and against medication therapy
in childhood anxiety disorders. Potential benefits and adverse side effects
of the anxiolytic drugs are considered. When information on children is
limited or unavailable, studies with adults are presented. Also noted are diagnostic issues concerning childhood anxiety disorders and why they affect treatment decisions and research. In addition, an effort is made to highlight the limitations of current knowledge, and suggestions for future
investigations are made.

Space limitations prevent this review from examining in detail the role
of nonpharmacological strategies in the treatment of childhood anxiety.

Multimodal treatment plans are often indicated, however, and the recent Practice Parameters for the Assessment and Treatment of Anxiety Disorders (American Academy of Child and Adolescent Psychiatry, 1993) presents this integrated approach. Two articles (Bemporad et al., 1993; Drobes and Strauss, 1993) provide excellent reviews of psychodynamic and behavioral treatments of childhood anxiety disorders. In addition, Kendall and colleagues (1991) detail cognitive-behavioral therapeutic approaches for anxious children. Since behavioral therapy is the treatment of choice for simple phobias, they are not included in this review of the pharmacological treatment of childhood anxiety disorders. This review also does not deal with anxiety that is secondary to medical illnesses or conditions, since the appropriate treatment is correction of the underlying medical condition. For a review of physical conditions that mimic anxiety disorders, the reader is referred to the Practice Parameters for Assessment and Treatment of Anxiety Disorders (American Academy of Child and Adolescent Psychiatry, 1993).

## BACKGROUND

The first edition of the *Diagnostic and Statistical Manual of Mental Disorders* (American Psychiatric Association, 1952) contained few references to childhood mental disorders in general, and virtually nothing about childhood disorders with anxiety as a prominent feature. *DSM-II* (American Psychiatric Association, 1968) introduced a section on behavioral disorders of childhood and adolescence and included two subcategories with significant anxiety features: "withdrawing reaction of childhood (or adolescence)" and "overanxious reaction of childhood (or adolescence)." However, the most significant change in nosology occurred with the publication of *DSM-III* (American Psychiatric Association, 1980). The *DSM-III* defined and described criteria for three anxiety disorders "usually first evident in infancy, childhood, or adolescence": separation anxiety, avoidant disorder and overanxious disorders. In addition, *DSM-III* categorized several other childhood disorders that often feature prominent anxiety symptoms, e.g., stuttering and elective mutism. Another important feature of *DSM-III* was that it specifically recognized that "adult" anxiety disorders—such as obsessive-compulsive disorder (OCD), panic attacks, posttraumatic stress disorder (PTSD), and phobias—could begin in childhood. These changes paralleled interest in research about childhood anxiety, which addressed issues of more accurate diagnosis and appropriate treatments.

Nosological advances continued in *DSM-III-R* (American Psychiatric Association 1987), which modified some individual criteria to emphasize that all "adult" anxiety disorders can be diagnosed in childhood. It did not introduce any new diagnostic categories. In *DSM-IV* (American Psychiatric Association, 1994), overanxious disorder was deleted and most children who previously fit these criteria now will be classified as having generalized anxiety disorder with childhood onset. Avoidant disorder of childhood also has been dropped and replaced by childhood-onset social phobia (social anxiety disorder). Separation anxiety disorder, which reflects developmental issues unique to children, was retained. Thus, the trend in *DSM-IV* is to emphasize the continuity between anxiety disorders in children and adults, except where developmental issues preclude this approach.

## *Effect of Changing Nosology on Psychopharmacology Research*

While the widespread use of standardized criteria has eliminated some methodological problems in child psychopharmacology research, others have appeared. Because the *DSM* criteria and diagnostic categories are still evolving, investigators are faced with a moving target when planning new research efforts. An excellent example of this is overanxious disorder, which appeared as "overanxious reaction of childhood (or adolescence)" in *DSM-II*, was significantly modified and reclassified in *DSM-III*, and was eliminated in *DSM-IV* in favor of generalized anxiety disorder of childhood onset. Given its turbulent life, it is little wonder that few investigators have attempted pharmacological studies of overanxious disorder and that no medication trials are available which meet the *DSM-IV* criteria for childhood-onset generalized anxiety disorder.

Although improvements in nosology facilitated treatment of pediatric disorders, they resulted in significant difficulties in applying earlier work to current diagnostic categories. Investigators initially focused on readily observable anxious behaviors, such as school refusal, because there were no systematic diagnostic criteria. Several early drug studies (Frommer, 1967; Gittelman-Klein and Klein, 1971, 1973, 1980) focused on school refusal. Typically, school refusal and associated studies are discussed with childhood anxiety disorders, especially separation anxiety disorder (Bernstein, 1990; Leonard and Rapoport, 1991). Yet, it is clear that children with school refusal are a heterogenous group and could represent, for example, simple phobia for school, social phobia, or conduct disorder. Bernstein et al. (1990) found that 65% of children with school refusal met criteria for both a depressive disorder and an anxiety disorder; 23% met criteria for a depressive disorder only; 12% had depressive and anxiety symptoms without meeting criteria for any disorder; and *none* met criteria for an anxiety disorder *alone*. In another study, "significant depression" was diagnosed in 22 (45%) of 51 children suffering from school phobia (Kolvin et al., 1984). Thus, one must cautiously extrapolate results of early medication studies in children with school refusal to current anxiety disorders of children.

The advent of standardized diagnostic criteria has raised issues about how to deal with anxiety symptoms that do not appear to fit a specific diagnostic category or are associated with a subgroup of patients with a nonanxiety diagnosis. Should such symptoms be a focus of pharmacological treatment or not, and if so, what are the appropriate medications? As an example, autistic children had been reported to respond poorly to tricyclic antidepressants (Campbell, 1975; Campbell et al., 1971), yet Gordon and coworkers (1992, 1993) reported that clomipramine was effective for both stereotypic behaviors and generalized autistic symptoms in a pair of controlled trials.

Comorbidity of anxiety disorders with other childhood psychiatric disorders, particularly depression, needs further research attention. Studies of depressed children, many (60% to 80%) of whom also had anxiety disorders, have not found antidepressants to be efficacious (Geller et al., 1992; Ryan et al., 1986). This raises the issue of whether children with comorbid anxiety and depression may be less responsive to tricyclics. This is consistent with work by Ryan et al. (1986), who found that adolescents with depression and separation anxiety disorder had a poorer response to imipramine than those with depression alone. It would also be in keeping with adult studies which find patients with comorbid anxiety and depression to be treatment resistant (Akiskal, 1990; Black and Noyes, 1990; Foa et al., 1987; Roose et al., 1986).

### Obstacles to Research on Childhood Anxiety Disorders

Even if the "perfect" classification of childhood anxiety disorders and related conditions were developed and confirmed, psychopharmacological research in this area would be hindered by economic, structural, and ethical limits.

The pharmaceutical industry remains one of the major funding sources for pharmacological studies in the United States. There is little incentive for the industry to conduct premarketing or postmarketing controlled treatment trials in children, since they are very expensive and raise liability concerns. This, coupled with the fact that medications are available (even if not approved by the Food and Drug Administration for this use) to the pediatric patient by prescription, provides little incentive for the pharmaceutical companies to develop safety and efficacy data specifically for children.

Research is also limited by a paucity of trained researchers. A 1989 survey of child psychiatry faculty in the United States (Shapiro et al., 1991) identified 95 "limited commitment researchers" and 45 "researchers." Of the latter group, only 10 identified psychopharmacology or other somatic treatments as an area of research interest, and 7 identified anxiety disorders as a diagnostic category of research interest. Clearly, this would suggest that the number of child psychopharmacologists focusing on anxiety disorders is very small.

Any research with children raises special ethical concerns, largely because of their developmental immaturity and consequent reliance on adults to make "informed consent." Federal Regulations (US Department of Health and Human Services, 1991) govern research (receiving federal funding) with children and are generally applied for all research with children. These regulations err in favor of providing protection to children and place numerous restrictions on such research, particularly that which involves treatments or procedures with "more than minimal risk." Depending on interpretation by local institutional review boards, blood sampling, biological studies, and even psychological testing can be considered "more than minimal risk" and may be prohibited unless there is direct benefit to a specific child. Furthermore, any proposed treatment which involves "more than minimal risk" must be expected to be superior to that which is currently approved. Thus, pediatric drug trials must follow adult clinical studies and approval. These restrictions make it unlikely that attempts will be made to develop any novel medications specifically targeted toward childhood anxiety disorders.

### Early Research with Anxious Children

The earliest report of pharmacotherapy of anxious children was by Fish (1960). On the basis of Fish's open trials of various medications in a diverse outpatient population, diphenhydramine was recommended for the treatment of childhood anxiety symptoms. However, a subsequent double-blind, placebo-controlled study of diphenhydramine in a heterogeneous group of pediatric inpatients did not support its efficacy (Korein et al., 1971).

Chlordiazepoxide (Librium®) was introduced in the United States in the early 1960s. Shortly thereafter, Krakowski (1963) published a small open trial that suggested chlordiazepoxide was effective as a treatment for anxiety associated with a variety of "emotional disturbances" in children. Kraft (1965) described similar results in a larger open trial with a heterogeneous patient population but found the greatest improvement in a subgroup of children with school phobia. Of note, a paradoxical reaction consisting of hyperactivity, dyscontrol, and rage was observed in 10% of these patients. This dyscontrol reaction has continued to be problematic. A double-blind, crossover trial by Frommer (1967) found chlordiazepoxide plus phenelzine superior to phenobarbital as a treatment for children with depression and/or phobic symptoms.

To our knowledge, there is only one other early drug trial for pediatric anxiety. Equivocal results were obtained in a double-blind, crossover study that compared diazepam with placebo as a treatment for anxiety symptoms in 12 hospitalized children and adolescents, 2 of whom had schizophrenia and the remainder, psychoneurosis (Lucas and Pasley, 1969). Neither schizophrenic patient completed the study, and a third child also was withdrawn. For the nine patients who finished the trial, combined symptom ratings (including anxiety and tension) slightly favored diazepam, whereas clinical ratings slightly favored placebo. Anxious older adolescents seemed to respond better to diazepam in this study.

## PHARMACOTHERAPHY OF SPECIFIC ANXIETY DISORDERS

### Obsessive-Compulsive Disorder

From a pharmacological standpoint, OCD is probably the best studied of all pediatric anxiety disorders and the condition currently most amenable to drug therapy. The serotonin reuptake blocking drugs, such as clomipramine, fluoxetine, sertraline, and fluvoxamine, have been found to be effective in controlled trials of adults with OCD. Systematic trials of clomipramine and fluoxetine demonstrate pediatric safety and efficacy, and anecdotal evidence exists for the newer agents (Leonard et al., 1993a).

Clomipramine's efficacy for pediatric OCD has been demonstrated clearly in double-blind studies comparing it to placebo (DeVeaugh-Geiss et al., 1992; Flament et al., 1985) and desipramine (Leonard et al., 1989). In the study by Flament and colleagues (1985), nearly 75% of children had a moderate to marked response to clomipramine within 5 weeks of treatment of doses between 100 and 200 mg/day (approximately 3 mg/kg per day). Not only was this degree of improvement replicated in a later study with a crossover design, but some degree of relapse occurred in two thirds of patients who received clomipramine first and then switched to desipramine, even though they had received clomipramine therapy for only 5 weeks (Leonard et al., 1989). The improvement appears to be sustained in most cases, but clomipramine is clearly a treatment and not a cure. When patients who had received long-term maintenance treatment with clomipramine were blindly switched to desipramine for 2 months, almost all (90%) relapsed, indicating that most patients require continued clomipramine treatment (Leonard et al., 1991), especially since for many it is a chronic disorder (Leonard et al., 1993b).

A recent double-blind crossover trial suggests that fluoxetine (fixed dose of 20 mg/day) also may be useful in childhood and adolescent OCD (Riddle et al., 1992). This study found a 44% decrease in obsessive-compulsive symptoms (as measured by the Children's Yale-Brown Obsessive Compulsive Scale [CY-BOCS]) with fluoxetine, versus a 27% decrease with placebo. This improvement on the CY-BOCS did not reach statistical significance, possibly because of a small sample size. On another measure (Clinical Global Impression Scale for OCD), however, there was a significant and favorable change from baseline for the fluoxetine-treated group compared with the group receiving placebo. A double-blind, parallel-group design study of 11 Tourette's syndrome patients with obsessive-compulsive symptoms (but not necessarily OCD) did not find a significant difference between fluoxetine and placebo, although only 4 patients completed the active medication treatment phase (Kurlan et al., 1993).

Fluvoxamine has been reported to be effective for OCD in studies with adults (Goodman et al., 1989, 1990; Jenike et al., 1990b), and it produced a significant decline in symptom severity on Y-BOCS scores in a recent open trial with 14 adolescents with OCD (Apter et al., 1994). Controlled trials with fluvoxamine in children are ongoing but at the time of this writing, the results are not yet available. Sertraline (Chouinard et al., 1990; Jenike et al., 1990a) has also been reported to be effective in adult patients with OCD, although currently there are no published controlled trials in children. There are, however, ongoing trials at several sites. Anecdotal reports suggest that it is well tolerated and effective in the younger age group, although there are no published reports available to substantiate this.

### Separation Anxiety and School Refusal

**Tricyclics.** Four placebo-controlled studies have examined the efficacy of tricyclic antidepressants for separation anxiety or school refusal associated with separation anxiety. In a double-blind study, Gittelman-Klein and Klein (1971, 1973, 1980) randomized 45 children with "school phobia" to receive either placebo or 100 to 200 mg of imipramine per day for 6 weeks. Both groups of children also received behaviorally oriented psychotherapy. Imipramine was superior to placebo in terms of the number of children returning to school (81% for imipramine versus 47% for placebo) and symptom improvement (as measured by self-report, parents, and clinicians). Klein et al. (1992) attempted unsuccessfully to replicate their earlier findings in 20 children with separation anxiety, for whom prior behavioral treatment had failed. It is unclear why this more recent study did not find imipramine superior to placebo. Possible explanations are smaller sample size or a different population. All the original patients had school phobia, whereas those in the latter study had separation anxiety, with or without school phobia. Another difference was that children in the second study had previously failed to respond to behavioral treatment, whereas those in the initial trial received behavior therapy as part of the study.

Berney and colleagues (1981) treated 51 school-phobic children (aged 9 to 14 years) with clomipramine or placebo. They failed to demonstrate a difference between the two treatments, although this may have been due to their patient population (44% also had depressive symptoms) or inadequate clomipramine doses (40 to 75 mg/day). Bernstein et al. (1990) compared alprazolam and imipramine as treatments for school refusal in a pair of studies. In the open study with 17 patients, two thirds of those completing alprazolam or imipramine trials had moderate to marked global improvement of their anxiety symptoms. Results were less clear in the double-blind, placebo-controlled study with 24 patients. On the Anxiety Rating for Children, there was a significant difference in posttreatment scores (calculated as change from baseline) in favor of active medication (alprazolam or imipramine), with similar trends noted on depression rating scales. However, analysis of covariance failed to show any differences between treatment groups. It is unknown whether a larger sample size might have resulted in significant differences. Thus, after four controlled studies involving 140 children, the best that can be said is that tricyclic antidepressants may be helpful in some cases of separation anxiety disorder and school refusal, but definitive proof is lacking.

**Benzodiazepines.** Not long after the introduction of benzodiazepines, D'Amato (1962) described an open trial of chlordiazepoxide (10 to 30 mg/day) for school refusal in children between 8 and 11 years of age. Eight of 9 children treated with the medication returned to school within 2 weeks, whereas only 2 of 11 treated with psychosocial methods returned to school within 2 weeks. In another large series of open trials, chlordiazepoxide (30 to 60 mg/day) was of benefit to 53 of 130 children and adolescents (7 to 17 years of age) with a variety of anxiety disorders. The greatest improvement was in the school-phobic group, where 77% improved (Kraft, 1965), but systematic ratings were not used. All of these studies found a low rate of side effects secondary to chlordiazepoxide, with drowsiness and dizziness being the most common. Biederman (1987) recently reported success using clonazepam (0.5 to 3 mg/day) in an open trial to treat two children with separation anxiety disorder and one child with overanxious disorder, all with panic-like symptoms. Eighteen children and adolescents with separation anxiety responded favorably to an open trial of alprazolam (0.5 to 6.0 mg/day), although ratings by teachers and children were less encouraging than those by parents and psychiatrists (Kutcher et al., 1992).

In one of the few controlled studies of benzodiazepines for childhood anxiety disorders, Graae et al. (1994) studied 15 children (aged 7 to 13 years) with a variety of anxiety disorders (14 had separation anxiety disorder as one of their diagnoses) in a double-blind, crossover trial comparing 4 weeks of placebo to 4 weeks of clonazepam (up to 2 mg/day). Twelve children, 11 of whom had separation anxiety, completed the study. One child dropped out for nonstudy reasons and two others dropped out because they experienced marked disinhibition while taking clonazepam. Clonazepam was not found to be superior to placebo on Brief Psychiatric Rating Scale or Clinical Global Impression Scale ratings, but six (50%) of the children who completed the study no longer met criteria for an anxiety disorder at the end of the study. Ten children had side effects while taking clonazepam (most experienced drowsiness or irritability and concurrent oppositional behavior). Although these side effects were usually mild, two children subsequently dropped out because of these effects.

### *Generalized Anxiety Disorder with Childhood Onset (Formerly Overanxious Disorder)*

Generalized anxiety disorder has received little attention from pediatric psychopharmacologists. The aforementioned open trial of clonazepam in one child (Biederman, 1987) was promising. A double-blind study of 30 children and adolescents with avoidant or overanxious disorder found no difference between alprazolam (up to 0.04 mg/kg per day, mean daily dose of 1.57 mg) and placebo (Simeon et al., 1992). Patients with overanxious disorder appeared to be even less responsive to alprazolam than was the group as a whole. Thus, further study is necessary before one can reach a conclusion about the efficacy of the benzodiazepines for generalized anxiety in children. An open trial of fluoxetine (10 to 60 mg/day, mean 25.7 mg/day) in 21 children and adolescents with overanxious disorder plus a variety of other anxiety disorders, but not OCD or panic disorder, has recently been published (Birmaher et al., 1994). Seventeen patients had moderate to marked improvement, and the severity of anxiety was reduced from marked to mild on the Clinical Global Impression Scale. These promising results with fluoxetine need to be pursued via placebo-controlled trials.

Buspirone has recently been reported to be effective for generalized anxiety disorder in open trials. A 13-year-old boy with overanxious disorder and school refusal was successfully treated with buspirone, 10 mg/day (Kranzler, 1988). In an open-label study of adolescents with overanxious disorder or generalized anxiety disorder, ratings on the Hamilton Anxiety Scale decreased significantly after 6 weeks of buspirone therapy (15 to 30 mg/day) (Kutcher et al., 1992). These open trials suggest that controlled trials are merited.

### Panic Disorder

Despite reports clearly documenting that panic disorder can have its onset in childhood (Black and Robbins, 1990), there are no systematic psychopharmacological studies to evaluate efficacy. The clinician must extrapolate from adult data and interpret case studies.

**Tricyclics and benzodiazepines.** While several well-controlled studies have demonstrated that tricyclic antidepressants and benzodiazepines are effective treatments for panic disorder in adults (see reviews by Hollander et al., 1988, and Klerman, 1992), there are no such studies in children and adolescents. Case reports suggest that tricyclic antidepressants (imipramine or desipramine) (Black and Robbins, 1990; Garland and Smith, 1990) are effective for panic disorder in children and adolescents. Ballenger and colleagues (1989) reported that three children with panic disorder and agoraphobia responded to either imipramine alone ($n = 1$) or in combination with alprazolam ($n = 2$).

Clonazepam has also been reported to be useful for panic disorder. Biederman (1987) reported that three prepubertal children with panic-like symptoms responded to clonazepam. In an open trial, four adolescents (aged 16 to 19 years) with panic disorder reported a decrease in frequency of attacks and less anxiety when treated with clonazepam, 1.0 to 2.0 mg/day (Kutcher and Mackenzie, 1988). The same group also has reported encouraging preliminary results of a double-blind study of adolescents with panic disorder (Kutcher et al., 1992). Of the 12 patients studied to date, 80% of those treated with clonazepam were moderately to markedly improved on the Clinical Global Impression Scale, whereas only 20% of the placebo group experienced a similar change. Both the frequency of panic attacks and the severity of anxiety symptoms decreased. Side effects of clonazepam were minimal, although irritability and restlessness caused one subject to withdraw from the study.

**Other medications.** No controlled studies have examined the efficacy of propranolol for panic disorder in children and adolescents, but Jorrabchi (1977) reported it to be helpful in treating pediatric hyperventilation syndrome, a possible variant of panic disorder. Fourteen treatment-resistant patients were given 30 to 60 mg/day of propranolol and 13 improved within a week of starting medication. However, eight relapsed during the 5 days after propranolol was discontinued.

### Childhood-Onset Social Phobia (Formerly Avoidant Disorders of Childhood)

Most children who would have met *DSM-III-R* criteria for avoidant disorder of childhood now meet *DSM-IV* criteria for social phobia. According to *DSM-IV*, social phobia is a disorder in which there is a persistent fear of situations in which the patient is exposed to public scrutiny; in addition, the patient may fear acting in a way that will be humiliating or embarrassing. The social phobia may be circumscribed and involve only a few situations, e.g., speaking in public, taking a test, or playing music at a recital, or it may be of the generalized type such that it includes most social situations (American Psychiatric Association, 1994). The generalized type of social phobia may correspond more closely to avoidant disorder of childhood, whereas the circumscribed variant may include severe cases of performance anxiety. It is not clear whether the two types of social phobia exist on a continuum or they represent distinct syndromes.

A recent case report suggests buspirone was beneficial in an adolescent with social phobia and mixed personality disorder (Zwier and Rao, 1994), but obviously controlled trials are required. There have been only two controlled medication studies including patients with avoidant disorder. Using a double-blind random assignment design, Simeon et al. (1992) compared alprazolam (up to 0.04 mg/kg per day) and placebo for the treatment of avoidant or overanxious disorder in 30 children and adolescents. There was no significant difference between the two treatment groups, although patients treated with alprazolam seemed to have a slightly greater improvement. More recently, Black and Uhde (1994) reported a 12-week, double-blind, placebo-controlled trial of fluoxetine in 15 children and adolescents with elective mutism and either social phobia or avoidant disorder. Improvements were noted by parents, teachers, and clinicians with both treatments. There was only a significant difference, favoring fluoxetine, on parents' ratings of mutism change and global change. The small sample size in this study (only six children completed active therapy) and the limited effect observed mean that the definitive study in this area remains to be done.

Pharmacological treatment of generalized social phobia in adults includes β-blockers, benzodiazepines, and monoamine oxidase inhibitors (MAOIs). Phenelzine, atenolol, and placebo were compared as treatments for social phobia in a double-blind trial with 74 adults, 56 of whom had generalized social phobia and 18 of whom had discrete social phobia (Liebowitz et al., 1992). For the group as a whole, the response rate for phenelzine was 64%, significantly greater than that for atenolol (30%) or placebo (23%), with similar findings in the subgroup with generalized social phobia. Gelernter and colleagues (1991) compared the efficacy of phenelzine, alprazolam, and placebo in a parallel design, with 15 adult patients (one quarter had generalized social phobia) receiving each medication. On the basis of blinded clinician ratings, patients had greater improvement (on the Work and Social Disability Scale) while receiving phenelzine than did those receiving alprazolam or placebo. After a blinded medication taper, patients who had been receiving phenelzine (compared with those who had been receiving placebo) remained significantly improved, whereas those who had been receiving alprazolam did not.

More recently, in an open trial of 14 adult patients with generalized social phobia, 10 were found to have a moderate to marked improvement while receiving fluoxetine, 20 to 100 mg/day (Black et al., 1992). These results suggest that generalized social phobia may respond well to MAOIs and possibly to fluoxetine and other serotonin specific reuptake inhibitors (SSRIs). Unfortunately, the child psychiatrist is left with extrapolating from the adult data. We hope that the SSRIs will prove effective when studied systematically, as they offer practical advantages over the MAOIs. Clearly, a great deal of work remains to be done in this area with both children and adults.

### Specific Social/Performance Anxiety Disorders

Results of studies in adults for specific social anxiety disorders, e.g., performance anxiety, are mixed. Noyes (1988) reviewed 11 controlled trials that compared the efficacy of single doses of β-blockers, including propranolol, to placebo or diazepam in the treatment of performance anxiety associated with music performances, public speaking, and examinations. Two studies, both using mepindolol (a β-receptor antagonist), failed to produce a subjective response and failed to improve performance. The other nine studies all demonstrated improvement as judged by either subjective response, or performance, or both. Two studies dealing with examination performance may be of particular interest to child psychiatrists. In one, Krishnan (1976) gave undergraduates with "exam nerves" either oxprenolol (a β-blocker) or diazepam. Students receiving the β-blocker had a greater improvement in test scores than those receiving diazepam, even though the students receiving diazepam thought they had performed better. Drew et al. (1985) found a single dose (120 mg) of propranolol significantly improved examination performance, with the greatest benefit seen in the subjects with the greatest anxiety. In general, most of the benefit seen with β-blockers appears to be due to a reduction in autonomically mediated symptoms of anxiety, i.e., palpitations and tremor, not a decrease in subjective feelings of anxiety (Noyes, 1982; Noyes, 1988). These studies are more difficult to extrapolate to children, as it is uncommon to treat children for a specific performance anxiety.

## PTSD and Reactive Attachment Disorder of Childhood

PTSD can be diagnosed in the pediatric age group and in young children who have been abused or neglected before 5 years of age. It may be diagnosed along with reactive attachment disorder of childhood (American Psychiatric Association, 1987). One variant of reactive attachment disorder is characterized by excessive social inhibition and may include anxiety symptoms such as avoidance and hypervigilance. It is currently unclear whether or not there is a relationship between reactive attachment disorder and childhood anxiety and whether or not medications are of any value. Given the prevalence of child abuse and neglect, this is an area that merits research.

Despite the frequency of PTSD in children, there has been only one report of the use of medications for pediatric PTSD. Famularo and colleagues (1988) used propranolol to treat 11 agitated, hyperaroused children with PTSD secondary to physical or sexual abuse. This was an open study using an off-on-off design with a 2-week period during which the medication was gradually increased to a maximum of 2.5 mg/kg per day, a 2-week period on the final dose of propranolol, and then a 1-week period during which the propranolol was tapered off. Three children could not tolerate the maximum dose of propranolol but did tolerate lower doses. While receiving propranolol, the children had significantly fewer PTSD symptoms compared to the periods before or after this medication. Controlled trials of propranolol in pediatric PTSD have not yet been published and clinically, the treatment is often symptom focused.

Research on pharmacological treatments for PTSD in adults has been driven by the large number of Vietnam veterans with this condition, although recent work has begun to examine other types of trauma victims. A recent review of this adult literature (Silver et al., 1990) noted the predominance of case reports and open trials. In the absence of pervasive comorbid conditions, the authors recommended tricyclic antidepressants as the initial psychopharmacological treatment, with subsequent therapy dependent on the patient's symptoms and initial response. Other medications they suggest as helpful include MAOIs (especially for refractory depression), lithium augmentation of tricyclics (for refractory depression and anger), carbamazepine (for flashbacks), propranolol (for significant distress on reexposure and for persistent autonomic arousal), clonidine (for persistent autonomic arousal), benzodiazepines (for sleep disturbance), and trazodone (for sleep disturbance). More recently, buspirone was reported to be helpful in three adults with PTSD (Wells et al. 1991). Without controlled trials in adults, it is difficult to make recommendations for treatment in children.

### Selective Mutism (Elective Mutism)

Selective mutism (formerly elective mutism in *DSM-III-R*) is included in this review because there is speculation that it may be a childhood model of social phobia (Black and Uhde, 1992, 1994; Crumley, 1990; Golwyn and Weinstock, 1990; Leonard and Topol, 1993). As is often true with relatively rare conditions, little information is available on the use of medications in selective mutism. A 7-year-old girl with a 2-year history of elective mutism and "associated shyness" was successfully treated with the MAOI, phenelzine (Golwyn and Weinstock, 1990). A small, double-blind, placebo-controlled trial of fluoxetine in 15 children and adolescents with elective mutism plus social phobia or avoidant disorder (Black and Uhde, 1994) was discussed in this review under childhood-onset social phobia.

## DISCUSSION

In summary, this review of the systematic pharmacological trials for childhood anxiety disorder revealed only 13 controlled studies: 5 for OCD, 4 for social refusal/separation anxiety disorder, and 4 for avoidant/overanxious disorder or mixed diagnostic groups. This is surprisingly limited given that studies of children and adolescents have reported rates of anxiety disorders between 8% and 9% in community samples (Berenson, 1993).

OCD is the anxiety disorder that has been studied most extensively in childhood. There is good evidence that clomipramine is effective for this condition, and some evidence supports fluoxetine's efficacy. Separation anxiety and school phobia have also been well studied. Results of these investigations have been mixed but suggest imipramine and the benzodiazepines may be helpful. Less is known about the pharmacotherapy of other childhood anxiety disorders. Open trials with buspirone have suggested efficacy for overanxious disorder, yet the controlled trial with alprazolam did not. Panic disorder is just beginning to receive attention in pediatric patients, and preliminary anecdotal reports with imipramine and alprazolam are encouraging. Similarly, case reports of successful treatment of avoidant disorder with alprazolam suggested it may be effective. However, this was not substantiated by the controlled trial. The efficacy of propranolol for pediatric PTSD, which was suggested by one open study, requires additional study. The development of the new class of medications, the SSRIs, are promising in terms of a better-tolerated side effect profile and evidence of efficacy for a variety of disorders in adults. Their application in children merits investigation.

In conclusion, research on pharmacological treatments for childhood anxiety disorders remains in its infancy, with few trials using placebo controls, double-blind design, adequate medication doses, and/or well-defined, homogeneous patient populations. Thus, clinicians treating anxious children are left without systematic treatment guidelines. Unfortunately, it seems likely that economic, structural, and ethical factors will continue to limit work in this area. Nevertheless, efforts should be made to establish the effectiveness of pharmacotherapy for these troubling pediatric disorders.

## REFERENCES

Akiskal HS (1990), Toward a clinical understanding of the relationship of anxiety and depressive disorders. In: *Comorbidity of Mood and Anxiety Disorders*, Maser JF, Cloninger CR, eds. Washington, DC: American Psychiatric Press, pp 597–607

Allen AJ, Rapoport JL, Swedo SE (1993), Psychopharmacologic treatment of childhood anxiety disorders. *Child Adolesc Psychiatr Clin North Am* 2:795–817

American Academy of Child and Adolescent Psychiatry (1993), AACAP official action: practice parameters for the assessment and treatment of anxiety disorders. *J Am Acad Child Adolesc Psychiatry* 32:1089–1098

American Psychiatric Association (1952), *Diagnostic and Statistical Manual of Mental Disorders, 1st edition*. Washington, DC: American Psychiatric Association

American Psychiatric Association (1968), *Diagnostic and Statistical Manual of Mental Disorders, 2nd edition (DSM-II)*. Washington, DC: American Psychiatric Association

American Psychiatric Association (1980), *Diagnostic and Statistical Manual of Mental Disorders, 3rd edition (DSM-III)*. Washington, DC: American Psychiatric Association

American Psychiatric Association (1987), *Diagnostic and Statistical Manual of Mental Disorders, 3rd edition-revised (DSM-III-R)*. Washington, DC: American Psychiatric Association

American Psychiatric Association (1994), *Diagnostic and Statistical Manual of Mental Disorders, 4th edition (DSM-IV)*. Washington, DC: American Psychiatric Association

Apter A, Ratzoni G, King RA et al. (1994), Fluvoxamine open-label treatment of adolescent inpatients with obsessive-compulsive disorder of depression. *J Am Acad Child Adolesc Psychiatry* 33:342–348

Ballenger JC, Carek DJ, Steele JJ, Cornish-McTighe D (1989), Three cases of panic disorder with agoraphobia in children [see comments]. *Am J Psychiatry* 146:922–924

Bemporad JR, Beresin E, Rauch PK (1993), Psychodynamic theories and treatment of childhood anxiety disorders. *Child Adolesc Psychiatr Clin North Am* 2:763–777

Berenson CK (1993), Evaluation and treatment of anxiety in the general pediatric population: a clinician's guide. *Child Adolesc Psychiatr Clin North Am* 2: 727–747

Berney T, Kolvin I, Bhate SR et al. (1981), School phobia: a therapeutic trial with clomipramine and short-term outcome. *Br J Psychiatry* 138:110–118

Bernstein GA (1990), Anxiety disorders. In: *Psychiatric Disorders in Children and Adolescents*. Garfinkel BD, Carlson GA, Weller EB, eds. Philadelphia: Saunders, pp 64–83

Bernstein GA, Garfinkel BD, Borchardt CM (1990), Comparative studies of pharmacotherapy for school refusal. *J Am Acad Child Adolesc Psychiatry* 29:773–781

Biederman J (1987), Clonazepam in the treatment of prepubertal children with panic-like symptoms. *J Clin Psychiatry* 48(suppl):38–42

Birmaher B, Waterman GS, Ryan N et al. (1994), Fluoxetine for childhood anxiety disorders. *J Am Acad Child Adolesc Psychiatry* 33:993–999

Black B, Robbins DR (1990), Panic disorder in children and adolescents. *J Am Acad Child Adolesc Psychiatry* 29:36–44

Black B, Uhde TW (1992), Case study: elective mutism as a variant of social phobia. *J Am Acad Child Adolesc Psychiatry* 31:1090–1094

Black B, Uhde TW (1994), Treatment of elective mutism with fluoxetine: a double-blind, placebo-controlled study. *J Am Acad Child Adolesc Psychiatry* 33:1000–1006

Black B, Uhde TW, Tancer ME (1992), Fluoxetine for the treatment of social phobia. *J Clin Psychopharmacol* 12:293–295

Black DW, Noyes R Jr (1990), Comorbidity and obsessive-compulsive disorder. In: *Comorbidity of Mood and Anxiety Disorders*, Maser JD, Cloninger CR, eds. Washington, DC: American Psychiatric Press, pp 305–316

Campbell M (1975), Pharmacotherapy in early infantile autism. *Biol Psychiatry* 10:399–423

Campbell M, Fish B, Shapiro T, Floyd A Jr (1971), Imipramine in preschool autistic and schizophrenic children. *J Autism Child Schizophr* 1:267–282

Chouinard G, Goodman W, Greist J et al. (1990), Results of a double blind placebo controlled trial of a new serotonin uptake inhibitor, sertraline, in the treatment of obsessive-compulsive disorder. *Psychopharmacol Bull* 26:279–284

Crumley FE (1990), The masquerade of mutism (letter). *J Am Acad Child Adolesc Psychiatry* 29:318–319

D'Amato G (1962), Chlordiazepoxide in management of school phobia. *Dis Nerv Sys* 23:292–295

DeVeaugh-Geiss J, Moroz G, Biederman J et al. (1992), Clomipramine hydrochloride in childhood and adolescent obsessive-compulsive disorder: a multicenter trial. *J Am Acad Child Adolesc Psychiatry* 31:45–49

Drew PJT, Barnes JN, Evans SJW (1985), The effect of acute beta-adrenoceptor blockade on examination performance. *Br J Clin Pharmacol* 19:783–786

Drobes DJ, Strauss CC (1993), Behavioral treatment of childhood anxiety disorders. *Child Adolesc Psychiatr Clin North Am* 2:779–793

Famularo R, Kinscherff R, Fenton T (1988), Propranolol treatment for childhood posttraumatic stress disorder, acute type. A pilot study. *Am J Dis Child* 142:1244–1247

Fish B (1960), Drug therapy in child psychiatry: pharmacological aspects. *Compr Psychiatry* 1:212–227

Flament MF, Rapoport JL, Berg CJ et al. (1985), Clomipramine treatment of childhood obsessive-compulsive disorder. A double-blind controlled study. *Arch Gen Psychiatry* 42:977–983

Foa EB, Steketee G, Kozak MJ, Dugger D (1987), Effects of imipramine on depression and obsessive-compulsive symptoms. *Psychiatry Res* 21:123–136

Frommer EA (1967), Treatment of childhood depression with antidepressant drugs. *Br Med J* 1:729–732

Garland EJ, Smith DH (1990), Case study: panic disorder on a child psychiatric consultation service. *J Am Acad Child Adolesc Psychiatry* 29:785–788

Gelernter CS, Uhde TW, Cimbolic P et al. (1991), Cognitive-behavioral and pharmacological treatments of social phobia: a controlled study. *Arch Gen Psychiatry* 48:938–945

Geller B, Cooper TB, Graham DL, Fetner HH, Marsteller FA, Wells JM (1992), Pharmacokinetically designed double-blind placebo-controlled study of nortriptyline in 6- to 12-year-olds with major depressive disorder. *J Am Acad Child Adolesc Psychiatry* 31:34–44

Gittelman-Klein R, Klein DF (1971), Controlled imipramine treatment of school phobia. *Arch Gen Psychiatry* 25:204–207

Gittelman-Klein R, Klein DF (1973), School phobia: diagnostic considerations in the light of imipramine effects. *J Nerv Ment Dis* 156:199–215

Gittelman-Klein R, Klein DF (1980), Separation anxiety in school refusal and its treatment with drugs. In: *Out of School*, Hersov L, Berg I, eds. New York: Wiley, pp 321–341

Golwyn DH, Weinstock RC (1990), Phenelzine treatment of elective mutism: a case report. *J Clin Psychiatry* 51:384–385

Goodman WK, Price LH, Delgado PL et al. (1990), Specificity of serotonin reuptake inhibitors in the treatment of obsessive-compulsive disorder. Comparison of fluvoxamine and desipramine [see comments]. *Arch Gen Psychiatry* 47:577–585

Goodman WK, Price LH, Rasmussen SA, Delgado PL, Heninger GR, Charney DS (1989), Efficacy of fluvoxamine in obsessive-compulsive disorder. A double-blind comparison with placebo. *Arch Gen Psychiatry* 46:36–44

Gordon CT, Rapoport JL, Hamburger SD, State RC, Mannheim GB (1992), Differential response of seven subjects with autistic disorder to clomipramine and desipramine. *Am J Psychiatry* 149:363–366

Gordon CT, State RC, Nelson JE, Hamburger SD, Rapoport JL (1993), A double-blind comparison of clomipramine, desipramine, and placebo in the treatment of autistic disorder. *Arch Gen Psychiatry* 50:441–447

Graae F, Milner J, Rizzotto L, Klein RG (1994), Clonazepam in childhood anxiety disorders. *J Am Acad Child Adolesc Psychiatry* 33:372–376

Hales RE, Yudofsky SC (1987), *The American Psychiatric Press Textbook of Neuropsychiatry*. Washington, DC: American Psychiatric Press

Hollander E, Liebowitz MR, Gorman JM (1988), Anxiety disorders. In: *The American Psychiatric Press Textbook of Psychiatry*, Talbott JA, Hales RE, Yudofsky SC, eds. Washington, DC: American Psychiatric Press, pp 443–491

Jenike MA, Baer L, Summergrad P, Minichiello WE, Holland A, Seymour R (1990a), Sertraline in obsessive-compulsive disorder: a double-blind comparison with placebo. *Am J Psychiatry* 147:923–928

Jenike MA, Hyman S, Baer L et al. (1990b), A controlled trial of fluvoxamine in obsessive-compulsive disorder: implications for a serotonergic theory [see comments]. *Am J Psychiatry* 147:1209–1215

Jorrabchi B (1977), Expressions of the hyperventilation syndrome in childhood. *Clin Pediatr (Phila)* 16:1110–1115

Kendall PC, Chansky TE, Freidman M et al. (1991), Treating anxiety disorders in children and adolescents. In: *Child and Adolescent Therapy: Cognitive-Behavioral Procedures*, Kendall PC, ed. New York: Guilford Press, pp 131–164

Klein RG, Koplewicz HS, Kanner A (1992), Imipramine treatment of children with separation anxiety disorder. *J Am Acad Child Adolesc Psychiatry* 31:21–28

Kleman GL (1992), Treatments for panic disorder. *J Clin Psychiatry* 53(suppl): 14–19

Kolvin I, Berney TP, Bhate SR (1984), Classification and diagnosis of depression in school phobia. *Br J Psychiatry* 145:347–357

Korein J, Fish B, Shapiro T, Gehner EW, Levidon L (1971), EEG and behavioral effects of drug therapy in children: chlorpromazine and diphenhydramine. *Arch Gen Psychiatry* 24:552–563

Kraft I (1965), A clinical study of chlordiazepoxide used in psychiatric disorders of children. *Int J Neuropsychiatry* 1:433–437

Krakowski AJ (1963), Chlordiazepoxide in treatment of children with emotional disturbances. *N Y State J Med* 63:3388–3392

Kranzler H (1988), Use of buspirone in an adolescent with overanxious disorder. *J Am Acad Child Adolesc Psychiatry* 27:789–790

Krishnan G (1976), Oxprenolol in the treatment of examination stress. *Curr Med Res Opin* 4:241–243

Kurlan R, Como PG, Deeley C, McDermott M, McDermott MP (1993), A pilot controlled study of fluoxetine for obsessive-compulsive symptoms in children with Tourette's syndrome. *Clin Neuropharmacol* 16:167–172

Kutcher SP, Mackenzie S (1988), Successful clonazepam treatment of adolescents with panic disorder. *J Clin Psychopharmacol* 8:299–301

Kutcher SP, Reiter S, Gardner DM, Klein RG (1992), The pharmacotherapy of anxiety disorders in children and adolescents. *Psychiatr Clin North Am* 15:41–67

Leonard HL, Lenane MC, Swedo SE (1993a), Obsessive compulsive disorder. *Child Adolesc Psychiatr Clin North Am* 2:655–666

Leonard HL, Rapoport JL (1989), Anxiety disorders in childhood and adolescence. In: *Review of Psychiatry*, Vol 8, Tasman A, Hales RE, Frances AJ, eds. Washington, DC: American Psychiatric Press, pp 162–179

Leonard HL, Rapoport JL (1991), Separation anxiety, overanxious, and avoidant disorders. In: *Textbook of Child and Adolescent Psychiatry*, Wiener JM, ed. Washington, DC: American Psychiatric Press, pp 311–322

Leonard HL, Swedo SE, Lenane MC et al. (1991), A double-blind desipramine substitution during long-term clomipramine treatment in children and adolescents with obsessive-compulsive disorder. *Arch Gen Psychiatry* 48:922–927

Leonard HL, Swedo SE, Lenane MC et al. (1993b), A 2- to 7-year follow-up study of 54 obsessive-compulsive children and adolescents. *Arch Gen Psychiatry* 50:429–439

Leonard HL, Swedo SE, Rapoport JL et al. (1989), Treatment of obsessive-compulsive disorder with clomipramine and desipramine in children and adolescents. A double-blind crossover comparison. *Arch Gen Psychiatry* 46:1088–1092

Leonard HL, Topol D (1993), Elective mutism. *Child Adolesc Psychiatr Clin North Am* 2:695–708

Liebowitz MR, Schneier F, Campeas R et al. (1992), Phenelzine vs atenolol in social phobia: a placebo-controlled comparison. *Arch Gen Psychiatry* 49:290–300

Lucas AR, Pasley FC (1969), Psychoactive drugs in the treatment of emotionally disturbed children: haloperidol and diazepam. *Compr Psychiatry* 10:376–386

Noyes R Jr (1982), Beta-blocking drugs and anxiety. *Psychosomatics* 23:155–170

Noyes R Jr (1988), Beta-adrenergic blockers. In: *Handbook of Anxiety Disorders*, Last CG, Hersen M, eds. New York: Pergamon Press, pp 445–459

Riddle MA, Scahill L, King RA et al. (1992), Double-blind, crossover trial of fluoxetine and placebo in children and adolescents with obsessive-compulsive disorder. *J Am Acad Child Adolesc Psychiatry* 31:1062–1069

Rodriguez A, Rodriguez M, Eisenberg L (1959), The outcome of school phobia: a follow-up study based on 41 cases. *Am J Psychiatry* 116:540–544

Roose SP, Glassman AH, Walsh BT, Woodring S (1986), Tricyclic nonresponders: phenomenology and treatment. *Am J Psychiatry* 143:345–348

Ryan ND, Puig-Antich J, Cooper T et al. (1986), Imipramine in adolescent major depression: plasma level and clinical response. *Acta Psychiatr Scand* 73:275–288

Shapiro T, Mrazek D, Pincus HA (1991), Current status of research activity in American child and adolescent psychiatry: part I. *J Am Acad Child Adolesc Psychiatry* 30:443–448

Silver JM, Sandberg DP, Hales RE (1990), New approaches in the pharmacotherapy of posttraumatic stress disorder. *J Clin Psychiatry* 51(suppl):33–38

Simeon JG, Ferguson HB, Knott V et al. (1992), Clinical, cognitive, and neurophysiological effects of alprazolam in children and adolescents with overanxious and avoidant disorders. *J Am Acad Child Adolesc Psychiatry* 31:29–33

US Department of Health and Human Services (1991), Code of Federal Regulations, Title 45: Public Welfare, Part 46: Protection of Human Subjects, Subpart D: Additional DHHS Protections for Children Involved as Subjects in Research, Sections: 46.401–46.409. Washington, DC: US Government Printing Office

Wells BG, Chu CC, Johnson R et al. (1991), Buspirone in the treatment of posttraumatic stress disorder. *Pharmacotherapy* 11:340–343

Zwier KJ, Rao U (1994), Buspirone use in an adolescent with social phobia and mixed personality disorder (cluster A type). *J Am Acad Child Adolesc Psychiatry* 33:1007–1011

# 18

# Practical Guidelines for the Assessment and Treatment of Selective Mutism

Sara P. Dow

*National Institute of Mental Health, Bethesda, Maryland*

Barbara C. Sonies, Donna Scheib, Sharon E. Moss

*National Institutes of Health*

Henrietta L. Leonard

*National Institute of Mental Health, Bethesda, Maryland*

**Objective:** *To provide practical guidelines for the assessment and treatment of children with selective mutism, in light of the recent hypothesis that selective mutism might be best conceptualized as a childhood anxiety disorder.* **Method:** *An extensive literature review was completed on the phenomenology, evaluation, and treatment of children with selective mutism. Additional recommendations were based on clinical experience from the authors' selective mutism clinic.* **Results:** *No systematic studies of the phenomenology of children with selective mutism were found. Reports described diverse and primarily noncontrolled treatment approaches with minimal follow-up information. Assessment and treatment options for selective mutism are presented, based on new hypotheses that focus on the anxiety component of this disorder. Ongoing research suggests a role for behavior modification and pharmacotherapy similar to the approaches used for adults with social phobia.* **Conclusion:** *Selectively mute children deserve a comprehensive evaluation to identify primary and comorbid problems that might require*

Reprinted with permission from the *Journal of the American Academy of Child and Adolescent Psychiatry*, 1995, Vol. 34, No. 7, 836–846. Copyright © 1995 by the American Academy of Child and Adolescent Psychiatry.

*treatment. A school-based multidisciplinary individualized treatment plan is recommended, involving the combined effort of teachers, clinicians, and parents with home- and clinic-based interventions (individual and family psychotherapy, pharmacotherapy) as required.*

Selective mutism is a disorder of childhood characterized by the total lack of speech in at least one specific situation (usually the classroom), despite the ability to speak in other situations. Recently there has been a shift in the etiological views on selective mutism, deemphasizing psychodynamic factors and instead focusing on biologically mediated temperamental and anxiety components (Black and Uhde, 1992; Crumley, 1990; Golwyn and Weinstock, 1990; Leonard and Topol, 1993). Reports in the literature, in addition to our clinical work, suggest that selective mutism may be the manifestation of a shy, inhibited temperament, most likely modulated by psychodynamic and psychosocial issues and in some cases associated with neuropsychological delays (developmental delays, speech and language disabilities, or difficulty processing, social cues) (Figure 1). Although systematic study of this hypothesis is still needed, cognitive-behavioral treatment interventions, in addition to pharmacotherapy, have become more common than traditional psychodynamic approaches. The intent of this article was to provide practical guidelines for the assessment and treatment of selective mutism based on our clinical experience along with reports from the literature.

## BACKGROUND

### History and Definition

In the latter part of the 19th century, Kussmaul (1877) described a disorder in which people would not speak in some situations, despite having the ability to speak. Kussmaul named this disorder "aphasia voluntaria," thereby emphasizing what he thought was a voluntary decision not to speak. When Tramer (1934) observed the same symptoms, he called the problem "elective mutism," with the belief that these children were "electing" not to speak. The most recent edition of the *Diagnostic and Statistic Manual of Mental Disorders (DSM-IV)* (American Psychiatric Association, 1994) has adopted a new term: "selective mutism." The change from "elective" to "selective" (implying that the children do not speak in "select" situations) is consistent with new theories of etiology that deemphasize oppositional behavior and instead focus more on anxiety issues. The diag-

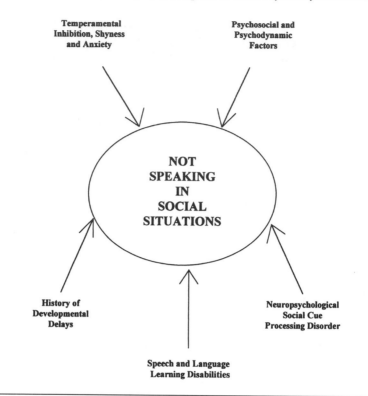

**Figure 1.** Factors that may influence speech and social inhibition.

nosis of selective mutism, however, revolves around only one primary symptom: "consistent failure to speak in specific social situations ... despite speaking in other situations" (American Psychiatric Association, 1994, p. 115). Additional criteria require that the symptom last at least 1 month, be severe enough to interfere with educational or occupational achievement, and not be due to another problem (such as insufficient knowledge of the language, a communication disorder, pervasive developmental disorder, schizophrenia, or another psychotic disorder). Despite these criteria, the population of children with selective mutism remains heterogeneous, which could complicate treatment recommendations.

### Differential Diagnosis

Since speech inhibition can be a secondary symptom of many other psychiatric disorders (including pervasive developmental disorder, schizophrenia, and severe mental retardation), differential diagnosis for selective mutism can be complex (American Psychiatric Association, 1994). When a communication disorder is present, distinguishing between symptoms that are secondary to speech and language problems and those that are suggestive of selective mutism may be even more difficult. Although speech and language deficits can cause speech inhibition (Lerea and Ward, 1965), several authors have reported that speech and language problems can also exist comorbidly with selective mutism (Kolvin and Fundudis, 1981; Wilkins, 1985; Wright, 1968).

## Epidemiology

Selective mutism has been described as a rare disorder, affecting fewer than 1% of school-age children, but little systematic research has been done to support this estimate. Using fairly strict diagnostic criteria, Fundudis and colleagues (1979) identified two selectively mute children in a survey of 3,300 seven-year-olds in Newcastle, U.K., a rate of 0.06%. In contrast, Brown and Lloyd (1975) reported a much higher prevalence of 0.69% (42/6,072 children). However, this estimate was obtained after only 8 weeks of school, and 56 weeks later, the rate had fallen to 0.02% (1/6,072 children).

## Etiology

Etiological explanations for selective mutism have varied widely (Leonard and Dow, 1995). Some have explained it as a response to family neurosis, usually characterized by overprotective or domineering mothers and strict or remote fathers (Browne et al., 1963; Meijer, 1979; Meyers, 1984; Parker et al., 1960; Pustrom and Speers, 1964). Others have suggested that the symptom could be a manifestation of unresolved psychodynamic conflict (Elson et al., 1965; Youngerman, 1979). In addition, some have reported that it may develop as a reaction to trauma, such as sexual abuse or early hospitalization (MacGregor et al., 1994). Divorce, death of a loved one, and frequent moves have also been postulated to play a role in symptom development.

In the more recent literature, authors have noted a resemblance between selectively mute children and socially phobic adults (Black and Uhde, 1992; Crumley, 1990; Golwyn and Weinstock, 1990; Leonard and Topol, 1993). Crumley (1990) reported the case of a 29-year-old man who had been selectively mute at age 8 1/2 years. The man remembered being afraid to speak for fear that he "might say or do the wrong thing" (Crumley, 1990,

p. 318). He also described experiencing "sudden episodes of intense anxiety" and physical symptoms that were suggestive of panic (shortness of breath, palpitations, dizziness) when he was placed in a situation where speech was expected. As an adult, the patient still had anxiety in social situations and often would not initiate conversation for fear that he would "say the wrong thing and embarrass myself" (Crumley, 1990, p. 319). Crumley speculated that the patient's problems with social phobia might have been related to his initial elective (selective) mutism symptoms.

Black and Uhde (1992) described a selectively mute girl who had told her mother that she was reluctant to speak because "her voice sounded funny and she did not want others to hear it" (Black and Uhde, 1992, p. 1090). Her family psychiatric history was remarkable for paternal public-speaking anxiety and maternal childhood shyness. Boon (1994) reported the case of a 6-year-old girl who did not speak to adults. She explained her inability to speak by saying, "my brain wouldn't let me; my voice sounds strange" (Boon, 1994, p. 283). The girl's father was in treatment for panic disorder, and her paternal grandfather had had an anxiety disorder. Boon (1994, p. 283) speculated that research on the pharmacotherapy of selective mutism ". . . likely will support the view that elective mutism is an anxiety/OCD spectrum disorder."

## *Phenomenology*

Several authors found selective mutism to be more prevalent in females than males (Hayden, 1980; Wergeland, 1979; Wilkins, 1985; Wright, 1968). However, others found the disorder only slightly more frequent in females (Brown and Lloyd, 1975; Kolvin and Fundudis, 1981), and some found no sex difference (Parker et al., 1960). Onset is usually insidious, with parents reporting that the child "has always been this way" (Hayden, 1980; Kolvin and Fundudis, 1981; Leonard and Topol, 1993; Wright, 1968; Wright et al., 1985), but the diagnosis is often not made until the child enters kindergarten or first grade and verbal skills become more essential (5 to 6 years old).

Nearly all descriptions of selectively mute children in the literature have included some reference to their shyness, inhibition, or anxiety. Some have described them as ". . . particularly sensitive, shy, afraid of everything strange or new . . ." (Wergeland, 1979, p. 219), others called them "unduly timid and sensitive" (Morris, 1953, p. 667), and others reported "shy, timid, clinging behavior away from home" (Hayden, 1980, p. 128). One author went so far as to characterize them as not only shy, but actually "socially inept" (Friedman and Karagan, 1973, p. 250). Our clinical experience with selectively mute children has suggested that anxiety may play a much larger role than previously acknowledged, and these reports support such a hypothesis.

A wide variety of comorbid psychiatric problems have been described in children with selective mutism. Kolvin and Fundudis (1981) reported an increased incidence of elimination problems (as high as 42% for enuresis and 17% for encopresis, versus 15% and 2% for controls). Others found obsessive-compulsive features (Hayden, 1980; Kolvin and Fundudis, 1981; Wergeland, 1979), school phobia (Elson et al., 1965; Parker et al., 1960; Pustrom and Speers, 1964; Wright, 1968), and depression (Wilkins, 1985).

Although there have been no reports of systematic speech and language assessment, several authors have noted speech delays or problems among selectively mute children. Kolvin and Fundudis (1981) reported that the 24 selectively mute children in their study began speaking significantly later than 102 matched controls (27.3 months versus 21.9 months; no *p* value given). In addition, half (12/24) of these same selectively mute children had immaturities of speech at the time of evaluation, whereas only 9% (9/102) of the normal controls had any such problems. Wilkins (1985) reported that 6 (25%) of the 24 selectively mute children he studied had a delayed onset of speech and 2 (8.3%) had speech problems at the time of evaluation, while no such problems were found in any of the controls. Wright (1968) found articulation problems in 5 (21%) of his 24 patients, one of whom was dysarthric. Of note, these authors measured speech problems only and gave no reports of linguistic ability. Preliminary data from comprehensive speech and language assessments of selectively mute children evaluated in our clinic reveal that just less than one half had mild to moderate expressive or receptive language delays severe enough to warrant intervention (unpublished data). It appears that the rate of speech and language delays in the selectively mute population (and the impact of such delays) merits further investigation.

## ASSESSMENT

Any child who is being considered for a diagnosis of selective mutism should have a comprehensive evaluation to rule out other explanations for the mutism and to assess comorbid factors. An individualized treatment plan can then be developed.

### *Parental Interview*

Since most selectively mute children will not speak to clinicians, an interview with the parent or guardian of the child can provide essential information (Table 1).

TABLE 1
Assessment of Selectively Mute Children

| Areas | Parental Interview | Clinical Interview |
|---|---|---|
| Symptoms | • Type of onset (insidious, sudden)<br>• Past treatments and efficacy<br>• Where and to whom the child will speak | • Observations from interacting with the child |
| Social interaction | • Ability to make and keep friends<br>• Extent and pattern of participation in social activities<br>• Degree of shyness/inhibition in familiar and foreign settings<br>• Individuals to whom child will speak<br>• Ability to communicate needs | • Observations of temperament made during interaction with child (shy? anxious? inhibited? interactive?) |
| Psychiatric | • Detailed assessment of psychiatric symptoms (use of a structured interview is preferred by some)<br>• Family history of psychiatric problems and excessive shyness<br>• Temperament during developmental stages | • Mental status examination |
| Medical | • Child's medical history, including illnesses or hospitalizations<br>• Prenatal and perinatal history<br>• Developmental history<br>• Family medical history | • Physical examination, (including screening for neurological or oral-sensorimotor problems) |
| Audiological | • Frequency of otitis media<br>• Any reported concerns about hearing problems | • Peripheral sensitivity (pure-tone and speech stimuli)<br>• Tympanometry and acoustic reflex (for middle ear) |
| Academic and cognitive | • Review of academic achievement (grades, teacher reports) | • Standardized tests of cognitive skills and achievement |
| Speech and language | • Reported complexity and fluency of child's speech at home<br>• Nonverbal communication (gestures, etc.)<br>• Any history of speech and language delays<br>• Detailed description of child's speech production, language use and comprehension<br>• Discussion of environmental influences on language learning (bilingualism, etc.) | • Receptive language: assess using standardized tests<br>• Expressive language: assess using audiotape and standardized testing, if possible (note lengh of utterances grammatical complexity, tone of voice)<br>• Speech: assess using audiotape (note fluency, pronunciation, rhythm, stress, inflection, pitch, volume) |

A description of the child's symptom history, particularly onset (sudden or insidious), may help establish the diagnosis of selective mutism. Any patterns of behavior that are not characteristic of selective mutism, such as not talking to immediate family members, abrupt cessation of speech in one environment, or absence of speech in all settings, raise concerns about other neurological or psychiatric problems (e.g., autism, aphasia). A history of neurological insult, developmental delays, neuropsychological deficits, and/or atypical speech and language difficulties (such as problems with prosody) could be suggestive of Asperger's disorder, right hemisphere deficit disorder, or social emotional learning disabilities, rather than selective mutism (Voeller, 1986; Weintraub and Mesulam, 1983). Children with these disorders often have symptoms of shyness and social isolation and thus may appear similar to selectively mute children, but research suggests that their symptoms are based on an inability to process social cues.

Also of interest is the degree to which the child is verbally and nonverbally inhibited. Some selectively mute children are shy and anxious in unfamiliar environments, while others will interact in some way even if they will not speak (perhaps by nodding their head or smiling). Targeted questions about the child's verbal and nonverbal interaction, relationships with friends, and anxiety in social situations can be revealing. The child's social interaction outside of school, such as in a restaurant or on the telephone, should also be explored.

A structured diagnostic interview, such as the Diagnostic Interview for Children and Adolescents-Parent version (Herjanic and Campbell, 1977) or the Schedule for Affective Disorders and Schizophrenia for School-Age Children-Epidemiologic Version (Orvaschel and Puig-Antich, 1987) can be helpful for assessment of comorbid psychiatric symptoms. Pervasive developmental disorder, schizophrenia, and mental retardation can cause speech inhibition and thus might rule out a diagnosis of selective mutism.

Academic ability should also be discussed. Because it is difficult to evaluate children with selective mutism via traditional testing, minor learning disabilities may be overlooked. Parent and teacher comments, academic reports, and standardized testing results can all be helpful to evaluate the child's skills and determine whether further testing is indicated.

Reviewing the child's medical history is essential because physical problems might underlie the child's mutism. Neurological injury or delay can result in speech and language problems or social skills deficits, both of which can exacerbate speech inhibition. In addition, some authors have reported that early hospitalizations or abuse may play a role in the development of selective mutism (MacGregor et al., 1994). Hearing should also be checked (particularly if the child has a history of frequent ear infections), since hearing problems are sometimes associated with learning and language delays.

Family history of selective mutism, extreme shyness, or anxiety disorders (social phobia, panic disorder, obsessive-compulsive disorder) may put the child at risk for developing similar problems and should be thoroughly explored with the parents. In addition, a complete family history of any psychiatric or medical diagnoses, including response to treatment, can be helpful.

Evaluation of speech and language ability is essential. Factors that might have influenced a child's language development, such as a parent with identified speech and language problems, or a lack of adequate exposure to the language (as in some bilingual homes), should be considered. Inadequate or confusing language exposure may result in expressive problems, and additional practice may be necessary for the child to function at normal levels. Other questions should focus on the child's ability to communicate his or her needs, both verbally and nonverbally. Descriptions of the complexity and quality of language (mean length of utterance, range of vocabulary, use of difficult verb tenses and complicated grammar) can help one evaluate expressive language ability. Pragmatic language abilities, such as turn-taking in conversation, understanding of nonverbal communicative cues, and so on, should also be explored. Other questions might focus on the child's speech production (voice, fluency, resonance, rate, and rhythm), to identify phonological problems. It can also be helpful to have parents provide an audiotape of the child speaking at home (as detailed later), because few children with selective mutism will actually speak to clinicians.

Many checklists have been used to assess speech and language ability, including the Classroom Communication Checklist (Ripich and Spinelli, 1985), the Interpersonal Language Skills Checklist (McConnell and Blagden, 1986), and the Environmental Language Inventory (MacDonald, 1978). We adapted these scales to create the National Institutes of Health Parent Checklist (Sonies et al., 1993; available upon request), which augments information provided by standardized speech and language testing. In this questionnaire, parents are asked to respond to statements regarding the expressive, receptive, and pragmatic abilities of their child, indicating frequency (never, rarely, sometimes, frequently, or always). This checklist, or others, can be used to supplement standardized speech and language testing.

### Child Assessment

Interviewing the child is a crucial part of the assessment as it allows the clinician to directly observe the severity and nature of the child's mutism, as well as to pursue any concerns raised by the parents (Table 1).

Temperament, quality of interaction, and ability to communicate verbally and nonverbally can all be observed during the interview with the child. As most selectively mute children will not talk to the clinician, other forms of nonverbal communication (playing, drawing) may be used to assess anxiety or shyness in social situations. Some selectively mute children will avoid eye contact and withdraw from social situations, while others are more interactive and will smile, giggle, and nod answers to questions, even if they will not speak.

A review of the physical examination will ensure that the child has no medical problems that could potentially complicate the clinical picture. Oral sensory and motor ability should be evaluated, with particular note to any orofacial abnormalities that might interfere with articulation. Neurological difficulties, as evidenced by drooling, grimacing, muscular asymmetry, tongue and lip weakness, abnormal gag reflex, or impaired sucking or swallowing, can be relevant because they may impede the movements necessary for normal speech.

Auditory testing should be completed to ensure that hearing difficulties are not contributing to the mutism. Several studies have shown that even mild audiological impairments can have a negative effect on speech and language development (Fundudis et al., 1979). General tests of peripheral sensitivity (using both pure-tone and speech stimuli) are usually adequate to detect problems. In addition, tympanometry and acoustic reflex testing can be used to assess middle ear function.

Standardized psychological testing may be necessary to confirm parental and teacher reports of the child's cognitive abilities, particularly because many of these children are difficult to assess academically. While learning disabilities are rarely the cause of mutism, they could exacerbate the problem. Tests of intellectual capacity (which measure components of memory, attention, reasoning, and judgment) can be invaluable toward obtaining a measure of the child's potential level of functioning. Many different tests are available, but the performance section of the WISC-R (Wechsler, 1974) and Raven's Colored Progressive Matrices (Raven, 1976) were found to be good measures of cognitive ability in our selective mutism clinic since children were not required to respond orally.

A formal speech and language evaluation, including components of receptive language, expressive language, and phonology, is an essential part of the assessment. While speech and language are closely tied, they are separate entities and thus require different types of assessment. Speech is ". . . the activity of articulating speech sounds," while language involves higher cortical functioning: ". . . the communication of thoughts by the use of meaningful units combined in a systematic way" (Bishop, 1994, p. 556). A complete evaluation of the child's ability will utilize several different approaches, combining standardized testing with information obtained from the parents, as well as an audiotape of the child speaking at home.

Most of the children referred to our selective mutism clinic had never received formal speech and language testing, perhaps in part because of a misconception that nonverbal children cannot be evaluated for speech and language functioning. Several tests of receptive language ability that can be administered to nonverbal subjects are available. The Peabody Picture Vocabulary Test (Dunn and Dunn, 1981) is useful as an initial screening for receptive language problems, since it can be administered nonverbally and it has been standardized for children as young as 2 years old. To evaluate more complex receptive ability, one could use a variety of other tests, including (but not limited to) the Token Test for Children (DiSimoni, 1978), the Test for Auditory Comprehension of Language-Revised (Woolfolk, 1985), the Test of Language Development (Hammil and Newcomer, 1982), and the Detroit Test of Learning Aptitude-Primary (Hammil and Bryant, 1986). For less responsive or immature children, the Utah Test of Language Development (Mecham and Jones, 1989) or the Preschool Language Scale-3 (Zimmerman et al., 1991) might be more appropriate.

A prerecorded audiotape of the child speaking at home can be used to evaluate phonological ability, including length of utterances, grammatical construction, tone of voice, and response to verbalizations. In addition, one should be alert for any abnormalities of rhythm, stress, inflection, pitch, or volume. Speech defects have been noted to cause speech inhibition in some cases and thus could exacerbate the symptoms of selective mutism (Lerea and Ward, 1965).

## TREATMENT

Treatment for selective mutism has for a long time been considered difficult; some have described the disorder as "intractable." Many different approaches have been used to treat this disorder, including a variety of behavioral techniques, psychodynamic approaches, family therapy, speech therapy, and most recently pharmacological intervention (for reviews, see Cline and Baldwin, 1994; Kratochwill, 1981; Tancer, 1992). Unfortunately, the majority of treatment reports have been in case study format, many with only a single subject. While case studies may be helpful to describe a new approach or intervention, generalizing from such reports can be problematic. In many of these reports, procedures were not sufficiently described to allow for replication, outcome measures were not objective or standardized, alternative explanations for symptom remission were not explored, and unsuccessful cases were not reported (Wells; 1987).

Some authors have attempted to increase validity using a more systematic case study approach, the "single-case experimental design" (Bauermeister and Jemail, 1975; Cunningham et al., 1983). For example, objective symptom measures (such as number of words spoken per hour) have been used to quantify outcome, and treatment results have been compared to baseline. A few authors have even used multiple baselines (home, school, other settings). However, single-case experimental design is still limited by small sample size, and systematic trials with larger groups are needed. Only two controlled studies of treatment for selective mutism were found in the literature, one using behavioral therapy (Calhoun and Koenig, 1973) and the other using pharmacotherapy (using fluoxetine) (Black and Uhde, 1994). Both studies reported success in the treated group, as detailed in later sections.

### Behavioral

Behavioral interventions, based on principles of learning theory, have been the most frequently used treatment for selective mutism. Reed (1963) was one of the first to suggest that mutism could be a learned behavior and thus might respond to behavioral techniques such as reinforcement and stimulus fading. He hypothesized that mutism developed either as a means of getting attention or as an escape from anxiety. Treatment was thus directed at extinguishing all reinforcement for the mutism, while simultaneously bolstering self-confidence and decreasing anxiety (Reed, 1963).

There have been many subsequent attempts to use behavioral techniques to encourage speech in selectively mute children (the reader is referred to Cunningham et al., 1983; Labbe and Williamson, 1984; and Sanok and Ascione, 1979, for reviews). However, the only controlled study of behavioral therapy to date was that of Calhoun and Koenig (1973), which involved eight selectively mute children. In this study, children were randomly assigned to treatment or control groups, and data (number of words per 30 minutes) were collected by trained observers at baseline, posttreatment, and follow-up. Although treatment was not described in sufficient detail to assess or replicate, it appeared to consist of teacher and peer reinforcement of verbal behavior. Subjects who received active treatment were found to have significantly more vocalizations than untreated subjects 5 weeks after the start of treatment ($p < .01$), but improvement was not significant at follow-up 1 year later ($p < .10$).

In addition to this controlled study, there are numerous case reports of behavioral treatment for selective mutism. Most authors used some type of reinforcement for speaking, often combined with an absence of reinforcement for the mute behavior. Some also used punitive measures (forcing the child to sit in the corner, splashing the child with water), but these may have a tendency to increase a child's anxiety and thus would not be recommended. Stimulus fading, a technique similar to the "desensitization" used to treat social phobia, has also been reported to be an effective approach, particularly when combined with reinforcement (the reader is referred to Heimberg and Barlow, 1991, for a review of cognitive-behavioral therapy for social phobia in adults). In stimulus fading, therapists set simple goals and then gradually increase the difficulty of the task. For example, Scott (1977) used this approach with a 7-year-old girl, gradually adding new people into a room in which the girl was speaking. Three months after the end of treatment, Scott reported that, although she ". . . will always be a shy child and will possibly experience difficulty in communication . . . the problem of mutism no longer exists" (Scott, 1977, pp. 269–270).

Other authors have reported on the effectiveness of techniques such as "shaping" to initiate speech in the school setting (Austad et al., 1980). Shaping is a procedure in which the therapist reinforces mouth movements that approximate speech until true speech is achieved. "Self-modeling," a technique in which the child watches videotaped segments of himself or herself performing desired behaviors (speaking, interacting), has also been tried with some success, though only with case studies (Dowrick and Hood, 1978; Pigott and Gonzales, 1987).

## Psychodynamic

While insight-oriented psychodynamic therapy was at one time the preferred treatment for selective mutism, cognitive-behavioral approaches are now being used with increasing frequency. Psychodynamic theory characterizes mutism as a manifestation of intrapsychic conflict, and treatment is focused on identifying and resolving such underlying conflicts. The treatment process can be time consuming, particularly if the child will not speak, and as a result many psychodynamic therapists have utilized art or play to facilitate communication and expedite therapy (Landgarten, 1975).

## Family Therapy

In older reports, family pathology was often postulated to be a causal factor in the development of selective mutism (Goll, 1979; Lindblad-Goldberg, 1986; Meijer, 1979; Meyers, 1984; Pustrom and Speers, 1964). Authors described patterns of interaction in the family which seemed to encourage the child's mutism and thus prevent resolution of the symptom (Meyers, 1984). Family therapy was used to identify and treat such dysfunctional patterns. Although no systematic research has been done using family therapy as the primary intervention for selective mutism, reports suggest that this approach can be effective in some cases (Goll, 1979).

More recently, clinicians have not seen the child's symptom as a result of family pathology, but rather they have tried to involve family members in the design and implementation of a treatment plan. However, if family problems are identified that may be having an impact on the child's symptoms, a more traditional, insight-oriented family treatment approach could be appropriate.

### Pharmacotherapy

There are a few recent reports of pharmacological treatment for selective mutism, all using medications which have been helpful for social phobia (selective serotonin reuptake inhibitors). Golwyn and Weinstock (1990) described a 7-year-old girl with elective mutism and "associated shyness" who responded to phenelzine (up to 2 mg/day) with improvement noted as early as 6 weeks. She progressed from not speaking a word at school to being able to talk freely to teachers, peers, and therapists. Her father had panic disorder and had responded to phenelzine. Black and Uhde (1992) described a 12-year-old girl with elective mutism and social anxiety who responded to fluoxetine (20 mg/day): she was able to speak freely with adults and peers at school, and the response was maintained at 7 months. Boon (1994) reported "positive effects" in the fluoxetine treatment of a 6-year-old selectively mute girl but did not provide details.

Black and Uhde (1994) recently completed a 12-week trial of fluoxetine in children with elective mutism (placebo-controlled, parallel design). The six children taking active medication showed significant improvement on some ratings of mutism and anxiety but not on others, and subjects in both groups were still judged to be symptomatic at the conclusion of the study. Although interesting and somewhat promising, these results suggest that perhaps a longer trial, a more individualized dosage schedule, or combined intervention should be considered. In obsessive-compulsive disorder, a combination of pharmacotherapy and behavioral intervention is the treatment of choice (Leonard et al., 1994). Several investigators are currently studying the efficacy of serotonin reuptake inhibitors for the treatment of selective mutism, specifically fluoxetine and fluvoxamine. A medication trial should be considered if anxiety is a prominent factor or if symptoms have been resistant to other treatment attempts.

### Speech Therapy

Several authors have noted an increased prevalence of speech and language problems in the selectively mute population (Kolvin and Fundudis, 1981;

Wilkins, 1985; Wright, 1968). Smayling (1959) was the first to use speech therapy as the primary intervention for selective mutism, speculating that "speech defects, while not demonstrably the sole etiological factor, were causally related to the mutism" (p. 58). In Smayling's report, six selectively mute children who had some degree of speech or language disability were treated with half-hour sessions of speech therapy two to three times per week until the problems were resolved (2 to 21 months). Therapists intentionally avoided mentioning the mutism or discussing the child's feelings, instead focusing on articulation and language training. Once the speech problems had been corrected, five of the six children began to speak in school. Strait (1958) also used speech therapy, but in conjunction with behavioral modification techniques such as reinforcement. Though both Smayling and Strait studied children with identified speech and language problems, it is likely that any selectively mute child could benefit from structured language practice.

### School-Based Multidisciplinary Individualized Treatment Plan

An effective individualized treatment program could be implemented in the school environment, with the coordinated efforts of parents, clinicians, and teachers. The goal of a treatment program should be to decrease the anxiety associated with speaking while encouraging the child to interact and communicate (Table 2).

Interventions that could be easily carried out by the classroom teacher include separating the class into small groups and identifying supportive peers. In some cases, an alternate means of communication (such as cards or gestures) might initially be necessary to allow the child to communicate basic needs. Any such system should be kept simple, however, so the child will still have incentive to communicate verbally.

Behavioral approaches can be helpful for encouraging the child to interact both verbally and nonverbally. At the start of a behavioral program, expectations should be kept low, perhaps rewarding the child for behaviors that he or she has already mastered or that are within reach. Once the child has gained confidence in his or her ability, the difficulty of the desired behavior can be increased. For example, one might begin by rewarding the child for whispering a single word and gradually increase the expectations until the child is saying the word in a normal volume. The type of reward could also be chosen according to the child's preferences (favorite candy, social praise, etc.). Once the child has become comfortable speaking in one environment, attempts can be made to generalize speech to other individuals or environments, using techniques such as stimulus fading.

TABLE 2
School-Based Multidisciplinary Intervention

| Goals | Specific Interventions |
|-------|------------------------|
| Decrease anxiety | • Child should not be forced to speak<br>• Keep child in regular classroom unless special needs other than selective mutism supersede<br>• Less emphasis on verbal performance (play nonverbal games)<br>• Encourage relationships with peers<br>• Cognitive-behavioral interventions: desensitization with relaxation<br>• Coordinate school-based program with out-of-school interventions (individual and family psychotherapy, pharmacotherapy) |
| Increase nonverbal communciation | • Set up system for alternate means of communication (symbols, gestures, cards)<br>• Small-group situations<br>• Facilitate peer relationships |
| Increase social interaction | • Identify compatible peers for play in and out of school<br>• Small-group situations<br>• Activities that do not require verbal skills<br>• Activities that encourage social skills |
| Increase verbal communication | • Structured behavioral modification plan: positive reinforcement for interactive and communicative behaviors, eventually reinforcement for speech<br>• Speech and language therapy to develop linguistic skills<br>• Pragmatically based language practice |

The assistance of a speech therapist could be helpful in the development of a behavioral program for selective mutism, even if no specific speech and language impairments have been identified. Some selectively mute children have reported that they are afraid they will say the wrong thing or that their voice sounds funny, and speech and language practice could help such children gain confidence in their linguistic ability. Treatment might focus on perfecting pronunciation skills, increasing comprehension, and learning pragmatic skills, such as turn-taking during conversation. Practicing real-life interchanges until they have become automatic and less stressful might eventually help reduce a child's social inhibitedness.

## SUMMARY

This article was developed in response to questions raised by families, clinicians, and educators in the course of evaluating selectively mute children in our clinic. Although ongoing studies of phenomenology and treatment were not yet completed, it was thought that there was an urgent need for practical information regarding assessment and treatment. Teachers and parents had asked how to treat these children and had questioned the appropriateness of special educational placements, yet no literature was available to assist them and many of the clinicians they turned to were unfamiliar with this disorder.

In our opinion, any child referred for selective mutism deserves a comprehensive assessment that addresses neurological, psychiatric, audiological, social, academic, and speech and language concerns. In the past, many of these children have not received complete assessments, either because clinicians believed they were untestable due to lack of verbal response or because clinicians deemed such assessments unnecessary. Our experience has been that it is not only possible to evaluate these children, but it is essential. Such evaluations can play an important role in identifying primary and comorbid issues and in developing appropriate treatment. Cognitive-behavioral, psychodynamic, pharmacological, and speech and language treatment approaches could all be integrated to decrease anxiety and to encourage speech and social interaction. Further systematic research will be required to evaluate the comparative effectiveness of these approaches.

## REFERENCES

American Psychiatric Association (1994), *Diagnostic and Statistical Manual of Mental Disorders, 4th edition (DSM-IV)*. Washington, DC: American Psychiatric Association

Austad LS, Sinninger R, Stricken A (1980), Successful treatment of a case of elective mutism. *Behavior Therapist* 3:18–19

Bauermeister JJ, Jemail JA (1975), Modification of "elective mutism" in the classroom setting: a case study. *Behav Ther* 6:246–250

Bishop DVM (1994), Developmental disorders of speech and language. In: *Child and Adolescent Psychiatry: Modern Approaches*, Rutter M, Taylor E, Hersov L, eds. Oxford, England: Blackwell Scientific Publications, pp 546–568

Black B, Uhde TW (1992), Elective mutism as a variant of social phobia. *J Am Acad Child Adolesc Psychiatry* 31:1090–1094

Black B, Uhde TW (1994), Fluoxetine treatment of elective mutism: a double-blind, placebo-controlled study. *J Am Acad Child Adolesc Psychiatry* 33: 1000–1006

Boon F (1994), The selective mutism controversy. *J Am Acad Child Adolesc Psychiatry* 33:283

Brown JB, Lloyd H (1975), A controlled study of children not speaking at school. *Assoc Workers Maladjusted Child* 3:49–63

Browne E, Wilson V, Laybourne PC (1963), Diagnosis and treatment of elective mutism in children. *J Am Acad Child Psychiatry* 2:605–617

Calhoun J, Koenig KP (1973), Classroom modification of elective mutism. *Behav Ther* 4:700–702

Cline T, Baldwin S (1994), *Selective Mutism*. London: Whurr Publishers

Crumley FE (1990), The masquerade of mutism. *J Am Acad Child Adolesc Psychiatry* 29:318–319

Cunningham CE, Cacaldo MF, Mallion C et al. (1983), A review and controlled single case evaluation of behavioral approaches to the management of elective mutism. *Child Fam Behav Ther* 5:25–49

DiSimoni F (1978), *The Token Test for Children*. Boston: Teaching Resources Corporation

Dowrick PW, Hood M (1978), Transfer of talking behaviours across settings using faked films. In: *New Zealand Conference for Research in Applied Behavioural Analysis*, Glynn EL, McNaughton SS, eds. Auckland, NZ: University of Auckland Press

Dunn LM, Dunn LM (1981), *Peabody Picture Vocabulary Test-Revised*. Circle Pines, MN: American Guidance Services

Elson A, Pearson C, Jones CD, Schumacher E (1965), Follow up study of childhood elective mutism. *Arch Gen Psychiatry* 13:182–187

Friedman R, Karagan N (1973), Characteristics and management of elective mutism in children. *Psychol Sch* 10:249–254

Fundudis T, Kolvin I, Garside R (1979), *Speech Retarded and Deaf Children: Their Psychological Development*. London: Academic Press

Goll K (1979), Role structure and subculture in families of elective mute children. *Fam Process* 18:55–68

Golwyn DH, Weinstock RC (1990), Phenelzine treatment of elective mutism: a case report. *J Clin Psychiatry* 51:384–385

Hammil DD, Bryant BR (1986), *The Detroit Test of Learning Aptitude-Primary.* Austin, TX: Pro-ED

Hammil DD, Newcomer PL (1982), *The Test of Language Development.* Austin, TX: Pro-ED

Hayden TL (1980), Classification of elective mutism. *J Am Acad Child Psychiatry* 19:118–133

Heimberg RG, Barlow DH (1991), New developments in cognitive-behavioral therapy for social phobia. *J Clin Psychiatry* 5211 (suppl):21–30

Herjanic B, Campbell W (1977), Differentiating psychiatrically disturbed children on the basis of a structured psychiatric interview. *J Abnorm Child Psychol* 5:127–135

Kolvin I, Fundudis T (1981), Elective mute children: psychological, development, and background factors. *J Child Psychol Psychiatry* 22:219–232

Kratochwill TR (1981), *Selective Mutism: Implications for Research and Treatment*, Hillsdale, NJ: Erlbaum

Kussmaul A (1877), *Die Störungen der Sprache.* Leipzig: FCW Vogel

Labbe EE, Williamson DA (1984), Behavioral treatment of elective mutism: a review of the literature. *Clin Psychol Rev* 4:273–294

Landgarten H (1975), Art therapy as a primary mode of treatment for an elective mute. *Am J Art Ther* 14:121–125

Leonard HL, Dow SP (1995), Selective mutism. In: *Anxiety Disorders in Children and Adolescents*, March J, ed. New York: Guilford Press, pp 235–250

Leonard HL, Swedo SE, Allen AJ, Rapoport JL (1994), Obsessive-compulsive disorder. In: *International Handbook of Phobic and Anxiety Disorders in Children and Adolescents*, Ollendick TH, King NJ, Yule W, eds. New York: Plenum Press, pp 207–221

Leonard HL, Topol DA (1993), Elective mutism. *Child Adolesc Psychiatr Clin North Am* 2:695–707

Lerea L, Ward B (1965), Speech avoidance among children with oral-communication defects. *J Psychol* 60:265–270

Lindblad-Goldberg M (1986), Elective mutism in families with young children. In: *Treating Young Children in Family Therapy*, Vol 18, Combrinck Graham L, ed. Rockville, MD: Aspen Publications, pp 31–42

MacDonald J (1978), *Environmental Language Inventory.* San Antonio, TX: Psychological Corporation

MacGregor R, Pullar A, Cundall D (1994), Silent at school: elective mutism and abuse. *Arch Dis Child* 70:540–541

McConnell N-, Blagden C (1986), *Interpersonal Language Skills Checklist.* East Moline, IL: LinguiSystems

Mecham MJ, Jones JD (1989), *The Utah Test of Language Development-3*. Austin, TX: Pro-ED

Meijer A (1979), Elective mutism in children. *Isr Ann Psychiatry Relat Discip* 17:93–100

Meyers SV (1984), Elective mutism in children: a family systems approach. *Am J Fam Ther* 22(4):39–45

Morris JV (1953), Cases of elective mutism. *Am J Ment Defic* 57:661–668

Orvaschel H, Puig-Antich J (1987), *Schedule for Affective Disorders and Schizophrenia for School-Age Children: Epidemiologic Version*. Medical College of Pennsylvania, Eastern Pennsylvania Psychiatric Institute

Parker EB, Olsen TF, Throckmorton MC (1960), Social case work with elementary school children who do not talk in school. *Soc Work* 5:64–70

Pigott HE, Gonzales FP (1987), Efficacy of video tape self-modeling in treating an electively mute child. *J Clin Child Psychol* 16:106–110

Pustrom E, Speers RW (1964), Elective mutism in children. *J Am Acad Child Psychiatry* 3:287–297

Raven JC (1976), *The Colored Progressive Matrices*. London: HK Lewis

Reed G (1963), Elective mutism in children: a reappraisal. *J Child Psychol Psychiatry* 4:99

Ripich D, Spinelli (1985), Classroom Communication Checklist. In: *School Discourse Strategies*, Ripich D, Spinelli, eds. San Diego: College Hill

Sanok RL, Ascione FR (1979), Behavioral interventions for elective mutism: an evaluative review. *Child Behav Ther* 1:49–67

Scott E (1977), A desensitisation programme for the treatment of mutism in a seven year old girl: a case report. *J Child Psychol Psychiatry* 18:263–270

Smayling JM (1959), Analysis of six cases of voluntary mutism. *J Speech Hear Disord* 24:55–58

Sonies BC, Scheib D, Moss S (1993), *National Institutes of Health Parent Checklist*. Bethesda, MD: National Institutes of Health

Strait R (1958), A child who was speechless in school and social life. *J Speech Hear Disord* 23:253–254

Tancer NK (1992), Elective mutism. In: *Advances in Clinical Child Psychology*, Vol 14, Lahey BB, Kazdin AE, eds. New York: Plenum Press, pp 265–288

Tramer M (1934), Elektiver Mutismus bei Kindern. *Z Kinderpsychiatr* 1:30–35

Voeller K (1986), Right-hemisphere deficit syndrome in children. *Am J Psychiatry* 143:1004–1009

Wechsler D (1974), *Manual for the Wechsler Intelligence Scale for Children-Revised*. New York: The Psychological Corporation

Weintraub S, Mesulam M (1983), Developmental learning disabilities and the right hemisphere. *Arch Neurol* 40:463–468

Wells K (1987), Scientific issues in the conduct of case studies: annotation. *J Child Psychol Psychiatry* 28:783–790

Wergeland H (1979), Elective mutism. *Acta Psychiatr Scand* 59:218–228

Wilkins R (1985), A comparison of elective mutism and emotional disorders in children. *Br J Psychiatry* 146:198–203

Woolfolk EC (1985), *The Test for Auditory Comprehension of Language-Revised.* Allen, TX: DLM Teaching Resources

Wright HH, Miller MD, Cook MA, Littman JR (1985), Early identification and intervention with children who refuse to speak. *J Am Acad Child Psychiatry* 24:739–746

Wright HL (1968), A clinical study of children who refuse to talk in school. *J Am Acad Child Psychiatry* 7:603–617

Youngerman J (1979), The syntax of silence: electively mute therapy. *Int Rev Psychoanal* 6:283–295

Zimmerman IL, Steiner VG, Pond RE (1991), *The Preschool Language Scale-3.* New York: The Psychological Corporation

# 19

# Pemoline Effects on Children with ADHD: A Time-Response by Dose-Response Analysis on Classroom Measures

**William E. Pelham, Jr.**
*University of Pittsburgh and Western Psychiatric Institute and Clinic, Pittsburgh*

**James M. Swanson**
*University of California, Irvine*

**Mary Bender Furman**
*University of California, Irvine*

**Heidi Schwindt**
*University of Pittsburgh*

**Objective:** *To evaluate the dose-response by time-response characteristics of pemoline (Cylert®) on dependent measures of behavior and academic performance in a laboratory classroom.* **Method:** *After a 2-week baseline, a double-blind crossover design was used to compare placebo, 18.75 mg, 37.5 mg, 75 mg, and 112.5 mg of pemoline, q.a.m., with each dose administered for 1 week. Medication was given at 9:00 A.M., and performance was measured beginning immediately and beginning 2, 4, and 6 hours after ingestion. The dependent measures included number of math problems completed correctly, teacher-recorded*

Reprinted with permission from the *Journal of the American Academy of Child and Adolescent Psychiatry*, 1995, Vol. 34, No. 11, 1504–1513. Copyright © 1995 by the American Academy of Child and Adolescent Psychiatry.

The authors thank the Hospital for Sick Children, Toronto, Research Institute and Abbott Laboratories, Canada, for their support during this study, and Abbott Laboratories, U.S.A., for support of manuscript preparation. The first author was supported in part by grants AA06267, DA05605, MH40567, MH45576, and MH48157 during the writing of this paper.

*rates of on-task behavior and noncompliance, and teacher rat-
ings on an Abbreviated Conners Teacher Rating Scale.* **Results:**
*There were linear effects of medication, with pemoline doses
greater than 18.75 mg having an effect beginning 2 hours after
ingestion and lasting through the seventh hour after ingestion.*
**Conclusions:** *Results are contrasted with widespread mis-
beliefs regarding pemoline's time course and efficacy.*

The most common form of treatment for children with attention-deficit
hyperactivity disorder (ADHD) is medication with one of the CNS psychostimulant drugs, methylphenidate (MPH), dextroamphetemine, or pemoline. Of these, MPH is by far the most commonly used, accounting for
90% of the medication given to children who have ADHD (Safer and
Krager, 1984), with pemoline and *d*-amphetamine used far less frequently.
Although it is generally considered effective in ameliorating acutely the
symptoms of ADHD, the brief time course of the standard preparation of
MPH limits its usefulness. MPH has a behavioral half-life of 3 hours with
a curvilinear time course in which peak effects are obtained by 2 hours after
ingestion and generally disappear 2 to 3 hours later (Pelham et al. 1987;
Solanto and Conners, 1982; Swanson et al., 1978). Thus, MPH is typically
administered with breakfast and again at lunch to provide adequate coverage for children's behavior during school hours. The practical effect of the
time course of MPH is that a child who takes medication with breakfast and
at lunchtime, a very common dosage regimen, is affected very little by
MPH during the midday hours when morning medication is wearing off
and before afternoon medication has taken effect. Thus, during some times
when he or she may need medication the most (e.g., unstructured school
periods such as the lunchroom and the midday recess), the typical child
medicated with standard MPH is for all practical purposes unmedicated or
undermedicated. Furthermore, many schools refuse to administer or super-
vise the administration of midday doses of MPH, and many children who
have ADHD are embarrassed at having to take medication at school (Safer
and Krager, 1994; Sleator et al., 1982), both conditions leading to poor
compliance with midday dosing of standard preparations of short-acting
stimulants. In addition, if medication coverage is needed for afternoon
times (e.g., after-school playtime, after-school homework), then a third
dose of standard MPH is needed, typically administered right after school.

As a result of these problems, considerable interest has been directed toward CNS stimulants that have a long-acting effect on children with
ADHD, thus avoiding the problematic time course and other difficulties associated with midday dosing of standard MPH. Dextroamphetamine has

been available for some time in a timed-release form. In one study of the efficacy of Dexedrine Spansules® (DS), Brown et al. (1980) reported that DS had a later peak plasma level that lasted longer than standard dextroamphetamine, but that the clinical response time appeared to be shorter. Pelham et al. (1990) showed that the behavioral effects of DS lasted at least 9 hours. However, *d*-amphetamine is regarded as having a higher side effect profile than MPH, limiting its desirability (Dulcan, 1986; Safer and Allen, 1976).

Ritalin SR® was designed to exert an effect equivalent to two 10-mg tablets of Ritalin®, given 4 hours apart; however, the time course of Ritalin SR® appears to be quite variable. In one study, it did not affect some behaviors until 3 hours after ingestion, and it began to lose its effects on some measures 5 hours after ingestion (Pelham et al., 1987). Furthermore, individual responsiveness to SR-20 is highly variable compared to standard MPH both across children and within children across time (Pelham et al., 1987, 1990). Thus long-acting forms of both dextroamphetamine and MPH have shortcomings that mitigate their usefulness.

In contrast to the standard preparations of MPH and dextroamphetamine, pemoline has a longer half-life (Collier et al., 1985; Sallee et al., 1985, 1992) and a longer effective span of action (Pelham et al., 1990). It would appear to be a logical choice for those seeking a long-acting stimulant. However, it is used far less often than MPH—in only 2% of medicated children in one survey (Safer and Krager, 1984)—and has been studied much less extensively. In clinical settings practitioners anecdotally report that pemoline does not appear to have the same beneficial effects that MPH does, and these clinical impressions carry over to professional recommendations (e.g., Barkley, 1990; Dulcan, 1986; Wilens and Biederman, 1992). However, it is not clear whether this is due to a lack of efficacy of the drug or from the manufacturer's recommendations regarding how the medication is to be prescribed.

For example, the recommended pemoline dosing regimen is to begin with the lowest possible dose, 37.5 mg, and increase doses in 18.75-mg increments at weekly intervals until an effective dose is reached (Abbott, 1994). The package insert states that clinical improvement with Cylert® is gradual and that it may take *3 or 4 weeks* before the drug has a therapeutic effect (Abbott, 1994). These recommendations are repeated by professionals in recent reviews (e.g., Wilens and Biederman, 1992), as well as influential formularies (American Society of Hospital Pharmacists, 1994). Furthermore, for years after pemoline was introduced to the market, the manufacturer recommended beginning doses of 18.75 mg and noted that *6 to 8 weeks* may be required before a therapeutic effect was apparent.

If 18.75- or 37.5-mg doses of pemoline are insufficient to produce substantive improvement in most children with ADHD, one practical consequence of these recommendations is that children with ADHD who are given pemoline will be given ineffective dosages for several weeks. Indeed, it now appears likely that practitioners who have followed these recommendations regarding pemoline dosing may have unwittingly prescribed subtherapeutic doses and may have discontinued medication before an effective dose was reached, thereby contributing to the perception that pemoline is less effective than other stimulants. That possibility is given clear support by the few empirical studies that have been conducted with pemoline.

Conners and Taylor (1980) compared pemoline and MPH in an 8-week, between-group study. At mean daily doses of 60.6 mg q.a.m. for pemoline and 22.0 mg in two divided doses for MPH, both medications were superior to placebo, with teacher ratings as the main dependent measure. Pemoline was slightly but not significantly less efficacious than MPH during the 8-week study, but surprisingly the effects of pemoline maintained for 2 weeks after medication termination, while those of MPH dissipated immediately, as expected. Similarly surprising was the finding that parents rated MPH as slightly more effective than pemoline. Given that parent ratings are based on a child's after-school and evening behavior, the expectation had been that pemoline might be rated as more effective than MPH by parents. Despite its beneficial effects on parent and teacher ratings, pemoline was not found to affect performance on standard cognitive tasks such as the Matching Familiar Figures Task or the Continuous Performance Task. Finally, the effects of dose on response were not evaluated systematically in this study; instead children were individually titrated to the mean doses noted above. It is possible that the slightly superior effects of MPH resulted from a more effective dose than was utilized with pemoline.

In another study, Stephens et al. (1984) compared the effects of 1.9 mg/kg pemoline and 0.3 mg/kg MPH on two learning tasks—nonsense spelling and paired-associates. In a crossover design, children were tested on the second of two consecutive days of medication administration at 1 hour postingestion for MPH and 2 hours postingestion for pemoline. Results revealed equivalent beneficial effects of pemoline (mean dose = 55.7 mg) and MPH (mean dose = 8.7 mg) on the two cognitive tasks. These results imply (1) that no time further than 2 days is needed to obtain behavioral effects with pemoline that are as great as those obtained with MPH and (2) that pemoline *does* have beneficial effects on cognitive tasks when tested 2 hours after ingestion at a sixfold greater dose than MPH tested 1 hour after ingestion (cf. Conners and Taylor, 1980).

A study that compared pemoline (56.25 mg) with 10 mg of DS, SR-20, standard MPH (10 mg b.i.d.), and placebo confirmed this finding regarding a maximum of 2 days required for onset for a variety of measures of behavior and academic performance (Pelham et al., 1990). With drug condition randomized over single days for DS, SR-20, MPH, and placebo and randomized over triplets of days for pemoline, the effects of pemoline q.a.m. on the second and third days of consecutive administration were identical with those of MPH b.i.d., SR-20 q.a.m., and DS q.a.m. on the first day of administration. Furthermore, the time courses of the long-acting preparations were similar, with effects being evident on a continuous performance task 1 hour after ingestion and still present 8 hours later. It is interesting that there were considerable individual differences in responsiveness to the medications, with pemoline being recommended for children's ongoing treatment more frequently than either MPH or SR-20.

Finally, this study yielded important information about the behavioral equivalence of these medications. Because the group mean drug effects were identical, it can be concluded that the drug doses were behaviorally equivalent, meaning that q.a.m. pemoline dosing must occur at 6 times that of a single MPH dose given b.i.d. (or t.i.d.) to have the same effect. Given that 10 mg is the most commonly administered dose of MPH, 56.25 mg would be expected to be a common dose of pemoline. However, with current dosing recommendations, that dose would not be reached until the second week of treatment at the earliest, and under previous guidelines until the third week.

Although this study and Stephens et al. (1984) suggested that pemoline needs 2 days of consecutive administration before a behavioral effect is obtained, other investigators have reported similar results with a single acute dose. Both Collier et al. (1985) and Sallee et al. (1992) found similar results when examining the pharmacodynamics of an acute dose of 2.0 mg/kg pemoline (median dose was 56.25 mg for Sallee et al.). Sallee et al. found a mean time to peak plasma concentration of 2.3 hours, which remained the same when assessed again after 3 weeks of medication. As did Pelham et al. (1990), Sallee et al. reported that effects of pemoline were detectable within 1 hour after ingestion, although it is noteworthy that Sallee assessed the effect after the first dose given rather than after the second or third dose.

Thus, what little research is available contradicts the prevailing beliefs, as well as the manufacturer's recommendations, regarding pemoline. It appears that pemoline has an acute effect rather than the gradual one widely believed. It also appears that doses considerably higher than 18.75 or 37.5 mg are needed to have an effect—the mean dose used in all previous studies was approximately 56.25 mg. However, with the exception of the two pharmacodynamic studies cited above, no published information is available regarding higher doses, even though the maximum dose recommended by Abbott is 112.5 mg. Indeed, the pattern of differences among and omissions in extant studies highlight the lack of knowledge concerning the dose effects and time course of pemoline and emphasize the need for a study to examine these characteristics of the drug. The purpose of the present investigation was to study the effects on a variety of dependent measures of different doses of pemoline administered to children with ADHD in a hospital classroom setting. The study was designed in such a way that the first 7 hours of the time course for pemoline could be determined for each of four doses ranging from 18.75 to 112.5 mg.

We hypothesized that the effects of pemoline would be acute, detectable within 2 hours, and persisting linearly throughout the duration of the 7-hour assessment period. In addition, we expected to find pemoline to be efficacious in both behavioral and cognitive domains of functioning, with maximum therapeutic results being obtained at doses higher than those typically initiated in clinical settings. Finally, we predicted that individual response to pemoline would be comparable with rates of response found with MPH.

## METHOD

### Subjects

Subjects were selected from among referrals from primary physicians for diagnostic and medication evaluations to the Child Development Clinic of the Department of Neurology of the Hospital for Sick Children in Toronto. The clinic physicians referred children with attention deficit disorder (ADD) diagnosed according to *DSM-III* (this study was conducted prior to the publication of *DSM-III-R*). Twenty-eight children, 22 boys and 6 girls, whose ages ranged from 5 to 12 years with a median age of 8 years 10 months, participated in the study. All children had a diagnosis of ADD, 23 with and 5 without hyperactivity, according to *DSM-III* criteria. A checklist (Swanson, Nolan, and Pelham [SNAP] Checklist) that was developed to assess *DSM-III* criteria was completed by each child's parent and teacher. Each child's mother and teacher also rated him or her on the Abbreviated Conners Rating Scale (Goyette et al., 1978). The mean mother rating was 16.8 (SD = 6.5), and the mean teacher rating was 19.5 (SD = 8.0). Diagnosis was made by the second author on the basis of parent ratings, teacher ratings, and a parent interview that consisted of the *DSM-III* symptoms of ADD. The parent interview consisted of asking the child's parent to respond "yes" or "no" regarding the presence of each of the *DSM-III* symptoms of ADD. Children with mental retardation were screened out during the referral process. Twelve children were enrolled in special classes for emotionally handicapped or learning-disabled children for some portion of their school days, while the remainder were mainstreamed.

## Procedure

During each week of the 7-week study, each child spent one school day in an outpatient clinic at the hospital, and the other four school days in the regular school placement. The initial 2 weeks of the 7-week study were baseline weeks. During the remaining 5 weeks, in a double-blind crossover design, placebo, 18.75 mg, 37.5 mg, 75 mg, and 112.5 mg of pemoline were compared. Two children (one of the youngest and one of the oldest) did not tolerate the highest dose of pemoline. Therefore, they received 56.25 mg and 75 mg as their two highest doses. Each dose was administered once a day (before breakfast) for 6 days at home, and at the hospital on 1 day at 9:00 A.M. (at least 1 hour after breakfast). The order of the five doses was counterbalanced using a Latin square. Children received each dose for 1 week, from Sunday through the following Saturday.

Five groups of children were established, and each group came to the hospital on the same day of the week for the 7 weeks of the study. Four of the groups consisted of five or six boys grouped according to age and grade, and the fifth group consisted of six girls whose ages ranged from 6 to 12 years. On their assigned day, children arrived at the hospital at 8:30 A.M. and spent the first 30 minutes of the day completing pretest measures. At 9:00 A.M., the children received their medication.

After the warm-up period, the daily schedule was broken into four 1-hour testing sessions, starting at 9:00 A.M. (ingestion), 11:00 A.M., 1:00 P.M., and 3:00 P.M., during which children's behavior and performance were assessed. During each assessment period, half of the subjects worked on academic tasks in a small classroom with one teacher, while the other children completed the Paired Associate Learning task (Swanson et al., 1978) in individual testing sessions for 30 minutes; the subjects then switched places for the final 30 minutes. After the third assessment period, the children completed a spelling post-test.

The academic tasks consisted of a 16-minute period during which the children worked on math problems that were matched to their current ability. Each child had four pages of problems to complete and was given 4 minutes to work on each page. The teacher gathered the papers and recorded accuracy and productivity for later analysis. While the children worked on the math problems, the teacher observed the children and recorded on-task behavior. For 15 minutes, the teacher glanced at the children one time per minute and assessed whether the children were on-task. An independent observer coded on-task behavior during one of the assessment periods each day for reliability purposes (the average percentage agreement was 80%). During the remainder of the 30-minute classroom period, children studied their assigned spelling words for that day. For the entire 30 minutes of each classroom period, the teacher tracked the number of commands she gave and the number of times that children failed to comply with a command.

There were no behavioral contingencies for academic work or behavior in the classroom. However, children who were severely disruptive were placed in time out for periods of 5 to 15 minutes. After the last classroom period, the teacher completed an Abbreviated Conners Teacher Rating Scale (ACTRS) (Goyette et al., 1978) that covered the entire day on each of the children. Because of their common use in medication studies, these ACTRS ratings serve as a standardized measure of response to medication.

The dependent measures for this investigation included the number of math problems completed correctly in each 16-minute period, teacher-recorded rates of on-task behavior (the percentage of the 15 checks on which the child was on-task), teacher-recorded frequency counts of noncompliance during each class, and teacher ratings on the ACTRS. Performance on the Paired Associate Learning task, spelling, and other tasks completed in the hospital, as well as measures gathered on other days in the children's regular school settings, will be reported elsewhere.

## RESULTS

A series of five (dose: placebo, 18.75 mg, 37.5 mg, 75 mg, 112.5 mg) × four (time since ingestion: 0 hours, 2 hours, 4 hours, 6 hours) analyses of variance with orthogonal decomposition was performed on the measures of arithmetic problems correct, on-task behavior, and noncompliance. When the interactions of time since ingestion and dose were significant, analyses (orthogonal decompositions) of simple effects were conducted to assess the time course of each dose. For these analyses, the effect of time since ingestion reflects the effect of drug, since ingestion occurred at 9:00 A.M. and dependent measures were evaluated at 2 to 3, 4 to 5, and 6 to 7 hours later. Results are shown in Tables 1, 2, and 3 and in Figures 1 through 3. Table 1 shows the means for each dose (collapsed over the 2-, 4-, and 6-hour assessments) on each dependent measure and reveals increasing effects with

TABLE 1
Means (and Standard Deviations) for the Dependent Variables as a Function of Dose

| Dependent Measures | Placebo | 18.75 mg | Dose 37.5 mg | 75.0 mg | 112.5 mg |
|---|---|---|---|---|---|
| Arithmetic Correct[a] | 50.4 | 56.0 | 68.2 | 71.5 | 75.0 |
| | (45.6) | (41.8) | (51.1) | (62.8) | (60.6) |
| On-Task Behavior[a] | 44.1 | 61.0 | 66.2 | 70.1 | 75.4 |
| | (20.5) | (21.0) | (21.3) | (25.7) | (19.4) |
| Noncompliance[a] | 4.6 | 2.8 | 2.7 | 2.3 | 1.3 |
| | (3.6) | (2.5) | (2.8) | (2.9) | (1.6) |
| ACTRS | 16.4 | 13.2 | 12.4 | 8.6 | 7.1 |
| | (7.0) | (5.4) | (7.5) | (6.1) | (5.1) |

*Note:* ACTRS = Abbreviated Conners Teacher Rating Scale.
[a] Averaged across the 11:00 A.M., 1:00 P.M., and 3:00 P.M. assessments.

TABLE 2

*F* Values for the Dependent Variables as a Function of Dose and Time

| Measure | F Values for Dose | | | F Values for Time | | | F Values for Dose × Time | | |
|---|---|---|---|---|---|---|---|---|---|
| | Main[a] | Linear[b] | Cubic[b] | Main[c] | Linear[b] | Quadratic[b] | Main[d] | Linear, Linear[b] | Linear, Quadratic[b] |
| Arithmetic Correct | 3.42** | 12.02*** | | 8.84‡ | 13.68*** | 6.48** | 2.80*** | 21.52† | |
| On-Task Behavior | 10.23‡ | 31.57‡ | | 4.44*** | 10.63*** | | 3.53† | 31.24‡ | |
| Noncompliance | 5.08† | 12.39*** | 5.42* | 11.27‡ | 20.38† | 7.04** | 3.69‡ | 11.92*** | 12.01*** |
| ACTRS | 13.24‡ | 56.92‡ | | e | e | e | e | e | e |

*Note:* ACTRS = Abbreviated Conners Teacher Rating Scale.

[a] $F(4, 108)$.

[b] $F(1, 27)$.

[c] $F(3, 81)$.

[d] $F(12, 324)$.

[e] These cells do not apply because the ACTRS was completed only once daily.

* $p < .05$; ** $p < .025$; *** $p < .001$; † $p < .01$; ‡ $p < .0001$.

TABLE 3
Simple Effects of Time at Each Dose

| Measure | Placebo | 18.75 mg | 37.5 mg | 75.0 mg | 112.5 mg |
|---|---|---|---|---|---|
| | | *F* Values for Time | | | |
| Arithmetic Correct | | | 4.60 | 8.21† | 6.99† |
| On-Task Behavior | 3.28* | | 3.27* | 4.71*** | 6.11† |
| Noncompliance | | | 7.05† | 13.92‡ | 7.12† |

*Note: F*(3, 81). The effect of time is the effect of medication, as effects were monitored from ingestion through 7 hours postingestion.
* $p < .05$; ** $p < .025$; *** $p < .01$; † $p < .001$; ‡ $p < .0001$.

increasing dose. As Table 2 reveals, the linear effects of dose were highly significant for all three dependent measures. The linear components of the dose by time interaction were significant for all three dependent measures. As Figures 1 through 3 illustrate, the interactions reflect the fact that the effects of dose became greater over time, the effect that would be expected if

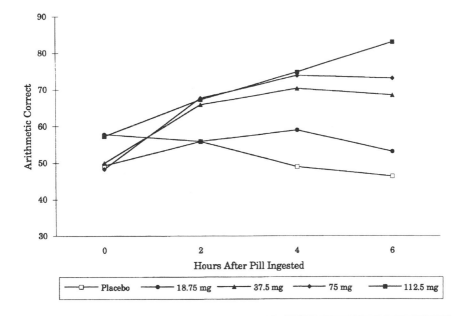

**Figure 1.** Arithmetic problems correct as a function of dose and time.

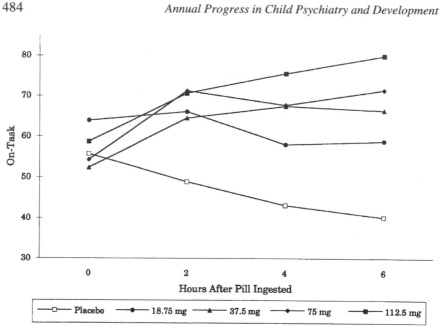

**Figure 2.** On-task behavior as a function of dose and time.

---

there were no drug effect immediately following ingestion (at 9:00 A.M.) and increasing effects as pemoline began to take effect 2, 4, and 6 hours later.

To investigate these significant interactions, the simple effects of time at each level of dose were conducted (Table 3). These analyses reflect the time course and therefore the effect of each dose. As shown in Table 3, the effects were highly significant for all doses at 37.5 mg or above. There were no significant effects of time at the 18.75-mg dose, indicating that this dose had no effect on the classroom measures. The effect of time at the placebo level of dose for on-task behavior reflects the significant *decrease* in on-task behavior over the course of the daily assessments.

An analysis of variance assessing the effect of dose was performed on the teacher ratings on the ACTRS. As shown in Table 2, this analysis of variance showed a main effect of dose that was accounted for by the linear component. Teacher ratings decreased steadily with increasing dosage of pemoline (Table 1).

Side effects were monitored on the laboratory day by the laboratory classroom teacher. Table 4 presents the percentage of children judged as exhibiting side effects by dose as reported as either moderate or severe by

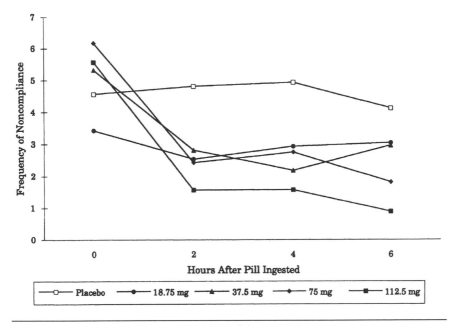

**Figure 3.** Noncompliance as a function of dose and time.

the laboratory teacher. As the table shows, side effects were minimal at all doses, with side effects being reported most often on placebo.

At the end of the study, the treating clinicians (J.M.S. and each child's pediatrician in the Neurology Clinic) made a determination based on all available information regarding whether Cylert® should continue to be used in the child's ongoing treatment. It was determined that 25 of the 28 children were favorable responders to pemoline, and their treatment was continued.

## DISCUSSION

The main findings of the study are as follows: (1) pemoline has clear beneficial effects on measures of classroom behavior and academic performance, and the effects are comparable with those reported in studies of MPH; (2) pemoline has an onset of behavioral action on these measures within 2 hours postingestion when it has been given between 2 and 5 consecutive days; (3) pemoline's effects on classroom measures last for at least 7 hours postingestion; (4) pemoline's effects in the dose range from 18.75

## TABLE 4
### Percentages of Children Rated as Showing Side Effects by Medication Condition

| Side Effects Measured | | Medication Condition | | | |
|---|---|---|---|---|---|
| | Placebo | 18.75 mg Pemoline | 37.5 mg Pemoline | 75.0 mg Pemoline | 112.5 mg Pemoline |
| Crabby, touchy | 19 | 21 | 10 | 10 | 0 |
| Whiny | 6 | 11 | 14 | 5 | 0 |
| Worried | 5 | 5 | 0 | 5 | 5 |
| Fearful | 0 | 5 | 0 | 0 | 0 |
| Anxious | 20 | 10 | 5 | 0 | 11 |
| Withdrawn | 10 | 5 | 0 | 5 | 16 |
| Dull | 10 | 0 | 4 | 5 | 6 |
| Drowsy | 10 | 10 | 0 | 5 | 0 |
| Tearful | 0 | 0 | 5 | 10 | 0 |
| Tired | 10 | 5 | 10 | 0 | 0 |
| Jittery | 43 | 15 | 14 | 5 | 11 |
| Restless | 50 | 30 | 39 | 19 | 12 |
| Stomachache | 5 | 0 | 0 | 0 | 6 |
| Headache | 5 | 0 | 0 | 0 | 11 |
| Muscle ache | 0 | 5 | 0 | 0 | 0 |
| Vomiting | 0 | 0 | 0 | 0 | 0 |
| Rash | 0 | 0 | 0 | 0 | 0 |
| Weakness | 0 | 0 | 0 | 0 | 0 |
| Dry mouth | 0 | 0 | 0 | 0 | 11 |
| Fainting | 0 | 0 | 0 | 0 | 0 |
| Eye twitches | 0 | 0 | 0 | 0 | 0 |
| Tics (frequent muscle jerks) | 0 | 0 | 5 | 0 | 0 |
| Biting fingernails | 5 | 0 | 5 | 0 | 6 |
| Repetitive tongue movements | 5 | 0 | 0 | 10 | 0 |
| Picking (at skin or clothes) | 0 | 5 | 13 | 0 | 0 |
| Distortion of vision | 0 | 0 | 0 | 0 | 0 |

*Note:* Evidence of a side effect is defined as endorsement of either "moderate" or "severe" on a 4-point scale (none, mild, moderate, or severe).

mg to 112.5 mg are linear, although there are minimal effects of the lowest dose; (5) side effects of pemoline were minimal and were not associated with increasing dose; and (6) clinical response to pemoline was present in as high a percentage of subjects as has been reported elsewhere for MPH and *d*-amphetamine. These findings are consistent with the previously reported studies of pemoline but are in contrast to the widespread belief among both practitioners and academicians that pemoline has a delayed onset of 3 or more weeks and is not efficacious for children with ADHD.

These results are consistent with earlier pemoline studies in several respects. Given that the effects of pemoline in the classroom are immediate, the study lends indirect support to the previous reports of immediate action in pharmacodynamic studies (Collier et al., 1985; Sallee et al., 1992). Stephens et al. (1984) and Sallee et al. also reported beneficial effects on laboratory measures of learning of single acute doses (of 1.9 and 2.0 mg/kg, respectively) with time courses (in Sallee et al.) and effects similar to those we report herein. The present results extend those reports to classroom measures of on-task behavior, noncompliance, and arithmetic performance (as well as to teacher ratings, although time course was not measured for that measure). Numerous studies have revealed beneficial MPH effects on measures of arithmetic performance in the classroom (see Carlson and Bunner, 1993, for a review). These findings are the first to show that pemoline has similar effects. Pelham et al. (1985) used exactly the same methodology to examine MPH (0.15, 0.3, and 0.6 mg/kg) effects on arithmetic performance in a laboratory classroom setting. When the findings for pemoline for this study are compared directly to MPH effects (mean doses were 4.2, 8.7, and 17.5 mg of MPH) in Pelham et al. (1985), the results are quite comparable (see Pelham, 1986, for a graphic comparison). Indeed, when the effects on arithmetic in the present study and paired associate learning, continuous performance, and nonsense spelling in previous studies are considered as a whole, the beneficial effects of pemoline on cognition in children with ADHD appear to be the same as for MPH (see Rapport and Kelly, 1991, for a review of MPH effects on cognition in ADHD).

As Pelham et al. (1990) previously reported in an acute dosing study, 56.25 mg of pemoline q.a.m. has effects on classroom seatwork completion and classroom rule-following that were equivalent (for the subjects as a group) to those of 10 mg of MPH b.i.d., SR-20 q.a.m., and 10 mg of DS q.a.m. The present findings extend those to measures of on-task behavior, noncompliance with teacher requests, and arithmetic performance, none of which were measured in the previous study. Furthermore, the present results measured teacher perceptions on the ACTRS across the day from 9:00 until 4:00, a time period that is more typical of a school day than the 60-

minute classroom that Pelham et al. (1990) used, and the present study yielded considerably larger drug effects on the ACTRS—a reduction from 16 to 7—than Pelham et al. reported—a reduction from 4 to 2. The pemoline effects on the ACTRS ratings and the on-task measures reported herein are quite comparable with those that have been reported in similar studies for comparable doses of MPH (e.g., see Rapport et al., 1985, 1986).

The time course analyses revealed similar effects for all three classroom dependent measures, as Figures 1 through 3 reveal. The dose effects were accounted for primarily by their linear components. As Table 3 and Figures 1 through 3 illustrate, 18.75 mg had no effect, while the effects of each higher dose began to be apparent 2 hours after ingestion and increased over the next 4 to 5 hours, with performance improving incrementally and linearly with increasing doses and with time after ingestion. The 112.5-mg dose had the highest level between 3:00 and 4:00, when the lower doses had reached plateaus.

On-task behavior showed time course effects similar to those for noncompliance and arithmetic with one exception. The significant dose × time interaction reflects a pattern wherein unmedicated subjects' on-task behavior decreased over the course of the day, while on-task behavior increased steadily over time with all doses of pemoline except for 18.75 mg. On this measure, pemoline not only improved performance relative to placebo but also prevented a substantial decline in performance over the course of 7 hours postingestion.

As Figure 3 illustrates, the significant interactions on the measure of noncompliance reflect the facts that subjects' rates of noncompliance were unchanged over time given placebo and 18.75 mg, while doses of pemoline from 37.5 through 112.5 produced improvement in compliance that was clearly evident at 2 hours postingestion and did not decrease substantially thereafter. Again, the highest dose of pemoline was most effective at reducing subjects' rates of noncompliance (see also Table 1).

It is interesting to compare the dose × time graphs for arithmetic problems and noncompliance with regard to potentially different time courses for different behaviors. The magnitude of the effects are similar and the quadratic components of the time by dose interaction are similar for arithmetic and noncompliance. At the same time, the effect of dose appears to be more linear for arithmetic correct than for noncompliance. Perhaps pemoline affects behavioral inhibition more quickly than it affects attention or learning. Although there have long been speculations regarding the differential effects of dose on different domains of functioning (e.g., Pelham, 1986; Rapport and Kelly, 1991; Sprague and Sleator, 1977), there has been little discussion of whether the time course of these effects may differ (see, however, Solanto and Conners, 1982, for another possible example dealing with MPH). Pelham et al. (1987) reported a similar finding when evaluating SR-20—that is, a more delayed onset for a continuous performance task than on counselor ratings of behavior on the ACTRS. Given that the time courses of the long-acting medications in particular are important to understand to ensure adequate medication coverage throughout the day, additional research focused on dose-response by time-response questions would appear useful.

It is worth emphasizing that these pemoline effects contradict widespread misperceptions regarding the drug's time course and efficacy. The findings reported herein clearly document that the drug is efficacious; it had acute effects comparable with those reported elsewhere for MPH, and all but three children were found to be responders and continued to take the medication. Pelham et al. (1990) reported a suggestion of a differentially positive individual responsiveness to pemoline compared with the other two long-acting agents. The findings also support previously reported results from measures of blood level and laboratory tasks documenting that pemoline has an effective time of onset of 2 hours. As Stephens et al. (1984) demonstrated, pemoline effects on two laboratory learning tasks measured at 2 hours postingestion are identical with MPH effects on the same tasks measured 1.5 hours postingestion.

We suspect that the reason that clinicians believe that pemoline has a considerably slower onset of effects is that they are beginning the medication at dosages that are too low to yield effects comparable with what is seen with MPH. Certainly, the present results show that 18.75 mg is an ineffective dose for children of elementary school age (mean age of just under 9 years). Previous studies have shown that 56.25 to 61 mg of pemoline q.a.m. produces effects equivalent to 9 to 11 mg of MPH b.i.d. (Conners and Taylor, 1980; Pelham et al., 1990; Stephens et al., 1984). Therefore, a dose of 37.5 mg of pemoline, which is the manufacturer's recommended starting dose, is roughly equivalent to 5 to 7 mg of MPH b.i.d., which would be considered by most to be a *low* dose of MPH for a typical 9-year-old (the approximate mean age of children in this study). The most common dose of MPH that is administered in clinical settings is 10 mg, given two or three times per day, and MPH is often started at a 10-mg dose, or at the least quickly titrated to that level, yielding maximum therapeutic effects. In contrast, it would take 2 or 3 weeks before a comparable dose of pemoline is reached if 37.5 were the starting dose and it were adjusted weekly in 18.75-mg increments—exactly the pattern clinicians observe. Our clinical work has involved starting pemoline with doses at 37.5 (for lower weight) or 56.25 (for higher weight) and adjusting upward in a matter of days rather than weeks (e.g., 2 or 3 days per dose). Such a dosing regimen is no more likely to produce side effects than a weekly dose adjustment and provides more immediate salutary effects than the regimen currently recommended and widely used. Indeed, rapid titration to a clinically effective dose is widely agreed to be a procedural requirement for MPH dosing, and the present results suggest that the same should be true for pemoline.

The side effects reported in Table 4 are similar to those reported in previous studies of pemoline's side effects (e.g., Conners and Taylor, 1980; Pelham et al., 1990), but the present study extends previous results to a dose-response analysis. As others have reported (e.g., Barkley et al., 1990), many *behavioral* side effects such as jitteriness and restlessness are reported more often on placebo than on drug conditions. The majority of side effects reported by teachers were described as mild. No side effect was more likely to be reported at a level greater than mild for any dose of pemoline relative to placebo. Of note is that this was true for tongue movements, eye twitches, and tics, all of which have been described anecdotally in extant literature as more common with pemoline than MPH. That was not supported in this empirical study. Parent side effect ratings of sleep disturbances are not reported in this article, but Conners and Taylor (1980) showed pemoline's effects on sleep problems to be comparable with those of twice-daily MPH.

It should be noted that liver enzyme tests were not given in this study because of its brevity. Elevations in liver enzymes were *reported* in 1% to 3% of children taking pemoline in early studies (Page et al., 1974) and in current discussions of drug regimens (Weiss and Hechtman, 1993). However, the *actual rate* of elevations in clinical practice appears to be no greater than one tenth of these rates (F.R. Sallee, personal communication, February 1995). Although apparently unrelated to symptoms of liver functioning and reversible upon pemoline discontinuation, current recommendations are that assessment of liver function should be conducted initially and at 6-month intervals for patients on maintenance pemoline regimens.

These results add to the studies that have shown efficacy of a long-acting stimulant preparation, in this case pemoline. Although it is widely believed that the long-acting preparations including pemoline are not as efficacious as short-acting stimulant preparations, these data add to the literature that shows that pemoline has effects comparable with those of standard MPH on ecologically valid measures of classroom functioning. It is noteworthy that the time course analyses confirm that a single dose of pemoline (37.5 to 112.5 mg) lasts at least 7 hours, with the highest dose not peaking until that time. If a young adolescent boy with ADHD who would otherwise take 20 mg of MPH t.i.d. were to take a single morning dose of

112.5 mg of pemoline, it would likely provide all-day coverage of school behavior and performance, as well as coverage of after-school, homework time. An increasing number of middle school children and adolescents with ADHD will not take medication at school because of embarrassment or school policy (Safer and Krager, 1994), highlighting the particular advantage of a long-acting preparation for older children and adolescents with ADHD. Indeed, given that prescriptions for long-acting preparations are increasing differentially for adolescents (Safer and Krager, 1988a,b, 1994) and that no research has directly examined the effects of long-acting preparations, including pemoline, in ADHD adolescents, such research is warranted.

Finally, we should note that we combined children with diagnoses of ADD with and without hyperactivity in this study. Because subjects were not blocked on that variable prior to random assignment to order, we could not analyze for differential drug effects as a function of diagnosis. However, Barkley et al. (1991) have shown that ADHD effects are comparable in children with and without hyperactivity, and we should expect the same to be true for pemoline.

## REFERENCES

Abbott (1994), *Package insert for Cylert*. Abbott Park, IL: Abbott Laboratories, USA

American Society of Hospital Pharmacists (1994), *AHFS Drug Information*. Bethesda, MD: American Society of Hospital Pharmacists, Inc

Barkley RA (1990), *Attention Deficit Hyperactivity Disorder: A Handbook for Diagnosis and Treatment*. New York: Guilford

Barkley RA, DuPaul GJ, McMurray MB (1991), Attention deficit disorder with and without hyperactivity: clinical response to three doses of methylphenidate. *Pediatrics* 87:519–531

Barkley RA, McMurray MB, Edelbrock CS, Robbins K (1990), Side effects of methylphenidate in children with attention deficit hyperactivity disorder: a systematic, placebo-controlled investigation. *Pediatrics* 86:184–192

Brown GL, Ebert MH, Mikkelsen EJ, Hunt RD (1980), Behavior and motor activity response in hyperactive children and plasma amphetamine levels following a sustained release preparation. *J Am Acad Child Psychiatry* 19:225–239

Carlson CL, Bunner MR (1993), Effects of methylphenidate on the academic performance of children with attention-deficit hyperactivity disorder and learning disabilities. *Sch Psychol Rev* 22:184–198

Collier CP, Soldin SJ, Swanson JM, MacLeod SM, Weinberg F, Rochefort JG (1985), Pemoline pharmacokinetics and long term therapy in children with attention deficit disorder and hyperactivity. *Clin Pharmacokinet* 10:269–278

Conners CK, Taylor E (1980), Pemoline, methylphenidate, and placebo in children with minimal brain dysfunction. *Arch Gen Psychiatry* 37:922–932

Dulcan MK (1986), Comprehensive treatment of children and adolescents with attention deficit disorders: the state of the art. *Clin Psychol Rev* 6:539–569

Goyette CH, Conners CK, Ulrich RF (1978), Normative data on revised Conners parent and teacher rating scales. *J Abnorm Child Psychol* 6:221–236

Page JG, Bernstein JE, Janicki RS, Michelli FA (1974), A multi-clinic trial of pemoline in childhood hyperkinesis. In: *Clinical Use of Stimulant Drugs in Children*, Conners CK, ed. Amsterdam: Excerpta Medica, pp 98–123

Pelham WE (1986), The effects of psychostimulant drugs on learning and achievement in children with attention-deficit hyperactivity disorders and learning-disabilities. In: *Psychological and Educational Perspectives on Learning Disabilities*, Torgesen JK, Wong B, eds. New York: Academic Press, pp 259–295

Pelham WE, Bender ME, Caddell J, Booth S, Moorer S (1985), The dose-response effects of methylphenidate on classroom academic and social behavior in children with attention deficit disorder. *Arch Gen Psychiatry* 42:948–952

Pelham WE, Greenslade KE, Vodde-Hamilton MA et al. (1990), Relative efficacy of long-acting CNS stimulants on children with attention deficit-hyperactivity disorder: a comparison of standard methylphenidate, sustained-release methylphenidate, sustained-release dextroamphetamine, and pemoline. *Pediatrics* 86:226–237

Pelham WE, Sturges J, Hoza J, Schmidt C, Bijlsma J, Moorer S (1987), Sustained release and standard methlyphenidate effects on cognitive and social behavior in children with attention deficit disorder: *Pediatrics* 80:491–501

Rapport MD, DePaul GJ, Stoner G, Jones JT (1986), Comparing classroom and clinic measures of attention deficit disorder: differential, idiosyncratic, and dose-response effects of methylphenidate. *J Consult Clin Psychol* 54:334–341

Rapport MD, Kelly KL (1991), Psychostimulant effects on learning and cognitive function: findings and implications for children with attention deficit hyperactivity disorder. *Clin Psychol Rev* 11:61–92

Rapport MD, Stoner G, DuPaul GJ, Birmingham BK, Tucker S (1985), Methylphenidate in hyperactive children: differential effects of dose on academic, learning, and social behavior. *J Abnorm Child Psychol* 13:227–244

Safer DJ, Allen RP (1976), *Hyperactive Children: Diagnosis and Management*, Baltimore: University Park Press

Safer DJ, Krager JM (1984), Trends in medication treatment of hyperactive school children. In: *Advances in Learning and Behavioral Disabilities*, Vol 3, Gadow KD, ed. Greenwich, CT: JAI Press, pp 125–149

Safer DJ, Krager JM (1988a), A survey of medication treatment for hyperactive/inattentive students. *JAMA* 260:2256–2258

Safer DJ, Krager JM (1988b), Trends in medication treatment of hyperactive school children: results of six biannual surveys. *Clin Pediatr (Phila)* 22: 500–504

Safer DJ, Krager JM (1994), The increased rate of stimulant treatment for hyperactive/inattentive students in secondary schools. *Pediatrics* 94:462–464

Sallee FR, Stiller R, Perel J (1992), Pharmacodynamics of pemoline in attention deficit disorder with hyperactivity. *J Am Acad Child Adolesc Psychiatry* 31: 244–251

Sallee FR, Stiller R, Perel J, Bates T (1985), Oral pemoline kinetics in hyperactive children. *Clin Pharmacol Ther* 37:606–609

Sleator EK, Ullman RK, von Neumann A (1982), How do hyperactive children feel about taking stimulants and will they tell the doctor? *Clin Pediatr (Phila)* 21:474–479

Solanto MV, Conners CK (1982), A dose-response and time-action analysis of autonomic and behavioral effects of methylphenidate in attention deficit disorder with hyperactivity. *Psychophysiology* 19:658–667

Sprague RL, Sleator E (1977), Methylphenidate in hyperkinetic children: differences in dose effects on learning and social behavior. *Science* 198:1274–1276

Stephens R, Pelham WE, Skinner R (1984), The state-dependent and main effects of pemoline and methylphenidate on paired-associates learning and spelling in hyperactive children. *J Consult Clin Psychol* 52:104–113

Swanson J, Kinsbourne M, Roberts W, Zucker K (1978), Time-response analysis of the effect of stimulant medication on the learning ability of children referred for hyperactivity. *Pediatrics* 61:21–29

Weiss G, Hechtman LT (1993), *Hyperactive Children Grown Up: ADHD in Children, Adolescents, and Adults.* New York: Guilford

Wilens TE, Biederman J (1992), The stimulants. *Psychiatr Clin North Am* 41: 191–222

# 20

# Efficacy of Methylphenidate for Attention-Deficit Hyperactivity Disorder in Children with Tic Disorder

Kenneth D. Gadow, Jeffrey Sverd, Joyce Sprafkin, Edith E. Nolan, and Stacy N. Ezor

*State University of New York, Stony Brook*

**Background:** *The findings from case reports and patient questionnaire surveys have been interpreted as indicating that administration of stimulants is ill-advised for the treatment of attention-deficit hyperactivity disorder in children with tic disorder.* **Methods:** *Thirty-four prepubertal children with attention-deficit hyperactivity disorder and tic disorder received placebo and three dosages of methylphenidate hydrochloride (0.1, 0.3, and 0.5 mg/kg) twice daily for 2 weeks each, under double-blind conditions. Treatment effects were assessed using direct observations of child behavior in a simulated (clinic-based) classroom and using rating scales completed by the parents, teachers, and physician.* **Results:** *Methylphenidate effectively suppressed hyperactive, disruptive, and aggressive behavior. There was no evidence that methylphenidate altered the severity of tic disorder, but it may have a weak effect on the frequency of motor (increase) and vocal (decrease) tics.* **Conclu-**

Reprinted with permission from *Archives of General Psychiatry*, 1995, Vol. 52, 444–455. Copyright © 1995 by the American Medical Association.

*This study was supported in part by a research grant from the Tourette Syndrome Association Inc, Bayside, NY, and US Public Health Service grant MH 45358 from the National Institute of Mental Health, Bethesda, Md.*

*Methylphenidate placebos were supplied by Ciba-Geigy Pharmaceutical Co, Summit, NJ.*

*We thank Joseph Schwartz, PhD, for assisting us with the data analyses, Linda Volkersz for conducting clinic evaluations, and Michele J. De Angelis and Michael V. De Angelis for providing pharmacy services. We are particularly indebted to the courageous families who made this study possible.*

**sion:** *Methylphenidate appears to be a safe and effective treatment for attention-deficit hyperactivity disorder in the majority of children with comorbid tic disorder.*

In spite of a relatively long and productive history of research on stimulant drug therapy for childhood behavior disorders, controversies remain, and none is more divisive than its appropriateness for the treatment of attention-deficit hyperactivity disorder (ADHD) in children with comorbid tic disorder. Historically, Bradley[1] was one of the first investigators to note that some children with behavior disorders who were receiving clinical doses of amphetamine "gave evidence of increased emotional tension by . . . accentuation of ticlike motor activities" (eg, nail biting, hair pulling, and nose picking). Later, Mattson and Calverly[2] described a case of drug-induced involuntary movements (lip smacking, grimacing, and eyelid twitching) in an 8-year-old boy who was treated with 5 mg of dextroamphetamine sulfate. Early studies of children treated with methylphenidate hydrochloride, which is currently the most widely prescribed drug for hyperactivity and/or ADHD,[3] also found that this stimulant significantly increased fingernail biting[4] and induced tics in a small percentage of subjects.[5] Golden[6] reported the first case of apparent methylphenidate-induced Tourette syndrome (TS) in a 9-year-old hyperactive boy. After 8 weeks of treatment, a variety of motor and vocal tics suddenly developed in the child and did not abate after administration of medication (10 mg, twice a day) was terminated. Additional cases have been described.[7,8]

Early case reports of stimulant drug therapy specifically for the treatment of tic disorder indicated limited efficacy and tic exacerbation in some individuals.[9–12] As an aside, it is noteworthy that these early reports also note that tic exacerbation is associated with almost all psychotherapeutic drugs,[9] which is an accurate description of currently popular medications as well.[13] The past two decades have witnessed a flurry of case reports, some of which were controlled drug evaluations,[11,14,15] questionnaire surveys, and chart reviews, that question the safety of stimulants for the treatment of ADHD in children with tic disorder.[16,17] Briefly, the findings from questionnaire surveys and chart reviews suggest increased tics associated with stimulant medication in 40% to 50% and 10% to 30% of patients, respectively. Controlled studies that employed multiple challenge doses provided the most compelling evidence of tic exacerbation in specific individuals.[11] Perhaps the most influential proscription against stimulant drug therapy was a case review study by Lowe et al[18] of patients who were treated in university and community-based clinics that concluded "motor tics or diagnosed TS in a child should be a contraindication to the use of stimulant medication for alleviation of hyperactive symptoms." Much less attention was given to a literature review by Shapiro and Shapiro[16] that appeared about the same time and that noted the methodological problems and logical inconsistencies in the existing literature that is interpreted as supporting stimulant tic induction and/or exacerbation hypotheses. The relatively common co-occurrence of hyperactivity and tic disorder in children who are referred for psychiatric evaluation of behavioral disturbance[19-22] makes this controversy a significant issue in child psychiatry.

The debate over the safety and efficacy of stimulants for inattentive and/or disruptive behaviors in children with tic disorder has been further complicated by a major controversy over the pleiotropic manifestations of the TS diathesis. Children with TS experience a variety of behavioral, affective, and cognitive disabilities, and there is much disagreement as to which are intrinsic to the tic disorder (ie, phenocopies of other childhood disorders) and which are comorbidities.[17,23-26] For example, it was once argued that the attention deficits and disruptive behaviors seen in children with tic disorder are phenocopies of true ADHD and oppositional defiant disorder and/or conduct disorder, respectively, and that stimulants were ineffective for their clinical management.[27]

Response to stimulant medication also has played an important role in theory formulation concerning the neuropathologic characteristics of tic disorder. Most notable was the observation that stimulants exacerbated tics in some individuals,[11,14,15] which supported hyperdopaminergic dysfunction as a probable cause of tic expression.[24,28] Alternatively, evidence suggesting that the effect of stimulants on tics is heterogeneous and that some patients even experience tic amelioration[29-32] has led to more complex theories of dopaminergic involvement in the pathogenesis of tic disorder. For example, Comings[29] and Comings and Comings[30] suggested that early exposure to stimulant medications in children at risk for the development of TS might delay the onset of tics by preventing secondary hypersensitization of subcortical dopamine pathways, which results from genetically caused hypofunction of mesocortical dopamine pathways. Friedhoff[33] hypothesized that following transient worsening of tics on initial exposure to methylphenidate, the drug may induce a reduction in dopamine receptor sensitivity, resulting in tic amelioration, whereas others[34,35] suggested the corollary theory that stimulants might reduce the long-term severity of TS symptoms by desensitizing catecholamine receptors.

Although the findings from controlled studies of stimulants in children with ADHD and tics or compulsive behaviors are encouraging,[32,36-39] this existing research is limited both in scope (relatively small patient samples) and in diagnostic clarity. The following is a report of the safety and efficacy of methylphenidate in a relatively large sample of children with ADHD and a diagnosed tic disorder. Participants were assigned at random to various sequences of placebo and three dosages of methylphenidate under double-blind conditions. To be eligible for the study, ADHD had to be a primary reason for seeking clinical services.

## SUBJECTS AND METHODS

### Subjects

The subjects were 34 children (31 boys and three girls) between the ages of 6 years 1 month and 11 years 11 months, who were referred for evaluation to the Tic Disorders Clinic, Stony Brook, NY, by a clinician who specialized in the treatment of patients with tic disorders (J. Sverd) or to a child psychiatry outpatient service (Table 1). The diagnostic procedure included child and parent clinical interviews and a battery of psychometric instruments for assessing ADHD symptoms and tics. The study sample included 11 children who were described in preliminary reports.[37,39]

Prior to the children's enrollment in the study, parents were warned repeatedly of the possible risk of irreversible tic exacerbation as a result of stimulant treatment and were required to sign a written statement consenting to their child's participation. Once enrolled in the study, each child was monitored very closely. Parents had telephone access to clinicians (home and office) day and night for the duration of the drug evaluation, and the school was alerted to the possibility of tic exacerbation and the importance of immediate notification of changes in clinical status.

**Acceptance criteria.** Potential subjects had to meet *DSM-III-R*[40] diagnostic criteria for ADHD and either chronic motor tic disorder or Tourette disorder (established on the basis of a clinical interview with the parent) and, in general, be above the cutoff on two of three parent- and teacher-completed hyperactivity and/or ADHD behavior rating scales. The ADHD measures that were part of the diagnostic evaluation included the Abbreviated Teacher Rating Scale (ATRS)/Abbreviated Parent Rating Scale (APRS),[41] the Inattention-Overactivity With Aggression (IOWA) Conners Teacher's Ratings Scale,[42] The Conners (48-item) Parent Rating Scale,[43] the Mothers' Objective Method for Subgrouping (MOMS) checklist,[44] and the parent and teacher versions of the Stony Brook Child Psychiatric Checklist-3R.[45] All

TABLE 1
Patient Characteristics at Diagnosis*

| Characteristics | No. of Patients | Mean (SD) |
|---|---|---|
| Age | 34 | 8 y 10 mo (1 y 11 mo) |
| IQ | 28 | 105.9 (13.7) |
| Age at onset of tics | 23 | 5 y 7 mo (2 y 7 mo) |
| Race/ethnicity, No. (%) | 34 (100) | NA |
| White | 29 (85) | NA |
| Hispanic | 3 (9) | NA |
| Asian | 1 (3) | NA |
| Black | 1 (3) | NA |
| Research Diagnostic Criteria, No. (%) | 34 (100) | NA |
| Tourette syndrome, definite | 22 (65) | NA |
| Tourette syndrome by history | 11 (32) | NA |
| Chronic multiple motor tics | 1 (3) | NA |
| Hyperactivity/ADHD measures (cutoff score) | | |
| Parent ADHD measures | | |
| Stony Brook ADHD index (>7) | 32 | 9.9 (2.4) |
| Conners hyperactivity index (>15) | 33 | 18.1 (4.6) |
| MOMS hyperactivity subscale (>2) | 34 | 4.1 (1.2) |
| Teacher ADHD measures | | |
| Stony Brook ADHD index (>7) | 30 | 9.8 (3.6) |
| ATRS (>15) | 31 | 20.0 (6.0) |
| IOWA Conners I-O subscale (>6) | 33 | 11.4 (3.0) |
| Tic measures | | |
| Physician tic scale | | |
| YGTSS | 34 | |
| Total motor tic score | | 13.8 (3.3) |
| Total phonic tic score | | 10.6 (3.8) |
| Overall impairment rating | | 18.0 (12.5) |
| Global severity score | | 42.3 (17.0) |
| TS-CGI | 22 | 3.6 (0.7) |
| STSS | 22 | 2.9 (1.3) |
| Videotape tic counts | 33 | |
| Motor tics | | 18.9 (12.6) |
| Vocal tics | | 0.3 (0.7) |
| Commorbidities, aggression (cutoff score) | | |
| IOWA Conners aggression scale (>3) | 33 | 7.4 (4.9) |
| MOMS aggression subscale (>2) | 34 | 2.7 (1.9) |
| Special education, No. (%) | 34 (100) | NA |
| Full time (self contained) | 9 (26) | NA |
| Part time (resource room) | 14 (41) | NA |
| None | 11 (32) | NA |

TABLE 1 (*Continued*)

| Characteristics | No. of Patients | Mean (SD) |
|---|---|---|
| Family history tics/motor habits, No. (%) | 32 (100) | NA |
| A first-degree relative | 30 (94) | NA |
| Both biological parents | 16 (50) | NA |

\* ADHD indicates attention-deficit hyperactivity disorder; MOMS, Mothers' Objective Method for Subgrouping; ATRS, Abbreviated Teacher Rating Scale; IOWA, Inattention-Overactivity With Aggression; I-O, inattention-overacting; YGTSS, Yale Global Tic Severity Scale; TS-CGI, Tourette Syndrome–Clinical Global Impression Scale; STSS, Shapiro Tourette Syndrome Severity Scale; and NA, not applicable.

but two participating children were above the cutoff on at least two of three parent measures of hyperactivity and/or ADHD, and 26 were above the cutoff on at least two of three teacher measures.

The tic measures completed by one of us (J. Sverd) at the diagnostic evaluation included the Yale Global Tic Severity Scale,[46] the Tourette Syndrome-Clinical Global Impression Scale,[23(pp55–78)] the Shapiro Tourette Syndrome Severity Scale,[17] and the Tourette Syndrome Unified Rating Scale.[47] Each child also was videotaped during a 15-minute simulated classroom observation session during which the number of motor and vocal tics emitted was recorded. Briefly, our subjects' tic symptoms ranged from mild to severe (Table 1). All children met research diagnostic criteria[48,49] for either TS (definite or by history) or chronic multiple motor tic disorder (definite). The terms "definite" and "by history" were defined as follows: definite meant that motor and/or phonic tics must be witnessed by a reliable examiner directly at some point in the illness or be recorded by videotape or cinematography, and by history meant that tics were witnessed by a reliable family member or close friend and the description of tics as demonstrated are accepted by a reliable examiner. At least two reliable examiners in different settings witnessed motor tics in all of our subjects. A subsample of parents (n = 22) were asked to evaluate the current status of their children's motor and vocal tics, respectively: less severe than usual (10%, 20%), average severity (76%, 70%), or more severe than usual (14%, 10%).

**Comorbidities.** The Diagnostic Interview for Children and Adolescents-Revised[50,51] was administered to the mothers (parent version) and children (child version) (n = 21; 18 boys and three girls) and confirmed the diagnosis of ADHD in all cases. Most (81%) of the interviewed patients were comorbid for either oppositional defiant disorder (n = 15) or conduct disorder (n = 2). The number of children above the clinical cutoff on the aggression subscale of the IOWA Conners Teacher's Rating Scale and the MOMS aggression subscale was 23 and 20, respectively (Table 1). More than one third (n = 8) also met diagnostic criteria (best estimate diagnosis based on the child and parent Diagnostic Interview for Children and Adolescents-Revised and child self-report) for an anxiety disorder (overanxious disorder, separation anxiety disorder, or simple phobia) and/or depressive or dysthymic disorder. Three children met diagnostic criteria for obsessive-compulsive disorder.

**Medication history.** Children were not excluded from participation in the study if they had prior experience with stimulant drug therapy or if such therapy purportedly had exacerbated their tics. Thirteen of the children had a prior history of drug therapy for either ADHD (n = 8) or ADHD and TS (n = 5): 10 received stimulants; four, antipsychotic drugs; two, clonidine; and two, alprazolam. Seven children were receiving medication at the time of referral. In the case of stimulants (n = 5), the minimum washout period was 1 week. The washout period for the children who were receiving an antipsychotic drug (pimozide) or clonidine was 3 and 2 weeks, respectively. Of the 10 children who were treated previously with stimulants, undocumented tic exacerbation was reported by parents in four children, and tic onset after drug exposure was reported in two children.

**Rejection criteria.** Children who met one or more of the following criteria were excluded from consideration for the study: were believed to be too severely ill (dangerous to self or others); tics were the major clinical management concern; were psychotic or mentally retarded (IQ < 70); or had a seizure disorder, major organic brain dysfunction, major medical illness, medical or other contraindication to medication (other than tics), or pervasive developmental disorder.

## *Medication*

Subjects received placebo and three dosages of methylphenidate hydrochloride (0.1 mg/kg [mean ± SD, 4.4 ± 1.5 mg], 0.3 mg/kg [mean, 9.0 ± 3.3 mg], and 0.5 mg/kg [mean ± SD, 14.0 ± 3.9 mg]) for 2 weeks each. For ease of administration, individual doses in milligrams were rounded off to the nearest 2.5 mg (0.1-mg/kg dosage) or 5 mg (0.3- and 0.5-mg/kg dosages). The upper limit for the 0.5-mg/kg dosage was 20 mg. Dose schedules were counterbalanced and assigned on a random basis. When the 0.5-mg/kg dosage was not preceded by a low-dose condition, the child was gradually built up to the moderate dose. Medication was administered twice daily, approximately 3 5 hours apart, 7 days a week. In most cases, the morning dose was given by parents before the child left for school, and the noon dose was administered by the school nurse. Medication and identically matching placebos were dispensed to the parents and school nurses in dated, sealed envelopes at 2-week intervals. Parents and nurses were asked to return unused medication envelopes, which allowed us to assess compliance. Medication was administered under double-blind conditions (i.e., no one involved in the clinical management of the patient, data collection, or interaction with the school knew the identity of the treatment conditions). Given the possibility of a medical emergency, one investigator (K.D.G.) had access to the dosage code.

## Procedure

Once the medication evaluation began, each child with ADHD and at least one parent (typically the mother, who was designated as the respondent for all of the clinical assessments) were required to come to the clinic at 2-week intervals for clinical evaluation and to receive the next 2-week allotment of medication. During the clinical evaluation, the parent was interviewed by the clinician (J. Sverd), and the child's clinical status was determined. The parent was asked to complete separate rating scales for the child's ADHD and tic symptoms. The clinician also briefly interviewed the child, observed tics, and assessed weight, heart rate, and blood pressure.

Following the physician's evaluation, children were required to complete work activities in a simulated classroom, during which time they were videotaped for 15 minutes through a one-way window. Clinic observations were conducted approximately 1.25 hours after drug ingestion.

A subsample of children (n = 28) completed a computerized version of the Continuous Performance Task (CPT) approximately 1.75 hours after drug ingestion. The CPT was first administered as part of the diagnostic evaluation. Prior to testing, the examiner demonstrated the task, gave the child a practice trial, and reminded him or her what the target was. The examiner remained in the room during testing, sat approximately 1.2 m behind the child, and engaged in a task while the child completed the CPT.

In addition to the rating scales that the parent completed as part of the clinic interview, parents were asked to provide behavioral, side effect, and tic ratings for each weekend. The parent completed one set of ratings for their child's behavior during the morning and early afternoon on Saturday and Sunday.

Teachers completed behavioral, side effect, and tic ratings for each subject's behavior 2 days per week for the duration of the drug evaluation.

## Measures

**Physician evaluations.** The tic measures (completed by J. Sverd) included the Yale Global Tic Severity Scale and the Tourette Syndrome Unified Rating Scale, which were completed for the entire sample, and the Global Tic Rating Scale (GTRS),[52,53] the Tourette Syndrome-Clinical Global Impression Scale, and the Shapiro Tourette Syndrome Severity Scale, which were added to the assessment battery for the last 22 subjects. Four subscales from the Yale Global Tic Severity Scale were used the total motor tic score, the total phonic tic score, the overall impairment rating, and the global severity score. Three tic scales from the Tourette Syndrome Unified Rating Scale were administered: the Shapiro Symptom Checklist (total number of tics), the tic count (number of tics observed in 2 minutes during quiet conversation with the patient), and the LeWitt Disability Scale. The latter is a global symptom severity-impairment scale that assesses tics and tic-related features (eg, compulsive actions, obsessive thoughts, ritualistic behaviors, anxiety spells, disruptive behavior disorders, and attention deficits).

Obsessive-compulsive symptoms were evaluated using two scales from the Tourette Syndrome Unified Rating Scale. Parents were first asked five screening questions about the presence of obsessions and compulsions using the Obsessive-compulsive Disorder Screen, and then they evaluated the severity of these symptoms with the Clinical Global Impression Scale–Obsessive-compulsive Disorder.[23(pp55–78)] Because neither of these scales pertain to specific symptoms, they must be considered global assessment instruments.

### Simulated classroom.

The playroom procedure developed by Routh and Schroeder[54] and modified by Roberts et al[55] and Milich and colleagues[56] was used to assess the effect of medication on tics. In this study, we used only the 15-minute restricted academic period. In the restricted academic setting, the child is instructed to complete worksheets and not to play with toys on an adjacent table. Worksheet items are similar to those on the coding subtest of the Wechsler Intelligence Scale for Children-Revised. Clinic sessions were videotaped to facilitate ease of scoring. For this study, videotapes were coded for the presence of motor and vocal tics. However, the latter were so infrequent that they precluded meaningful data analysis. The 15-minute observation sessions were divided into 180 five-second intervals, and tics were coded as either present or not present in each interval. Prior to coding the medication conditions, two experienced raters (J Sprafkin and S N.E.)

reviewed a list of the child's known tics and coded the baseline (diagnostic) session. The two coders plus a third judge (K.D.G.) then met and reached a consensus on the identity of each tic (tic inventory). If interrater reliability for the baseline session was below criterion ($\kappa < 0.60$), the baseline tape was recoded until the minimum reliability criterion was met. The four drug trials were then evaluated by the primary coder, and two randomly selected trials were scored by the secondary coder to assess reliability. Although the coders used the tic inventory as a guide, any new tics that emerged during the drug evaluation were also coded. The overall $\kappa$ for the drug trials was 0.70 (range, 0.41 to 0.77).

**Continuous performance task.** The CPT used in this study was a computerized version developed by Halperin et al,[57] in which the child is instructed to press the space bar whenever the letter $A$ follows the letter $X$ on the screen. The CPT generates three measures (inattention, impulsivity, and dyscontrol) that are uncorrelated with each other and IQ. This version of the CPT has been shown to have good test-retest reliability, to correlate with teacher ratings of inattention, to be sensitive to stimulant drug effects, and to distinguish children with ADHD from controls.[58,59]

**Parent and teacher ratings.** The Conners[41] ATRS contains 10 items rated on a four-point scale (0 indicates not at all; 3, very much) that are summed to generate a total score. A factor analysis of the ATRS revealed two factors[60]: factor 1 refers to behaviors generally considered to be symptoms of hyperactivity, and factor 2 assesses emotional lability. The addition of five items to the ATRS permitted the determination of the inattention-overactivity and aggression subscale scores of the IOWA Conners Teacher's Rating Scale.[42] The IOWA Conners Teacher's Rating Scale has been shown to differentiate between the behavioral dimensions of hyperactivity and aggression and demonstrates adequate reliability and sensitivity to stimulant drug effects.[42,61-65] The ATRS was completed by the teacher 2 days per week for the child's behavior during school for each week of the dose-response evaluation.

Parents used the Conners APRS[41] to evaluate their child's behavior during morning and early afternoon on Saturday and Sunday. During their biweekly clinic evaluations, they also completed the MOMS for their child's behavior during the previous week. The MOMS contains 10 (hyperactivity and/or ADHD) symptoms arranged in a checklist format. The mother simply checks whether or not each item characterizes her child (1 indicates checked; 0, unchecked). The MOMS generates a hyperactivity scale score and an aggression scale score, both of which demonstrate convergent and divergent validity.[44]

The Peer Conflict Scale[65-67] was used by parents and teachers to assess aggressive interactions with other children. The Peer Conflict Scale shows adequate test-retest reliability and convergent validity with direct observations of negativistic behaviors.[65]

Parents and teachers recorded their perceptions of changes in tic status on the GTRS according to the same schedule as the behavior rating scales. Both parents and teachers were made aware of the behaviors and vocalizations that were considered tics during the diagnostic phase of the patient evaluation. Our own research shows the GTRS to be reliable.[53]

Parents and teachers evaluated adverse drug reactions using the Stimulant Side Effects Checklist (SSEC).[66,68] The SSEC contains 13 side effect items rated on a four-point scale (0 indicates not at all; 3, very much). Individual items are grouped to form three indexes of drug effects: the mood index, the attention-arousal index, and the somatic complaints index. One item pertains to abnormal movements.

### Statistical Analyses

The teacher- and parent-completed rating scale scores were first analyzed using a two-way (bahavior by scale) repeated measures analysis of variance (ANOVA). Measures were grouped according to respondent (parent or teacher) and domain (ADHD behaviors or side effects). Both type of scale and dosage (placebo, 0.1 mg/kg, 0.3 mg/kg, or 0.5 mg/kg) were within-subjects factors. The data sets for a few children were incomplete because care providers did not complete the ratings. (Unless noted otherwise, all reported significant main effects are also significant using the Greenhouse-Geisser correction.) Tests for trend were also conducted to provide information about the form of the relation between doses of methylphenidate and the dependent variable. To localize the source of statistically significant dose effects, post hoc Newman-Keuls tests were performed to assess differences between doses in the rate of occurrence of specific behaviors.

**Tics.** The tic data were first analyzed using two-way (tic measure by dose) repeated measures ANOVAs; separate analyses were conducted for each respondent (observer, parent, or teacher). Given our concern about the possibility of making a type II error (i.e., erroneously concluding that methylphenidate did not have an adverse effect on tics), follow-up repeated measures ANOVAs were performed on each respondent category even when the main effect of dose was not significant.

A power analysis (using published estimates of $r = .5$ to $.8$ for the 3-week stability [autocorrelation] of direct observations and ratings of tic frequency and severity)[69] indicated that a sample of 34 subjects provided 80% power to detect treatment effects of 0.33 SDs or larger assuming the stability equals 8. If the stability is as low as .5, an effect of at least 0.50 SDs could be detected with 80% power.

**Multivariate analyses of variance.** Separate two-way multivariate ANOVAs were conducted for the behavior rating scales for each of the three sets of raters (teachers, parents, and physician). Unless indicated otherwise, univariate ANOVAs were conducted only when the results of these analyses indicated that there was a significant main effect of dose ($P < .01$, using the Wilks' λ criterion).

# RESULTS

## ADHD Symptoms

**Teacher ratings.** Analyses of the teacher behavior rating scale data revealed a significant main effect of behavior ($F[5,140] = 54.76, P < .0001$) and dose ($F[3,90] = 34.74, P < .0001$). The behavior-by-dose interaction was also significant ($F[15,450] = 20.57, P < .0001$). Follow-up repeated measures ANOVAs were performed on each of the teacher rating scales (Table 2). Dose effects were significant for all of the teacher rating scales of hyperactivity, oppositionality, and aggressivity. Symptom severity decreased with each increment in dose, with the corresponding tests for linear trend being significant for each scale. For the inattention-overactivity subscale, the cubic trend was also significant ($F[1,30] = 4.87, P = .04$). In general, there was a dramatic diminution of symptom severity with the 0.1-mg/kg dosage, little change in ratings of symptom severity (plateau) with the 0.3-mg/kg dosage, and continued but more modest additional improvement with the 0.5-mg/kg dosage. Post hoc analyses revealed that, with the exception of factor 2 of the ATRS, there were statistically significant differences between placebo and all three drug dosages and between dosages of 0.1 mg/kg and 0.5 mg/kg (Table 3) but no significant differences between dosages of 0.1 mg/kg and 0.3 mg/kg. It is noteworthy that comparisons between placebo and the 0.1-mg/kg dosage indicate a diminution in symptom severity of at least 30% on most measures of ADHD symptoms.

TABLE 2

Untransformed Means (SDs), Analyses of Variance, and Tests for Trend for Behavior Rating Scales and CPT and for Dosage of Methylphenidate*

| | Placebo | Methylphenidate Hydrochloride | | | F Ratio | P | Trend Tests |
|---|---|---|---|---|---|---|---|
| | | 0.1 mg/kg | 0.3 mg/kg | 0.5 mg/kg | | | |
| **Teacher ratings** | | | | | | | |
| ATRS | | | | | | | |
|   Factor 1 | 14.2 (4.6) | 10.0 (7.0) | 9.3 (6.4) | 7.1 (5.4) | 18.91 | .0001 | L |
|   Factor 2 | 11.4 (3.8) | 7.9 (5.3) | 7.1 (4.5) | 5.7 (4.1) | 20.59 | .0001 | L |
| | 2.9 (2.1) | 2.2 (2.4) | 2.2 (2.6) | 1.4 (1.8) | 5.94 | .001 | L |
| IOWA Conners | | | | | | | |
|   I-O scale | 8.7 (3.1) | 6.2 (3.9) | 5.8 (3.7) | 4.6 (3.3) | 18.7 | .0001 | L, C |
|   Aggression scale | 4.3 (3.7) | 2.6 (3.4) | 2.3 (3.5) | 1.4 (2.0) | 13.49 | .0001 | L |
|   Peer Conflict Scale | 5.2 (4.9) | 3.6 (5.3) | 2.7 (5.0) | 1.7 (2.5) | 8.94 | .0001 | L |
| **Parent Ratings** | | | | | | | |
| APRS | 11.8 (7.3) | 8.6 (5.0) | 10.2 (5.4) | 7.8 (4.6) | 4.45 | .006 | L, C |
| MOMS | | | | | | | |
|   Hyperactivity scale | 2.8 (1.6) | 2.7 (1.6) | 2.6 (1.3) | 2.0 (1.5) | 4.17 | .008 | L |
|   Aggression scale | 2.4 (2.0) | 1.9 (1.7) | 1.9 (1.7) | 1.5 (1.7) | 3.90 | .002 | L |
|   Peer Conflict Scale | 5.6 (4.9) | 4.3 (4.5) | 4.5 (4.1) | 3.0 (3.3) | 3.50 | .02 | L |
| **CPT** | | | | | | | |
|   Inattention | 7.5 (5.7) | 6.0 (5.2) | 5.6 (6.0) | 5.2 (6.1) | 2.80 | .045 | L |
|   Impulsivity | 2.1 (3.1) | 2.8 (4.5) | 1.2 (1.6) | 1.8 (4.8) | 1.83 | .15 | NA |
|   Dyscontrol | 7.0 (9.4) | 4.2 (5.9) | 2.5 (2.8) | 2.2 (5.4) | 5.89 | .001 | L, Q |

* CPT indicates Continuous Performance Task; ATRS, Abbreviated Teacher Rating Scale; IOWA, Inattention-Overactivity With Aggression; I-O, inattention-overactivity; APRS, Abbreviated parent Rating Scale; L, significant linear trend; C, significant cubic trend; NA, not applicable; and Q, significant quadratic trend.

TABLE 3
Mean Group Differences Between Treatment Conditions for Observations,
Rating Scales, and CPT*

| Behavior Category | Placebo vs 0.1 mg/kg | Placebo vs 0.3 mg/kg | Placebo vs 0.5 mg/kg | 0.1 mg/kg vs 0.5 mg/kg |
|---|---|---|---|---|
| Teacher rating scales | | | | |
| ATRS | 4.18† | 4.94† | 7.14† | 2.96‡ |
| Factor 1 | 3.48† | 4.31† | 5.73† | 2.25‡ |
| Factor 2 | 0.64 | 0.67 | 1.43‡ | 0.79 |
| IOWA Conners I-O subscale | 2.59‡ | 2.93‡ | 4.19† | 1.60‡ |
| IOWA Conners aggression subscale | 1.71‡ | 2.05† | 2.92† | 1.21‡ |
| Peer Conflict Scale | 1.58‡ | 2.49† | 3.51† | 1.93‡ |
| Parent rating scales | | | | |
| APRS | 3.16‡ | 1.62 | 4.01† | 0.85 |
| MOMS hyperactivity subscale | 0.11 | 0.23 | 0.84‡ | 0.73‡ |
| MOMS aggression subscale | 0.47 | 0.53 | 0.93‡ | 0.46 |
| Peer Conflict Scale | 1.27 | 1.08 | 2.58† | 1.31 |
| CPT | | | | |
| Inattention | 1.56 | 1.93 | 2.35‡ | 0.79 |
| Dyscontrol | 2.79 | 4.49† | 4.76† | 1.97 |
| Physician tic ratings observations | | | | |
| Shapiro Symptom Checklist, vocal tics | 1.07‡ | 0.14 | 0.55 | 0.52 |
| 2-Minute tic count, motor tics | 1.99 | 3.63 | 5.70‡ | 3.71 |
| Teacher GTRS tic ratings | | | | |
| Frequency of motor tic index | 0.31 | 0.59 | 0.90‡ | 0.59 |
| Frequency of vocal tics index | 0.54† | 0.54† | 0.56† | 0.02 |
| Tic severity index | 0.25 | 0.52 | 0.76‡ | 0.51 |

* Dosages are for methylphenidate hydrochloride. CPT indicates Continuous Performance Task; ATRS, Abbreviated Teacher Rating Scale; IOWA, Inattention-Overactivity With Aggression; I-O, inattention-overactivity; APRS, Abbreviated Parent Rating Scale; MOMs, Mothers' Objective Method for Subgrouping; and GTRS, Global Tic Rating Scale.
  † $P < .01$ using Newman-Keuls test.
  ‡ $P < .05$ using Newman-Keuls test.

**Parent ratings.** Analyses of these data revealed a significant main effect of dose (F[3,72] = 4.66, $P$ = .005). Follow-up repeated measures ANOVAs were performed, and dose effects were significant for all scales (Table 2). Post hoc analyses revealed significant differences between the 0.5-mg/kg dosage and placebo for all scales (Table 3). Even the placebo and the 0.1-mg/kg dosage comparison was significant for the APRS. Trend analyses indicated a significant linear function for the hyperactivity (F[1,29] = 7.15, $P$ = .012) and aggression (F[1,29] = 21.17, $P$ < .0001) subscales of the MOMS, the Peer Conflict Scale (F[1,27] = 4.59, $P$ = .04), and the APRS (F[1,31] = 6.90, $P$ = .01). The cubic function was also significant for the APRS (F[1,31] = 5.84, $P$ = .02) and was marginally significant for the Peer Conflict Scale (F[1,27] = 3.73, $P$ = .06).

**Continuous performance task.** Repeated measures ANOVAs were conducted for each of the three CPT scores (n = 28) and the four treatment conditions (Table 2). There were significant dose effects for both the inattention and the dyscontrol measures. Tests for trend indicated significant linear functions: inattention (F[1,27] = 7.54, $P$ = .01) and dyscontrol (F[1,27] = 8.59, $P$ = .007). Performance improved with increasing dose. The quadratic function was also significant for the dyscontrol measure (F[1,27] = 5.16, $P$ = .03). Post hoc comparisons between placebo and the 0.5-mg/kg dosage were significant for both measures, as was the comparison between placebo and the 0.3-mg/kg dosage for the dyscontrol score (Table 3).

**Severity of tic symptoms and behavioral drug response.** To examine the possibility that the response to medication may have been affected by the severity, frequency, or number of tics (as determined at diagnosis), subjects were separated into two groups on the basis of median splits for each tic variable: severity (Yale Global Tic Severity Score), frequency (number of tics observed during the 15-minute videotaping session in the clinic), and the total number of different tics (Shapiro Symptom Checklist from the Unified Tourette Syndrome Rating Scale). Separate three-way repeated measures ANOVAs with two within-subject factors (behavior and dose) and one between-subjects factor (group) were conducted for the behavior ratings scales for each of the three sets of raters (teachers, parents, and physician). The results of these analyses did not reveal a single statistically significant dose-by-group interaction.

*Frequency and Severity of Tics*

**Physician evaluations.** A 9×4 (scale-by-dose) repeated measures ANOVA conducted on the tic scale scores revealed a significant main effect of scale

(F[8,224] = 302.97, $P$ < .0001), a marginally significant main effect of dose (F[3,84] = 2.69, $P$ = .06), and a significant scale-by-dose interaction (F[24,672] = 1.85, $P$ = .009). (A multivariate ANOVA of the physician measures was not significant.) The means, SDs, and repeated measures ANOVAs for each tic scale are presented in Table 4. (With the exception of the LeWitt Disability Scale, increasing mean values indicate a worsening in tic status.) There was little evidence that methylphenidate exacerbated tics. This was also the case using the three physician scales (the Shapiro Tourette Syndrome Severity Scale, the Tourette Syndrome—Clinical Global Impression Scale, and the GTRS) that were added to the assessment battery. The only indication of tic worsening was the physician's 2-minute motor tic count. A linear trend provided a good fit to the data (F[1,32] = 5.98, $P$ < .02). The frequency of motor tics was significantly higher when the children received the 0.5-mg/kg dosage than when they received placebo (Table 3). The number of different vocal tics (Shapiro Symptom Checklist) exhibited during the previous week as reported by the parent to the physician was also dose-dependent, with the rate when the children received the 0.1-mg/kg dosage being significantly lower that that when they received placebo or the 0.3-mg/kg dosage. There was no main effect of dose or scale-by-dose interaction when the latter two scales were excluded from the analyses.

Exploratory analyses that were conducted on the component scales of the Yale Global Tic Severity Scale revealed a marginally significant phonic tics score (F[3,90] = 2.70, $P$ = .05), with lower levels of vocal tics when the children received medication: placebo (mean score, 1.68), 0.1-mg/kg dosage (mean score, 1.25), 0.3-mg/kg dosage (mean score, 1.58), and 0.5-mg/kg dosage (mean score, 1.64).

The physician's global assessment of obsessive-compulsive symptoms (Clinical Global Impression Scale–Obsessive-compulsive Disorder) also did not show drug effects (F[3,84] = 0.86, $P$ = .46).

**Simulated classroom.** Although the frequency of motor tics was slightly higher in each of the three dose conditions compared with the placebo condition (Table 4), there was no significant effect of dose.

**Teacher ratings.** Analyses of teacher ratings of tic frequency and severity on the GTRS indicated a main effect of dose (F[3,87] = 4.52, $P$ = .006). Follow-up ANOVAs indicated a significant dose effect for the frequency of vocal tic index (Table 4). Vocal tics were rated as less frequent for the three medication conditions compared with the placebo condition (Table 3), and a linear function provided a good fit to the data (F[1,29] = 8.20, $P$ = .008). Post hoc comparisons between placebo and all three doses of methylphenidate were significant.

## TABLE 4
### Means (SDs) and Analyses of Variance for Observation and Ratings of Motor and Vocal Tics*

| Measure | Placebo | Methylphenidate Hydrochloride | | | F Ratio | P | Trend Tests |
| --- | --- | --- | --- | --- | --- | --- | --- |
| | | 0.1 mg/kg | 0.3 mg/kg | 0.5 mg/kg | | | |
| Physician ratings | | | | | | | |
| YGTSS | | | | | | | |
| Total motor tics | 11.6 (4.0) | 12.3 (3.8) | 11.9 (4.5) | 12.0 (4.2) | .057 | .64 | NA |
| Total phonic tics | 7.9 (4.7) | 6.7 (5.8) | 7.5 (3.9) | 8.6 (6.7) | 2.04 | .11 | NA |
| Overall impairment rating | 9.1 (9.5) | 10.3 (8.8) | 12.4 (10.9) | 10.3 (10.6) | 0.86 | .46 | NA |
| Global severity score | 28.3 (15.9) | 29.3 (15.6) | 31.9 (17.4) | 29.1 (16.5) | 0.43 | .73 | NA |
| Tourette Syndrome Unified Rating Scale | | | | | | | |
| Shapiro Symptom Checklist | | | | | | | |
| No. of motor tics | 11.6 (6.5) | 11.5 (5.3) | 11.6 (5.7) | 11.7 (6.2) | 0.02 | .997 | NA |
| No. of vocal tics | 3.2 (2.7) | 2.1 (2.8) | 3.3 (3.4) | 2.6 (3.3) | 3.22 | .03 | NS |
| Motor tic count | 9.4 (7.1) | 11.3 (10.4) | 13.0 (12.0) | 15.0 (14.8) | 2.96 | .04 | L |
| Vocal tic count | 0.4 (0.8) | 0.5 (1.6) | 0.7 (2.0) | 0.60 (0.9) | 0.60 | .60 | NA |
| LeWitt Disability Scale | 67.6 (11.5) | 69.4 (9.7) | 70.6 (11.4) | 72.4 (9.7) | 2.19 | .09 | NA |
| STSSS | 1.7 (0.9) | 1.9 (0.9) | 1.9 (1.2) | 1.9 (1.2) | 0.48 | .69 | NA |
| Teacher ratings, GTRS | | | | | | | |
| Motor tic index | 2.8 (2.6) | 2.5 (2.6) | 2.2 (2.1) | 1.9 (2.0) | 2.68 | .05 | L, C |
| Vocal tic index | 1.3 (1.2) | 0.7 (0.8) | 0.7 (1.0) | 0.7 (1.0) | 5.66 | .001 | L |
| Tic severity index | 2.0 (2.0) | 1.8 (2.2) | 1.5 (2.0) | 1.3 (1.7) | 2.68 | .05 | L |
| Parent ratings, GTRS | | | | | | | |
| Motor tic index | 2.4 (1.7) | 2.5 (1.8) | 2.4 (1.7) | 3.3 (2.5) | 2.24 | .09 | NA |
| Vocal tic index | 1.2 (1.1) | 1.1 (1.1) | 1.1 (1.3) | 1.2 (1.1) | 0.19 | .90 | NA |
| Tic severity index | 1.6 (1.7) | 1.9 (2.0) | 1.9 (2.5) | 2.2 (2.6) | 0.70 | .55 | NA |
| Clinic observations | | | | | | | |
| Motor tic frequency | 18.1 (13.3) | 22.2 (17.8) | 20.7 (18.0) | 21.3 (18.0) | 0.69 | .56 | NA |

* YGTSS indicates Yale Global Tic Severity Score; STSSS, Shapiro Tourette Syndrome Severity Score; GTRS, Global Tic Rating Scale; NA, not applicable; NS, no significant trend; L, significant linear trend; and C, significant cubic trend.

There were marginally significant dose effects for the frequency of motor tics index and the tic severity, index (Table 4). Ratings of motor tic frequency and tic severity improved with methylphenidate treatment. Post hoc comparisons between placebo and the 0.5-mg/kg dosage were significant for both indexes (Table 3). Linear trend functions were significant for both indexes, but the cubic function was also significant for the frequency of motor tics index (F[1,29] = 5.40, $P$ = .03).

**Parent ratings.** Analyses of the parent ratings of tic frequency and severity as measured on the GTRS did not reveal a main effect of dose (Table 4). Descriptively, mean ratings of motor tic frequency ($P$ = .09) and tic severity were higher for the 0.5-mg/kg dosage compared with the other treatment conditions.

In an effort to examine the possibility that tic exacerbation may be manifest as a rebound effect, a subsample of parents (n = 21) also were asked during their children's biweekly clinic evaluation to compare their children's tics during the evening (on the weekend) with tic status during the day (1 indicates more severe; 2, about the same; and 3, less severe). The mean ratings for all four treatment conditions were virtually identical for both motor (F[3,60] = 0.41, $P$ = .75) and vocal (F[3,60] = 1.76, $P$ = .17) tics. Descriptively, for the placebo condition, six children were rated as having motor tics that are more severe in the evening, and two, as having less severe tics in the evening. With the 0.5-mg/kg dosage, six children were rated as having more severe tics in the evening, but of these, only one was not so rated when receiving placebo.

**Severity of tic symptoms and drug response.** To examine the possibility that response to medication may have been affected by the severity, frequency, or number of tics (as determined at diagnosis), subjects were separated into two groups on the basis of median splits for each tic variable on the aforementioned tic measures. Separate three-way repeated measures ANOVAs with two within-subject factors (behavior and dose) and one between-subjects factor (diagnostic tic status) were conducted for the behavior rating scales for each of the three sets of raters (teachers, parents, and physician). The results of these analyses did not reveal a single statistically significant ($P$ < .05) interaction between dose and diagnostic tic status.

## Adverse Drug Reactions

**Teacher ratings.** There was a statistically significant effect of dose (F[3,90] = 3.56, $P$ = .02), behavior (F[2,60] = 8.00, $P$ < .001), and behavior-by-dose interaction (F[6,180] = 2.94, $P$ = .009) for the teacher-completed SSEC ratings. In general, SSEC ratings were more favorable for methylphenidate conditions than for the placebo condition, but only the ANOVA for the mood index was significant (F[3,93] = 6.01, $P$ < .001). Post hoc comparisons indicated that 0.5 mg/kg ratings were significantly ($P$ < .01) lower than placebo and 0.1 mg/kg ratings, and a linear function provided a good fit to the data (F[1,30] = 9.92, $P$ = .004).

**Parent ratings.** The analysis of the main effect of dose for the parent-completed SSEC ratings was not significant, but the main effect of behavior (F[3,87] = 12.56, $P$ < .0001) and the behavior-by-dose interaction (F[9,261] = 2.28, $P$ = .02) were. Similar to the teacher ratings, the mean parent SSEC ratings were generally lower for the drug conditions compared with the placebo condition, but only the ANOVA for the somatic complaints index was significant (F[3,87] = 4.88, $P$ = .004). Somatic complaints were significantly ($P$ < .01) more severe with the 0.5-mg/kg dosage compared with placebo. A linear function provided a good fit to the data (F[1,29] = 10–66, $P$ = .003).

**Physician evaluations.** Repeated measures ANOVAs were conducted for heart rate, blood pressure, and weight measurements for the four treatment conditions. Dose effects were evident only for heart rate (F[4,84] = 3.68, $P$ = .008). The rate for the 0.5-mg/kg dosage (mean ± SD, 93.5 ± 13.9) was significantly ($P$ < .05) higher than that for placebo (mean ± SD, 85.5 ± 10.0).

## COMMENT

All of the children in the study showed dramatic clinical improvement consequent to methylphenidate treatment, there were no nonresponders. Administration of methylphenidate was highly effective in the amelioration of inattentive, disruptive, and aggressive behaviors in children with ADHD and comorbid tic disorder as assessed by teacher- and parent-completed behavior rating scales and a computer-presented CPT evaluation in the clinic. These findings are consistent with the results of numerous studies of hyperactive children and/or children with ADHD.[70,71] It is noteworthy that treatment with the 0.1-mg/kg dosage resulted in significant improvement in teacher ratings of symptom severity. Credit for documenting the efficacy of relatively low dosages of methylphenidate (0.1 mg/kg) in short-term clinical trials goes to Werry and Sprague,[72] who showed that treatment effects even could be measured with teacher-completed behavior rating scales. Others also have reported significant treatment effects for the

0.1-mg/kg dosage on activity level.[73] Trend analyses of most dependent measures indicated dose effects to be linear, which lends additional support to previous investigations.[74,75] However, the magnitude of clinical improvement associated with the 0.3-mg/kg dosage compared with the 0.5-mg/kg dosage was generally trivial for many children. The 0.5-mg/kg dosage was associated with more side effects, but fortunately they were generally of limited clinical significance.

Even more gratifying than the finding that methylphenidate was effective for the management of ADHD behaviors in this clinical population is the compelling evidence that supports its relatively benign impact on the severity of tics. During the course of this short-term drug evaluation, physician, teacher, and parent ratings were in uniform agreement that methylphenidate did not lead to a worsening in the severity of the children's tic disorder. In fact, teacher ratings actually suggest improvement in the severity (and frequency) of motor and vocal tics when children were receiving methylphenidate compared with placebo. Although it may be tempting simply to dismiss this finding as a positive halo effect, at this juncture, such an interpretation is definitely premature.

The data pertaining to methylphenidate's effect on the frequency of motor tics are mixed. Detailed examination of videotapes of children performing an academic task for 15 minutes in a simulated classroom did not reveal any drug-related changes in tic frequency, which is consistent with caregiver ratings. However, the findings from the physician's 2-minute tic count of motor tics did indicate a statistically significant tic exacerbation with the 0.5-mg/kg dosage, which is consistent with our report on the initial sample of subjects.[39] Given the number of tic measures and the negative findings from the simulated classroom observations, this could be a spurious finding. However, it is also possible that stimulant medication interacts with specific somatic (eg, level of arousal) and environmental variables to produce tic exacerbations in certain situations, a hypothesis that warrants further study. For example, the children were present in the room as the physician interviewed the parent about changes in tic status, and occasionally, some even performed mock tics in response to specific questions when the physician was interviewing the parent. Most children were aware that the physician was observing them for tics during the tic-count procedure. Curiously, direct observations of these same children in public school settings did reveal a statistically significant increase in the frequency of occurrence of motor tics in the classroom with the 0.1-mg/kg dosage, but the magnitude of tic exacerbation was relatively small.[76] Furthermore, tic worsening was not observed in the lunchroom or on the playground and, according to teacher and parent reports, was evidently beyond the detection of care providers.

It is extremely difficult to determine whether changes in the observed frequency of tics in the physician's office or the simulated classroom represent true drug-induced tic exacerbation in specific individuals or simply natural fluctuations in tic frequency over time. (Unfortunately, the mean duration of cycles of waxing and waning is not known.) The fact that the frequency of motor tics emitted during the simulated classroom sessions conducted at diagnosis and when the children were receiving placebo differed by at least 0.5 SD (diagnostic) in 61% of the children does not bode well for the former interpretation. In other words, given the moderately high reliability of this type of assessment,[77] this finding indicates a great deal of instability over time (several weeks) and provides strong support for the natural waxing and waning in the frequency of tic symptoms during the course of a short-term drug study.

The tendency for methylphenidate to have a beneficial effect on vocal tics is inconsistent with our findings for motor tics. It is possible that parents inadvertently considered impulsive ADHD vocalizations when they reported vocal tics to the physician. Research on stimulant drugs and vocal behavior is contradictory, indicating both increased[78] and decreased[79–81] verbal productivity. However, as with other drug-induced changes in the behavior of hyperactive children and/or children with ADHD, these seemingly discrepant findings probably can be explained in terms of differences in task demands and setting characteristics. Although direct observations of the frequency of tic occurrence in the school setting also support a modest treatment-related suppression of vocal tics,[76] at this point, it is premature to draw any firm conclusions about the effect of methylphenidate on vocal tics.

The possibility that methylphenidate treatment may be associated with changes in the frequency but not the perceived severity of motor tics (at least in terms of behavior exhibited in the physician's office) has important assessment implications. In the clinical setting, it may be prudent to overlook insignificant changes in tic frequency, especially when alternative interventions carry a greater risk of behavioral or somatic toxic effects. Alternatively, the failure of clinician-completed tic rating scales to detect changes in the frequency of tic occurrence could obfuscate attempts to determine the cause of tic disorders, as in the case of a differential response to drugs.[33]

The generalizability of the findings from this study are subject to several qualifications. First, our data pertain to observed treatment effects over an 8-week period and therefore cannot address the issue of tic exacerbation as a function of long-term drug exposure. Although we have not had to terminate methylphenidate treatment for any of the children in this study for this reason, until the follow-up study in progress is completed, we are unable to comment with certainty about the potential risks of maintenance therapy. Second, our study was not designed specifically to address the issue of stimulant-induced tic exacerbation in individual children but rather to examine critically the notion that these drugs are contraindicated for the study population as a whole. To address adequately the individual drug reactions, we believe that specific treatment conditions should be repeated during the course of the evaluation.[82] Third, our findings pertain only to children with ADHD and with tics that are of mild to moderate severity and that occur frequently enough to be observed during 15-minute intervals. We specifically avoided children whose tics could only change in one direction on our dependent measures (i.e., very mild cases could only get worse; severe cases could only get better). Fourth, although this study was not designed to address the possible exacerbation of comorbid anxiety and mood disorders, neither the global obsessive-compulsive disorder measure nor the LeWitt Disability scale showed a worsening of symptoms. The teacher-completed SSEC mood index actually indicated improvement in affect with methylphenidate administration, which is consistent with the findings of studies using caregiver and child self-report measures.[83] Finally, the use of a crossover design may have resulted in contamination of the placebo condition by prior exposure to medication (protracted carry-over effects). However, comparison of the frequency of tic occurrence (simulated classroom) between baseline and placebo conditions for children who received placebo first (n = 8) and last (n = 9) indicated a small decrease in tics for both groups. This finding, combined with the absence of statistically significant rebound effects (daytime vs evening parent ratings) or tolerance (2 vs 6 weeks of drug exposure),[76] strongly suggests that this is not an issue.

Our findings also touch on theories pertaining to the neuropathologic causes of tic disorders. For example, dopamine receptor sensitivity modification theory[33] suggests that on initial exposure to methylphenidate, hyperdopaminergic receptors may be stimulated further to produce tic exacerbation in some patients. On continued exposure to this dopamine agonist, a reduction in dopamine sensitivity results. This, in turn, leads to the amelioration of tic symptoms. If this is true, tic exacerbation should occur at a higher rate during the early part of the dose evaluation than during the latter part. Our data indicate that this is not the case.[76] Another theory suggests that tic disorder and ADHD are both a result of a genetic deficit that causes an imbalance in mesencephalic-mesolimbic dopamine pathways, which leads to hypofunction of mesocortical dopamine pathways and disinhibition and hypersensitivity of subcortical dopamine pathways.[29] This theory predicts that psychostimulant treatment should ameliorate hyperactivity without adversely affecting tic status,[24] and our findings with regard to the severity of tic symptoms are consistent with this theory. Additional considerations that might explain the absence of tic exacerbation consequent to exposure to clinical doses of methylphenidate are the following: first, differential effects of dopamine on striatal outputs may be involved in differential clinical effects of exogenously administered drugs,[84] and second, evidence exists for a complex interaction of a number of neurotransmitter systems in the pathogenesis of hyperkinetic movement disorder and TS.[24,28,84-87]

In summary, the findings from this investigation indicate that methylphenidate is an effective treatment for ADHD and negativistic behaviors in children with ADHD and tic disorder. In spite of an intense effort using a lengthy battery of tic assessment measures, numerous evaluators, and a variety of settings, we were unable to document statistically or clinically significant adverse effects on the severity of tics pursuant to methylphenidate drug therapy. Nevertheless, the frequency of observed motor tic occurrence in the public school classroom was shown to be higher when patients received a low dose (0.1 mg/kg) of methylphenidate hydrochloride than when they received placebo.[76] Methylphenidate appears to have a differential effect on ADHD and motor and vocal tics, which suggests structural polymorphism in the neurochemical mechanisms and anatomical substrates involved in the genesis of tics and other pleiotropic manifestations of the TS diathesis. The findings from this study should not be interpreted as indicating that methylphenidate is universally benign with regard to tic exacerbation. Evidence from a multiple challenge study suggests that it can have an adverse effect on tics in specific children,[14] albeit, even with reliable and valid assessment procedures, it is often extremely difficult to determine whether methylphenidate is the cause of observed changes in tic frequency or severity.[13,32,54,82] Furthermore, it bears repeating that all psychotherapeutic drugs are capable of inducing or exacerbating comorbid conditions. Finally, this study does not address the possibility that tic exacerbations might result from longer-term drug exposure, but preliminary findings from our ongoing maintenance therapy study indicate that this is not a clinical issue in most cases.

## REFERENCES

1. Bradley C. Benzedrine and Dexedrine in the treatment of children's behavior disorders. *Pediatrics*. 1950;5:24–36.
2. Mattson RH, Calverty JR. Dextroamphetamine sulfate—induced dyskinesias. *JAMA*. 1968;204:400–402.

3. Gadow KD. Prevalence of drug therapy. In: Werry JS, Aman M, eds. *Practitioner's Guide to Psychoactive Drugs for Children and Adolescents.* New York, NY Plenum Publishing Corp; 1993:57–74.

4. Conners CK, Eisenberg L. The effects of methylphenidate on symptomatology and learning in disturbed children. *Am J Psychiatry.* 1963;120:458–464.

5. Weiss G, Minde K, Douglas V, Werry J, Sykes D Comparison of the effects of chlorpromazine, dextroamphetamine, and methylphenidate on the behavior and intellectual functioning of hyperactive children. *Can Med Assoc J.* 1971;104:20–25.

6. Golden GS. Gilles de la Tourette's syndrome following methylphenidate administration. *Dev Med Child Neurol.* 1974;16:76–78.

7. Golden GS. The effect of central nervous system stimulants on Tourette syndrome *Ann Neurol.* 1977;2:69–70.

8. Pollack MA, Cohen NL, Friedhoff AJ. Gilles de la Tourette's syndrome: familial occurrence and precipitation by methylphenidate therapy. *Arch Neurol.* 1977;34:630–632.

9. Abuzzahab FS, Anderson FO. Gilles de la Tourette's syndrome cross-cultural analysis and treatment outcome. In: Abuzzahab FS, Anderson FO, eds. *Gilles de la Tourette's Syndrome.* St Paul, Minn, Mason Publishing Co; 1976; 1:71–79.

10. Kelman DH, Gilles de la Tourette's disease in children: a review of the literature. *J Child Psychol Psychiatry.* 1965;6:219–226.

11. Meyerhoff JL, Snyder SH. Gilles de la Tourette's disease and minimal brain dysfunction: amphetamine isomers reveal catecholamine correlates in an affected patient. *Psychopharmacologia.* 1973;29:211–220.

12. Singer K. Gilles de la Tourette's disease *Am J Psychiatry* 1963;120:80–81.

13. Gadow KD, Sverd J. Stimulants for ADHD in child patients with Tourette's syndrome: the issue of relative risk *J Dev Behav Pediatr.* 1990;11:269–271.

14. Caine ED, Ludlow CL, Polinsky RJ, Ebert MH. Provocative drug testing in Tourette's syndrome: *d-* and *l*-amphetamine and haloperidol. *J Am Acad Child Psychiatry.* 1984;23:147–152.

15. Feinberg M, Carroll BJ. Effects of dopamine agonists and antagonists in Tourette's disease. *Arch Gen Psychiatry.* 1979;36:979–985.

16. Shapiro AK, Shapiro E. Do stimulants provoke, cause or exacerbate tics and Tourette's syndrome? *Compr Psychiatry.* 1981;22:265–273.

17. Shapiro AK, Shapiro ES, Young JG, Feinberg TE. *Gilles de la Tourette Syndrome* 2nd ed New York, NY: Raven Press: 1988.

18. Lowe TL, Cohen DJ, Detior J, Kremenitzer MW, Shaywitz BA. Stimulant medications precipitate Tourette's syndrome. *JAMA.* 1982;247:1729–1731.

19. Comings DE, Comings BG. A controlled study of Tourette syndrome, I: attention-deficit disorder, learning disorders, and school problems. *Am J Hum Genet.* 1987;41:701–741.

20. Conners CK. Symptom patterns in hyperkinetic, neurotic, and normal children. *Child Dev.* 1970;41:667–682.

21. Munir K, Biederman J, Knere D. Psychiatric comorbidity in patients with attention deficit disorder: a controlled study. *J Am Acad Child Adolesc Psychiatry* 1987;26:844–848.

22. Sverd J, Curley AD, Jandorf L, Volkersz L. Behavior disorder and attention deficits in boys with Tourette syndrome. *J Am Acad Child Adolesc Psychiatry.* 1988;27:413–417.

23. Cohen DJ, Bruun RD, Leckman JF, eds *Tourette's Syndrome and Tic Disorders.* New York, NY: John Wiley & Sons Inc; 1988.

24. Comings DE. *Tourette Syndrome and Human Behavior.* Duarte, Calif: Hope Press; 1990.

25. Kurlan R, ed. *Handbook of Tourette's Syndrome and Related Tic and Behavioral Disorders.* New York, NY: Marcel Dekker Inc; 1993.

26. Sverd J. Clinical presentations of the Tourette syndrome diatheses. *J Multihandicapped Pers.* 1989;2:311–326.

27. Golden GS. Tics and Tourette syndrome. *Hosp Pract (Off Ed).* 1979;14:91–93, 96–97, 100.

28. Anderson GM, Pollak ES, Chatterjee D, Leckman JF, Riddle MA, Cohen DJ. Postmortem analysis of subcortical monoamines and amino acids in Tourette syndrome. In: Chase TN, Friedhoff AJ, Cohen DJ, eds. *Tourette Syndrome: Genetics, Neurobiology, and Treatment.* New York, NY: Raven Press; 1992; 58:123–133.

29. Comings DE. A controlled study of Tourette syndrome, VII: summary: a common genetic disorder causing disinhibition of the limbic system. *Am J Hum Genet* 1987;41:839–866.

30. Comings DE, Comings BG. Tourette's syndrome and attention deficit disorder with hyperactivity: are they genetically related? *J Am Acad Child Psychiatry.* 1984;23:138–146.

31. Erenberg G, Cruse RP, Rothner AD. Gilles de la Tourette's syndrome: effects of stimulant drugs. *Neurology.* 1985;35:1346–1348.

32. Sverd J, Gadow KD, Paolicelli LM. Methylphenidate treatment of attention-deficit hyperactivity disorder in boys with Tourette's syndrome. *J Am Acad Child Adolesc Psychiatry.* 1989;28:574–579.

33. Friedhoff AJ. Receptor maturation in pathogenesis and treatment of Tourette syndrome In: Friedhoff JA, Chase TN, eds. *Gilles de la Tourette Syndrome.* New York, NY: Raven Press, 1982;35:133–140.

34. Price RA, Leckman JF, Pauls DL, Cohen DJ, Kidd KK. Gilles de la Tourette's syndrome: tics and central nervous system stimulants in twins and nontwins. *Neurology.* 1986;36:232–237.

35. Waserman J, Lal S, Gauthier S, Gilles de la Tourette's syndrome in monozygotic twins. *J Neurol Neurosurg Psychiatry.* 1983;46:75–77.

36. Borcherding BG, Keysor CS, Rapoport JL, Elia J, Amass J Motor/vocal tics and compulsive behaviors on stimulant drugs: is there a common vulnerability. *Psychiatry Res.* 1990;33:83–94.

37. Gadow KD, Nolan EE, Sverd J. Methylphenidate in hyperactive boys with co-morbid tic disorder, II: short-term behavioral effects on school settings. *J Am Acad Child Adolesc Psychiatry.* 1992;31:462–471.

38. Konkol RJ, Fischer M, Newby RF. Double-blind, placebo-controlled stimulant trial in children with Tourette's syndrome and attention-deficit hyperactivity disorder. *Ann Neurol.* 1990;28:424. Abstract.

39. Sverd J, Gadow KD, Nolan EE, Sprafkin J, Ezor SN. Methylphenidate in hyperactive boys with comorbid tic disorder, I: clinic evaluations. In: Chase TN, Friedhoff AJ, Cohen DJ, eds. *Tourette Syndrome: Genetics, Neurobiology, and Treatment.* New York, NY: Raven Press; 1992;58:271–281.

40. American Psychiatric Association. *Diagnostic and Statistical Manual of Mental Disorders, Revised Third Edition.* Washington, DC: American Psychiatric Association; 1987.

41. Conners CK. Rating scales for use in drug studies with children. *Psychopharmacol Bull.* 1973;9(special issue):24–84.

42. Loney J, Millich R. Hyperactivity, inattention, and aggression in clinical practice. In: Wolraich M, Routh DK, eds. *Advances in Developmental and Behavioral Pediatrics.* Greenwich, Conn: JAI Press Inc; 1982;3:113–147.

43. Goyette CH, Conners CK, Ulrich RF. Normative data on revised Conners Parent and Teacher Rating Scales. *J Abnorm Child Psychol.* 1978;6:221–236.

44. Loney J. A short parent scale for subgrouping childhood hyperactivity and aggression. Presented at the Annual Meeting of the American Psychological Association; August 1984; Toronto, Ontario.

45. Gadow KD, Sprafkin J. *Stony Brook Child Psychiatric Checklist-3R.* Stony Brook: Dept of Psychiatry, State University of New York-Stony Brook; 1987.

46. Leckman JF, Riddle MA, Hardin MT, Ort SI, Swartz KL, Stevenson J, Cohen DJ. The Yale Global Tic Severity Scale: Initial testing of a clinic-rated scale of tic severity. *J Am Acad Child Adolesc Psychiatry.* 1989;28:566–573.

47. Kurlan R, Riddle M, Como P. *Tourette Syndrome Unified Rating Scale.* Bayside, NY: Tourette Syndrome Association Inc; 1988.

48. Tourette Syndrome Workshop Committee on Classification and Rating Scales. *Report of the Tourette Syndrome Workshop on Definitions of Tic Disorders.* Bayside NY: Tourette Syndrome Association Inc; 1988.

49. Kurlan R. Tourette's syndrome: current concepts. *Neurology.* 1989;39:1625–1630.

50. Reich W, Welner Z. *Diagnostic Interview for Children and Adolescents: Revised Version for Children Ages 6–12 (DSM-III-R Version).* Saint Louis, Mo: Division of Child Psychiatry, Washington University; 1988.

51. Reich W, Welner Z. *Diagnostic Interview for Children and Adolescents: Revised Parent Version for Children Ages 6–17 (DSM-III-R Version).* Saint Louis, Mo: Division of Child Psychiatry, Washington University; 1988.

52. Gadow KD, Paolicelli LM. *Global Tic Rating Scale.* Stony Brook Dept of Psychiatry, State University of New York-Stony Brook; 1986.

53. Nolan EE, Gadow KD, Sverd J. Observations and ratings of tics in school settings. *J Abnorm Child Psychol.* 1994;22:579–593.

54. Routh DK, Schroeder CS, Standardized playroom measures as indices of hyperactivity. *J Abnorm Child Psychol.* 1976;4:199–207.

55. Roberts MA, Ray RS, Roberts RJ. A playroom observational procedure for assessing hyperactive boys. *J Pediatr Psychol.* 1984;9:177–191.

56. Millch R, Loney J, Landau S. Independent dimensions of hyperactivity and aggression: a validation with playroom observational data. *J Abnorm Psychol.* 1982;91:183–198.

57. Halperin JM, Wolf LE, Pascualyaca DM, Newcorn JH, Healey JM, O'Brien JD, Morganstein A, Young JG. Differential assessment of attention and impulsivity in children. *J Am Acad Child Adolesc Psychiatry.* 1988;27:326–329.

58. Halperin JM, Matier K, Bedl G, Sharma V, Newcorn JH. Specificity of inattention, impulsivity, and hyperactivity to the diagnosis of attention-deficit hyperactivity disorder. *J Am Acad Child Adolesc. Psychiatry* 1992;31:190–196.

59. Matler K, Halperin JM, Sharma V, Newcorn JH, Sathaye N. Methylphenidate response in aggressive and non-aggressive ADHD children: distinctions on laboratory measures of symptoms. *J Am Acad Child Adolesc Psychiatry.* 1992;31:219–225.

60. Epstein MH, Cullinan D, Gadow KD. Teacher ratings of hyperactivity in learning disabled, emotionally disturbed and mentally retarded children. *J Special Educ.* 1986;20:219–229.

61. Atkins MS, Pelham WE, Licht MH. The differential validity of teacher ratings of inattention/overactivity and aggression. *J Abnorm Child Psychol.* 1989; 17:423–436.

62. Halperin JM, O'Brien JD, Newcorn JH, Healey JM, Pascualvaca DM, Wolf LE, Young JG. Validation of hyperactive aggressive and mixed hyperactive/aggressive childhood disorders: a research note. *J Child Psychol Psychiatry.* 1990;31:455–459.

63. Milch R, Fitzgerald G. Validation of inattention/overactivity and aggression ratings with classroom observations. *J Consult Clin Psychol.* 1985;53:139–140.

64. Milich R, Landau S. Teacher ratings of inattention/overactivity and aggression: cross validation with classroom observations. *J Clin Child Psychol.* 1988;17:92–97.

65. Nolan EE, Gadow KD. Relation between ratings and observations of stimulant drug response in hyperactive children. *J Clin Child Psychol.* 1994;23:78–90.

66. Gadow KD. A school-based medication evaluation program. In: Matson JL, ed *Handbook of Hyperactivity in Children*. Needham Heights, Mass: Allyn & Bacon; 1993;186–219.

67. Gadow KD. *Peer Conflict Scale*. Stony Brook Dept of Psychiatry, State University of New York-Stony Brook; 1986.

68. Gadow KD. *Stimulant Side Effects Checklist*. Stony Brook: Dept of Psychiatry, State University of New York-Stony Brook, 1986.

69. Goetz CG, Tanner CM, Wilson RS, Carroll VS, Como PG, Shannon KM. Clonidine and Gilles de la Tourette's syndrome: double-blind study using objective rating methods. *Ann Neurol.* 1987;21:307–310.

70. Barkley RA. *Attention Deficit Hyperactivity Disorder: A Handbook for Diagnosis and Treatment*. New York, NY: Guilford Press; 1990.

71. Gadow KD. *Hyperactivity, Learning Disabilities, and Mental Retardation*. Austin, Tex: PRO-ED; 1986, 1.

72. Werry JS, Sprague RL. Methylphenidate in children: effects of dosage. *Aust N Z J Psychiatry.* 1974;8:9–19.

73. Solanto MV. Behavioral effects of low-dose methylphenidate in childhood attention deficit disorder: implications for a mechanism of stimulant drug action. *J Am Acad Child Psychiatry.* 1986;25:96–101.

74. Douglas VI, Barr RG, Amin K, O'Neill ME, Britton BG. Dosage effects and individual responsivity to methylphenidate in attention deficit disorder. *J Child Psychol Psychiatry.* 1988;29:453–475.

75. Rapport MD, Stoner G, DuPaul GJ, Kelly K, Tucker SB, Schoeler T. Attention deficit disorder and methylphenidate, multilevel analysis of dose-response effects on children's impulsivity across settings. *J Am Acad Child Adolesc Psychiatry.* 1988;27:60–69.

76. Gadow KD, Nolan EE, Sverd J, Sprafkin J. School observations of ADHD children with tic disorder effects of methylphenidate treatment. *J Dev Behav Pediatr.* In press.

77. Chappell PB, McSwiggan-Hardin MT, Scahill L, Rubenstein M, Walker DE, Cohen DJ, Leckman JF. Videotape tic counts in the assessment of Tourette's syndrome, stability, reliability, and validity. *J Am Acad Child Adolesc Psychiatry.* 1994;33:386–393.

78. Creager RO, Van Riper C. The effect of methylphenidate on the verbal productivity of children with cerebral dysfunction. *J Speech Hear Res.* 1967;10: 623–628.

79. Ludlow CL, Rapoport JL, Bassich CJ, Mikkelson EG. Differential effects of dextroamphetamine on language performance of hyperactive and normal boys In: Knights RM, Bakker DJ, eds. *Treatment of Hyperactive and Learning Disordered Children*. Baltimore, Md: University Park Press; 1980:185–205.

80. Barkley RA, Cunningham CE, Karlsson J. The speech of hyperactive children and their mothers: comparison with normal children and stimulant drug effects. *J Learning Disabilities*. 1983;16:105–110.

81. Whalen CK, Collins BE, Henker B, Alkus SR, Adams D, Stapp J. Behavior observations of hyperactive children and methylphenidate (Ritalin) effects in systematically structured classroom environments: now you see them, now you don't. *J Pediatr Psychol*. 1978;3:177–187.

82. Sprafkin J, Gadow KD. Four purported cases of methylphenidate-induced tic exacerbation: methodological and clinical doubts. *J Child Adolesc Psychopharmacol*. 1993;3:231–244.

83. Gadow KD. Pediatric psychopharmacotherapy: a review of recent research. *J Child Psychol Psychiatry*. 1992;33:153–195.

84. Albin RL, Young AB, Penney JB. The functional anatomy of basal ganglia disorders. *Trends Neurosci*. 1989;12:366–375.

85. Young AB, Penney JB. Biochemical and functional organization of the basal ganglia. In: Jankovic J, Tolosa E, eds. *Parkinson's Disease and Movement Disorders*. Baltimore, Md: Urban & Schwarzenberg; 1988:1–11.

86. Haber SN, Wolfer D. Basal ganglia peptidergic staining in Tourette syndrome: a follow-up study. In: Chase TN, Friedhoff AJ, Cohen DJ, eds. *Tourette Syndrome: Genetics, Neurobiology, and Treatment*. New York, NY: Raven Press; 1992;58:145–150.

87. McConville BJ, Norman AB, Vogelson MH, Erenberg G. Sequential use of opioid antagonists and agonists in Tourette's syndrome. *Lancet*. 1994; 343–601.

# Part VI

# SPECIAL ISSUES

In the last decade, the number of children conceived by reproductive technologies has increased substantially. Golombok, Cook, Bish, and Murray are among the first authors to document the effects of new reproductive technologies on parenting and children's socioemotional development. They present a well-conceived study using four groups: in vitro fertilization (the child is genetically related to both parents), donor insemination (the child is genetically related to the mother but not the father), naturally conceived child, and adopted at birth child (genetically related to neither parent). The groups were not matched for social class or child age. The children were between four and eight years old. It is worth noting that children with congenital problems were eliminated from the study. The authors do not say if these children were overrepresented in any group.

A variety of measures were used. Quality of parenting was assessed via an interview technique. Ratings of warmth, emotional involvement, and quality of mother-child interaction and father-child interaction were completed. Child psychiatric disorder was assessed using a standardized interview and the Rutter Scales for teacher and mother. Additional measures obtained with the children were The Separation Anxiety Test for representations of attachment relationships, the Family Relations Test for positive feelings between child and mother and child and father, and the Perceived Competence Scale for Young Children.

Findings indicated a higher incidence of marital problems and maternal anxiety and depression for those with a naturally conceived child. Mothers of IVF children were rated higher on warmth and amount of interaction than mothers with a naturally conceived child. Despite the differences on the parenting variables, there were no differences between groups for any of the child measures. The authors speculate that there were no differences on child outcomes because in nondysfunctional families, raised levels of warmth may not result in even greater well-being for the child. Alternatively group differences for the children's measures may have not been detected because of weaknesses in the measures. It also seems possible that parents who have endured difficult procedures to have children could be reluctant to describe anxieties or concerns, thus, presenting as better parents. Interestingly, imbalance in genetic relationships between the parent and child did not appear to disrupt the parenting process. The authors also mention the important issue of telling children about their origins, a topic worthy of another paper. This is an impressive early effort to understand the implications of reproductive technology on parenting and on child development.

The next paper in this section, the Identity of Mixed Parentage Adolescents, explores a rarely-addressed topic. Which ethnic group do children identify with when they have one Caucasian and one African parent. Many social service organizations and professional social work associations have been concerned about allowing interracial adoption or foster care. They have claimed that children reared by a parent of a different ethnicity will not be comfortable with or knowledge about their own ethnicity. In contrast, advocates of transracial fostering refute that the stability that a home with potentially loving parents can provide is more important than the color of the parent's skin. Data collected by Tizard and Phoenix address these issues indirectly by studying a sample of "mixed parentage" children raised by their own parents. The children were all black/white being raised by either a single parent or two parents. Mixed parentage children are still quite rare. In Britain where this study was conducted, the Census indicated that less than 1% of children are of mixed black and white origin.

The goal of this study was to determine the racial identities, friendship patterns and cultural allegiances of the mixed parentage adolescents. Previous studies have primarily used self-referred samples. The authors found a more representative sample by going directly to schools. Fifty-eight teenagers, 14 to 18 year olds were interviewed individually. The majority of the semistructured interviews were conducted by black female interviewers. Data on social class were collected to examine its effects on identity.

Results indicated that few of the teens identified themselves as white, some identified themselves as black, and the majority of the teens referred to themselves by a term indicating their mixed parentage, such as half and half, mixed or brown. When asked about friendships, most of the sample felt comfortable with blacks and whites, but more teens had a close white friend than a close black friend and a white boyfriend or girlfriend. The authors were surprised to find that teens living with a single white parent only were more strongly affiliated with black people and those living with a black parent were more strongly affiliated with white people. Additionally, the type of school attended was an important variable for affiliation. Children attending multiracial and public schools were more strongly affiliated with black people.

In sum, only a few of the teens seemed confused about their racial identity. Most felt they were accepted by both whites and blacks. Having a positive racial identity was not associated with having a black parent. Rather, attending a multiracial school which provided opportunities for associating with a black and mixed peer group seemed to be important in helping teens establish a healthy identity. A methodological issue noted by the authors is that the race of the interviewer influenced the responses of the teens.

This study is an interesting attempt to describe the attitudes and affiliations of mixed parentage children. Longitudinal or cross-sectional studies would illuminate some of the questions highlighted by this study. For example, are younger children more uncomfortable about their mixed parentage? How does that resolve itself as the children reach the teen years and are attempting to consolidate their identity in numerous areas? This study has important implications for transracial adoption and social work policy. Results indicate that opportunities to participate in multiracial schools and peer groups are more important for fostering healthy racial identities than same-race parents.

The third paper in this section describes the cognitive and emotional functioning of orphanage children and of refugee children living in families. It is one of numerous papers published in recent years describing the plight of children orphaned by political upheaval or wars. In third world countries, group care is usually the only alternative for the millions of orphaned children. As stated in the Rutter paper (Chapter 5), attachment theory has resulted in more awareness of children's needs in residential settings.

In this study Wolff, Tesfai, Egasso, and Aradom, sought to determine whether group care was a viable alternative for children without families. The authors compared children living in a large institution with children living with at least one parent in a refugee camp. The children were from an African country, Eritrea, that has been at war with Ethopia for over 25 years. The orphanage had been reorganized, incorporating modern principles of child development and appropriate group care, shortly before the study began. The refugees were also living under difficult circumstances but were with a parent in a self-contained household.

Measures obtained were of social-emotional development (Behavior Screening Questionnaire), nonverbal intelligence (Leiter, Token, and Ravens), language (receptive, expressive and pragmatics), and physical status. There were 74 children in each group ranging from four to seven years. Children with physical and neurological handicaps or obvious mental retardation were not chosen for the study. Results indicated few behavioral differences among the two groups with more enuresis and aggression toward peers among orphan children and more irrational fears among refugee children. On the cognitive measures, the children in the orphanage scored higher. Language data were limited but did not appear to differ by group.

The authors conclude that the minimal behavioral symptoms and the advanced cognitive performance of the orphans compared to children living in refugee families indicates that it is possible to provide humane group care for children. They cite previous studies that indicated emotional difficulties in the young children who were living in the institution prior to its reorganization. In part the brief questionnaire measure of socioemotional development may not have captured feelings of anxiety, depression or loss in these children. In addition the measure of behavioral symptoms was obtained from an interview with the caretakers who may have minimized problems in their charges. The authors discuss the findings as supporting Bowlby's theory of the effect of permanent separation from parents and notions of psychological vulnerability and responses to stress at a young age.

The last paper is on ethical issues in conducting biological psychiatry research with children. A working group was convened by the National Institutes of Mental Health to examine the ethical issues involved in biological research. This paper is a summary of the issues considered and the recommendations made by this group. The article starts with a caution about historical abuses that occurred in the area of behavioral genetics; views on determinism in mental disorders are similar. The federal research safeguards for children are presented. The Working Group declares that children are overprotected by restrictive rules. One example is that drug studies are difficult to obtain approval for with children. As a result 80% of the drugs prescribed for children have the clause "not to be used in children." The group concludes that any risk assessment must include the risk of not having data for clinical decisions.

Issues such as a reexamination of minimal risk, an assessment of risk–benefit ratio for invasive procedures, informed consent, and the use of normal controls are discussed. Research is cited indicating that by age 9 children have enough cognitive capacity to participate in an informed decision about research. This leads to the recommendation that children 12 or older should be able to consent to research on their own and that children between the ages of 7 and 12 should be able to consent and have parental assent. This is the reverse of current procedure.

The authors discuss the need to include normal controls in studies. They propose that adolescents, at least, should be allowed to consent (as an altruistic motion) even if they do not stand to benefit directly from the research. However, the authors question whether it would ever be acceptable to expose normal controls to the use of PET or MRI procedures. Another issue discussed is the use of financial inducements or nonmonetary inducements such as pleasing the investigator who is also the child's therapist. For this later situation, they suggest bringing in a neutral clinician to assess the situation.

Finally, the handling of unexpected knowledge obtained during a study and the special risks already inherent in being from a particular social group are discussed.

In sum, this thoughtful paper raises important considerations for both researchers and clinicians. Both groups need the information obtained from biological psychiatry but children both with and without mental disorders need protection as well. Further dialogue is suggested among ethicists, clinicians, researchers, and policy makers.

# 21

# Families Created by the New Reproductive Technologies: Quality of Parenting and Social and Emotional Development of the Children

**Susan Golombok, Rachel Cook, Alison Bish, and Clare Murray**
*City University, London*

*The creation of families by means of the new reproductive technologies has raised important questions about the psychological consequences for children, particularly where gamete donation has been used in the child's conception. Findings are presented of a study of family relationships and the social and emotional development of children in families created as a result of the 2 most widely used reproductive technologies, in vitro fertilization (IVF) and donor insemination (DI), in comparison with control groups of families with a naturally conceived child and adoptive families. The quality of parenting was assessed using a standardized interview with the mother, and mothers and fathers completed questionnaire measures of stress associated with parenting, marital satisfaction, and emotional state. Data on children's psychiatric state were also obtained by standardized interview with the mother, and by questionnaires completed by the mothers and the children's teachers. The children were administered the Separation Anxiety Test, the Family Re-*

Reprinted with permission from *Child Development*, 1995, Vol. 66, 285–298. Copyright © 1995 by the Society for Research in Child Development, Inc.

We are grateful to Karin Grossmann, Mark Hamilton, Loius Hughes, Michael Humphrey, Brian Lieberman, John Parsons, David Quinton, Marjorie Rutter, Michael Rutter, Robert Winston, and their colleagues, as well as to Sheila Fell, Tayside Regional Council, Strathclyde Regional Council, and Surrey Social Services for their involvement in the study. The research was funded by the Medical Research Council.

*lations Test, and the Pictorial Scale of Perceived Competence
and Social Acceptance. The results showed that the quality of
parenting in families with a child conceived by assisted conception is superior to that shown by families with a naturally
conceived child. No group differences were found for any of
the measures of children's emotions, behavior, or relationships
with parents. The findings are discussed in terms of their implications for understanding the role of genetic ties in family functioning and child development.*

In recent years a rapidly increasing number of children have been conceived by the new reproductive technologies. These include in vitro fertilization (IVF) in which the child is genetically related to both parents, donor
insemination (DI) in which the child is genetically related to the mother but
not the father, and egg donation in which the child is genetically related to
the father but not the mother. When both egg and sperm are donated, the
child is not genetically related to either parent. This latter group of children
are similar to adopted children in that they are genetically unrelated to both
parents, but differ in that the parents experience a pregnancy and develop
a relationship with the child from birth. In the case of surrogacy, the child
may be genetically related to neither, one, or both parents depending on the
use of a donated egg and/or sperm. As Einwohner (1989) points out, it is
possible for a child to have five parents—the egg donor, the sperm donor,
the birth mother, and the two social parents whom the child knows as
mother and father.

A major concern arising from the creation of these new types of family
has been the psychological consequences for children of originating from
donated gametes and thus being genetically unrelated to one or both social
parents. It has been suggested that a missing genetic link between the child
and a parent may pose a threat to the relationship between the nongenetic
parent and the child (Warnock, 1984). More specifically, it has been argued
that it is the secrecy surrounding donor insemination and egg donation that
may undermine family relationships, and that children conceived by gamete donation may feel confused about their identity (Clamar, 1989;
Daniels & Taylor, 1993; Snowden, 1990; Snowden, Mitchell, & Snowden,
1983). Children may also feel deceived by their parents if they eventually
discover the facts about their conception.

As the majority of children conceived by gamete donation are not told
about their origins (Amuzu, Laxova, & Shapiro, 1990; Klock & Maier,
1991), any difficulties they may experience cannot be attributed to the
overt knowledge that they are genetically unrelated to one or both parents.

Instead, conception by gamete donation would only be expected to have negative consequences for the resulting child to the extent that the lack of genetic ties interferes with parent-child relationships. It is well established that children's social and emotional development is fostered within the context of parent-child relationships (Darling & Steinberg, 1993; Maccoby, 1992). Interactions characterized by parental warmth, responsiveness, and sensitivity to the child's needs (Ainsworth, Blehar, Waters, & Wall, 1978; Bowlby, 1969, 1988), in combination with firm control (Baumrind, 1989), are generally believed to promote positive development in the child. It seems, therefore, that difficulties in the social and emotional development of children created by gamete donation are most likely to arise where this method of conception interferes with the process of interaction between the parents and the child.

More general concerns that are related to the use of the new reproductive technologies, but not to gamete donation per se, have also been raised. For example, it has been suggested that couples who have not come to terms with their infertility may experience difficulties in relating to their children (Burns, 1990). This has been reported to be a problem for some adoptive parents (Brodzinsky, 1987; Humphrey & Humphrey, 1988). It may be expected, therefore, that family relationships may be disrupted where one or both partners continue to feel distressed about their own or their partner's infertility after the birth of the child. In addition, while some couples find that the experience of infertility has no deleterious effect on their marriage, for others the stress of infertility as well as the stressful nature of the procedures involved in infertility treatment result in marital difficulties (Cook, Parsons, Mason, & Golombok, 1989). A common feature of the new reproductive technologies is the alienation of the father from the process of conception, which in itself may put a strain on the marriage. For couples whose relationship difficulties persist, problems are likely to develop for the child (Cox, Owen, Lewis, & Henderson, 1989; Howes & Markman, 1989).

The aim of the present study was to examine the quality of parent-child relationships and the social and emotional development of children in families created as a result of the two most common new reproductive methods, IVF and DI, and to compare these families with two control groups: a group of families with a naturally conceived child and a group of adoptive families, the alternative option for infertile couples who wish to become parents. Studying these families provides an opportunity to examine the role of genetic ties in family functioning and child development. Families with a child conceived by egg donation were not included, as only a small number of very young children had been born as a result of this technique when the investigation began.

## METHOD

*Subjects*

Forty-one families with a child conceived by IVF and 45 families with a child conceived by DI were obtained through infertility clinics throughout the United Kingdom. The control groups of 43 families with a naturally conceived child and 55 families with a child adopted at birth were recruited through the records of maternity wards and adoption agencies, respectively. All of the children were between 4 and 8 years of age. Children with major congenital abnormalities, children who had experienced obstetric or perinatal complications that were thought likely to involve brain damage or risk of persisting disability, and children of a multiple birth were not included in the study.

As the total UK population of IVF children in this age range at the time of study was estimated to be less than 200, all IVF families with a child of 4 years or older at each of the four participating clinics who met the inclusion criteria were asked to take part. The response rate was 95%. The other groups of families were matched as closely as possible for the age and sex of the child and the age and social class of the parents. The response rates for DI, adoptive, and naturally conceived families were 62%, 76%, and 62%, respectively.

There was a similar proportion of boys and girls in each group of families. A significant difference between groups was found for age of the child, $F(3, 180) = 9.82, p < .001$. The adopted children were oldest, aged 6 years on average, and the youngest were the DI children, with a mean age of $5\frac{1}{2}$ years. Similarly, a significant group difference was found for the age of the mothers, $F(3, 180) = 8.45, p < .001$, but not fathers. In line with their children, the adoptive mothers were the oldest (mean age 40 years) and the DI mothers were the youngest (mean age 36 years). The average age of the fathers was 41 years. There was also a significant difference between groups for social class as measured by the father's occupation, $\chi^2 = 18.56, p < .05$, with the naturally conceived families receiving the highest ratings and the DI families the lowest. The large majority of families in each group were middle class. The groups did not differ significantly in family size, although there was a trend toward fewer children in the assisted reproduction families, $\chi^2 = 20.98, p < .06$. For children who had siblings, there was a significant group difference for birth order of the target child, $\chi^2 = 19.46, p < .01$, reflecting a greater number of eldest children in the donor insemination families. Although complete matching was not achieved, the group differences that were identified for age of the child and the mother, and for social class, were not large. Where a significant relationship was identified between any of these three demographic measures and a dependent variable, analysis of covariance was used.

All of the parents were contacted in the first instance by a letter from the clinic or adoption agency. Those who agreed to participate were visited at home on two occasions by a researcher trained in the study techniques. On the first visit, data were collected from the mother by interview, and from both parents by questionnaire. Most of the fathers and some of the mothers returned their questionnaires by post, and completed questionnaires were obtained from 95% of mothers and 76% of fathers. Eighty-six percent of parents whose child was at school gave permission for the teacher to receive a questionnaire, and 86% of these were returned. In order to maintain confidentiality and minimize bias, the teachers were not informed about the precise nature of the research. Instead, they were told that the child was participating in a general study of child development. On the second visit, data were collected from the child using a battery of standardized tests. Assessments were carried out with 85% of the children.

## Measures

**Parents' marital and psychiatric state.** A standardized interview was administered to the mother to obtain systematic information relating to the psychiatric state of the parents. Both the mother and the father completed the Golombok Rust Inventory of Marital State (Rust, Bennun, Crowe, & Golombok, 1988; Rust, Bennun, & Golombok, 1990), a questionnaire measure of the quality of the marital relationship for which a score of around 30 represents an average marriage, and a score of greater than 40 indicates severe marital difficulties. The Trait Anxiety Inventory (Spielberger, 1983) and the Beck Depression Inventory (Beck & Steer, 1987) were also completed by both parents to assess anxiety and depression, respectively. All three of these instruments have been shown to have good reliability and to discriminate well between clinical and nonclinical groups.

**Quality of parenting.** The quality of parenting was assessed by standardized interview with the mother using an adaptation of the technique developed by Quinton and Rutter (1988). This procedure has been validated against observational ratings of mother-child relationships in the home, demonstrating a high level of agreement between global ratings of the quality of parenting by interviewers and observers (concurrent validity, $r = 0.63$). The interview, which was tape-recorded, lasted for around $1\frac{1}{2}$ hours and was conducted with the mother alone. Detailed accounts were obtained of the child's behavior and the parents' response to it. The mothers were asked to describe the child's daily routine, focusing on waking, meal times, leaving for school/day-care, returning home, mother's and father's play activities with the child, and bedtime. Information was obtained on the parents' handling of any problems associated with these areas, and particular attention was paid to parent-child interactions relating to issues of control and the child's fears and anxieties. Four overall ratings of the quality of parenting were made taking into account information obtained from the entire interview: (1) *warmth* was rated on a 6-point scale ranging from 0 ("none") to 5 ("high"). This rating of the mother's warmth toward the child was based on the mother's tone of voice and facial expression when talking about the child, spontaneous expressions of warmth, sympathy and concern about any difficulties experienced by the child, and enthusiasm and interest in the child as a person. (2) *Emotional involvement* was rated on a 5-point scale from 0 ("little or none") to 4 ("extreme"). This rating took account of the extent to which the family day was organized around the child; the extent to which the needs or interests of the child were placed before those of other family members; the extent to which the mother was overconcerned, overprotective, or inhibited the child from age-appropriate independent activities; the extent to which the mother was willing to leave the child with other caretakers; and the extent to which the mother had interests or engaged in activities apart from those relating to the child. (3) *Mother-child interaction* and (4) *father-child interaction* were each rated on a 5-point scale ranging from 0 ("very poor") to 4 ("very good"). These ratings of the quality of interaction between the parent and the child were based on mothers' reports of the extent to which the parent and the child enjoyed each other's company, wanted to be with each other, spent time together, enjoyed joint play activities, and showed physical affection to one another, as well as the extent to which the parent took responsibility for caregiving and disciplining the child. While the validity of mothers' reports of father-child interaction has not been established using observational ratings of father-child relationships, a correlation of 0.4 was found between mothers' reports of father-child interaction and fathers' reports of the child being difficult to manage as measured by the *difficult child* subscale of the Parenting Stress Index (Short Form). This gives some evidence for the validity of the mothers' reports of father-child interaction, particularly in view of the differences between these two constructs. Twenty-seven randomly selected interviews were coded by a second interviewer who was "blind" to family type in order to calculate interrater reliabilities. Pearson product-moment coefficients for warmth, emotional involvement, mother-child interaction, and father-child interaction were found to be 0.75, 0.63, 0.72, and 0.69, respectively.

The short form of the Parenting Stress Index (PSI/SF) (Abidin, 1990) was administered to both parents to provide a standardized assessment of stress associated with parenting for mothers and fathers. This measure produces a total score of the overall level of parenting stress an individual is experiencing, as well as the three subscale scores of *parental distress* (feelings of parental incompetence, stresses associated with restrictions on lifestyle, conflict with the child's other parent, lack of social support, and depression), *parent-child dysfunctional interaction* (the parent's perception that the child does not measure up to expectations and that interactions with the child are not reinforcing), and *difficult child* (the behavioral characteristics of children that make them easy or difficult to manage). Test-retest reliability for this instrument has been shown to be high over a 6-month period. Concurrent and predictive validity has been demonstrated for the full-length questionnaire, and the short form has been reported to correlate very highly with the full-length version.

**Children's emotions, behavior, and relationships.** The child's psychiatric state was assessed using a standardized interview with the mother with well-established reliability and validity (Graham & Rutter, 1968). Detailed descriptions were obtained of any behavioral or emotional problems shown by the child. These descriptions of actual behavior, which included information about where the behavior was shown, severity of the behavior, frequency, precipitants, and course of the behavior over the past year, were transcribed and rated "blind" to the knowledge of family type by an experienced child psychiatrist. Psychiatric disorder, when identified, was rated according to severity and type. The presence of behavioral or emotional problems in the children was also assessed using the Rutter "A" scale, which is completed by the child's mother, and the Rutter "B" scale, which is completed by the child's teacher. An overall score of psychiatric state is obtained from each scale. Both questionnaires have been shown to have good interrater and test-retest reliability, and to discriminate well between children with and without psychiatric disorder (Rutter, Cox, Tupling, Berger, & Yule, 1975; Rutter, Tizard, & Whitmore, 1970).

An adaptation of the Separation Anxiety Test (Klagsbrun & Bowlby, 1976) was administered to the children to assess their internal representations of their attachment relationships with parents. The test consists of a series of six photographs of a same-sex child experiencing separation from the parents. Three photographs depict mild separations (i.e., saying goodnight) and three depict severe separations (i.e., parents go on vacation for 2 weeks). The child is asked what the child in the picture would feel and what the child in the picture would do on separation. A coding scheme for these data has been developed by Grossmann and Grossmann (1991). Each child obtains a total score of security of attachment representation that takes account of affectivity (the degree to which the child attributes negative emotions, such as sadness or anger, to the child in the picture), coping (the degree to which the child attributes a coping response, such as an action that will help master the situation, to the child in the picture), and expression (the degree to which the child shows a facial expression and tone of voice that are appropriate to the verbal response). Ratings of affectivity and coping are each made on a 5-point scale according to standard criteria, with a high score representing high affectivity and high coping, respectively. Expression is rated on a 3-point scale, with a high score representing an appropriate expression. An overall score is then calculated for each picture that takes account of the appropriateness of the affectivity and coping according to the type of separation depicted (i.e., mild vs. severe), as well as the expression rating. Finally, a total score is obtained for each child that incorporates the responses to all six pictures. This coding scheme has been validated for 6-year-olds against these children's attachment to the mother and the father in the laboratory at 1 year of age. Significantly more children who had been classified as securely attached at 1 year responded appropriately to at least one picture in terms of affectivity, coping, and expression than children who had been classified as insecurely attached at 1 year (Grossmann & Grossmann, 1991). This was true of 100% of securely attached children, compared with 40% of insecurely attached children. In the present investigation, the testing session was not videotaped, so that ratings of expression could not be made. For this reason, the coding scheme was modified to include only the ratings of affectivity and coping. A total score was obtained for each child ranging from 0 (representing very insecure attachment) to 12 (representing very secure attachment). To calculate interrater reliability, data from 60 randomly selected children were coded by a second interviewer who was "blind" to family type. A Pearson product-moment coefficient of 0.76 was obtained.

A modified version of the Family Relations Test (Bene & Anthony, 1985) was also administered to obtain a standardized assessment of the children's feelings about their parents. The child chose an imaginary mother and father from a set of cut-out figures, and these were placed in front of the child, together with a neutral figure, "Mr. Nobody." The child was then given a set of cards with an emotional message printed on each (e.g., "[child] thinks you are nice"), and was asked to give each card to the person for whom they felt it was most appropriate. The test was scored to produce a measure of positive feelings and a measure of negative feelings from the child to each parent, and a measure of positive feelings and a measure of negative feelings from each parent to the child. Acceptable test-retest reliability has been demonstrated, and validation studies have shown the test to discriminate between clinical and nonclinical groups of children (Bean, 1976; Kaufman, Weaver, & Weaver, 1972; Philip & Orr, 1978). Children's responses to the test have also been shown to reflect independent assessments of both mothers' and fathers' feelings toward them (Bene & Anthony, 1985). Significantly more children whose mothers had been categorized as "accepting" (according to data obtained from interviews with the mother by a rater who was "blind" to the child's test responses) attributed predominantly positive feelings to their mother than children whose mother had been categorized as "neglecting." Similarly, a small group of children whose fathers had been described by social workers or by the mother as hostile, punitive, or disliking of them were found to attribute predominantly negative feelings to their father when administered the test. In the present investigation, the scores were combined to give two global ratings for each child: (1) *positive feelings between child and mother* [(positive feelings to mother + positive feelings from mother) − (negative feelings to mother + negative feelings from mother)], and (2) *positive feelings between child and father* [(positive feelings to father + positive feelings from father) − (negative feelings to father + negative feelings from father)]. The higher the score, the more positive the feelings.

Each child was administered the Pictorial Scale of Perceived Competence and Social Acceptance for Young Children (Harter & Pike, 1984). This is a measure of children's perceptions of their cognitive and physical competencies, and of their perceptions of acceptance by their mother and by peers, all of which have been shown to be associated with the development of self-esteem in later childhood. A score is obtained for each of the following subscales: (1) *cognitive competence*, (2) *physical competence*, (3) *maternal acceptance*, and (4) *peer acceptance*. The higher the score, the more positive the child's feelings of competence and social acceptance. Satisfactory internal consistency has been demonstrated, with coefficient $\alpha$ values ranging from 0.85 to 0.89 for the different age groups of children studied. The scale has been shown to discriminate between groups of children in predicted ways, for example, between peer acceptance and length of time at a school, and between perceived cognitive competence and academic achievement at school, indicating that it is a valid measure.

## RESULTS

### Parent's Marital and Psychiatric State

Almost all of the parents were married (four couples with a naturally conceived child were cohabiting). Only two sets of parents in the IVF, DI, and naturally conceived groups, and one set of adoptive parents, had separated. With respect to the quality of the parents' marital relationship, group differences in GRIMS scores were found for mothers, $F(3, 160) = 3.25$, $p < .05$, and fathers, $F(3, 136) = 3.12$, $p < .05$, indicating a greater incidence of marital difficulties among couples with a naturally conceived child. A significant difference in anxiety level as assessed by the Trait Anxiety Inventory was found for mothers, $F(3, 170) = 3.92$, $p < .01$, and fathers, $F(3, 135) = 4.46$, $p < .01$. Depression, as assessed by the Beck Depression Inventory, also differed between groups for mothers, $F(3, 168) = 4.06$, $p < .01$, but not for fathers. These group differences reflect higher levels of anxiety and depression among parents with a normally conceived child (see Table 1). Few mothers had received treatment for psychiatric disorder, or had been prescribed psychotropic medication. While this was also true for fathers, a group difference in the proportion who had received psychiatric treatment was shown, $\chi^2 = 18.87$, $p < .05$. Five fathers with a naturally conceived child had received psychiatric treatment, whereas none of the other fathers had ever sought psychiatric help.

### Quality of Parenting

Group comparisons of the global ratings of quality of parenting (warmth, emotional involvement, mother-child interaction, and father-child interaction) and the Parenting Stress Index (Short Form) scores for mothers and fathers were conducted using MANOVA. Wilks's lambda was significant, $F(18, 365) = 2.35$, $p < .002$, showing an overall difference in quality of parenting between groups. The following contrast analyses were then carried out using one-way ANOVAs to address specific questions (see Table 2; Figure 1): (1) *Assisted Reproduction versus Naturally Conceived* (AR vs. NC). This contrast examines whether families with a child conceived by assisted reproduction (IVF and DI) are different from families with a naturally conceived child. (2) *Assisted Reproduction versus Adoptive* (AR vs. A). This contrast examines whether families with a child conceived by assisted reproduction (IVF and DI) are different from families with an adopted child. (3) *In Vitro Fertilization versus Donor Insemination* (IVF vs. DI). This contrast determines whether IVF and DI families differ from each other, and thus examines the consequences of one parent being genetically unrelated to the child. (4) *In Vitro Fertilization versus Adoptive* (IVF vs. A). This contrast between IVF and adoptive families also has implications for understanding the importance of genetic relationships. It addresses the question of whether families matched for the desire to have children differ according to whether or not the children are genetically re-

TABLE 1

Comparison Between IVF, DI, Adoptive, and Naturally Conceived Families on Mothers' and Fathers' Test Scores

| | IVF | | | DI | | | ADOPTIVE | | | NATURALLY CONCEIVED | | | F | p |
|---|---|---|---|---|---|---|---|---|---|---|---|---|---|---|
| | N | $\bar{X}$ | SE | N | $\bar{X}$ | SE | N | $\bar{X}$ | SE | N | $\bar{X}$ | SE | | |
| Marital state, mothers ...... | 35 | 25.9 | 1.9 | 40 | 26.6 | 1.8 | 53 | 22.1 | 1.6 | 36 | 29.8 | 1.9 | 3.25 | <.05 |
| Marital state, fathers ........ | 30 | 25.9 | 1.7 | 35 | 24.7 | 1.6 | 50 | 22.9 | 1.3 | 25 | 30.2 | 1.9 | 3.12 | <.05 |
| Trait anxiety, mothers ...... | 38 | 36.7 | 1.3 | 42 | 35.1 | 1.3 | 55 | 37.5 | 1.1 | 39 | 41.4 | 1.3 | 3.92 | <.01 |
| Trait anxiety, fathers ........ | 30 | 35.9 | 1.4 | 35 | 36.7 | 1.3 | 49 | 35.2 | 1.1 | 25 | 42.2 | 1.6 | 4.46 | <.01 |
| Depression, mothers ........ | 37 | 5.5 | .8 | 42 | 4.4 | .7 | 55 | 4.4 | .6 | 38 | 7.8 | .8 | 4.06 | <.0 |
| Depression, fathers .......... | 30 | 5.0 | .7 | 35 | 4.6 | .6 | 51 | 4.5 | .5 | 25 | 6.8 | .8 | 1.96 | N.S. |

NOTE.—Table shows sample size, mean, standard error, F, and significance levels of one-way ANOVAs for mothers' and fathers' scores on the Golombok Rust Inventory of Marital State, the Spielberger Trait Anxiety Inventory, and the Beck Depression Inventory.

## TABLE 2
### Comparison Between IVF, DI, Adoptive, and Naturally Conceived Families on Parenting Meaures

| | IVF | | | DI | | | Adoptive | | | Naturally Conceived | | | | | Contrasts | | | | |
|---|---|---|---|---|---|---|---|---|---|---|---|---|---|---|---|---|---|---|---|
| | N | $\bar{X}$ | SE | N | $\bar{X}$ | SE | N | $\bar{X}$ | SE | N | $\bar{X}$ | SE | F | p | AR vs. NC[a] | AR vs. A[a] | IVF vs. DI[b] | IVF vs. A[b] | DI vs. A[b] |
| Mother's warmth to child | 41 | 4.0 | .16 | 45 | 3.8 | .15 | 54 | 3.6 | .14 | 43 | 3.4 | .15 | 2.91 | <.05 | p < .01 | N.S. | N.S. | p < .05 | N.S. |
| Mother's emotional involvement with child | 41 | 2.3 | .11 | 45 | 2.4 | .10 | 54 | 2.1 | .09 | 43 | 1.9 | .10 | 4.37 | <.01 | p < .001 | N.S. | N.S. | N.S. | N.S. |
| Mother-child interaction | 41 | 3.3 | .10 | 45 | 3.3 | .10 | 54 | 3.1 | .09 | 43 | 3.0 | .10 | 2.60 | <.05 | p < .05 | N.S. | N.S. | N.S. | N.S. |
| Father-child interaction | 40 | 2.9 | .12 | 44 | 2.8 | .12 | 53 | 2.8 | .11 | 40 | 2.3 | .12 | 4.70 | <.01 | p < .001 | N.S. | N.S. | N.S. | N.S. |
| Total PSI/SF score, mother | 38 | 68.2 | 2.4 | 42 | 63.7 | 2.3 | 55 | 66.7 | 2.0 | 39 | 73.8 | 2.4 | 3.18 | <.05 | p < .01 | N.S. | N.S. | N.S. | N.S. |
| Parental distress | 39 | 24.1 | 1.0 | 42 | 20.5 | .9 | 55 | 21.7 | .8 | 39 | 26.2 | 1.0 | 6.90 | <.001 | p < .01 | N.S. | p < .01 | N.S. | N.S. |
| Parent-child dysfunctional interaction | 38 | 18.6 | .7 | 42 | 18.0 | .7 | 55 | 19.2 | .6 | 39 | 20.1 | .7 | 1.51 | N.S. | ⋮ | ⋮ | ⋮ | ⋮ | ⋮ |
| Difficult child | 39 | 25.7 | 1.1 | 42 | 24.9 | 1.0 | 55 | 25.7 | .9 | 39 | 27.4 | 1.1 | .92 | N.S. | ⋮ | ⋮ | ⋮ | ⋮ | ⋮ |
| Total PSI/SF score, father | 29 | 70.1 | 2.8 | 35 | 71.1 | 2.5 | 51 | 65.2 | 2.1 | 25 | 75.2 | 3.0 | 2.64 | <.05 | N.S. | N.S. | N.S. | N.S. | N.S. |
| Parent distress | 30 | 23.4 | 1.1 | 35 | 23.5 | 1.0 | 51 | 21.8 | .8 | 25 | 27.5 | 1.2 | 4.44 | <.01 | p < .01 | ⋮ | N.S. | N.S. | N.S. |
| Parent-child dysfunctional interaction | 29 | 20.0 | .9 | 35 | 19.8 | .8 | 51 | 18.6 | .7 | 25 | 20.2 | 1.0 | .73 | N.S. | ⋮ | ⋮ | ⋮ | ⋮ | ⋮ |
| Difficult child | 29 | 26.7 | 1.3 | 35 | 27.3 | 1.2 | 51 | 24.7 | .9 | 25 | 27.5 | 1.4 | 1.42 | N.S. | ⋮ | ⋮ | N.S. | ⋮ | ⋮ |

NOTE.—Table shows sample size, mean, standard error, F, significance levels, and contrasts of one-way ANOVAs for scores of mother's warmth to child, mother's emotional involvement with child, mother-child interaction, father-child interaction, and mothers' and fathers' total and subscale PSI/SF scores.

[a] User contrast.

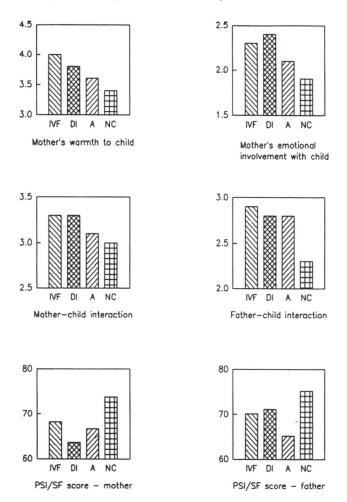

**Figure 1.** Mean scores for measures of parenting quality for IVF, DI, adoptive, and naturally conceived families.

lated to their parents. (5) *Donor Insemination versus Adoptive* (DI vs. A). This contrast examines whether DI families with a child who is genetically unrelated to one parent (the father) are different from families where the child is adopted and thus genetically unrelated to both parents. It addresses the question of whether it is better for children to be genetically related to at least one parent than none, or better for them to be genetically unrelated to both parents than just one to prevent an imbalance in the relationship between each parent and the child. As no significant relationships were found between age of the child, age of the mother, or social class on any of the measures of quality of parenting, these demographic variables were not entered into the analyses as covariates.

A significant difference was found between groups for warmth, $F(3, 179) = 2.91, p < .05$. Contrast analyses showed that mothers with a child conceived by assisted reproduction expressed greater warmth toward their child than mothers with a naturally conceived child (User Contrast [AR vs. NC], $p < .01$). There was no significant difference in expressed warmth to the child according to type of assisted reproduction (IVF vs. DI). Whereas adoptive mothers did not differ in expressed warmth to the child from DI mothers, they did show less warmth than IVF mothers (Fisher's LSD comparison, $p < .05$).

The groups also differed in the level of mothers' emotional involvement with the child, $F(3, 179) = 4.37, p < .01$. Mothers of children conceived by assisted reproduction showed greater emotional involvement than mothers with a naturally conceived child (User Contrast [AR vs. NC], $p < .001$), with no difference between IVF and DI mothers. The level of emotional involvement shown by mothers of adoptive children was similar to that of IVF and DI mothers.

Group differences were found for mother-child interaction, $F(3, 179) = 2.60, p < .05$, and father-child interaction, $F(3, 173) = 4.7, p < .01$. Both mothers (User Contrast [AR vs. NC], $p < .05$) and fathers (User Contrast [AR vs. NC], $p < .001$) of children conceived by assisted reproduction showed greater interaction with their children than mothers and fathers of naturally conceived children. There was no difference in the quality of interaction between IVF and DI mothers, or between IVF or DI fathers, and adoptive mothers and fathers did not differ significantly from the mothers and fathers of children conceived by assisted reproduction techniques.

Stress associated with parenting as assessed by total Parenting Stress Index (Short Form) scores was found to differ between groups for mothers, $F(3, 170) = 3.18, p < .05$, and fathers, $F(3, 136) = 2.64, p < .05$. Analyses of the subscale scores showed that the group difference for total Parenting Stress Index (Short Form) scores reflected a difference in the parental distress subscale for both mothers, $F(3, 171) = 6.90, p < .001$, and fathers, $F(3, 137) = 4.44, p < .01$, with parents of naturally conceived children reporting significantly greater levels of distress than parents whose children were conceived by assisted reproduction (User Contrast for mothers [AR vs. NC], $p < .01$, and User Contrast for fathers [AR vs. NC], $p < .01$). A difference was also found between IVF and DI mothers for this subscale (Fisher's LSD comparison, $p < .01$), with IVF mothers reporting more distress than DI mothers. No significant differences in parental distress were found among IVF, DI, and adoptive fathers.

Factor analysis of the four parenting variables derived from the interview (warmth, emotional involvement, mother-child interaction, and father-child interaction) and the Parenting Stress Index (Short Form) scores for mothers and fathers yielded a first factor with an eigenvalue of 2.57, accounting for 43% of the variance. The loadings of the six variables on this factor ranged from 0.54 to 0.79.

In order to establish whether the group differences relating to quality of parenting may be explained by group differences in parents' anxiety, depression, and marital satisfaction, the ANOVAs contrasting assisted reproduction families with naturally conceived families (AR vs. NC) were repeated with mothers' and fathers' Trait Anxiety Inventory scores, Beck Depression Inventory scores, and Golombok Rust Inventory of Marital State scores as covariates. A significant group difference remained for all of the variables apart from mothers' stress associated with parenting (warmth $F = 4.42$, $p < .05$; emotional involvement $F = 7.16$, $p < .01$; mother-child interaction $F = 5.53$, $p < .05$; father-child interaction $F = 6.56$, $p < .01$; parenting stress—mothers $F = 1.28$, N.S.; parenting stress—fathers $F = 4.13$, $p < .05$).

## Children's Emotions, Behavior, and Relationships

Only eight children in the entire sample were rated as showing psychiatric disorder. Of these, two were IVF children (one with developmental disorder and one with conduct disorder), one was a DI child (with conduct disorder), three were adopted (two with conduct disorder and one with mixed conduct/emotional disorder), and two were naturally conceived (one with conduct disorder and one with mixed conduct/emotional disorder). Group comparisons of children's total "A" scale and "B" scale scores were conducted using one-way analyses of covariance, with age of the child and social class, respectively, as a covariate. In line with the ratings of psychiatric disorder, no significant differences between groups were found for these questionnaire measures of emotional and behavioral problems (see Table 3). Overall, the children's "A" scale and "B" scale scores were closely comparable to general population norms for 8-year-olds (Richman, Stevenson, & Graham, 1982; Stevenson, Richman, & Graham, 1985; Taylor, Sandberg, Thorley, & Giles, 1991).

Group comparisons of children's scores for the Separation Anxiety Test, the Family Relations Test, and the Pictorial Scale of Perceived Competence and Social Acceptance were conducted using one-way analyses of variance. The age of the child, age of the mother, and social class were not found to be significantly related to any of these measures and thus were not entered into the analyses as covariates. As shown in Table 3, no significant

TABLE 3

Comparison Between IVF, DI, Adoptive, and Naturally Conceived Families
on Children's Test Scores

| | IVF | | | DI | | | ADOPTIVE | | | NATURALLY CONCEIVED | | | | |
|---|---|---|---|---|---|---|---|---|---|---|---|---|---|---|
| | $N$ | $\bar{X}$ | SE | $N$ | $\bar{X}$ | SE | $N$ | $\bar{X}$ | SE | $N$ | $\bar{X}$ | SE | $F$ | $p$ |
| A scale[a] | 36 | 8.5 | .79 | 41 | 8.1 | .74 | 51 | 9.2 | .67 | 37 | 9.2 | .78 | .48 | N.S. |
| B scale[b] | 28 | 3.5 | .74 | 21 | 2.3 | .86 | 44 | 3.2 | .59 | 34 | 4.6 | .67 | 1.62 | N.S. |
| Separation Anxiety Test | 30 | 5.3 | .32 | 37 | 4.8 | .29 | 49 | 5.5 | .25 | 39 | 4.9 | .28 | 1.15 | N.S. |
| Family Relations Test: | | | | | | | | | | | | | | |
| Positive feelings, mother | 30 | 4.5 | .83 | 37 | 4.1 | .75 | 49 | 4.8 | .65 | 39 | 5.2 | .73 | .38 | N.S. |
| Positive feelings, father | 30 | 2.0 | .89 | 35 | 2.8 | .82 | 49 | 4.1 | .69 | 39 | 2.7 | .78 | 1.25 | N.S. |
| Pictorial Scale of Perceived Competence and Social Acceptance: | | | | | | | | | | | | | | |
| Cognitive competence | 31 | 3.2 | .09 | 37 | 3.3 | .08 | 49 | 3.3 | .07 | 39 | 3.4 | .08 | .41 | N.S. |
| Physical competence | 31 | 3.2 | .09 | 37 | 3.3 | .08 | 49 | 3.2 | .07 | 39 | 3.2 | .08 | .07 | N.S. |
| Maternal acceptance | 31 | 2.9 | .09 | 37 | 2.8 | .09 | 40 | 2.8 | .07 | 39 | 2.9 | .08 | .67 | N.S. |
| Peer acceptance | 31 | 3.1 | .11 | 37 | 3.1 | .10 | 49 | 3.2 | .09 | 39 | 3.0 | .10 | .83 | N.S. |

NOTE.—Table shows sample size, mean, standard error, $F$, and significance levels of one-way ANOVAs for children's scores on the A scale, the B scale, the Separation Anxiety Test, the Family Relations Test, and the Pictorial Scale of Perceived Competence and Social Acceptance.
[a] With social class as a covariate.
[b] With age of child as a covariate.

differences between groups were found for any of these measures. The subscale scores obtained by children for the Pictorial Scale of Perceived Competence and Social Acceptance in the present investigation were similar to normative data for this measure. As modified versions of the Separation Anxiety Test and the Family Relations Test were used, it was not possible to compare the scores of children in the present investigation with published norms.

Factor analysis of the variables derived from the Separation Anxiety Test, the Family Relations Test, and the Pictorial Scale of Perceived Competence and Social Acceptance gave two factors with eigenvalues greater than 1. The first factor had an eigenvalue of 2.23, accounting for 32% of variance, and the second factor had an eigenvalue of 1.62, accounting for 23% of variance. Factor 1 comprised all of the variables for the Pictorial Scale of Perceived Competence and Social Acceptance with loadings ranging from 0.69 to 0.80. Factor 2 is explained by the two Family Relations Test variables, which had loadings of 0.89 and 0.86, respectively. The Separation Anxiety Test score was found to be independent of the other variables.

## DISCUSSION

Contrary to the concerns that have been raised regarding the potential negative consequences of the new reproductive technologies for family functioning and child development, the findings of this study indicate that the quality of parenting in families with a child conceived by assisted conception is superior to that shown by families with a naturally conceived child, even when gamete donation is used in the child's conception. Families with a child conceived by assisted reproduction obtained significantly higher scores on measures of mother's warmth to the child, mother's emotional involvement with the child, mother-child interaction, and father-child interaction. In line with these findings, mothers and fathers of naturally conceived children reported significantly higher levels of stress associated with parenting. No significant differences were found between IVF and DI parents for any of these measures, apart from greater parental distress among IVF than DI mothers. It is important to point out that the families with a naturally conceived child were selected from the general population and did not constitute a dysfunctional group. Thus the investigation shows that the assisted reproduction families were functioning extremely well, and not that the control group was experiencing difficulties. The adoptive mothers and fathers were very similar in quality of parenting to the mothers and fathers of children conceived by assisted reproduction.

In view of these findings, it is not surprising that children conceived by assisted reproduction did not obtain significantly poorer scores than naturally conceived children or adopted children for the assessments of psychiatric state, attachment relationships, feelings toward their mother and father, and perceived competence and social acceptance. Instead, given the greater commitment to parenting in the assisted reproduction families, it could perhaps be expected that they would have obtained significantly better scores on these assessments than their naturally conceived counterparts. Examination of the children's scores in relation to general population norms, where these were available, shows that the children in all types of families were generally functioning well. It seems, therefore, that in nondysfunctional families, raised levels of warmth and parental involvement do not result in even greater well-being for the child. Alternatively, group differences for the children's assessments may not have been detected due to weaknesses in the measures.

It is possible that biases involved in the sampling procedure may have influenced these results. In particular, the response rates of 62% for the DI and naturally conceived families may reflect a tendency for parents of DI and naturally conceived children who were experiencing difficulties to opt out of the investigation. The effect of this for families with a naturally conceived child would be an underestimate of the differences between these families and the other family types. For the DI families, however, the outcome would be a more positive view than is generally the case. Our impression from telephone conversations with some DI parents who declined to take part was not that they were experiencing problems, but that they had decided to keep the child's origins secret and were concerned that by participating in the study the secret may be jeopardized in some way. They also gave the impression of not wanting to be reminded of the lack of genetic relationship between the father and the child. The adoptive parents who refused to participate were concerned about information being fed back to the adoption agency. Interestingly, when the initial letter was modified to include a statement that no information would be passed on to the agency, the response rate for adoptive families increased from 69% to 87%.

A characteristic of parents whose child was conceived as a result of the new reproductive technologies is that they are generally older than first-time parents of a naturally conceived child. From the time that the couple first realize that they may have an infertility problem, many years may pass before they seek help, and then the process of diagnosis and treatment may take several more years before, if successful, a child is born. Typically, women undergoing assisted reproduction do not become mothers until they are in their mid-thirties, an age by which most mothers who do not have a history of infertility have given birth to more than one child. In order to match the different family types for the age of the parents and of the child, and because we wished the group of families with a naturally conceived child to be as representative as possible of the general population, about 40% of the children conceived by IVF and DI did not have siblings, compared with about 20% of the children in the naturally conceived and adoptive control groups. One possible explanation, therefore, for the greater commitment to parenting shown by the assisted reproduction parents in comparison with the control group of parents with a naturally conceived child is that these parents were highly involved with their children due to the absence of siblings. However, when the group of families with a naturally conceived child was subdivided according to the presence or absence of siblings, no significant differences were found for any of the measures of quality of parenting. In addition, no significant relationship was found between number of children in the family and the measures of quality of parenting, apart from a significant association between larger family size and greater stress associated with parenting reported by mothers ($r = 0.23$, $p < .01$), or between birth order and any of the variables relating to quality of parenting for those children who had siblings.

The findings suggest that genetic ties are less important for family functioning than a strong desire for parenthood. Whether the child was genetically unrelated to one parent, in the case of donor insemination, or genetically unrelated to both parents, in the case of adoption, the quality of parenting in families where the mother and father had gone to great lengths to become parents was superior to that shown by mothers and fathers who had achieved parenthood in the usual way. The similarity in parenting quality between DI and adoptive mothers and fathers shows that it does not seem to matter whether the child is genetically unrelated to one parent or two; an imbalance in genetic relationships between the parents and the child does not appear to disrupt the parenting process. Thus the suggestion that DI fathers would have difficulty in relating to their children is not supported by the results of this study.

There is growing pressure from both social policy makers and from those working in the field of assisted reproduction to tell children conceived by gamete donation about their origins (Daniels & Taylor, 1993). This practice has been encouraged by the American Fertility Society (1993), and it has now become law in the United Kingdom that nonidentifying information about the donor may be given at age 18. In Sweden, individuals conceived by gamete donation even have a right to identifying information, allowing them to contact the donor when they grow up. The move toward greater openness stems to a large extent from research on adoption which has demonstrated that, for some people at least, knowledge about genetic origins is important for the development of a clear sense of identity (Hoopes, 1990; Sants, 1964; Schechter & Bertocci, 1990; Triseliotis, 1973). Children conceived by gamete donation may also benefit from knowledge about their past. Snowden (1990), reporting on interviews with a small number of young adults who had been told that they had been conceived by donor insemination, found no evidence to suggest that they had been traumatized by this information, were unsure of their identity, or that the father-child relationship had been damaged. It is important to point out, however, that while adoptive families and families with a child conceived by gamete donation are similar in that the child is genetically unrelated to at least one parent, the two types of families differ not only in that usually one parent is a genetic parent but also, and perhaps more importantly, in that the child had not been born to a genetically related mother and then given up for adoption. The fact that a child has always been a wanted child may constitute a very important difference.

In the present study, all but one of the adopted children knew about their past. In contrast, none of the DI parents had told their child that he or she had been conceived using semen from an anonymous donor. Thus, for children aged 4–8 years at least, keeping the method of conception secret from the child does not appear to have a negative impact on family relationships. It is yet to be seen how many parents will decide to tell the children as they grow up, and whether difficulties will arise as issues of identity become more salient at adolescence. A discrepancy in attitudes exists between professionals and the parents themselves on the issue of secrecy. While there are generally accepted stories in our society to explain adoption, this is not the case for IVF or reproductive procedures involving gamete donation, making it difficult for parents to tell their children about the way in which they were conceived. Parents often fear that the child will respond negatively to being told and will reject them (Cook, Golombok, Bish, & Murray, in press). As so few parents are currently telling their children about their origins, it remains for future research to inform us about the consequences of telling or not telling children about how they were conceived. In the meantime, the picture these families present is one of positive interactions between parents and children. There is no evidence to suggest that the negative experience of involuntary childlessness results in persisting difficulties when these extremely wanted children eventually arrive.

# REFERENCES

Abidin, R. (1990). *Parenting Stress Index Test Manual.* Charlottesville, VA: Pediatric Psychology Press.

Ainsworth, M. D. S., Blehar, M. C., Waters, E., & Wall, S. (1978). *Patterns of attachment: A psychological study of the Strange Situation.* Hillsdale, NJ: Erlbaum.

American Fertility Society. (1993). Guidelines for therapeutic donor insemination: Sperm. *Fertility & Sterility, 59,* 1S–9S.

Amuzu, B., Laxova, R., & Shapiro, S. (1990). Pregnancy outcome, health of children, and family adjustment after donor insemination. *Obstetrics and Gynecology, 75,* 899–905.

Baumrind, D. (1989). Rearing competent children. In W. Damon (Ed.), *Child development today and tomorrow.* San Francisco: Jossey-Bass.

Bean, B. W. (1976). *An investigation of the reliability and validity of the Family Relations Test.* Unpublished doctoral thesis, University of Kansas.

Beck, A., & Steer, R. (1987). *The Beck Depression Inventory Manual.* San Diego, CA: Psychological Corp.

Bene, E., & Anthony, J. (1985). *Manual for the Family Relations Test.* Windsor, UK: NFER-Nelson.

Bowlby, J. (1969). *Attachment and loss: Vol. 1. Attachment.* London: Hogarth.

Bowlby, J. (1988). *A secure base: Clinical applications of attachment theory.* London: Routledge.

Brodzinsky, D. M. (1987). Adjustment to adoption: A psychosocial perspective. *Clinical Psychology Review, 7,* 25–47.

Burns, L. H. (1990). An exploratory study of perceptions of parenting after infertility. *Family Systems Medicine, 8,* 177–189.

Clamar, A. (1989). Psychological implications of the anonymous pregnancy. In J. Offerman-Zuckerberg (Ed.), *Gender in transition: A new frontier.* New York: Plenum.

Cook, R., Golombok, S., Bish, A., & Murray, C. (in press). Keeping secrets: A controlled study of parental attitudes towards telling about donor insemination. *Journal of Orthopsychiatry.*

Cook, R., Parsons, J., Mason, B., & Golombok, S. (1989). Emotional, marital and sexual problems in patients embarking upon IVF and AID treatment for infertility. *Journal of Reproductive and Infant Psychology, 7,* 87–93.

Cox, M. J., Owen, M. T., Lewis, J. M., & Henderson, V. K. (1989). Marriage, adult adjustment, and early parenting. *Child Development, 60,* 1015–1024.

Daniels, K., & Taylor, K. (1993). Secrecy and openness in donor insemination. *Politics and Life Sciences, 12,* 155–170.

Darling, N., & Steinberg, L. (1993). Parenting style as context: An integrative model. *Psychological Bulletin, 113,* 487–496.

Einwohner, J. (1989). Who becomes a surrogate: Personality characteristics. In J. Offerman-Zuckerberg (Ed.), *Gender in transition: A new frontier.* New York: Plenum.

Graham, P., & Rutter, M. (1968). The reliability and validity of the psychiatric assessment of the child: II. Interview with the parent. *British Journal of Psychiatry, 114,* 581–592.

Grossmann, K. E., & Grossmann, K. (1991). Attachment quality as an organizer of emotional and behavioral responses in a longitudinal perspective. In C. M. Parkes, J. Stevenson-Hinde, & P. Marris (Eds.), *Attachment across the life cycle.* London: Routledge.

Harter, S., & Pike, R. (1984). The pictorial scale of perceived competence and social acceptance for young children. *Child Development, 55,* 1969–1982.

Hoopes, J. L. (1990). Adoption and identity formation. In D. M. Brodzinsky & M. D. Schechter (Eds.), *The psychology of adoption.* Oxford: Oxford University Press.

Howes, P., & Markman, H. J. (1989). Marital quality and child functioning: A longitudinal investigation. *Child Development, 60,* 1044–1051.

Humphrey, M., & Humphrey, H. (1988). *Families with a difference: Varieties of surrogate parenthood.* London: Routledge.

Kaufman, J. M., Weaver, S. J., & Weaver, A. (1972). Family Relations Test responses of retarded readers: Reliability and comparative data. *Journal of Personality Assessment, 36,* 353–360.

Klagsbrun, M., & Bowlby, J. (1976). Responses to separation from parents: A clinical test for young children. *British Journal of Projective Psychology, 21,* 7–21.

Klock, S. C., & Maier, D. (1991). Psychological factors related to donor insemination. *Fertility & Sterility, 56*, 489–495.

Maccoby, E. E. (1992). The role of parents in the socialization of children. *Developmental Psychology, 28*, 1006–1017.

Philip, R. L., & Orr, R. R. (1978). Family Relations as perceived by emotionally disturbed and normal boys. *Journal of Personality Assessment, 42*, 121–127.

Quinton, D., & Rutter, M. (1988). *Parenting breakdown: The making and breaking of intergenerational links.* Aldershot: Avebury Gower.

Richman, N., Stevenson, J., & Graham, P. J. (1982). *Pre-school to school: A behavioral study.* London: Academic Press.

Rust, J., Bennun, I., Crowe, M., & Golombok, S. (1988). *The handbook of the Golombok Rust Inventory of Marital State.* Windsor, UK: NFER-Nelson.

Rust, J., Bennun, I., & Golombok, S. (1990). The GRIMS: A psychometric instrument for the assessment of marital discord. *Journal of Family Therapy, 12*, 45–57.

Rutter, M., Tizard, J., & Whitmore, K. (1970). *Education, health and behaviour.* London: Longman.

Rutter, M., Cox, A., Tupling, C., Berger, M., & Yule, W. (1975). Attainment and adjustment in two geographical areas: I. The prevalence of psychiatric disorder. *British Journal of Psychiatry, 126*, 493–509.

Sants, H. J. (1964). Genealogical bewilderment in children with substitute parents. *British Journal of Medical Psychology, 37*, 133–141.

Schechter, M. D., & Bertocci, D. (1990). The meaning of the search. In D. M. Brodzinsky & M. D. Schechter (Eds.), *The psychology of adoption.* Oxford: Oxford University Press.

Snowden, R. (1990). The family and artificial reproduction. In Bromham et al. (Eds.), *Philosophical ethics in reproductive medicine.* Manchester: Manchester University Press.

Snowden, R., Mitchell, G. D., & Snowden, E. M. (1983). *Artificial reproduction: A social investigation.* London: Allen & Unwin.

Spielberger, C. (1983). *The handbook of the State-Trait Anxiety Inventory.* Palo Alto, CA: Consulting Psychologists Press.

Stevenson, J., Richman, N., & Graham, P. (1985). *Journal of Child Psychology and Psychiatry, 26*, 215–230.

Taylor, E., Sandberg, S., Thorley, G., & Giles, S. (1991). The epidemiology of childhood hyperactivity. *Maudsley Monographs*, Vol. 33, Oxford: Oxford University Press.

Triseliotis, J. (1973). *In search of origins: The experiences of adopted people.* London: Routledge & Kegan Paul.

Warnock, M. (1984). *Report of the Committee of Inquiry into Human Fertilization and Embryology.* London: HMSO.

# 22

# The Identity of Mixed Parentage Adolescents

Barbara Tizard and Ann Phoenix

*Birbeck College, London*

*Theories about "black identity" are discussed in relation to a study of adolescents with one white and one African or African-Caribbean parent. Interview findings on their racial self-definition, attitudes to their mixed parentage, and allegiance to black and white people and cultures reveal a wide range of racial identities and cultural allegiances. Differences are related to type of school, social class, and the degree of politicisation of the young person's attitudes to race. The findings are discussed in relation to the issue of interracial adoption and fostering, and to recent debates about the concept of an "essential" black identity.*

## INTRODUCTION

People of mixed black and white parentage have in the past generally been regarded with hostility, contempt or pity by white people, because of fears that they would dilute "white blood" with the qualities of an inferior race. Reflecting this, the terms used for them until very recently always had offensive connotations of animal breeding—mulatto (Portuguese for a young mule), metis (French for a mongrel dog), half-breed, and half caste. We use

---

Reprinted with permission from the *Journal of Child Psychology and Psychiatry*, 1995, Vol. 36, No. 8, 1399–1410. Copyright © 1995 by the Association for Child Psychology and Psychiatry.

The authors would like to acknowledge the help of the Department of Health, who funded the research, the research interviewers, the teachers and young people in the schools where we worked, and Charlie Owen, for his as yet unpublished analyses of recent Census and Labour Force Survey data referred to in this article.

the term "of mixed parentage," to avoid the biological overtones of "mixed race", and in this article we use "black" to refer only to those with two African or African-Caribbean parents.

The status of mixed parentage people has varied widely. In some countries they were accorded an intermediate status by white people, as inferior to whites, but superior to black people. In some of these countries they have been numerous enough to form a viable community, with their own schools, newspapers, politicians and poets (Gist & Dworkin, 1972). In Brazil, where they form the majority of the population, mixed parentage is not a matter of opprobrium. The U.S.A. on the other hand, after the abolition of slavery, refused to recognise an intermediate "racial" group. People with "one drop of black blood" were classified as black, and the majority of states retained laws against intermarriage until after the end of the Second World War. It is probably because of this history that black-white marriages, although increasing, are still rare in the U.S.A. (Root, 1992).

In Britain, where until the mid 1950s the black population was very small and mainly male, intermarriage, although stigmatised, has always occurred, and has lately markedly increased (Coleman, 1985). The 1987–89 Labour Force Surveys showed that of "West Indians" under the age of 30 who were married or cohabiting, 27% of men and 28% of women had a white partner. As a consequence of this recent increase, the 1991 Census found that of all mixed white and black *people* in Britain, 45% are under the age of 10, compared with 15% of those with two black parents, and 12% of those with two white parents (Owen, in preparation). But the overall number of these children is still very small. The 1991 Census found that only 0.39% of British children aged 0–4, and 0.16% of those aged 15–19, were classified as of mixed black and white origin (Owen, in preparation).

The racial identity of people of mixed parentage has been discussed, mainly by sociologists, since the thirties in the U.S.A. (Park, 1931; Stonequist, 1937) and the fifties in Britain (Little, 1948; Collins, 1957). Stonequist's theory that they are "marginal men", rejected by both white and black people, and in consequence inevitably maladjusted, gained widespread acceptance. According to Stonequist, there were only two ways in which people of mixed parentage could escape from their tormented state: by joining the white group, if they could "pass" as white, with all the denial and betrayal this involved, or by identifying with the stigmatised black group.

Politically conscious black people have always argued that the latter course is the only acceptable one, and in the seventies in the U.S.A. and the eighties in Britain they raised the issue in relation to transracial adoption and fostering. A black Director of Social Services urged that mixed parentage children "are regarded as black by society and eventually the majority of such children will identify with blacks, except in instances where reality and self-image have not merged" (Small, 1986). He argued that mixed parentage children brought up by white people will fail to develop a positive black identity, suffer confusion, be rejected by white people, and also by black people "for not being black enough in culture and attitude". He went on to argue that the term "mixed race" is in any case inappropriate, since the majority of African-Caribbeans have some white ancestors, and differ from those of "mixed race" only in the time at which the mixture occurred.

These views on the identity of mixed parentage people, widely accepted by British professionals, have recently been challenged in the U.S.A. Following a marked increase of interracial marriages, especially between Japanese and white people, there are estimated to be one million "biracial" children in the U.S.A. During the eighties many organisations of biracial and multiracial people were set up, with the aim of affirming and celebrating their mixed origins. They argue that "marginality" has been created by forcing either/or choices on mixed parentage people, many of whom neither wish nor need to choose between their heritages. Instead, they prefer to include both in their identity (Root, 1992).

Empirical evidence on the identity of mixed parentage people is scanty. There are clinical reports of mixed parentage youth exhibiting identity confusion and low self esteem, but remarkably few studies of the racial identity of those who are not clinic cases. Such evidence as there is, casts doubt on the theory that mixed parentage people generally experience identity problems. An early study of American Jews, whose parents had immigrated from Eastern Europe, found that only a small minority felt isolated or torn between two cultures. Many maintained that they were comfortable with an identity as *both* Jewish and American (Antonovsky, 1956). Thirty years later Wilson (1987) explored the identity of 6–9-year-old British children with one white and one African or African-Caribbean parent, using photographs of black, white and mixed parentage children. She concluded that the majority regarded themselves as "half-and-half", and were quite happy with this intermediate identity. It is possible that identity problems are more common in adolescence, although a small U.S. nonclinical study of black-white "biracial" adolescents found few problems (Gibbs & Hines, 1992). However, in both this study and Wilson's the results may have been influenced by the sampling method, which involved recruiting subjects by "snowballing" from interracial organisations.

In the study reported below the authors attempted to obtain a more representative sample of mixed parentage adolescents through the school system. We were particularly interested in the influence of social class and gender, since these variables have, until very recently, been ignored in discussions of racial identity. The study was part of a larger one which included white adolescents and those with two black parents, and which also addressed aspects of social class and gender identity. The findings reported here concern the racial identities and cultural allegiances of the mixed parentage young people, in particular whether they identified as black or white, or felt marginal, i.e. not accepted by either white or black people, or confused about their identity, whether they felt allegiance to black or white culture, and whether those with black identities were most likely to feel positive about their racial identity. Other issues, including their experiences of racism, and their strategies for coping with it, are reported elsewhere (Tizard & Phoenix, 1993), as are the findings of interviews with a sample of their parents. The main findings on the black and white sample, and comparisons between these groups and the mixed parentage group, are reported elsewhere (Phoenix & Tizard, in press).

## METHOD

### *Subjects*

In an attempt to obtain a representative sample of young people the authors approached the Directors of the then Inner London Education Authority and four other authorities in the London area for permission to carry out our research in their secondary schools. Having received permission at this level, we were then able to seek permission from the heads of those schools which were within relatively easy reach of central London, other than a few schools which Directors had asked us not to approach because they were in difficulties, and one which was shortly to close. We explained that we wanted to interview fifth formers (aged 15–16) who had one white and one African or African-Caribbean parent, or two African-Caribbean parents, and an equal number of white students. Generally, the heads consulted their staff before making a decision.

We aimed to work in a variety of schools, both multiracial and predominantly white, to see whether these variables influenced outcomes. Our original aim was to interview 12 young people from each school we visited, a working class girl and boy, and a middle class girl and boy, from each of the three "racial" groups. This proved to be totally unrealistic. The predominantly white schools often had no black or mixed parentage students in our age group, and the multiracial schools sometimes had no middle class students of any colour in our age group. Mixed parentage students were particularly hard to find. As described above, they constitute a very small proportion of then age group. Whilst this proportion must be substantially larger in London (the statistics are not available) mixed percentage 15-year-olds would still form less than 1% of their age group. It was also very difficult to locate young black people from middle class families, since the middle class black population of an age to have adolescent children is very small in Britain.

We therefore, extended our search to all the large and medium sized independent (private) schools, listed in a handbook of such schools, in and around London. Those schools which did have black and mixed parentage students were often single sex, and did not usually have working class students.

Of the 85 local authority schools which were approached, 12 refused permission, 29 gave permission, and the rest either did not have black or mixed parentage students in our age range, or were so slow in answering letters and phone calls, consulting staff, governors, etc. that we finally abandoned them. Of the 84 independent schools approached, 28 refused permission, 29 both had suitable students and gave permission for the research, whilst the rest did not have any black or mixed parentage students in our age range, or were dilatory about making up their minds. The most frequent reasons for refusal were that they did not want their students to be distracted from school work, or that they had had too many researchers in the school lately, or that they thought that interviews about "race" would disturb or divide the students.

The final sample was made up of 101 white students, 89 black, and 58 of mixed percentage. This article is confined to data on the mixed parentage group, who were attending 32 different schools. So far as we knew, they comprised all the mixed parentage young people aged 14 or over in the schools we visited.

Table 1 shows that of the mixed parentage sample, most were aged 15 or 16. Seventy two per cent were girls. This disproportion in gender was in part because we found mixed parentage subjects, and received permission to work, in 13 independent girls' schools, but in only five independent boys' schools, but there was also a preponderance of girls in our sample from state schools. Half the sample attended independent schools, where there were usually at most only one or two students in the year of African or African-Caribbean origin, although there was often a substantial minority from Asian or Arab families. In contrast, the local authority schools in our sample were almost all racially very mixed.

Fifty seven per cent of the young people lived with both their parents, the next most frequent arrangement was to live with a single white mother. We categorised social class by the occupation of the father in two parent

TABLE 1
Sample Characteristics of Mixed Parentage Group

|  | N | % |
|---|---|---|
| Parental social class: |  |  |
| I and II | 35 | 64 |
| III. IV. V | 22 | 39 |
| Mother's origin: |  |  |
| Britain, Ireland, Europe (all but one white) | 43 | 74 |
| Caribbean (all black) | 11 | 19 |
| African (all black) | 4 | 7 |
| Father's origin: |  |  |
| Britain, Ireland, Europe (all but one white) | 18 | 31 |
| Caribbean (all black) | 25 | 43 |
| African (all black) | 15 | 26 |
| Child's age: |  |  |
| 14 years | 10 | 17 |
| 15–16 years | 39 | 67 |
| 17–18 years | 9 | 15 |
| Child's gender: |  |  |
| Female | 42 | 72 |
| Male | 16 | 28 |
| Type of school attended: |  |  |
| Independent | 32 | 55 |
| Local authority | 26 | 45 |
| Predominantly white | 34 | 59 |
| Multiracial | 24 | 41 |
| Family Structure: |  |  |
| Both parents | 33 | 57 |
| Single parent | 17 | 29 |
| Parent and step parent | 6 | 10 |
| Sister, family friend | 2 | 3 |
| Racial Composition of Family: |  |  |
| Two parents, black and white | 35 | 60 |
| Single white parent/white parent and white step parent | 16 | 28 |
| Single black parent/black parent and black step parent | 7 | 12 |

households, or in the case of single mothers, the mother. Sixty one per cent of the parents were in professional or managerial occupations (social class 1 or 2). Most fathers were black, most mothers, white. Seventy-two per cent of the sample lived with a black parent. Most of these young people lived with both their parents, but a small number lived with a black parent and black step parent, on a single black parent. The social class categorisation of those living with a black parent or with a white parent only, generally a single mother, was almost identical. Although some of our single mothers were living on benefit, more were professional women.

## Interviews

The interviews were semi-structured, made up of mostly open-ended questions, asked in a predetermined order with predetermined wording, although the interviewers were free to ask any additional questions they saw fit to clarify meanings. Almost all took place in schools, usually in an empty classroom. Seventy eight per cent of the interviews of the mixed parentage students were carried out by two black women, one of whom was one of the authors, the rest by two white women. The interviewers did five preliminary tape recorded "training interviews" each, with nonsample subjects, after which the tape recordings were used to discuss the conduct of the interview and the codings with one of the authors. Instead of relying on a one-off initial calculation of inter-rater reliability, we aimed at complete agreement throughout. That is, after initial training the interviews were subsequently coded by the interviewers from the tape-recordings, and then checked against the interview transcripts by one or other of the authors, who in cases of disagreement consulted each other. Ratings of positive, problematic and intermediate identity were made by the two authors in consultation. Whilst this was time consuming, it ensured that coding was always agreed upon by at least two people. The interviews, which included questions not reported here on gender and social class, usually lasted between an hour and an hour and a half, the maximum time available in a school setting.

## Variables

Most of the findings relate to answers to single questions, reported later in the text. In addition, the following four composite variables were used in the main statistical analysis. They were obtained by summing the scores to several questions. "*Holding more politicised attitudes*" was summed from whether the terms half-caste and coloured were not used; whether racism was described as coming only from white people; whether racist name-calling was said to be racist in all circumstances: whether they believed that if they were white their future would be easier, if black, more difficult. *Affiliation to white people* was summed from whether they had any, or mainly, white friends, and also close white friends, whether they were more comfortable with white people, whether they would prefer their future partner to be white, whether they would prefer to live in a white area, and whether they named any white people when asked whether they had any heroes or heroines. *Affiliation to black people* was a separate, corresponding score. *Affiliation to black youth culture* was summed from whether they expressed a preference for any form of black youth music, and black youth fashions, and listened to black radio stations. If one of the questions in these summed scores had not been asked of all subjects, usually because the interview had to be curtailed, the sample number for that score was reduced.

In the statistical analysis, for comparisons involving these summed scores the Kruskal-Wallis non-parametric one-way analysis of variance was used, for cross tabulations, the Pearson $\chi^2$.

## RESULTS

### Racial Self Definition

When asked if they ever described people as "black", all but two of the mixed parentage sample said that they did at times. However, when asked whom they included in the term, only 46% included mixed parentage people. The rest confined its use to those with two African or African-Caribbean parents. In answer to a later question directed at the mixed parentage sample only, about whether they regarded *themselves* as black, 39% said that they did, a further 10% said that they did in certain situations, whilst 49% said that they did not. Instead, these young people regarded themselves as "brown", "half and half", "mixed", or, as well as, or instead of these terms, "coloured". None identified themselves as white, but 10% said that they "sometimes felt white", or that they "felt more white than black". Eighty percent used an additional term to refer to their mixed ancestry, most often "half-caste" (43%) or "mixed race" (24%). None used "mixed parentage".

The term 'half-caste' was used more frequently, but not significantly so, by students coming from a working class family. Describing themselves as "black" was not related to social class, nor to living with a black parent. It was, however, strongly related to a set of attitudes about racism which we have called politicised (Table 2). There was also some evidence that calling themselves black was related to appearance, since, of the nine young people who looked south European, only one thought of themselves as black.

### Attitudes to Their Mixed Parentage

The great majority of the mixed parentage young people—86% said that they did not want to be another colour, although 51% said that in the past they had done so. Eighty one per cent said that they were pleased to be of

TABLE 2
Associations of Identity with Political Attitudes, Affiliation,
Parental Messages, and Type of School

|  | Statistics | $\chi^2$ | $p$ | $N$ |
|---|---|---|---|---|
| Thinking of self as black with more politicised attitudes | K–W* | 9.1 | .003 | 54 |
| Wanting to be another colour now with strength of affiliation to white people | K–W | 4.5 | .03 | 50 |
| Having a problematic identity with parents telling to be proud | Pearson $\chi^2$ | 6.9 | .03 | 56 |
| Having a positive identity with attending a multiracial school | Pearson $\chi^2$ | 3.6 | .06 | 56 |

\* Kruskal–Wallis one-way analysis of rank.

mixed parentage, and 77% said that they were proud of their mixed parentage. Later, to a slightly differently worded question, "How do you feel, now that you are 15 (or whatever age they were) about having one white and one black parent?" 76% again gave positive answers.

In answer to the question whether there was any way in which they would like to alter their appearance, the most frequent response was a wish to lose weight. No one said they wanted to look fairer, but about a fifth of the sample would have preferred in some respects to look like a white person, in that they wanted long hair they could toss or flick, or in one case, green eyes. The great majority, 75%, said they had no preference for marrying someone of a particular colour, the rest being about equally divided between a preference for a white or a black partner.

We assessed as having a definitely positive "racial" identity the 60% of the sample who said that they felt both pleased and proud to be of mixed parentage, and who, even it in the past they had wished to be another colour, no longer did so. We excluded anyone who, despite giving these answers to direct questions, made comments during the interview which suggested that they might be in any way anxious, confused or troubled about their parentage. We assessed a further 20% as having a problematic identity, in that they now wished to be another colour, and/or made spontaneous comments which suggested that they were unhappy or anxious about their parentage. We regarded their identity as "problematic", rather than negative, because all, to a varying extent, expressed contradictory feelings, for example, liking to be of mixed parentage because it was interestingly "different", but sometimes wishing to be white. The remaining 20% whilst not wishing to be another colour, were not definitely positive about their racial identity.

Having a positive racial identity was not associated with thinking of one-self as black, or with living with a black parent, or coming from a particular social class, or holding politicised views. There was a tendency for it to be associated with attendance at a multiracial school, whilst a problematic identity was associated with a strong affiliation to white people, and para-doxically, with reporting that their parents had told them to be proud of being black, or of mixed parentage (Table 2). A possible explanation for this latter finding is that parents who considered that their children were experiencing problems with their racial identities were more likely to at-tempt to boost their morale by telling them that they should be proud of their colour than those whose children seemed confident.

### Friendships and Allegiances

Two thirds of the sample said that they felt equally comfortable with white and black people, with rather more of the rest feeling uncomfortable with black people than white. And whilst 85% had a close white friend, only 42% had a close black friend; 27% had no black friends. Similarly, of those who said they had a boy or girl friend, 78% said that he or she was white, and only 44%, black. However, three quarters said that they had no colour preference for a marriage partner, and most said they they would prefer to live in a racially mixed area (68%) or that they had no preference about the racial mix of their area (19%).

We gave each of the young people two scores, for the strength of their affiliation to white and to black people (see Method section). Those most strongly affiliated to black people were those attending multiracial and state schools, and those living with a *white* parent only (Table 3). Those most strongly affiliated to white people were those attending mainly white and Independent schools, and those living with a *black* parent.

Flourishing black youth cultures have developed in British cities, fo-cused on new forms of music, each with its own subculture, ideology, and distinctive clothes style. Some form of black music was the favourite music of half the mixed parentage sample—the most popular kind was soul—a quarter of the white sample, and four fifths of the black sample. However, only 27% of the mixed parentage sample preferentially listened to black radio stations, and only 20% wore black youth styles. Those with the strongest allegiance to a black youth culture were those who attended mul-tiracial schools, and state schools, and who came from working class fam-ilies (Table 3). The great majority, 73%, thought of themselves as English

TABLE 3
Associations with Affiliation to Black and White People with Type of School,
Family Composition and Social Class

|  | $\chi^2$ | $p$ | $N$ |
|---|---|---|---|
| Affiliation to black people with attending multiracial schools | 14.0 | .000 | 49 |
| Affiliation to black people with attending state schools | 13.2 | .003 | 49 |
| Affiliation to black people with living with white parent(s) only | 4.9 | .03 | 49 |
| Affiliation to white people with attending mainly white schools | 7.4 | .006 | 51 |
| Affiliation to white people with attending independent schools | 6.2 | .02 | 51 |
| Affiliation to white people with living with black parent(s) | 5.5 | .02 | 51 |
| Affiliation to Black Youth Cultures with being working class | 5.7 | .02 | 51 |
| Affiliation to Black Youth Cultures with attending multiracial schools | 8.6 | .003 | 55 |
| Affiliation to Black Youth Cultures with attending state schools | 6.7 | .01 | 55 |

The values are derived from a Kruskal–Wallis one-way Anova.

or British, rather than as partly or wholly of the nationality of their black parent. For many, a stronger identity was a Londoner—65% of the mixed parentage sample said that they felt more of a Londoner than English or British, etc. usually because of its multiracial nature, and because they felt at ease in London.

**Interviewer effects.**  In order to see whether there was a tendency for different responses to be given to different interviewers, the responses of the young people, that is, their summed scores, their responses to the individual questions described above, and the ratings made of their identity as positive or otherwise were compared for three interviewers, two black and one white. The fourth, white interviewer was omitted because she did only two interviews with the mixed parentage sample. Only one significant difference was found. The young people were less likely to tell the white inteviewer that they used the term half-caste ($\chi^2 = 11.1, p = 004$). There was also a tendency, which did not reach significance ($\chi^2 = 5.5, p = 06$) for her to be less often told by the young people that they were pleased to be of mixed parentage. None of the other comparisons of responses approached significance.

**Gender effects.**  The sample characteristics and responses to questions of male and female students were compared as above. No significant differences were found.

## DISCUSSION

Just over half our sample identified themselves as "half and half", "mixed", or "brown", rather than black. This identity was somewhat fluid, since some of those who identified themselves as black subsequently referred to themselves as mixed, whilst some who identified themselves as mixed said that in certain situations they might think of themselves as black. Identifying as black was not related to living with a black parent. It was not related to attending a multiracial school, or to adhering to a black youth culture. There was some evidence that it was related to appearance. It was strongly associated with holding more politicised attitudes about racism. Young people in an all white school, for example, might identify as black when they became politicised, but have no black friends or interest in black youth cultures, whilst those attending multiracial schools might regard themselves as "mixed", but have both black and white friends and admire black styles of music.

A fifth of the sample expressed a feeling of "marginality", in that they said they would prefer to be white, or either white or black, or in one case, black, because they found it painful to stand out in both black and white company as "different"—an experience which others interpreted positively as feeling "interestingly unusual". Only two of these young people talked about themselves in terms which suggested identity confusion.

The majority of our sample were very positive about their mixed heritage. They stressed the advantages of being accepted by both black and white people, of seeing things from both perspectives, or of being "special". Others again saw their mixed family as a witness against racism, or viewed their mixed parentage as part and parcel of their love for their parents.

There are a number of reasons why mixed parentage adolescents today might view their parentage more positively than in the past. Racism has by no means disappeared, but open manifestations of it are considered "out of order" in some secondary schools and neighbourhood networks, whilst black youth cultures and styles are admired by sectors of white youth. Some mixed parentage girls were admired by both black and white students for their skin colour and ringlets, and there are now a few famous mixed parentage "role models", including glamorous fashion models. These factors, together with the increasing liberalisation of white attitudes, and the increasing number of black and white partnerships, make it likely that young people of mixed parentage suffer rejection less often than in the past.

It was not the case that having a positive racial identity was linked to having a black identity, or to living with a black parent. It tended, however, to be associated with attending a multiracial school, whilst wishing to be another colour was associated with having mainly white friends and the cultural tastes predominantly associated with white people. A black and mixed peer group, then, seemed more important than living with a black parent in helping the young people to feel positive about their racial identity.

Most of the young people had at times experienced racial abuse, and thus rejection, from white people, and in a minority of cases from black people also (Tizard & Phoenix, 1993), but, despite this, they tended to have closer links to white people than to black. Thus, whilst the majority said that they felt equally comfortable with white or black people, and the great majority had both black and white friends, twice as many had close white friends as had black. This was probably a result of limited opportunity, since more than half were attending schools with very few black students.

Paradoxically, those most affiliated to white people were more likely to live with a black parent, usually in a two parent setting, than those living with a white parent only. This finding is difficult to interpret, particularly since family type is confounded with colour—most single parents were white. Factors which we did not assess, such as the racial composition of the neighbourhood, parent-child relationships, or parental political views and attitudes to race, may have been involved.

The cultural allegiances of the young people were not related to the colour of the parent they lived with, but to their social class, and their peer group. Those who were enthusiastic adherents of black music and clothes styles were more likely to attend multiracial state schools and come from working class families.

Despite efforts to achieve a gender balance, 72% of our sample were girls. This was in part because 13 independent girls' schools, but only five boys', gave us permission to work in their schools, but the gender imbalance was also present in the state schools. It is particularly difficult to interpret because it was not present in the black sample, where only 54% were girls (Phoenix & Tizard, in press), so that hypotheses such as that school staff put fewer boys forward because they were seen as less desirable interviewees, or that boys are more often absent through truanting, are difficult to sustain. However, in fact there were no significant gender differences in any of the responses reported above. This could arguably be because the number of boys in the sample was so small, but we did find significant gender differences in the same sample in reported experiences of racism (Tizard & Phoenix, 1993).

There is some evidence, mainly from the USA, that both black and white people tend to give different answers to questions with a racial content, according to the colour of the interviewer (Schaeffer, 1980). For this reason we aimed to "colour match" interviewers and interviewees. Since we did not find any mixed parentage interviewers we decided to use black interviewers for the mixed parentage group. However, for logistical reasons 22% of the interviews had to be carried out by two white interviewers, one of whom was omitted from the analysis of interviewer effects because she did only two interviews with the mixed parentage sample. In the great majority of cases there was no difference in the proportions of different types of responses given to the three interviewers, but significantly fewer young people told the white interviewer that they used the term "half-caste". It is not possible to know whether this difference was due to her colour, her age (she was older than the other two) or to some other factor.

We do not wish to generalise from our study to all young people of mixed parentage. Identity is likely to vary with age—half the sample said that in the past they had wanted to be another colour, whilst only 14% said they did so now. From their accounts, developmental improvements in both their understanding of racial abuse and their ability to cope with it were involved in this change. Samples with a different social class and gender distribution, carried out in different parts of Britain, might reveal a different pattern of findings. But our study does reveal a wide variety of "racial" identities and cultural allegiances amongst our mixed parentage sample, some of the variation being related to social class, type of school, and politicised attitudes. There was no evidence that a "biracial" identity adversely affected wellbeing. But is a "biracial" identity, as has been argued, a false identity, since others would see the young people as black? This argument confuses two meanings of "black". The young people's appearance ranged from African-Caribbean to European, with some looking like Pakistanis, but most would be seen as black in the sense of not white. However, whilst not denying this reality, many, like many Asians, would also claim an identity that differed from that of African-Caribbeans, in this case, a bi-racial identity.

In any case, the assumption that there is a single, "essential" black culture and identity is now disputed. Some black theorists point to the need to recognise the extraordinary diversity of black identities and cultural practices. Young black people construct their ethnicity not only from their roots in the Caribbean and Africa, but also from their own individual experience of being British. This experience varies with gender, social class, and education, and nowadays includes the impact of global cultural practices. Hence, it is argued, the terms race and ethnicity, which tend to be used interchangeably, should be recognised as distinct and different categories, (Gilroy, 1992; Hall, 1992; Katz, 1995).

We believe that our study raises questions about some of the assumptions underlying social work policy. The assumption that mixed parentage children "need" to acquire a black identity and culture implicitly denigrates their mixed background, and denies their right to construct identities that are both black and white. It shapes not only social work policy but is enshrined in official statistics—the 1991 Census offers no "mixed" category, the nearest options being "Black other" or "Any other ethnic group". A second assumption is that the colour of foster or adoptive parents is of paramount importance in the development of a positive racial identity.

It would clearly be unacceptable to allow children to be fostered or adopted by anyone, whether white or black, who was hostile to, or even unenthusiastic about, one half of the child's inheritance. But our findings suggest that during adolescence, school, social class, and peer groups exert more influence on racial identities than the colour of their parents.

## REFERENCES

Antonovsky, A. (1956). Towards a refinement of the 'Marginal Man' concept. *Social Forces, 35*, 57–62.

Coleman, D. (1985). Ethnic intermarriage in Great Britain. *Population Trends, 40*, 4–10.

Collins, S. (1957). *Coloured minorities in Great Britain*. Guildford: Lutterworth Press.

Gibbs, J. & Hines, A. (1992). Negotiating ethnic identity. In M Root (Ed.), *Racially mixed people in America* (pp. 223–238) London: Sage Publications.

Gilroy, P. (1992). The end of antiracism. In J. Donald & A. Rattansi (Eds), *Race, culture and difference*, (pp. 49–61). London: Sage Publications.

Gist, N. P. & Dworkin, A. G. (1972) *The blending of races: marginality and identity in World perspective*. New York: John Wiley and Sons.

Hall, S. (1992). New ethnicities. In J. Donald & A. Rattansi (Eds), *Race, culture and difference* (pp. 252–258) London: Sage Publications

Katz, I (1995) Anti-racism and modernism. In M Yelloly & M Henkel (Eds), *Learning and teaching in social work. Towards reflective practice* (p. 120–135) London: Jessica Kingsley.

Little, K. (1948) *Negroes in Britain*. London: Routledge and Kegan Paul.

Owen, C. (in preparation) Mixed ethnic groups in the 1991 Census.

Park, R. (1931). The mentality of racial hybrids. *American Journal of Sociology, 36*, 534–551.

Phoenix, A. & Tizard, B. (in press). *The social identities of young Londoners*. London Routledge.

Root, M. (1992). Within, between, and beyond race. In M. Root (Ed.), *Racially mixed people in America* (pp. 3–11). London: Sage Publications.

Schaeffer, N. C. (1980). Evaluating race of interviewer effects in a national survey. *Sociological Methods and Research, 8,* 400–419.

Small, J. (1986). Transracial placements: conflicts and contradictions. In S. Ahmed, J. Cheetham & J. Small (Eds), *Social work with Black children and their families* (pp. 81–99). London: Batsford.

Stonequist, E. V. (1937). *The marginal man: a study of personality and culture.* New York: Russell and Russell.

Tizard, B. & Phoenix, A. (1993). *Black, white or mixed race? Race and racism in the lives of young people of mixed parentage* London: Routledge.

Wilson, A. (1987). *Mixed race children, a study of identity.* London: Allen and Unwin.

# 23

# The Orphans of Eritrea: A Comparison Study

**Peter H. Wolff**
*Children's Hospital, Boston*

**Bereket Tesfai**
*Ministry of Social Affairs, Asmara, Republic of Eritrea*

**Habtab Egasso**
*Ministry of Social Affairs, Asmara, Republic of Eritrea*

**Tesfay Aradom**
*Boston College, Chestnut Hill*

*The social-emotional state and cognitive development was compared between a group of 74 4–7-year-old Eritrean orphans and refugee children living in families. Both groups had been exposed to the chronic stresses of war and drought, and the orphans had, in addition, lost both parents to the violence of war, and were living in an overcrowded orphanage. Contrary to expectations, there were relatively few clinically significant differences between comparison groups. The orphans showed more behavioral symptoms of emotional distress, but performed at a more advanced level on cognitive and language performance measures. The findings suggest that when group care is child-centered, it can under some circumstances be a viable so-*

Reprinted with permission from the *Journal of Child Psychology and Psychiatry*, 1995, Vol. 36, No. 4, 633–644. Copyright © 1995 by the Association for Child Psychology and Psychiatry.

We gratefully acknowledge the financial support of a research grant from the William T. Grant Foundation, and additional support from Redd Barna, Norwegian Save the Children Foundation. The authors would also like to thank Gebremeskel Fessaha, Yemani Dawit and Berhane Zere of the Eritrean Ministry of Social Affairs, and the entire staff of the Solomuna Orphanage for their support and encouragement. Without their help, the study could not have been carried out.

*lution for unaccompanied children in countries where adoption
and foster care are not realistic alternatives.*

## INTRODUCTION

There is widespread consensus that permanent separation of young children from both parents at an early age exposes them to increased risk for
major psychiatric illnesses in later life (Bowlby, 1980; Crook & Eliot,
1980). However, epidemiological studies suggest that the relation between
the loss of parents at an early age and adult psychopathology is weak
(Ragan & McGlashan, 1986), and that the many disruptions in the social
life of children after the death of a parent, rather than the death itself, may
explain most of the long term consequences (Rutter, 1980). Finally, there
is evidence to indicate that considerable recovery from early psychological traumas is not only possible but common (Anthony, 1987; Garmezy,
1983, 1984; Werner & Smith, 1982); and that timely intervention can in
many cases protect children against the adverse consequences of early loss
(Rutter, 1980, 1981).

At the present time, thousands of children in Third World countries are
permanently separated from their parents and dislocated from their homes
due to the violence and social disorganization of war. In developed countries, the traditional solution of caring for unaccompanied infants and children was to place them in large orphanages, where many of them suffered
severe and sometimes irreversible physical and psychological damage
(Goldfarb, 1945; Spitz, 1949). Such experiences led to the general conclusion that the group rearing of abandoned children is inherently destructive
and incompatible with normal psychological development (Bowlby, 1958,
1960; WHO, 1951). Adoption and foster care were therefore identified as
the only humane remedies for unaccompanied children.

Yet, group care for unaccompanied children has improved considerably
over the past 30 years (Tizard & Hodges, 1978). On the other hand, some
investigators have questioned whether foster care necessarily serves the
best interest of young children (Gruber, 1978; Rein, Nutt & Weiss, 1974).
Perhaps most important in the context of this report, the majority of unaccompanied children are now concentrated in developing countries where
adoption and foster care are often not realistic solutions. Humanitarian relief agencies have estimated, for example, that over half a million children
in the Sudan, Ethiopia, Eritrea and Mozambique have been orphaned by recurrent wars in the Horn of Africa. The problem of caring for unaccompanied children is probably as great or greater in other regions of Africa, Central America, and Eastern Europe (Aboud, Samuel, Hadera & Abdulaziz,

1991; Allodi, 1980; Chimienti, Nasr & Khalifeh, 1989; Cliff & Noorma-homed, 1993; Gibson, 1989; Kinzie, Sack, Angell, Manson & Roth, 1986). Finding sufficient numbers of families to care for abandoned children as well as their own in these countries is at best a remote possibility, espe-cially if there is no tradition of taking in biologically unrelated children. When fostering has been attempted in such countries, the children often become the victims of abuse and neglect (Bledsoe, Ewbank & Isiugo-Abanihe, 1988; Isiugo-Abanihe, 1985).

Some kind of group care probably offers the best hope of survival for virtually millions of unaccompanied children in Third World countries that have been devastated by war. Therefore, the focus of debate and investi-gation must shift from weighing the relative advantages of adoption and foster care, to examining what kinds of group care will best serve the needs of unaccompanied children when technical and financial resources are al-ready strained to the limit.

As a point of departure for addressing this question, we compared the social emotional state and cognitive development of 4–7-year-old orphans living in a large institution and of accompanied children living with at least one parent in their own homes in a neighbouring refugee camp. The study was carried out in Eritrea—a country on the Horn of Africa that had been at war with Ethiopia for at least 28 years when the study began. Eritrea is about the size of Pennsylvania; it borders the Red Sea, and has a popula-tion of about 3 million.

Throughout the war, the Ethiopian Air Force controlled the skies over Eritrea so that the entire economic and social life had been forced under-ground (Pateman, 1990). The war had also displaced thousands of families from their villages and forced them to resettle in refugee camps distributed throughout the countryside, one of which was adjacent to the orphanage. The Solomuna Orphanage and Refugee Camp where these studies were conducted had therefore been hidden in the least accessible and deepest canyons of Northern Eritrea where the children were, however, exposed to some of the harshest living conditions in all of Eritrea.

The Solomuna Orphanage could accommodate only 500 of the many thousands of Eritrean children orphaned by the war. Two years before the comparison study, the 500 children were cared for by a staff of about 120 adults. Most of the staff had no previous experience in caring for children, had received no formal or in-service training in clinical child development and had no children of their own. In addition to looking after the great emo-tional needs of the children, the staff had to gather all of the scarce wood fuel for cooking, and all the water from distant wells, cook all the meals, wash the children as well as their clothing, and constantly guard them against possible exposure to military attack. For purposes of organizational efficiency, the dormitories were arranged so that the children in a tent were all of the same age. Because of a severe shortage of dormitories and beds, from 50 to 70 children lived in each tent, the bunk beds were arranged in rows without any space between them; and younger children slept four to a bed, older children two to a bed. No child care worker was permanently assigned to any group of children. Instead, the staff was systematically rotated through the different groups, so that each staff member would get to know all of the children.

Recognizing that the social organization and physical facilities of the orphanage were grossly inadequate, and that many of the children were suffering from severe physical and emotional deprivation, the Eritrean Department of Social Affairs (DSA) in 1986 asked several outside consultants to survey the orphanage and to make concrete recommendations on how to improve the lives of the orphans (Jareg, 1988; Wolff, 1986). On the basis of these recommendations, the DSA was able to modify the social organization of the orphanage and to reorient the attitudes of the staff, in spite of the constant threat of air raids, the shortage of trained personnel, and the lack of material resources.

When the comparison study was carried out 2 years later, the tents had been replaced with stone houses; there were fewer children in each dormitory; new staff had been appointed after carefully screening candidates for their sensitivity to the needs of children, and the ratio of child care workers to children had been increased. In addition, the staff had been relieved of most ancillary duties, and they had participated in programs of in-service training on clinical child development on a regular basis. A permanent surrogate parent lived with the children as the primary caretaker, and two assistant caretakers were permanently assigned to each dormitory group to help the house mother. Finally, the dormitories had been reorganized to include a balance of older and younger children; and older children assumed some responsibility for looking after and teaching younger children.

The comparison study began in 1990 after the changes described above had been implemented. Most of the data were collected while the war was in progress, but data collection was not completed until shortly after defeat of the Ethiopian Armies in 1991. Children from the neighbouring refugee camp were chosen as the comparison group. However, they were not a 'normal' control group, because they had also been displaced from their homes, lived under the constant threat of bombardment or ground attacks, were exposed to the same chronic food and water shortages as the orphans, and lacked adequate housing, sanitary and recreational facilities. Nevertheless, they seemed the most informative comparison group for this study, because the main group of differences were that the orphans had lost both parents and lived in an overcrowded institution, while the refugee children were living with at least one parent in their own homes. Moreover, a normal control group was essentially inaccessible in Eritrea during the war.

## METHODS AND PROCEDURES

### *Research Personnel*

Two Eritrean members of the research team from the DSA assigned to the Solomuna orphanage had previous experience in clinical field research, were fluent in local languages, were fully conversant with the cultures and also had the trust of the refugee families. They collected all the data on children in the orphanage and refugee camp. The other two investigators had experience in developmental research but were only superficially acquainted with conditions in Eritrea. The four investigators met in several 2–3 week planning sessions at the orphanage to refine and practice the research protocol until they had achieved a satisfactory level of interobserver reliability on formal tests.

### *Samples*

The few children in either site who suffered from major physical handicaps, neurological disorders or frank mental retardation, were excluded before samples were selected. Thereafter, the age distribution of children for the sample was chosen to reflect the age distribution of the orphanage in general. To control for possible differences in the social conditions of the various dormitories children were chosen in alphabetical order from eight different dormitories until a sample of about five girls and five boys from each dormitory had been identified. From this group, equal numbers of boys and girls were chosen for study, to make up a total of 74 orphans. Sample selection was therefore not random in a formal sense. Subsequently, the control sample of 74 refugee children was selected on a case-matched basis from the 650 families living in the refugee camp (see Table 1).

### *Measures*

Where possible, culture-fair standardized psychological tests were chosen to evaluate the children's developmental status. However, the number of such tests relevant to our purposes was limited, and it was necessary to modify several other standardized tests for use with children growing up in rural Eritrea. The children's conversational skills were examined from tape-recorded semi-structured dialogues between the children and investigators.

TABLE 1
Group Characteristics—Study Samples

|                                      | Orphans   | Refugees  |
| ------------------------------------ | --------- | --------- |
| Number                               | 74        | 74        |
| Sex (female/male)                    | 39/35     | 36/38     |
| Age                                  |           |           |
| Mean (*SD*)                          | 5.7 (0.9) | 5.7 (0.9) |
| Age Distribution (*N*)               |           |           |
| 4-years                              | 5         | 5         |
| 5-years                              | 34        | 31        |
| 6-years                              | 17        | 19        |
| 7-years                              | 18        | 19        |
| Mean length of stay at orphanage     | 2.7 (1.6) | *         |

* 70% of refugee children had either been born in the camp or had arrived there before the age of 3 months. All others had come before their second birthday.

### (A) Social-Emotional Development

Behavioral Screening Questionnaires (BSQ) for preschool children (Richman, Stevenson & Graham, 1975) were completed by the field investigators during interviews with the orphans' primary care takers and the refugee children's parents. The 25-item questionnaire sampled six major adaptive domains including eating, sleeping, psychosomatic complaints, quality of social interactions and language development.

### (B) Intelligence

(1) *The Letter International Intelligence Scale.* (Letter, 1969), which was developed for cross-cultural comparisons and testing verbally handicapped children, and had been standardized for children from 2 to 12 years.

(2) *The Raven Progressive Matrices. (Coloured Series; Raven, 1958).* This is used extensively in Europe and Africa as a culture-fair measure of general intellectual ability, but sometimes used as a test of spatial abilities in North America.

### (C) Language

(1) *Receptive language.* The short version of the Token test that includes 16 combinations of tokens at increasing levels of difficulty was used (McNeal & Prescott, 1978).

(2) *Language pragmatics*. Each child was interviewed individually by one of the field investigators who initiated dialogues with open ended questions and encouraged the children to tell stories. Conversations were conducted in the local languages, tape recorded, translated into English, and analyzed off line for conversational style, turn-taking and coherence of connected discourse.

(3) *Expressive language*. A standardized test of expressive language based on the confrontation naming of line drawings (Gardner, 1990) was modified by substituting three-dimensional objects for pictures. However, the number of available objects that Eritrean children might be expected to recognize was limited. Nearly all children scored at or near the ceiling, and the results will not be reported.

## *(D) Physical Status*

(1) Carefully maintained medical records provided information about the history of debilitating illnesses, nutritional status and the like of each child.

(2) The Extended Pediatric Examination for minor neurological signs (Touwen & Prechtl, 1970) and the Halstead-Reitan version of the Grooved Peg Board for children (Reitan, 1969) were administered. Results of the neurological examination were scored for total number of signs, as well as for the subtotals of "pathological" and "developmental" signs (Wolff, Gunnoe & Cohen, 1983). Performance on the pegboard was scored for the time to complete the task with the right hand and the left hand, as well as for the number of pegs dropped by each hand.

## RESULTS

Given the magnitude of the environmental stresses experienced by the orphans, the findings of greatest interest were (1) that the differences between the orphans and refugee children were less than had been anticipated on the basis of the first survey 2 years before the social reorganization of the orphanage; and (2) that not all of the differences were in the anticipated direction.

### *Social-Emotional Status*

As expected, the orphans exhibited more behavioral symptoms than refugee children. Group differences were first computed by an analysis of variance, with group (orphans, refugee children) and age (younger, older) as classifying variables, and total number of behavioral symptoms per child as the outcome variable. There was a main effect by group, $F(1, 141) = 14.6$, $p < .0001$, and a group $\times$ age interaction, $F(1, 141 = 9.78; p = .0024$, but no main effect by age. *Post hoc* comparisons indicated that only the younger orphans (4–5 years old) showed significantly more behavioral symptoms than refugee children ($p < .05$), whereas children in the older comparison groups did not differ. Because there was a weak correlation between chronological age and length of stay in the orphanage, the higher incidence of behavioral symptoms among younger orphans might have been related to the anxiety created by the unfamiliarity of the setting when they first arrived at the institution. The frequency of behavioral symptoms was therefore reanalyzed with length of stay in the orphanage as a co-variate. This analysis indicated that the higher incidence of behavioral symptom among younger orphans was related only to their chronological age.

The two groups differed in each behavioral domain (eating, sleeping, psychosomatic complaints, social interactions, language development, and habit patterns; see Table 2), but a detailed item analysis indicated that one or two specific symptoms in each domain accounted for most of the differences (Figure 1). For example, enuresis was the only specific symptom among the sleep disturbances that was significantly more common in orphans than refugee children ($\chi^2 = 21.2, p < .0001, df\ 1$). Although the orphans also had more difficulty falling or staying asleep, and some of them were sleepwalkers, the group differences were not statistically significant. Similarly, the orphans were more aggressive in their interactions with peers ($\chi^2 = 7.6, p < .02, df\ 1$), and adults ($\chi^2 = 7.3, p < .2, df\ 1$). On the other hand, and contrary to expectations, the refugee children had significantly more irrational fears about animals, the dark, strange noises and the like than orphans ($\chi^2 = 13.4, p < .001, df\ 1$). There were no sex differences on

TABLE 2
Standardized test results

|                                | Orphans      | Refugees     | P       |
| ------------------------------ | ------------ | ------------ | ------- |
| Behavioral inventory           | 8.47 (5.2)   | 5.77 (3.4)   | <.0001  |
| Raven matrices                 | 13.3  (3.6)  | 11.50 (3.0)  | <.0008  |
| Leiter international            | 6.0   (1.4)  | 5.6   (1.3)  | <.005   |
| Token test                     | 7.0   (4.8)  | 5.4   (4.0)  | <.0004  |
| Naming confrontation           | 22.9  (2.1)  | 23.3  (1.7)  | NS      |
| Neuromotor                     | 5.7   (4.8)  | 5.6   (5.8)  | NS      |
| Purdue peg board (R + L/2)     | 2.0   (1.5)  | 1.9   (1.5)  | NS      |

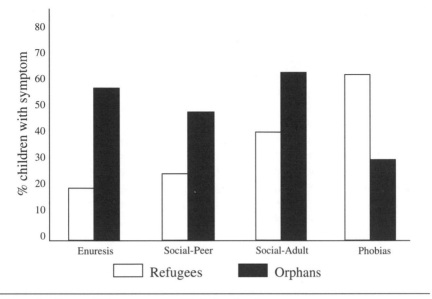

**Figure 1.** Group differences: specific behavioral symptoms.

any behavioral symptom except that enuresis was, as expected, more common in boys than girls.

### Intellectual and Language Development

Group differences in cognitive and language development were computed by similar analyses of variance, with group (orphans, refugees), sex, age and summary BSQ scores (above and below the median within group) as between subjects variable, and performance on individual language and cognitive tests as dependent measures.

**Leiter international scale.** In addition to the expected main effect by age ($F(1, 122) = 105.9, p = .0001$), there were main effects by group, ($F(1, 122) = 12.0, p = .0008$), and by BSQ scores, ($F(1, 122) = 4.1, p = .046$). Contrary to expectation, the orphans performed at a more advanced developmental level than refugee children. The frequency of behavioral symptoms was inversely correlated with performance on the Leiter scale. There were no main or interaction effects by sex.

**Raven matrices.** Aside from the expected main effect by age ($F(1, 116)$ = 12.6, $p$ = .0006), there was a main effect by group, ($F(1, 116)$ = 8.4, $p$ = .0045), and an age $\times$ group interaction, ($F(1, 116)$ = 6.61, $p$ = .011), but no main or interaction effects by BSQ score. The orphans performed at a more advanced level than refugee children, but these group differences were limited to 6–7-year-old children ($p$ < .05). There were no main or interaction effects by sex.

**Token tests.** In addition to the main effect by age, ($F(1, 120)$ = 89.7, $p$ = .0001), there was a main effect by group, ($F(1, 120)$ = 7.5, $p$ = .0004), and a group $\times$ age interaction ($F(1, 120)$ = 13.5, $p$ = .0001). Orphans performed at a more advanced level than refugee children, but these group differences were limited to 6–7-year-old children ($p$ < .05). There were no main or interaction effects by sex.

**Neuromotor status.** Age had expected main effects on the sum of minor neurological signs, ($F(1, 115)$ = 13.2, $p$ = .0004), and on performance speed of the Purdue Pegboard, ($F(1, 118)$ = 23.7, $p$ = .0001). The BSQ score also had a main effect on neuromotor status ($F(1, 115)$ = 6.5, $p$ = .011), but there were no main effects by group and no interaction effects. In both groups, children with more behavioral symptoms also exhibited more neuromotor signs. There were no main or interaction effects by group or sex on either set of neurological measures.

**Language pragmatics.** The war ended suddenly while the study was still in progress; and the refugee families were immediately returned to their villages, while the orphans were transferred to the capital in Asmara to await long term placement. Therefore, there was only enough time to record open ended conversations with 20 refugee children and 20 orphans; and under the time pressure of relocation, most of the recorded dialogues were not detailed enough for a planned quantitative socio-linguistic analyses. The available English transcripts did, however, suggest that the children in both groups understood the function of a dialogue and participated as conversational partners, appropriately alternating their roles as listener and speaker: they focused on the topic presented by the interviewer, and shifted focus when a new topic was introduced. The ideas expressed by children in the longer narratives were semantically coherent, and native speakers of Tigrinia who reviewed the tapes judged the sentence structure to be syntactically correct. In other words, none of the children exhibited significant deficits of communicative language.

## DISCUSSION

The finding that the orphans differed significantly from refugee children only on selected behavioral symptoms and that they outperformed the latter on cognitive tests, suggests that it is possible to provide humane group care for unaccompanied children that fosters their social and cognitive development, even when technical and material resources are severely limited. In view of the widespread signs and symptoms of emotional deprivation among children before the orphanage was reorganized (Jareg, 1988; Wolff, 1986), it is reasonable to conclude that the extensive social reorganization between 1988 and 1990 contributed in major ways to the apparent improvement in the social-emotional state of the orphans.

However, the study was carried out under conditions of active warfare. The measures were probably sensitive enough to exclude major developmental disorders or frank psychiatric disabilities, but they were global in character, had not been standardized on Eritrean populations, and may not have been sensitive to feelings of loss, depression, or anxiety which one might have expected among the orphans. Clinical observations suggested, for example, that the orphans still had great social-emotional needs and greedily latched onto strangers, although this expression of need had greatly diminished (see Wolff, Dawit & Zere, 1995). By contrast, the refugee children only took casual note of strangers, and returned to their games after waving a brief greeting. The refugee children were also not a "normal" control group, since they had been exposed to the same chronic environmental stresses as the orphans. Both groups may, therefore, have performed at a significantly lower level on cognitive and language tests and exhibited more behavioral symptoms than would Eritrean children growing up with their families under peace time conditions.

The greater prevalence of deviant behavior among orphans than refugee children is consistent with the hypothesis that permanent separation from both parents at an early age has a distinctly negative effect on social-emotional development (Bodman, 1941; Bowlby, 1980; Crook & Eliot, 1980). The finding that the youngest orphans in the group showed relatively more behavioral symptoms and were less advanced than older orphans relative to refugee children on cognitive measures is also consistent with the hypothesis that younger children are somewhat more vulnerable to psychological stress and deprivation than older children (Garmezy & Rutter, 1985; Jensen & Shaw, 1993; Lyons, 1987).

The relatively high incidence of nocturnal enuresis among the orphans relative to younger children in Western industrialized countries (Jenkins et al., 1980; Shaffer, 1985), may be related to their grief or anxiety (Lyons, 1987; Terr, 1991). However, enuresis was also more common among refugee children; and it is reported to be more prevalent in rural Ethiopian children who were studied under peacetime conditions (Giel & van Luijk, 1969) as well as in Israeli children who were raised in group settings (kibbutzim; Neubauer, 1965). The loss of both parents, and the psychological stresses of war may, therefore, not be the only factors that contributed to the high incidence of enuresis in the orphans.

Similarly, the more aggressive behavior of orphans may have been one expression of their anger or depression (Terr, 1991), but they lived in a very different social environment than the refugee children. The orphans generally played in groups closely supervised by child care workers with definite ideas about discipline, whereas the refugee children were free to play around the camp with little supervision, so that the opportunities for peer conflict and authority struggles with adults were considerably greater in the orphanage.

In view of the hypothesis that psychological trauma frequently leads to phobias in young children (Gibson, 1989; Terr, 1991; Ziv, Kruglanski & Shulman, 1974), one would have predicted that children who saw their parents killed would show more irrational fears than the refugee children. Yet, the opposite relationship was found. Eritreans familiar with the local culture suggested that the parents were much more concerned about the dangers of predatory animals and of natural phenomena such as thunder and lightning than the orphanage staff, and that they may have conveyed such fears either explicitly or implicitly to their children. Many refugee children were, in fact, afraid of animals or the dark, whereas the orphans sometimes organized excursions into the hills to hunt for snakes, and often ran errands in the dark.

The group differences in cognitive and language performance had not been expected, and may help to explain why the greater frequency of behavioral symptoms in the group of orphans was limited to a few circumscribed domains. Cognitive competence is thought to have an important protective effect on the ability to cope with psychological stresses, thereby reducing the differences in behavioral symptoms between comparison groups (Garmezy, 1984; Jensen & Shaw, 1993; Rutter, 1981).

The somewhat higher cognitive functioning of the orphans was probably not a result of differences in nutritional state, because both groups had received the same protein enriched supplementary diets; none of the children were significantly undernourished at the time of the study; and the groups did not differ in neuromotor status or fine motor skills. One possible reason for the orphans' higher level of cognitive performance may have been the differences in exposure to formal education. Before entering primary school, the orphans regularly attended kindergarten, while refugee children received no formal education until they entered primary school at the age of 6 or 7 years; therefore they relied primarily on informal teaching provided by their parents.

Moreover, the refugee children had spent nearly all of their lives in a totally isolated desert region of Eritrea, many of them having been born in the camp (see Table 1). By contrast, the orphans generally came to the orphanage when they were 3–4 years old, and may, therefore, have been exposed to an intellectually more stimulating social environment before being orphaned. However, almost no information was available about the early social experience of the orphans to test how early experiences might have contributed to the relatively higher cognitive performance of the orphans.

As a minimum, this descriptive study has demonstrated that it is sometimes possible to provide culturally appropriate and humane group care for relatively large numbers of orphans and other unaccompanied children in impoverished Third World countries where reunification with extended families, adoption, and foster care placement are not viable alternatives. However, the apparent success of Eritrean experience depended in part on the spirit of mutual cooperation that emerged in Eritrea during a protracted war of liberation that unified the population (Pateman, 1990), and that was probably transmitted by the orphanage staff to the children, giving them a sense of active participation (Jensen & Shaw, 1993; Rutter, 1981). The model of group care devised in Eritrea must first be adapted to local cultural traditions if it is to serve as a guideline in other war-torn Third World countries.

## REFERENCES

Aboud, F., Samuel, M., Hadera, A. & Abdulaziz, A. (1991). Intellectual social and nutritional status of children in an Ethiopian orphanage. *Social Science and Medicine, 33*, 1275–1280.

Allodi, F. (1980) The psychiatric effects of political persecution and torture on children and families of victims. *Canadian Mental Health, 28*, 8–10.

Anthony, E. J. (1987) Risk, vulnerability, and resilience: an overview. In E. J. Anthony & B. Cohler (Eds.), *The invulnerable child* (pp. 3–48). New York: Guilford Press.

Bledsoc, C., Ewbank, D. & Isiogo-Abanihe, U. (1988). The effect of child fostering in feeding practices and access to health services in rural Sierra Leone. *Social Science and Medicine, 27*, 627–637.

Bodman, F. (1941). War conditions and the mental health of the child. *British Medical Journal, 2*, 486–488.

Bowlby, J. (1958). The nature of the child's tie to his mother. *International Journal of Psychoanalysis, 39*, 350–373.

Bowlby, J. (1960). *Maternal care and mental health* Geneva: WHO (9th Printing).

Bowlby, J. (1980). *Attachment and Loss.* Vol. III. Loss. New York: Basic Books.

Chimienti, G., Nasr, J. A., & Khalifch, I. (1989). Children's reactions to war-related stress. *Social Psychiatry and Psychiatric Epidemiology, 24*, 282–287.

Cliff, J. & Noormahomed, A. R. (1993). The impact of war on children's health in Mozambique. *Social Science and Medicine, 36*, 843–848.

Crook, T. & Eliot, J. (1980). Parental death during childhood and adult depression. *Psychological Bulletin, 87*, 252–259.

Gardner, M. F. (1990). *Expressive one-word picture vocabulary test (Revised).* Novato, CA. Academic Therapy Publications.

Garmezy, N. (1983). Stressors of childhood. In N. Garmezy & M. Rutter (Eds), *Stress, coping and development in children* (pp 113–125). New York: Pergamon Press.

Garmezy, N. (1984). Stress-resistant children: The search for protective factors. In J. E. Stevenson (Ed), *Recent research in developmental psychopathology* (pp. 213–233) Oxford: Pergamon Press

Garmezy, N. & Rutter, M. (1985). Acute reactions to stress. In M. Rutter, L. A. Hersov (Eds), *Child and adolescent psychiatry* (pp. 152–176). Oxford: Blackwell Scientific Publications.

Gibson, K. (1989). Children in political violence. *Social Science and Medicine, 28*, 659–667.

Giel, R. & van Luijk, J. N (1969). Psychiatric morbidity in a small Ethiopian town. *British Journal of Psychiatry, 115*, 149–162.

Goldfarb, W. (1945). Effects of psychological deprivation in infancy and subsequent stimulation. *American Journal of Psychiatry, 102*, 18–33.

Gruber, A. R. (1978) *Children in foster care.* New York. Human Sciences Press.

Isiugo-Abanihe, U. (1985). Child fosterage in West Africa. *Population and Developmental Research, 11*, 3–73.

Jarcg, E. (1988) *Report on consultancy visit to Eritrea* Oslo. Redd Barna.

Jenkins, S., Bax, M. & Hart, H. (1980). Behavior problems in pre-school children. *Journal of Child Psychology and Psychiatry, 21*, 5–17.

Jensen, P. S. & Shaw, J. (1993). Children as victims of war current knowledge of the American Academy of Child and Adolescent Psychiatry. *Psychiatry, 32*, 697–708.

Kinzie, J. O., Sack, W. H., Angell, R. H., Manson, S. & Roth, B. (1986). The psychiatric effects of massive trauma on Cambodian children: I. The Children. *Journal of the American Academy of Child Psychiatry, 25*, 370–376.

Leiter, R. G. (1969). *Examiner's manual for the Leiter International Performance Scale.* Chicago: Stoelting.

Lyons, J. A. (1987). Post-traumatic stress disorder in children and adolescents: a review of the literature *Developmental and Behavioral Pediatrics, 8*, 349–356.

McNeal, M. R. & Prescott, T. E. (1978). Revised Token Test. Austin, TX: Pro-Ed.

Neubauer, P. B. (1965). *Children in collectives* Springfield, IL: C. C. Thomas.

Pateman, R. (1990) *Entrea: even the stones are burning.* Trenton, NJ: Red Sea Press.

Ragan, P. V. & McGlashan, T. H. (1986). Childhood parental death and adult psychopathology. *American Journal of Psychiatry, 143*, 153–157.

Raven, J. C. (1958). *Standard Progressive Matrices. Sets A, B, C, D, and E.* London: H. K. Lewis.

Rein, M., Nutt, T. E. & Weiss, H. (1974). Fostering family care: myth and reality. In A. L. Schorr (Ed.), *Children and decent people* (pp. 24–52). New York. Basic Books.

Reitan, R. M. (1969). *Manual for administration of neuropsychological test batteries for adults and children.* Indianapolis, IN. Author.

Richman, N., Stevenson, J. E. & Graham, P. J. (1975). Prevalence of behavior problems in 3-year-old children. An epidemiological study in a London borough *Journal of Child Psychology and Psychiatry, 16*, 277–287.

Rutter, M. (1980). The long term effects of early experiences. *Developmental Medicine and Child Neurology, 22*, 800–815.

Rutter, M. (1981). Stress, coping and development: some issues and some questions. *Journal of Child Psychology and Psychiatry, 22*, 323–356.

Shaffer, D. (1985). Enuresis. In M. Rutter & L. Hersov (Eds), *Child and adolescent psychiatry: modern approaches* (pp. 465–481). Oxford: Blackwell Scientific Publications.

Spitz, R. (1949). The role of ecological factors in emotional development. *Child Development, 20*, 145–155.

Terr, L. C. (1991). Childhood traumas: an outline and overview. *American Journal of Psychiatry, 148*, 10–20.

Tizard, B. & Hodges, J. (1978). The effect of early institutional rearing on the development of eight-year-old children. *Journal of Psychology and Psychiatry, 19*, 99–118.

Touwen, B. C. L. & Prechtl, H. F. R. (1970). *The neurological examination of children with minor nervous dysfunction* London. Spastics International/Heinemann.

Werner, E. E. & Smith, R. D. (1982). *Vulnerable but invincible: a study of resilient children* New York: McGraw-Hill.

Wolff, P. H. (1986). Report of First Eritrean International conference on primary health care. *War and the children of Eritrea.* Milan, Italy.

Wolff, P. H., Dawit, Y. & Zere, B. (1995). The Solomuna orphanage. A historical survey. *Social Science and Medicine, 40*, 1133–1139.

Wolff, P. H., Gunnoe, C. E. & Cohen, C. (1983). Associated movements as a measure of developmental age. *Developmental Medicine and Child Neurology, 25*, 417–429.

World Health Organization (1951). *Expert Committee on Mental Health, Report on the Second Session 1951. Technical Report Series #31.* Geneva: WHO Monographs.

Ziv, A., Kruglanski, A. W. & Shulman, S. (1974). Children's psychological reactions to wartime stress. *Journal of Personal Social Psychology, 30*, 24–30.

# 24

# Ethical Issues in Biological Psychiatric Research with Children and Adolescents

**L. Eugene Arnold and David M. Stoff**
*National Institute of Mental Health, Bethesda, Maryland*

**Edwin Cook, Jr.**
*University of Chicago*

**Donald J. Cohen**
*Yale Child Study Center*

**Markus Kruesi**
*University of Illinois, Urbana*

**Clinton Wright**
*Columbia University, New York*

**Jocelyn Hattab**
*Eitanim Hospital MH Center, Hadassah Medical School*

**Philip Graham**
*University of London*

**Alan Zametkin and F. Xavier Castellanos**
*National Institute of Mental Health, Bethesda, Maryland*

**William McMahon**
*University of Utah, Salt Lake City*

**James F. Leckman**
*Yale Child Study Center*

Reprinted with permission from the *Journal of the American Academy of Child and Adolescent Psychiatry*, 1995, Vol. 34, No. 7, 929–939.

The opinions expressed herein are the views of the authors and do not necessarily reflect the official position of the National Institute of Mental Health or any other part of the US Department of Health and Human Services.

583

**Objective:** *This article reviews, discusses, and elaborates considerations and recommendations summarized by the biological research working group at the May 1993 NIMH conference on ethical issues in mental health research on children and adolescents.* **Method:** *Notes from the conference were summarized and supplemented by a computer search of relevant literature. Drafts were circulated for comment to national and international experts, some of whom joined as coauthors.* **Results:** *Issues addressed include possible overprotection by policy makers and institutional review boards arising out of the recognition of children's special vulnerability without equal recognition of their need for research; the definition of minimal risk, which has often been equated with no risk in the case of children; assessment of the risk-benefit ratio; procedures for minimization of risk, such as improved technology, "piggybacking" onto clinical tests, and age-appropriate preparation; the difficulty of justifying risk for normal controls; age-graded consent; special considerations about neuroimaging; "coercive" inducement, both material and psychological; disposition of unexpected or unwanted knowledge about individuals, including the subject's right not to know and parent's right not to tell; and socioeconomic status and cultural/ethnic equity.* **Conclusions:** *The working group adopted a position of advocacy for children's right to research access while recognizing that this advocacy must be tempered by thoughtful protections for child and adolescent subjects.*

To mount effective prevention and treatment efforts for child and adolescent mental disorders will require thorough biological as well as psychosocial understanding of the disorders and of the children they afflict. Klin and Cohen (1994) describe how responsible clinical concern for the welfare of our patients might be said to impose an ethical imperative to conduct, or at least support, research, and, of course, to make sure it is done in an ethical manner. The 1989 Institute of Medicine report that spurred development of the National Plan for Research on Child and Adolescent Mental Disorders mentioned impediments to such research, including ethical and regulatory problems (Institute of Medicine, 1989, p. 172 ff.). On May 4–5, 1993, the National Institute of Mental Health convened a conference to examine ethical and regulatory issues in child and adolescent mental health research. One of the working groups at that conference was charged with examining issues impinging biological research. This article will summarize and elaborate that group's deliberations and recommendations. These touch on the issues of possible overprotection, the definition of minimal risk, assessment of risk-benefit ratio, risks of biological procedures, minimization of risk, normal controls, age-graded consent, special considerations about neuroimaging, "coercive" inducement, unexpected or unwanted knowledge about individuals, and socioeconomic, cultural, and ethnic issues.

## CAUTIONARY BACKGROUND AND HISTORY

Although this article emphasizes the research deprivation that children have suffered, we need to recall the historical context of abuses in which this has occurred. For example, Mann (1994) summarized historical concerns about behavioral genetics, one area related to biological mental health research: This burgeoning field struggles to escape the shadow of Nazi pseudoscientific justifications for anti-Semitism and genocide, which made eugenics so unrespectable that biologists for awhile abandoned the relationship of genes and behavior.

According to Mann (1994), most experts now agree that genes influence behavior (including disposition to mental disorders), but unfortunately, lay consumers of scientific information tend to translate this fact into "neurogenetic determinism," in which genes unilaterally determine behavior rather than interacting with the environment. (An example of interaction is phenylketonuria, in which genes interact with diet, and the genetic disorder is preventable by specific nurture.) For every person who believes that such research may help persons with mental problems, another fears that neurogenetic determinism will erode human dignity. Add to this concern the fact that abuses have occurred in the treatment of research subjects (and not only under Nazi auspices), and we can understand that those who are less than enthusiastic about the potential benefits of research have a basis for their opinion, a basis that needs to be taken seriously.

## SPECIAL PROTECTION FOR CHILDREN

Because of children's special vulnerability, society has established special legal and ethical protections for them in many situations, including research risk. This generally adds to the safeguards afforded by parents' natural protection. In fact, society sometimes implies that parents' judgment cannot be trusted to be protective enough and limits parents' rights to decide for their children in order to ensure additional protection. The special federal research safeguards for children include the following (45 Code of Federal Regulations [CFR], Subtitle A, Part 46, Subpart D, 10-1-91 Edition):

1. Both child assent and parent or guardian permission (in lieu of consent) are necessary.
2. Parents' or guardians' permission for research on their children may not be solicited or accepted unless one of the following pertains:
    A. The research has minimal risk (the degree of risk ordinarily encountered in daily life) or no risk.
    B. The research, though of greater than minimal risk, presents the prospect of direct benefit to the subjects great enough to justify the risk, and the risk-benefit ratio is at least as favorable as available alternatives.
    C. Though the risk is greater than minimal with no prospect of direct benefit, all of the following are true:
        i. The risk is a minor increase over minimal.
        ii. The intervention or procedure presents experiences reasonably commensurate with the subjects' actual or expected medical, dental, or other situations.
        iii. The intervention is likely to yield generalizable knowledge of vital importance for understanding or ameliorating the subjects' disorder.
    D. Research that the IRB finds presents a reasonable opportunity to understand, prevent, or alleviate a serious health problem of children receives a special approval by the Secretary of Health and Human Services.

Technically, the restrictions described apply only to federally supported research, but the federal requirement for an Institutional Review Board (IRB) in order to receive federal funding, coupled with the application of IRB review to all research at respective institutions, essentially brings all research under the purview of these regulations. The practical effect is that parents and guardians cannot give permission for some kinds of research on children to which competent adults could altruistically consent for themselves (Kopelman, 1989a,b; Laor, 1987). Furthermore, some IRBs interpret the regulations even more restrictively, adding another layer of "protection." In some cases, IRBs have equated *minimal risk* with *no risk* for children. This situation has some good points; children *should* have special protection; parents may not always have enough knowledge or sophistication to protect their children adequately; and it is better to err on the side of safety. However, some serious disadvantages for children and adolescents have emerged from the way this approach has played out, amounting to what we believe is overprotection.

## Overprotection

Children and adolescents may be overprotected by restrictive rules (or restrictive interpretations of rules) that deprive them of needed research. The tendency to abhor any research risk for children and adolescents (e.g., May, 1974; Ramsey, 1970, 1976, 1980, quoted by Laor, 1987) may interfere with adequately addressing their needs (Kopelman, 1989a). The dearth of research pertaining directly to children has long threatened to make them research orphans, inappropriately dependent on work done with adults (Shirkey, 1968). When new treatments are introduced after clinical trials only on adults, clinicians are forced to extrapolate to children. They are faced with a dilemma: either deprive children of the new treatment or subject them to the risk of an untested treatment that may or may not work the same as in adults. The clinical practicality is obvious. As a result, Mirkin (1975) reported that more than 80% of the drugs prescribed for children had in their prescribing information an "orphaning clause" such as "not to be used in children." The paradox is that children may need research results even more than adults do.

Treatments that are safe and effective in adults may be both, either, or neither in children. Even more importantly, a treatment that would be safe and effective in children may not always be effective in adults, so that research only on adults would miss its effectiveness. Etiologies of similar syndromes may also differ between childhood-onset and adult forms.

Animal models, although useful and desirable, also have limitations, perhaps more so for children and adolescents than for adults. For example, whereas children metabolize drugs faster than adults, in some experimental animals the adult animals metabolize faster than the young animals. Also, the relatively short juvenile stage of most animals may make them questionable analogies to humans for some mental disorders of children and adolescents. A problem shared with adult biological mental health research is that the key pharmacological properties of some receptors, such as $5\text{-HT}_{1B}$ receptors (e.g., Metcalf et al., 1992), differ in rodents and humans. Another problem is the unavailability of animal models for many children's mental health disorders.

A historical analogy offers a relevant lesson. After the thalidomide scare, there was active discouragement of including women of childbearing age in clinical trials of new drugs for more than a decade. However, once the drugs came on the market they were used in women of childbearing age in a non-studied fashion, posing a risk to more patients (or their fetuses) than if such patients had been included in controlled, well-monitored trials. And, of course, women were deprived of efficacy data to guide their treatment. This short-sighted policy has been reversed for women, who are expected to be included in research generally from now on (Ellis, 1994; Varmus, 1994). The consequences of not conducting research in children and adolescents might include the perpetuation or introduction of harmful practices, failure to discover etiology of illnesses, and failure to develop new treatments for psychiatric disorders of childhood and adolescence. Any risk assessment must include the risk of not having data for clinical decisions.

## DEFINITION OF MINIMAL RISK

One problem mentioned above is the definition of minimal risk, which Kopelman (1989b) has characterized as "pivotal." Unfortunately, some IRBs seem to interpret minimal risk as *not any risk*. A common-sense definition is needed, and is suggested by 45 CFR, Subtitle A, Part 46, Subpart A, 46.102(g) 10-1-91 Edition:

> "Minimal risk" means that the risks of harm anticipated in the proposed research are not greater, considering probability and magnitude, than those ordinarily encountered in daily life or during the performance of routine physical or psychological examinations or tests.

This seems to imply taking into consideration the everyday risks that parents and society routinely approve for children, such as bike riding, riding in a car, and even seasonally limited but otherwise daily activities like swimming or sledding. However, authorities are not clear about this. Kopelman (1989b) points out that the phrase "ordinarily encountered in daily life" can be interpreted three ways: "all the risks ordinary people encounter, or the risks all people ordinarily encounter, or the minimal risks all ordinary people ordinarily encounter." Nicholson (1986) has proposed a list of ordinary daily risks to which research risks can be compared in determining minimal risk. We endorse this as long as it is defined as a list of examples and not interpreted rigidly.

A question to be resolved is whether minimal risk should be defined the same for sick patients as for control subjects—whether the daily great risk of a serious disorder by comparison changes the estimation of minimal risk. It might be argued, for example, that patients who have daily exposure to electrolyte imbalance or malnutrition from an eating disorder or clinically need daily administration of risky drugs encounter more risk in daily life than normal controls. On the other hand, one could argue that their state of vulnerability from other risks makes them less able to tolerate an additional modicum of risk.

### Risk and Aversiveness

Although both aversiveness and risk represent potentially negative outcomes, a procedure can be risky without being aversive or uncomfortable, or can be aversive without being very risky (at least physically). For example, finger stick or venipuncture, universally acknowledged to carry minimal risk under sterile conditions, may be highly aversive to children (Fradet et al., 1990; Humphrey et al., 1992; Turkeltaub and Gergen, 1989). However, extreme aversiveness can constitute a psychological risk (adjustment disorder or posttraumatic stress disorder [PTSD]).

Furthermore, the aversiveness of a procedure is modified by a child's previous experience. A child who has learned to take clinically indicated spinal taps in stride through autohypnosis and recumbent games for a day may find little aversiveness in an additional spinal tap for research purposes. In fact, Kruesi et al. (1988) have found spinal taps to be no more aversive to children than attending school. On the other hand, a child who has had a catastrophic experience with a severe headache from a previous tap would be sensitized to fear and might experience the procedure as even more aversive than a naive subject. The obvious need for some individual evaluation of aversion-driven psychological risks is partly met by the requirement for child assent as well as parent permission: if the procedure is extremely aversive, assent will presumably not be given. The same procedure may be less aversive as part of a research protocol than when done as a routine clinical need because investigators typically invest time and effort in psychological preparation to maintain subject cooperation. Several authors (e.g., Castellanos et al., 1994; Jay et al., 1982) have documented that there is an opportunity to minimize the psychological risk of aversiveness by manipulating preliminary experience (rehearsal, role-playing, etc.). Thus in a well-run research protocol the psychological risk tends to be minimal.

### ASSESSMENT OF RISK-BENEFIT RATIO FOR INVASIVE BIOLOGICAL PROCEDURES

Risks should be broadly evaluated, considering known in vitro effects and in vivo effects in animals, adults, and other children and the effect of the technician's or clinician's skill on the risk. The database used for judgment about risk should include not only all available experimental findings, but also noncontrolled clinical and other observations. The assessment of risk-benefit ratio should also consider possibilities for improving the ratio by increasing benefits or decreasing risk or both.

A problem in extrapolating reports of adverse effects from clinical samples is that the clinical experience is often confounded by complicating factors, including the illness for which the clinical procedure was done. For example, an informal review of clinical studies of the side effects of lumbar puncture found the reports complicated by administration of cancer chemotherapy, spinal anesthesia, and contrast agents in the spinal canal, all of which could cause adverse effects that might be attributed to the lumbar puncture. Furthermore, inasmuch as the research procedure is carried out on a voluntary basis, it is unlikely to be done on those who anticipate the most distress from it; this probably reduces the psychological risk. An interesting related question concerns the subsequent effect on the child's later psychological reaction to the same test if it is clinically indicated: whether the child will tolerate it better because of success in the research administration or react to it more negatively because of being sensitized to the risks.

### Review of Risks of Biological Research Procedures

A literature search yielded few systematic studies about the physical or psychological risks of biological research procedures. Smith (1985) carried out a 1-year follow-up of a group of 7-year-old children who had had venipuncture for research purposes, and they found very few aftereffects. However, Turkeltaub and Gergen (1989), Fradet et al. (1990), and Humphrey et al. (1992) reported immediate (short-term) aversiveness and discomfort from similar clinical tests. Kruesi et al. (1988) found a postlumbar headache prevalence of 22% in child and adolescent psychiatric patients aged 6.5 to 19.8 years; this rate is comparable with that seen in adults. Similar results were found by Castellanos et al. (1994). Systematic follow-up of child and adolescent research subjects regarding both physical and emotional consequences would be of great value for future formal risk estimation.

## MINIMIZING RISK

Risks and fears should be minimized by limiting both the number and type of invasive tests. Responsible investigators have an obligation to do no more invasive tests than necessary to answer the central research questions and to devise designs that allow the minimum number of tests to suffice. A similar obligation pertains to the type and invasiveness of the test: perhaps a blood draw would suffice rather than a spinal tap, or urine rather than either. Tests that are less invasive should be devised; an example is the recent development of polymerase chain reaction, which enables genetic analysis from saliva rather than blood. Since risk and discomfort may be inversely proportional to the skill of the technician or clinician doing the procedure, the most skilled should be recruited to do research procedures. Another strategy for minimizing risk, of course, is to "piggyback" invasive tests on routine clinically indicated procedures: for example, taking an extra milliliter of spinal fluid or an extra 5 mL of blood for research purposes during a clinically indicated spinal tap or blood draw. Of course, this lower risk still requires informed consent and is justified only if a sufficient increment of biological information can be obtained for an approved investigation. Deciding the appropriate number and frequency of serial tests in a longitudinal study requires careful balancing of the value of incremental knowledge gained against the incremental risk for each repetition.

Another minimization of risk, or at least discomfort, involves carefully determining the value and hazards of preparatory procedures (e.g., fasting, special diets, resting) associated with the actual biological tests. The investigator must decide whether these are necessary for subject safety or merely for quality of test results. If the latter, the investigator must decide whether the increment of knowledge is worth the increment of subject discomfort.

Risk can be further minimized by implementation of procedures to prepare the subject and monitor consequences and aftereffects of biological tests (Castellanos et al., 1994; Jay et al., 1982; Kruesi et al., 1988). For example, Amiel (1985) devised a simple method of keeping children happily supine after a spinal tap: videotape movies. This reduced the risk of spinal headache. Children may have a lower or higher threshold for aversive stimuli than adults, or the effects of aversive stimuli may last a shorter or longer time. Some studies of children's thresholds and perceptions of aversive procedures could be useful.

## NEED FOR NORMAL CONTROLS

The argument for using "normal" (healthy) controls rests on the need for comparison norms for biological assays, challenges, and other tests. Without these, the test results from patients may be largely useless, and the research risk to patients proportionally "wasted." The argument against using normal controls is that they do not stand to benefit themselves from the results. When they are used, careful multistage screening designed to detect psychopathology is needed to ensure meaningful, truly normal or healthy, comparisons (Kruesi et al., 1990), and such carefully defined normal subjects would be least likely to benefit.

If the procedure poses more than minimal risk, current rules do not seem to allow child or adolescent normal controls to consent (i.e., to assent and have parents give permission for them). In a regulatory double bind, they are considered incapable of consenting for themselves, and their parents are not allowed to be altruistic on their behalf (i.e., permit altruistic participation). The question arises as to why adolescents should not be allowed to be altruistic (i.e., voluntarily undertake risk for the common good); it would reflect a developmental tendency detectable as early as preschool and reaching full flower in adolescence.

Of course, not all motivations for normal controls are altruistic. One child may find getting out of school for a day rewarding enough. Another may cherish the opportunity to impress peers. Yet another may be trying to feel special. There may even be neurotic motivation, such as guilt-motivated punishment seeking for assumed wrongdoing. The investigator needs to be alert to the motivation of the normal control subject and respond ethically to it.

## AGE-GRADUAL CONSENT

A system of more finely age-graded consent could empower adolescents to consent altruistically to moderate-risk protocols. The arguments against extending such consent empowerment below age 18 include the need to protect even adolescents from exploitation and the danger of a "slippery slope" if the age 18 lower limit is breached.

Nevertheless, Laor (1987) and Leikin (1993) suggest a continuous process of empowerment for consent paralleling the maturational process. One possibility might be increments of consent ability at the natural ages of cognitive ability increment. A considerable amount is now known about minors' understanding of the consent process, in addition to Piaget's (1958) basic work suggesting increments of ability at about 7 years and about puberty, when adult-like formal operations are attained. Lewis et al. (1978) found significant increases by grade level in awareness of risk, future consequences, wariness of individuals with vested interests, and need for independent professional advice. Keith-Spiegel and Maas (1981, quoted by Leikin, 1993) found that the reasoning of 9-year-olds about research risk is similar to that of adults. Weithorn and Campbell (1982) found that 14-year-olds show the same risk-benefit reasoning as 21-year-olds and that 9-year-olds reach the same conclusions through a different reasoning strategy. Lewis et al. (1978) found that 7- to 9-year-olds (but not 6-year-olds) asked all the relevant questions needed for an informed consent. Leikin (1993), after reviewing the literature, concluded that by age 9 children have enough cognitive capacity to *participate* in the decision (not to make it by themselves). Thus enough seems known about minors' understanding and judgment to justify more empowerment in the consent process, including the right to make some altruistic decisions.

Laor (1987), in fact, resolves the situation thus: " . . . every individual can achieve, and exercise, different levels of autonomy at different times. . . . The question as to who is or is not autonomous should be replaced by the questions of how much autonomy can/should be ascribed to/required of the individual in different circumstances, be the individual a child or an adult . . ." (pp. 131–132). He proposes that children aged 12 and older should be able to consent to research on their own (like adults); that between age 7 and 12 they can consent but parents' assent is also needed (the reverse of the current rules); and before age 7 parental consent is needed, whenever possible coupled with the child's assent. This recommendation was not adopted in 1977 by the American National Committee for the Protection of Human Subjects of Biomedical and Behavioral Research because of a lack of public consensus at the time (Grisso and Vierling, 1978; Laor, 1987; Melton, 1980). Maybe it is time to reconsider the recommendation, perhaps with some modification. For example, one expert who reviewed this manuscript thought that 14 would be a better age than 12 for adult-like consent, but otherwise endorsed Laor's proposal.

### Neutral Clinician to Ensure Understanding

Within such consent empowerment, of course, there will remain an obligation to make sure the child or adolescent understands the information provided. Because of wide individual variation, one cannot depend on the subject's age to ensure adequate understanding; even some adults have difficulty understanding the information at times. When the investigator is not the child's clinician (in the case of normal controls, the child's regular physician), it would be desirable for the two professionals to join in making sure the child understands the information provided. The participation of a neutral clinician whose only interest and responsibility are the child's welfare could help justify consent empowerment for younger children than are currently enfranchised. (If the investigator is the child's regular clinician, a neutral one could be recruited for the purpose.) Such a clinician would act as a counterbalance to the investigator's bias; it may be convenient for researchers to believe that children should be free to participate in research to a greater degree. The possibility of investigator self-serving blind spots makes a dialog with noninvestigator clinicians and other neutral parties essential, at least for policy formation. This seems to expect a lot of such neutral clinicians, who may need to be recruited from outside the research institution for this purpose to ensure neutrality. They should be paid for their time, perhaps through the IRB from the study budget; this expense would be justified if it makes a valuable but more-than-minimal-risk study ethically possible. Of course, cost and effort considerations would suggest that involvement of an additional clinician in day-to-day consent with individual child subjects is necessary and advisable only for research deemed to be of more than minimal risk by the IRB.

## SPECIAL RISKS ASSOCIATED
## WITH NEUROIMAGING TECHNOLOGY

Techniques for studying the brain have evolved rapidly during the past several decades, beginning with x-ray computed tomography (CT). Each type of imaging carries its own special risks. Though now almost obsolete, the history of CT scan use illustrates an interesting point about the concept of minimal risk and the impact of research on clinical risk: before systematic research, many clinicians routinely obtained such scans in developmental disorders such as autism; but research results and the careful thinking about risk and benefit associated with the informed consent process in research have led to a reduction in the number of clinical neuroimaging tests. Although magnetic resonance imaging (MRI) does not have the ionizing radiation risk that CT scans have, the potential risk of exposure to a high magnetic field cannot be measured accurately. In MRI studies, the greatest risk is probably sedation. Still, many IRBs have not allowed minors to participate in studies at the high magnetic fields (3 to 4 tesla) required to improve signal-to-noise ratio in functional MRI. Although functional MRI allows studying brain physiology without the ionizing radiation associated with positron emission tomography (PET) or single photon emission computed tomography (SPECT), it is not a currently viable method of studying neurochemistry or the receptors that are important in development and in pharmacological mechanisms of action.

There seems no question that with adequately informed assent from the subjects and informed permission of parents, PET studies of children and adolescents with severe mental disorders are ethical if designed to provide information that may benefit the affected children themselves. The question is whether it is ever acceptable for normal controls. The International Commission on Radiological Protection (IRCP) sets general public involuntary risk guidelines at 1 mSv per year (approximately 100 mrem), which is slightly above most background levels due to soil radioactivity and cosmic radiation at sea level. The IRCP sets occupational limits for whole body exposure at 50 mSv (5 rem) per year. In addition, a 30-mSv (3-rem) limit for exposure to any individual organ or tissue has been established by 21 CFR Ch. 1, Part 361.1. Considering even 17-year-old subjects less capable of consent, the IRCP and Food and Drug Administration have limited the exposure of normal children and adolescents as subjects to one-tenth the dose equivalent limit for adult research subjects. Under this guideline, with current detector systems for PET and longer acquisition times, some studies are feasible. To appreciate the stringency of this guideline, the risk from exposure to 3 mSv (one-tenth the adult limit of 30 mSv) is equivalent to the risk in 900 miles of highway driving (Huda and Scrimger, 1989).

## Efficiently Utilizing Radiation Safety Expertise

Studies with human subjects using ionizing radiation must be reviewed by both the local Radioactive Drug Review Committee (RDRC) and IRB throughout the research. RDRCs are composed of members with the expertise in radiation biology to assess the risk of exposure. This degree of expertise is often lacking on the IRB. It may be helpful to the IRB process for the RDRC to provide an estimate of risk of studies based on current knowledge of radiation biology for use by the IRB in considering the risk-benefit ratio of the study. A process of careful collaboration and consultation among researchers, RDRC, and IRB members is essential for a logical, unfragmented review with each party contributing their appropriate expertise and taking the appropriate responsibility.

## Sedation or Anesthesia for Imaging

Sedation of minors for imaging is a routine part of pediatric practice and is associated with low risk. For patients (not normal controls) the use of sedation in situations of no direct or immediate benefit requires careful justification but should not be categorically rejected, given the low risk. In view of the catastrophic nature of pervasive developmental disorders, childhood-onset schizophrenia, and similarly crippling disorders, this adjunct to imaging should not stand as a rigid impediment. Although anesthesiologists often argue that general anesthesia with intubation is safer than deep sedation, the added psychological impact will probably be unacceptable to most IRBs.

## INDUCEMENT

The possibility of "coercive inducement" poses the problem of determining how much is too large a compensation for the risk, discomfort, inconvenience, and lost time. Paradoxically, the greater the risk, the harder it is to justify a large subject compensation. This raises some ironic issues of fairness and justice: it seems that in fairness those who undergo greater risk should be rewarded with more compensation, but it is precisely in the high-risk situations that subjects need to be protected from undue inducement.

The same payment may be much more of an inducement for a poor subject than a wealthy one, but the inducement is not easily equalized because it does not seem fair to pay a poor subject less. The child's view of dollar amounts needs to be considered in any amount given directly to the child. For example, Keith-Spiegel and Maas (1976) found that minors aged 9 to 15 were more interested than adults in the compensation at the lower amounts. However, parents also need to be compensated for lost time from work and transportation costs. How generously parents are compensated may be an issue: a poor parent might be tempted to coerce the child into research for the compensation. Such exploitation would run counter to the usual expectation that the parent's judgment about the best interests of the child would protect the child from undue inducement. This presents a dilemma: Working middle-class parents should be reimbursed fairly for lost time from work, but this rate may verge on coerciveness for some poor families and it does not seem fair to pay poor or unemployed parents less.

It is understandable that some IRBs and even some ethics experts are tempted to dispose of such thorny decisions by banning compensation in child research, at least for the children themselves. Arguments against any compensation include avoidance of the dilemmas described above, ensuring that no coercion operates, and avoiding a differential recruitment of subjects of lower socioeconomic status (SES). Arguments for some compensation include fairness, recognition of the contributions made by the subjects and their parents, and avoiding a disproportionate burden on the working poor. It is the practice in some places to reimburse only transportation for the child and one parent. In fact, one of the authors of this article (P.G.) endorses that restriction. However, the majority of us propose that fair compensation at middle-class levels be offered when the study budget can afford it, and in high-risk studies where there is a concern about this being too tempting for the poorer subjects in the expected sample, some provision could be made for monitoring the consent process by a neutral clinician. Some ethicists suggest that there be no discussion about compensation until after consent in order to preclude any inducement. However, others believe that this might unfairly exclude some families who could not afford to take time off from work and pay transportation without some reimbursement. In practice, most IRBs take the position that knowledge about compensation is part of fully informed consent and many even require it to be in the consent form, at least for parents. (Some IRBs prohibit the child's being told about compensation given the parents.)

A recommendation not commonly followed is that none of the funding come from pharmaceutical companies or other interested parties (Small et al, 1994).

Paradoxically, insurance for injury during research, to which no one would object ethically, is an inducement not universally used despite general agreement about its desirability. This particular inducement, in fact, would make any research more ethical by reducing economic risk to the subject.

A nonmonetary inducement may occur when the sibling of a patient is used as normal control. The sib could be psychologically coerced by guilt and by the expectation to help the ill family member. A partial answer can come from observations such as those reported by Amiel (1985), who found that sibs of patients were enthusiastic about volunteering for a procedure involving two indwelling venous lines for a day, because it allowed them to share in the attention the sick sib had been getting and to satisfy their curiosity about what the patient had been going through.

Another nonmonetary inducement is the wish to please the investigator, especially if the investigator is also the child's therapist. There may be a fine line between cultivating an alliance and seductive trading on friendship. In a longitudinal study, there may be too much pressure for retention, with difficulty respecting the line between healthy, respectful expectation of fulfilling the agreement and manipulating guilt. A therapist or case manager not involved in the research can be one safeguard against undue inducement of this type. When the investigator is also the child's regular therapist, it might be advisable in high-risk research to invite a neutral clinician uninvolved in the study to monitor the child's voluntarism.

## UNEXPECTED OR UNWANTED KNOWLEDGE ABOUT INDIVIDUALS

Another special problem for biological procedures is disposition of unexpected or unwanted knowledge gained in the course of research, especially with normal controls. One example is the discovery of an untreatable disorder in a normal control. Another is the discovery of misattributed paternity in a genetic study where it means that the subject has not really inherited the high risk of a catastrophic dominant-gene disorder that he or she thinks he or she has. The arguments for telling the subject or family include their right to know and the avoidance of paternalism (protecting subjects and/or families from something they do not want or need protection from). The arguments for not telling include avoidance of harm, avoidance of irresponsibility (dumping the problem on the subject or family by a policy of telling all), and the subject's "right not to know" in genetic testing of nonpatients (Knoppers and Chadwick, 1994; Wertz et al., 1994). Age considerations should influence the decision: for example, a case of misattributed paternity might be handled quite differently with an oedipal 6-year-old than with a 16-year-old concerned about dating and desirability as a potential mate.

It appears desirable to discuss with the child and parents their wishes about possible contingencies before the results are known. Wertz et al. (1994) suggest that the minor should be the primary decision maker about being told things with no direct health benefits (i.e., no treatment or prevention possible) but that might be useful to the minor in making reproductive decisions. Of course, such a pretest discussion carries its own risks of arousing anxiety and curiosity unnecessarily, and it needs to be handled skillfully and reassuringly. There is also a place for general policy guidance from self-help groups for the respective disorders and from other nonresearch sources. Such groups could help formulate general guidelines about when and what subjects in various scenarios would like to be told. With no single good answer, decisions have to be made case by case.

A risk of unwanted knowledge increasingly noted by IRBs is an economic one: If a previously undiagnosed chronic disease or genetic propensity to it is found in the course of research, it could prevent the subject from getting medical (and possibly life) insurance in the future (Knoppers and Chadwick, 1994). Reportedly, some IRBs have interpreted this economic risk as more than minimal and have disapproved genetic protocols on this basis even though the other risks were acceptable. This particular risk is largely cultural artifact; it is not such a problem in the presence of universal health coverage or prohibition of exclusion for preexisting conditions. In the absence of such societal provisions, it seems that provision by the study budget of insurance against this risk could make all research more ethical and acceptable. It could be part of a more general insurance against injury as a research subject.

## CULTURAL, ETHNIC, AND SES ISSUES

In recruiting a sample, generalizability is an important consideration. Norms should reflect the general population, and a clinical sample should reflect the clinical population. This requires some attention to the SES and ethnic composition of the sample. Cultural and socioeconomic preferences, biases, opportunities, and confounds with exclusion criteria may skew a sample.

A special cultural/ethnic/SES problem for biological research concerns the fact that lower SES and one-parent families (more frequent in minority populations) may be less able to support the subject before, during, and after invasive procedures, which may put such subjects at higher risk. If subjects are chosen on the basis of minimizing risk, it may result in under-representation of some ethnic minorities, and certainly of the lower SES. This is an example of the protection versus equal opportunity dilemma. Exclusion could be either protection or paternalism, and inclusion could be equal opportunity or exploitation. This issue relates to the principle of "equity" in access to research mentioned by Knoppers and Chadwick (1994).

Some children in socioeconomic classes IV and V are already exposed to such a high degree of risk that some observers might consider it unacceptable to increase that degree of risk by adding to it the physical and emotional risks of being a research subject. For instance, the Working Group on Inequalities in Health (1980) found that British children in social class IV or V are already exposed to between five and seven times the risk of accidental death of children in social class I. It has also been suggested that research subjects of lower social class tend to be in research projects of greater risk than subjects from higher social classes. Barber et al. (1979) found that research projects with the possibility of considerable therapeutic benefit to the subject were most likely to be carried out on private patients, while projects of little or no therapeutic benefit were most likely to be carried out on welfare recipients. He also found the converse to be true: that projects in which the risks were relatively high compared to the possible benefits were twice as likely to be carried out on welfare recipients as projects with a more favorable risk-benefit analysis. It is not clear whether these general findings represent the specific situation of biological mental health research in children and adolescents.

This issue is important for biological research because of possible biological differences between ethnic groups in such things as drug response, toxicity, etc. If major ethnic groups are not represented in the sample, important findings could be missed that might be useful to the missing ethnic groups and to the advancement of clinical science. There has been official recognition of the need to ensure equal access to research and its fruits (Ellis, 1994; Varmus, 1994). This is another instance in which self-help support groups may be helpful. They could provide the extra support to allow full representation of minorities and lower SES subjects and assist with the longer preparation that might be necessary.

## Wards of the State

One social grouping of children who seem blatantly discriminated against in access to research opportunities are children who are wards of the state. These children frequently have a history of abuse and neglect and have a high rate of PTSD as well as other psychopathology. At this writing we know of no controlled studies in the United States of treatment (including psychosocial) in children with PTSD caused by abuse. Such research, as well as more basic research on the pathogenesis of PTSD, is needed. But investigators who attempt to recruit such subjects in many localities are hampered by onerous legal technicalities and the reluctance of authorities to "take a chance." This situation may have arisen from the opposite abuse in the past: occasionally using wards of the state, especially in institutions, as a convenience sample for research that could just as well have been carried out in the larger community. However, even the most stringent guidelines allow for the advisability of access to research on the special problems of the group in question. This common-sense distinction needs to be implemented by clear guidelines about types of research that should be encouraged with wards of the state, by education of public officials in those guidelines, and by legislative facilitation with appropriate safeguards. A similar argument might also be made regarding children in the juvenile justice system, who may have special research needs not being met.

## CONCLUSION

The working group that originated this article noted children's research needs not currently being met partly because of ethical and regulatory difficulties needing resolution. The working group and additional coauthors have adopted a position of advocacy for children's right to research access but also recognize that this advocacy must be tempered by thoughtful protections for child subjects within the historical context of subjects' rights. We are optimistic that a dialog among investigators, clinicians, ethicists, regulatory and review specialists, policy makers, community leaders, child advocates, and interested community groups can be initiated that will find an ethical way to provide equitable mental health research access for children and adolescents.

## REFERENCES

Amiel SA (1985), Pediatric research on diabetes: the problem of hospitalizing youthful subjects. *IRB Rev Hum Subj Res* 7:4–5

Barber B, Lally JJ, Makarushka JL, Sullivan D (1979), *Research on Human Subjects: Problems of Social Control in Medical Experimentation.* New Brunswick, NJ: Transaction Books, pp 53–57

Castellanos FX, Elia J, Kruesi MJP et al. (1994), Cerebrospinal fluid monoamine metabolites in ADHD boys. *Psychiatry Res* 52:305–316

Ellis GB (1994), *Inclusion of Women and Minorities in Research.* (OPRR Report 94-01). Bethesda, MD: NIH Office of Protection from Research Risks

Frader C, MacGrath PJ, Kay J, Adams S, Luke B (1990), A prospective survey of reaction to blood tests by children and adolescents. *Pain* 40:53–60

Grisso T, Vierling L (1978), Minors' consent to treatment: a developmental perspective. *Prof Psychol* 9:412–427

Huda W, Scrimger JW (1989), Irradiation of normal volunteers in nuclear medicine. *J Nucl Med* 30:260–264

Humphrey GB, Boon CMJ, van Linden van den Heuvell GFEC, van de Wiel HBM (1992), The occurrence of high levels of behavioral distress in children and adolescents undergoing routine venipunctures. *Pediatrics* 90:87–91

Institute of Medicine (1989), *Research on Children and Adolescents with Developmental, Behavioral, and Mental Disorders.* Washington, DC: National Academy Press

Jay SM, Elliot CH, Ozolins M, Olson RA, Pruitt SD (1982), Behavioral management of children's distress during painful medical procedures. *Behav Res Ther* 23:513–520

Keith-Spiegel P, Maas T (1981), Consent to research: are there developmental differences? *Proceedings of American Psychological Association*

Klin A, Cohen DJ (1994), The immorality of not knowing: the ethical imperative to conduct research in child and adolescent psychiatry. In: *Ethics in Child Psychiatry*, Hattab J, ed. Jerusalem, Israel: Gelfen Publishing House

Knoppers BM, Chadwick R (1994), The human genome project: under an international ethical microscope. *Science* 265:2035–2036

Kopelman LM (1989a), Children as research subjects. In: *Children and Health Care: Moral and Social Issues*, Kopelman LM, Moskop JC, eds. Boston: Kluwer Academic Publishers, pp 73–87

Kopelman LM (1989b), When is the risk minimal enough for children to be research subjects? In: *Children and Health Care: Moral and Social Issues*, Kopelman LM, Moskop JC, eds. Boston: Kluwer Academic Publishers, pp 89–99

Kruesi MJP, Lenane MC, Hibbs ED, Major J (1990), Normal controls and biological reference values in child psychiatry: defining normal. *J Am Acad Child Adolesc Psychiatry* 29:449–452

Kruesi MJP, Swedo SE, Coffey ML, Hamburger SD, Leonard H, Rapoport JL (1988), Objective and subjective side effects of research lumbar punctures in children and adolescents. *Psychiatry Res* 25:59–63

Laor N (1987), Toward liberal guidelines for clinical research with children. *Med Law* 6:127–137

Leikin S (1993), Minors' assent, consent, or dissent to medical research. *IRB Rev Hum Subj Res* 15:1–7

Lewis C, Lewis M, Ifekwunigue M (1978), Informed consent by children and participation in an influenza vaccine trial. *Am J Public Health* 68:1079–82

Mann CC (1994), Behavioral genetics in transition. *Science* 264:1687–1689

May WE (1974), Experimenting on human subjects. *Linacre Q* 41:238–252

Melton G (1980), Children's concepts of their rights. *J Clin Child Psychol* 9: 186–190

Metcalf MA, McGuffin RW, Hamblin MW (1992), Conversion of the human 5-HT$_{1D}$ beta serotonin receptor to the rat 5-HT$_{1B}$ ligand-binding phenotype of THR 355 site directed mutagenesis. *Biochem Pharmacol* 44:1917–1920

Mirkin BL (1975), Drug therapy and the developing human: who cares? *Clin Res* 23:106–113

Nicholson R (1986), *Medical Research with Children: Ethics, Law, and Practice.* Oxford, England: Oxford University Press, pp 82–86

Piaget J, Inhelder B (1958), *The Growth of Logical Thinking from Childhood to Adolescence.* New York: Basic Books

Ramsey P (1970), *The Passent as Person.* New Haven, CT: Yale University Press

Ramsey P (1976), The enforcement of morals: non-therapeutic research on children. *Hastings Cent Rep* 6:21–30

Ramsey P (1980), Unconsented touching and the autonomy absolute. *IRB Rev Hum Subj Res* 2:9–10

Shirkey HC (1968), Therapeutic orphans. *J Pediatr* 72:119–120

Small AM, Campbell M, Shay J, Goodman IS (1994), Ethical guidelines for psychopharmacological research in children. In: *Ethics and Child Mental Health*, Hattab J, ed. Jerusalem, Israel: Gefen Publishing House

Smith M (1985), Taking blood from children causes no more than minimal harm. *J Med Ethics* 11:127–131

Turkeltaub PC, Gergen PJ (1989), The risk of adverse reactions from percutaneous prick-puncture allergen skin testing, venipuncture, and body measurements: data from the second National Health and Nutrition Examination Survey 1976–80 (NHANES II). *J Allergy Clin Immunol* 84:886–890

Varmus H (1994), NIH guidelines on the inclusion of women and minorities as subjects in clinical research. *Fed Regist* 59:14508–14513

Weithorn L, Campbell S (1982), The competency of children and adolescents to make informed decisions. *Child Dev* 53:1589–1598

Wertz DC, Fanos JH, Reilly PR (1994), Genetic testing for children and adolescents. *JAMA* 272:875–881

Working Group on Inequalities in Health (1980), *Inequalities in Health.* Chairman: Sir D. Black, London: DHSS